BRADY
EMERGENCY CARE

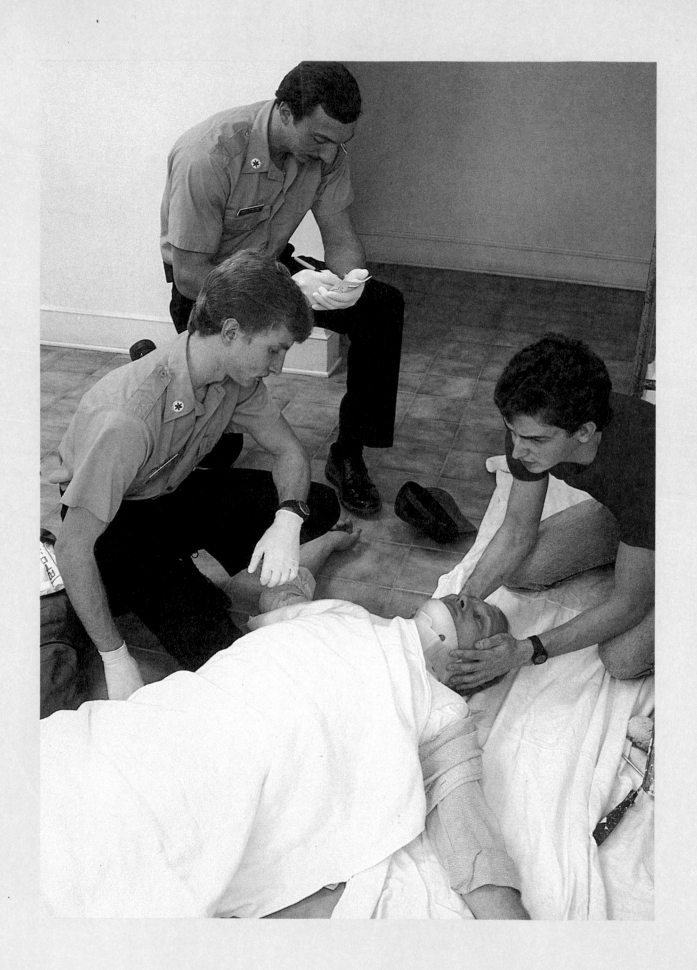

BRADY
BRADY
EMERGENCY CARE

FIFTH EDITION

Harvey D. Grant

Robert H. Murray, Jr.

J. David Bergeron

MEDICAL ADVISORS
Norman E. McSwain, Jr., M.D., F.A.C.S.
William R. Roush, M.D., F.A.C.E.P.

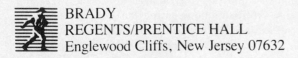
BRADY
REGENTS/PRENTICE HALL
Englewood Cliffs, New Jersey 07632

Library of Congress Cataloging-in-Publication Data

GRANT, HARVEY D., 1934–
   Emergency care / Harvey D. Grant, Robert H. Murray, Jr., J. David
Bergeron; medical advisors, Norman E. McSwain, Jr., William R.
Roush.—5th ed.
     p.   cm.
   "A Brady book."
   ISBN 0-89303-256-5
   1. Emergency medicine. 2. First aid in illness and injury. 3. Rescue
work.. 4. Emergency medical personnel. I. Murray, Robert H.,
1934– . II. Bergeron, J. David, 1944– . III. Title.
   [DNLM: 1. Allied Health Personnel. 2. Emergencies. 3. Emergency
Medical Services. 4. First Aid. WX 215 G762e)
RC86.7.G7 1990
616.02′5—dc20
DNLM/DLC   89–23191
for Library of Congress   CIP

NOTICE

It is the intent of the authors and publishers that this textbook be used as part of a formal Emergency Medical Technician course taught by a qualified instructor. The care procedures presented here represent accepted practices in the United States. They are not offered as a standard of care. EMT-level emergency care is to be performed under the authority and guidance of a licensed physician. It is the reader's responsibility to know and follow local care protocols as provided by the medical advisors directing the system to which he or she belongs. Also, it is the reader's responsibility to stay informed of emergency care procedure changes.

NOTE ON GENDER USAGE

Past attitudes have allowed our language to develop with the pronouns "he" and "his" being used in general to signify persons of either gender. For example, when describing the care for an injury to the upper limb, most people will say "his arm" even though 50% of the patients will probably be females. Our editors tell us that the repeated use of "he or she" is not proper in a long manuscript and the use of (s)he is incorrect in all cases.

Authorities in both professional journals and popular publications have stated that the "quick fix" approach should be discouraged. They recommend different sentence structures when appropriate and the traditional use of "he" and "his" when necessary. This is why you will find "he" often used when referring to the actions taken by an EMT. It is not the intent of the authors or the publisher to imply that women should not be EMTs or that they are any less professional than men in carrying out EMT-level care.

Editorial/production supervision: Tom Aloisi
Interior design: Judith A. Matz-Coniglio
Cover design: Ray Lundgren
Cover photo: George Dodson
Manufacturing buyer: Dave Dickey
Page layout: C. Hart Pelletreau and Karen Noferi

ISBN: 0-89303-256-5

ISBN: 0-89303-704-4   (Exam)

Prentice-Hall International (UK) Limited, *London*
Prentice-Hall of Australia Pty. Limited, *Sydney*
Prentice-Hall Canada Inc., *Toronto*
Prentice-Hall Hispanoamericana, S.A., *Mexico*
Prentice-Hall of India Private Limited, *New Delhi*
Prentice-Hall of Japan, Inc., *Tokyo*
Prentice-Hall of Southeast Asia Pte. Ltd., *Singapore*
Editora Prentice-Hall do Brasil, Ltda., *Rio de Janeiro*

TO THE STUDENT

A self-instructional workbook for this text is available through your college bookstore under the title *Self-Instructional Workbook for EMERGENCY CARE, Fifth Edition Revised*, by J. David Bergeron, with Allan Braslow, Ph.D. *EMT Review: Examination Preparation, 3rd Edition*, a comprehensive question and answer workbook correlated to this text (with sample examination), is also available. If not in stock, ask the bookstore manager to order a copy for you. If your course is being offered off-campus, ask your instructor where to obtain a copy. The *Workbook* and *Review Questions* can help you with course material by acting as a tutorial review and study aid.

Contents

4

Basic Life Support I: The Airway and Pulmonary Resuscitation

5

Basic Life Support II: CPR— Cardiopulmonary Resuscitation

6

Breathing Aids and Oxygen Therapy

7

Basic Life Support III: Bleeding and Shock

8

Injuries I: Soft Tissues and Internal Organs

9

Injuries II: Musculoskeletal Injuries—The Upper Extremities

10

Injuries II: The Lower Extremities

11

Injuries III: The Skull and Spine

12
Injuries III: Soft Tissue Injuries of the Head and Neck

13
Injuries IV: The Chest, Abdomen, and Genitalia

14
Medical Emergencies

15
Pediatric Emergencies

16
Childbirth

17
Burns and Hazardous Materials

18
Environmental Emergencies

SECTION ONE: Heat- and Cold-Related Emergencies

SECTION TWO: Water- and Ice-Related Accidents

19
Special Patients and Behavioral Problems

20
Triage and Disaster Management

26

Communications and Reports

27

Vehicle Rescue

CAPTIONS FOR SCANSHEETS

Dedication

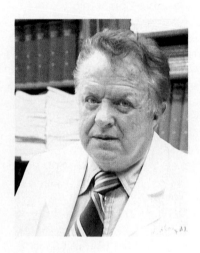

Dr. R Adams Cowley

The authors of *Emergency Care, 5th edition*, wish to dedicate this text to R Adams Cowley, M.D., the pioneer of emergency medical services and trauma patient care. Literally thousands of persons are alive today because Dr. Cowley remained persistent in his goal to treat trauma patients with a 24-hour system of specially trained emergency medical technicians, allied health workers, nurses, and physicians. He created the Maryland Institute for Emergency Medical Services and its internationally known Shock Trauma Center, providing the model for modern systems established to care for the critically ill and injured.

Dr. Cowley believed that there were too many "unnecessary deaths" associated with trauma. He viewed trauma as a disease, requiring specific approaches to care. The concept of the "golden hour" was Dr. Cowley's. He proved that the development of shock was responsible for many trauma-related deaths and, if the proper care to prevent or arrest the development of shock could be applied during the first hour after accidents, then the majority of trauma patients could be saved. In fact, the survival rate for patients at the Shock Trauma Center has grown from 40 percent at the time of its founding in the early 1960s to today's figure of 90 percent.

The dream of a trauma care network started in 1961 with a U.S. Army grant to open a two-bed clinical research unit at the University of Maryland. So impressive were the early results that the National Research Council gave $800,000 in 1963 for the renovation of a five-floor trauma treatment center at the hospital. Dr. Cowley worked with the Maryland State Police to utilize helicopters for the transport of trauma patients and was instrumental in the development of specialized training programs

The new Maryland Shock Trauma Center.

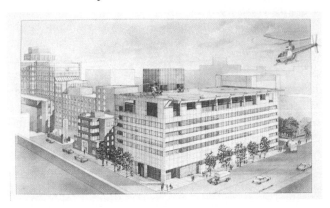

Jim Faulkner

for rescue and hospital personnel. This led the way to the creation of the first statewide Emergency Medical Services System in 1973, with the Shock Trauma Center serving as the primary hospital-based center of trauma care.

Dr. Cowley's development of emergency medical services continued until his retirement in the spring of 1989. His tenure as director of the Institute and the Maryland Shock Trauma Center has provided specialized medical training for hospital personnel, advanced pre-hospital emergency care training for emergency medical technicians, and a statewide telecommunications system. In 1989, the new Maryland Shock Trauma Center opened, providing Maryland with a state-of-the-art 138-bed facility for the care of the critically ill and injured.

At the time of his retirement, Dr. Cowley accepted the position of director of the University of Maryland-based Charles McC. Mathias, Jr. National Trauma Study Center. The Center is designed to be a worldwide source of information on trauma treatment. Certainly, it is to benefit from Dr. Cowley's standard of excellence.

Foreword

In 1795, the flying ambulance—a horse-drawn carriage staffed with trained medical personnel—was developed by Baron Larrey for Napoleon during his campaign in Prussia. Thus the era of prehospital care began. During the War between the States, Tripler and Letterman of the Army of the Potomac reintroduced these concepts, but little else was accomplished for almost another 100 years. Military conflicts, especially WW II, Korea, and Vietnam, demonstrated that non-physician technicians could improve the survival of trauma casualties by initiating treatment before the patient reached the hospital. Despite this experience, it was not until the mid-1960's that these lessons were applied to the general population when J. D. "Deke" Farrington and others developed the first EMT-A program for civilians. Since the establishment of the first EMT training program in the Chicago fire department, over one million individuals have been trained to the EMT-A level with more than one quarter of that number going on to Advanced Life Support levels. Today, EMS remains one of the fastest growing components of medical care in the United States.

This textbook on emergency care represents a new generation of EMS knowledge. Every effort has been made to ensure that the instructional material contained in this text is based on sound medical practice. It incorporates material from the National Standard Curriculum for EMT-A as developed by the U.S. Department of Transportation, as well as essential material from other courses including Prehospital Trauma Life Support, Basic Trauma Life Support, Advanced Cardiac Life Support, Pediatric Trauma Support, and Advanced Trauma Life Support. The skills and knowledge presented in this text provide the solid foundation needed to evaluate and manage the majority of emergencies encountered by the prehospital provider. Gaining this knowledge is not easy since it requires study, practice, and repetition.

The individual who becomes an EMT assumes responsibility for the life of the patient he agrees to manage. The EMT profession is like few other occupations in the world. Immediate critical decisions based on knowledge and judgment are required. EMTs do not have the opportunity to return to the textbook to determine appropriate patient care after arriving on the scene and before rendering care. They must have the knowledge and skill in their brain and hands before the patient is ever seen. Dedication to continuing education is required to keep knowledge current and patient management skills sharp. Individuals willing to accept the challenge of this demanding profession will find satisfaction if they are mentally prepared to provide the very best care possible.

Norman E. McSwain, Jr., M.D., F.A.C.S.
William R. Roush, M.D., F.A.C.E.P.

Preface

You are about to begin your training to become an emergency medical technician (EMT). EMT courses range from 100 to 130 hours in length, with the typical EMT course being 110 hours long. Regardless of the hours you spend in class, your course is most likely based on guidelines set by the Department of Transportation (DOT). This is not to say that there is one universal EMT course. Using the DOT guidelines as a foundation, physicians and instructors in your local Emergency Medical Services System have designed your course to meet specific needs of your community. The basic training is the same, but there are differences in each state as to what materials are presented.

This textbook takes into account some of the variations in emergency care procedures used in different states. That is why you will find alternative methods cited throughout the text. There are some procedures that vary so much that only the most common methods in use are discussed. For such cases, you will be directed to follow local protocols.

Why is there no one method of providing care for certain illnesses and injuries? First of all, there are cases where more than one procedure works. Your EMS System may have tested only one procedure and decided that it was efficient, easy to learn, and simple to use. A different EMS System may have tested a second method and had the same results. This means that you will be trained to use the methods in which your local EMS System has confidence based upon its own rigorous testing.

Methods change as studies are performed to find ways of improving care. Your EMS System may be conducting research on injuries to the extremities, while another EMS System is concentrating on injuries to the soft tissues of the face. As you can see, your course might contain more new information on the emergency care for a patient with a fractured limb, while a course in another EMS System could contain more on injuries to the eye. With time, each system will present its findings nationally and have its methods evaluated. Since this is an ongoing process, it is doubtful that any two EMS Systems will have the same training program.

One thing is certain: not all the methods you learn in your training will stay the same during your career as an EMT. You must keep up-to-date with local procedures. Your instructor will tell you how continuing education programs for EMTs are presented in your locality, the prehospital emergency care journals recommended by your EMS System, and any state- or locally-produced newsletters that are available to help the EMT stay current.

Who is the authority for your course? Your instructor. As new information is gained and new procedures are developed, your instructor is kept informed. Even new textbooks may not be 100% up-to-date; and, as we have explained, no textbook can cover the specific protocols for all 50 states. Should you have any questions about sources saying different things, ask your instructor. If this text takes one approach to an emergency and your instructor takes a different one, follow your instructor. We ask you to do this, not to please your instructor, but because a textbook cannot be easily changed to reflect up-to-the-minute information on all emergency care procedures.

Objectives and Skills

At the start of each chapter or section, you will find a list of objectives. These objectives tell you specifically what you should be able to do by the end of the chapter. The objectives used in this text are called behavioral or performance objectives. They state the things you should be able to do that can be measured by you and others to determine if you are learning the materials.

Each chapter or section also has a list of skills to inform you of what procedures you must be able to do as an EMT. In addition to these lists, there is a complete list of EMT skills in Chapter 1. Before you can become an EMT, you will have to pass a practical examination. Keep a close check on your ability to perform a given procedure as it is covered in your course. If you find you cannot do one of the skills listed for a chapter, see your instructor for additional help.

Terms

To become an EMT, you will have to be able to read and understand many medical terms. As an EMT, you will have to use these terms when communicating with other professionals in the EMS System. Each chapter has its own list of new terms. In addition, there is a section in the appendix to help you learn medical terminology. A full glossary of terms is provided at the end of the text.

When a medical term is used for the first time, a pronunciation guide will be given. For example, the medical term for referring to the chest is "thoracic." The first time this term is used, you will see the following:

thoracic (tho-RAS-ik)

The capital letters indicate the portion of the word that is to be emphasized. Since you will have to use medical terminology when speaking with other emergency care professionals, you should practice saying these words, and using them in conversations with your fellow students and your instructor.

Scansheets

There are many facts and procedures that are easier to learn if you can see them presented in one place, in a manner that allows for quick study. This is why we have developed scansheets for this textbook. A scansheet is a one- or multi-page method of covering a complete procedure of care, or reviewing essential information related to assessment and care. Many of the emergency care procedures covered

in this text are presented as scansheets. By looking at the illustrations and reading the text on a scansheet, you will be able to study most, if not all, of what you will need to know about the procedure being presented. Since all the information for a topic is usually shown on one or two pages, you will also be able to use a scansheet to help you with the practical training portions of your course.

Using This Textbook

As you read and study each chapter, you should:

1. Read the list of objectives found at the beginning of the chapter.
2. Be certain that you understand all the objectives before reading the chapter.
3. Read through the list of terms to familiarize yourself with the new terminology to be used in the chapter.
4. Read the chapter, keeping the list of objectives in mind. Pay close attention to the illustrations, charts, and lists.
5. Spend extra time on each scansheet. The information covered on a scansheet is very important.
6. Read through the summary at the end of the chapter.
7. After reading the chapter, go back over the list of objectives and see if you can accomplish each one. Use the list of objectives as a self-test.
8. Go back over the sections of the chapter that deal with the objectives you could not meet.
9. Read the list of skills and make certain that you can find all the procedures listed in the chapter or presented on scansheets that will allow you to practice during the laboratory portions of your course. Know what is required to carry out a procedure before you attend the lab.

How to Study

The responsibility for teaching is the teacher's and the responsibility for learning is that of the student. Since it is your responsibility to learn what your instructor teaches, you will have to study the materials presented in this text and in class. There is too much material presented in a short period of time to allow you to remember all that you hear, see, and read without well-organized periods of study.

Every person is unique. How a person studies is a very personal thing; different methods work for each individual. There are, however, some standard recommendations that you may find helpful:

- Always follow the directions given by your instructor and the objectives in this text. Otherwise, you may spend too much time on minor points and not enough on what is critical for the EMT to know.
- Take notes during your training. You should have lecture, reading, and practical laboratory notes.
- Have your own place to study, removed from other activities.
- Study by yourself until you are able to meet all the chapter objectives.
- After you have studied on your own, talk with fellow students and your instructor about what you have learned. These conversations will help you to retain what you have learned and will give you practice using medical terminology.
- When you do not understand something, ask your instructor. Other students in the course may not understand any more than you do. They also lack the experience your instructor will have.

Improving Future Training

Not all the ideas for better methods of training come from physicians, committees, and instructors. Some of the best ideas come from students who can tell us what areas of study caused them the most trouble. Other good ideas come from practicing EMTs who let us know what problems they face in the field.

Any student, practicing EMT, or instructor who has an idea on how to improve EMT training, this textbook, or the emergency care provided to patients should write to the authors in care of The Brady Telemarketing Department, Prentice Hall, Inc., Englewood Cliffs, NJ 07632.

Acknowledgments

Production

This is the Fifth Edition of the "yellow book." We would be amiss if we did not take the time to thank all those professionals who worked on each edition and give a special thanks to everyone who worked so hard on the Fourth Edition and the Fourth Edition, Revised. These individuals helped ensure a continuity of quality that is carried into the text's fifth edition.

The task of developing and producing a fifth edition is a complex and time-consuming job. The task was made a lot easier because of Claire Merrick from Brady. Claire believes in us, the book, and most importantly of all—the EMS System. When we needed resources, she found them; if we needed materials, she looked for them; in cases when the reviewers did not agree, she helped to settle the issues. We thank Claire for all her hard work and her sense of humor.

Our Senior Production Editor at Prentice Hall was Tom Aloisi. Tom was with us on the Fourth Edition. His ability to edit and coordinate text, art, photography, design, and paste-up is remarkable. He impressed us again and we hope to have his expert help in the future.

The level of professionalism at Prentice Hall is the highest. These individuals helped us in so many ways that we do not have enough space to list all that was done. It is fair to say that no manuscript can become a textbook without these dedicated persons. We would like to thank Barbara Cassel, Senior Managing Editor; Mary Carnis, Associate Managing Editor; Judy-Matz Coniglio, Designer; Charles Pelletreau, Page Makeup Coordinator; Karen Noferi, Page Makeup; Elaine Rusoff, Art Production Manager; Janet Schmid, Assistant Design Director; Joe DiDomenico, Art Director; and Bill Thomas, Copy Editor. Also, a special thanks to Claire Merrick's assistant, Harriet Tellem. She kept track of many things, including Claire.

The new color art was done by Network Graphics of Hauppauge, New York. They have done a remarkable job, keeping the Brady tradition of excellence in art alive. The new color photography was done by George Dodson at the Lightworks Studio in Stevensville, Maryland. George has worked with us on several editions, always providing what we need in the most interesting and instructionally sound shots. He was helped by Lou Jordan and Ron Schaefer. These two EMS career professionals found equipment, models, and locations. They directed the photo sessions to ensure technical accuracy. We admire the work that they and George produced.

A special thanks to Ron Schaefer and Beverly Sopp of the Maryland Institute for Emergency Medical Services for their help in gathering information on Dr. R Adams Cowley. We wish to thank Jim Faulkner for the photography used in the Dedication.

Medical Advisors

Over the years, procedures used in pre-hospital emergency care have become more complex. When everyone agrees on a given procedure, our work is made easier; however, this is less of a fact than it was in earlier editions. The three of us and Claire Merrick convinced Prentice-Hall that we needed physician-level help to settle some of the disagreements found in the field and to ensure accuracy in care procedures. Such expert help was given by Norman E. McSwain, Jr., M.D., F.A.C.S., Professor of Surgery, Department of Surgery, Tulane University Medical Center, New Orleans, Louisiana and William R. Roush, M.D., F.A.C.E.P., Department of Emergency Medicine, Akron City Hospital, Akron, Ohio and Associate Professor of Emergency Medicine, Northeast Ohio Universities, College of Medicine, Rootstown, Ohio. These two fine physicians went beyond the call of duty to help us with this project.

Reviewers

The reviewers for the Fifth Edition maintained the level of excellence we have experienced with reviews on the last five manuscripts. Their suggestions were most helpful and their ability to answer national and local questions on EMT-level care was of great importance in developing this edition. We thank each of them as individuals and collectively as a group of highly motivated EMS professionals.

Jane W. Ball, RN, DrPH
Pediatric EMS Training Program
Children's Hospital National Medical Center
Washington, D.C.

Frank T. Barranco, Sr., M.D.
Chief Fire Dept. Surgeon, Baltimore County Fire Dept.
Assistant Professor of Orthopaedic Surgery
Johns Hopkins University
Baltimore, MD

Gloria J. Bizjak, Assistant Coordinator
Upper & Lower Eastern Short Regions of Maryland Fire & Rescue Institute
University of Maryland
Berwyn Heights, MD

Kevin Brame, Fire Battalion Chief
Orange County Fire Department
Emergency Medical Services Program Manager
Member of the California State Fire Marshall Emergency Medical Services Curriculum Committee
Orange, CA

Allan Braslow, Ph.D., Pres.
Braslow & Associates
Greenwich, CT

Arthur J. DeMello
Past Director of Training-New York City EMS
Chief-Gerrittsen Beach Fire Department
Bayside, NY

Rod Dennison, B.S., EMT-P
Texas Dept. of Health
EMS Division
Temple, TX

Robert Dinetz
Supervisor, Curriculum Development and Training
Office of Emergency Medical Services
New Jersey Department of Health
Trenton, New Jersey

Martin Eichelberger, M.D.
Associate Professor of Surgery and Child Health
George Washington University
Director of Trauma Services and
Attending Surgeon Children's Hospital National Medical Center
Washington, D.C.

Michael J. Fagel
Lieutenant-EMT Coordinator at North Aurora Illinois Fire Dept.
EMT Instructor, Waubonsee Community College
Aurora, IL

Ann Hudgins, RN, BSN, EMT-P
Instructor-Emergency Medicine Education
University of Texas Southwestern Medical Center
Dallas, Texas

Bonnie Johnson, R-EMT, EMT-D
Meadowood County Area Fire Dept.
Keene, New Hampshire

Gary W. Jones, CRT
EMT-A/Rescue Instructor
Maryland Fire and Rescue Institute
University of Maryland
College Park, Maryland

Kevin Kraus, BS, EMT-P
New York State Disaster Preparedness Commission
Albany, NY

Norman E. McSwain, Jr., M.D., F.A.C.S.
Professor of Surgery
Department of Surgery
Tulane University Medical Center
New Orleans, LA

National Council of State EMS Training
Coordinators
Jefferson City, MO

William R. Roush, M.D., F.A.C.E.P.
Department of Emergency Medicine
Akron City Hospital-Akron Ohio
Associate Professor of Emergency Medicine
Northeast Ohio Universities, College of
  Medicine
Rootstown, Ohio

Sharron Silva, Ph.D.
Instructional Design Associate
American Red Cross National
  Headquarters
Washington, D.C.

Clark Staten, EMT-P, I/C
Adjunct Faculty: Triton Community College
River Grove, IL
Chicago Fire Department
Chicago, IL

BRADY
EMERGENCY CARE

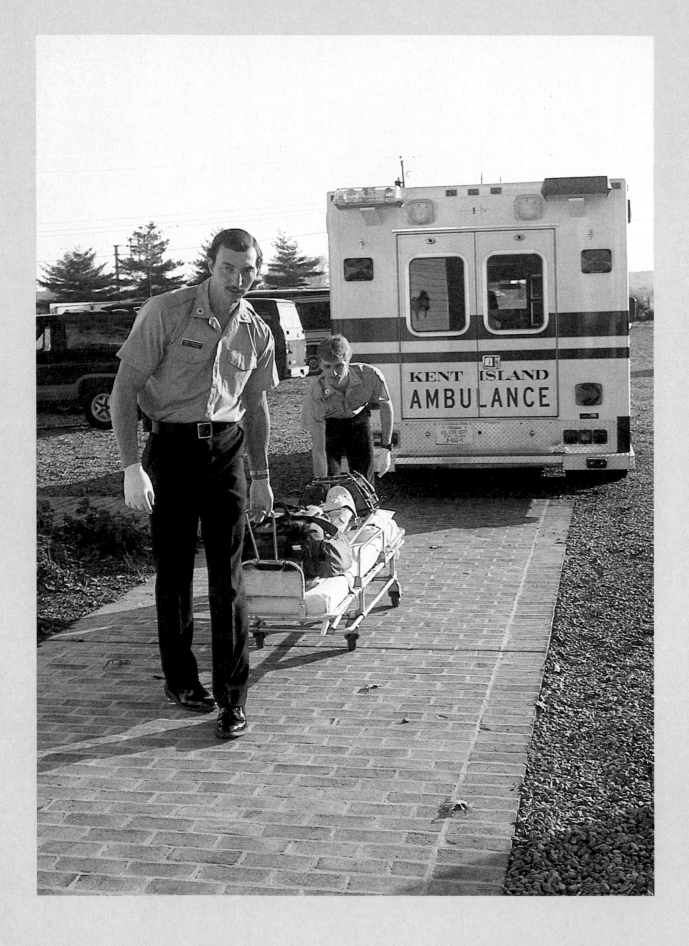

CHAPTER 1

The Emergency Medical Technician

OBJECTIVES   As an EMT, you should be able to:

1. Define *emergency medical services (EMS) system.* (p. 4 and pp. 10–11)
2. Define *emergency care.* (pp. 5–6 and p. 12)
3. Define *emergency medical technician (EMT).* (pp. 11–12)
4. List the NINE major duties of an EMT. (p. 12)
5. List some of the activities you may be called on to perform as part of your EMT duties. (p. 12 and p. 14)
6. Describe the desirable traits of an EMT. (p. 15)
7. Define *standard of care.* (p. 17)
8. State how the concept of negligence applies to EMT-level emergency care. (p. 17)
9. Define *abandonment.* (pp. 17–18)
10. Relate EMT responsibilities to Good Samaritan laws and the standard of care. (pp. 19–20)
11. Define *informed consent*, and distinguish between actual and implied consent. (pp. 18–19)
12. Distinguish between voluntary and involuntary consent. (p. 19)
13. Relate the laws governing patient consent and refusal of care to the child patient. (p. 18)
14. List SIX emergencies that may require you to file special reports. (pp. 20–21)
15. Describe the role and actions of an EMT when caring for a deceased person. (p. 21)
16. Describe three types of ambulances. (pp. 21–22)
17. Categorize the medical equipment, basic tools, and supplies used by the EMT. (pp. 22–23)

SKILLS   As an EMT, you should be able to:

1. Develop and display the desirable traits of an EMT.

2. Provide EMT-level care as defined by law and regulations.

TERMS you may be using for the first time:

Abandonment – to leave an injured or ill patient before the responsibility for care is properly transferred to someone of equal or superior training. The other person must accept the responsibility for care. Leaving the hospital without giving essential patient information to the staff is viewed by some courts and legal experts as a form of abandonment.

Actual Consent – consent given by the rational adult patient, usually in oral form, accepting emergency care. This must be informed consent.

Duty to Act – typically a local law that identifies which agencies have a legal responsibility to provide emergency care. If an EMT is a member of such an agency, he or she has a legal responsibility to render emergency care while on duty.

Emergency Care – at the EMT level this is usually the prehospital assessment and treatment of the sick or injured patient. This care is initiated at the emergency scene and is continued through transport and transfer to a medical facility. The physical and emotional needs of the patient are considered and attended to during care.

Emergency Medical Services (EMS) System – the complete chain of human and physical resources that provides patient care in cases of sudden illness and injury.

Emergency Medical Technician (EMT) – a professional-level provider of emergency care. This individual has received formal training and is appropriately certified. An EMT can be a paid career or a volunteer professional.

First Responder – a person who is part of the EMS System, having been trained in a First Responder course and, where it is policy, having the appropriate certification. Such an individual is trained below the level of the basic EMT.

Good Samaritan Laws – a series of laws, varying in each state, designed to provide limited legal protection for citizens and some health care personnel when they are administering emergency care. These laws require a person to act in good faith and provide care to the level of his or her training, to the best of his or her abilities. In some states, these laws do not apply to the paid EMT and may only apply to the volunteer when he or she is not on duty.

Implied Consent – a legal position that assumes an unconscious patient (or one so badly injured or ill that he cannot respond) would consent to receiving emergency care if he or she could do so. In some states, implied consent may apply to children when parents or guardians are not at the scene, to the developmentally disabled (e.g., mentally retarded), and to the mentally or emotionally disturbed.

Informed Consent – agreement by a rational adult patient to accept emergency care, after you state your name, the level of your training, what you believe may be the patient's condition, and what you plan to do. In many cases, informed consent does not exist unless the patient also knows the risks involved with the care procedures and the alternatives he or she has to accepting your care.

Morbidity – the occurrence of illness.

Mortality – the occurrence of death.

Negligence – at the EMT level this is the failure to provide the expected care at the standard of care. This improper care must lead to the injury or death of the patient if negligence is to be established.

Standard of Care – the minimum accepted level of emergency care to be provided as may be set forth by law, administrative orders, guidelines published by emergency care organizations and societies, local protocols and practice, and what has been accepted in the past (precedent). Each state or locality has its own standard of care.

THE EMERGENCY MEDICAL SERVICES SYSTEM

How It Began

Most of the techniques and procedures currently used in medicine have been developed since the 1940s. As developments in each new decade increase our scientific knowledge and lead to new techniques, many advances are carried over into the field of medicine. Today's hospitals are staffed by highly trained health care teams who use complex medical procedures, accurate methods of detecting disease, elaborate equipment, and new "wonder" drugs. This is a far cry from the hospital of the last century where most patients who entered expected to die.

The advantages of modern medicine are lost if the patient does not have access to them. Sudden illness or severe injury may cause irreversible damage or death unless appropriate care is initiated as soon as possible. The concept of providing professional-level care at the emergency scene and en route to the hospital is one of the newest advances in total patient care. The emergency medical services (EMS) system was developed to allow the emergency capabilities of the hospital to be used to begin care of the patient at the emergency scene.

Historians are unable to document specific systems for emergency patients before the 1790s. The need to provide care for battlefield casualties inspired the French to begin the transport of patients so they could be cared for by physicians away from the scene of battle. Care probably did not begin until the patients reached the physician. The concern for the suffering of soldiers on the battlefield continued into the next century, leading to the formation of what was to become the International Red Cross in 1863. This organization recognized that there was a responsibility to provide care for the wounded as soon as possible.

In the United States, emergency care also began during the time of war. A dedicated nurse, Clara Barton, started professional-level emergency care for the wounded during the Civil War. She was instrumental in the United States joining the International Red Cross, working from 1881 until 1905 to have Congress grant a charter for the American Red Cross. Her efforts, and the work of another nurse, Jane Delano, firmly established the American Red Cross. This organization's efforts to provide initial care for accident victims and those taken suddenly ill began to develop after World War II.

Ambulance services in the United States began in a few major cities at the turn of the century. Most were transport systems only, offering little or no emergency care. Smaller cities, towns, and rural areas did not begin to develop ambulance services until after World War II. Where services developed to provide emergency care with transport, the fire service was often the agency responsible for rendering care.

Medical teams in the Korean Conflict and the Vietnam War produced advances in the techniques and procedures used to care for injuries and the effects of injuries (trauma). These methods were modified and combined with those developed in the civilian sector to produce field emergency care procedures and the beginnings of specialized emergency medical centers (e.g., the Shock Trauma Unit at University Hospital in Baltimore).

During the mid 1960s, the National Academy of Sciences' National Research Council studied the problem of emergency care. Its intent was to establish standards for prehospital care. Modern emergency medical services began when it issued the following statement:

Employees or volunteer members of public and private organizations having a responsibility for the delivery of health services must be trained in and held accountable for administration of specialized care and delivery of the victims of acute illness or injury to a medical facility. This category of lay persons includes ambulance personnel, rescue squad workers, policemen, firemen, lifeguards, workers in first aid or health facilities of public buildings and industrial plants, attendants at sports events, civil defense workers, paramedic personnel, and employees of public or private health service agencies. Specialized training, retraining and accreditation of such persons necessitate development of training courses, manuals and training aids adequate to provide instruction in all emergency care short of that rendered by physicians or by paramedic personnel under their direct supervision.

Ambulance personnel are responsible for all lay emergency care from the time they first see the victim through transportation and delivery to care of a physician. They must therefore be able not only to appraise the extent of first aid rendered by others, but also to carry out what additional measures will make it safe to move the victim and minimize morbidity and mortality. They must operate the vehicle safely and efficiently; maintain communication between the scene of the emergency, traffic authorities, dispatchers, and emergency departments; render necessary additional care en route; and transmit records and reports to medical and other authorities. Although the emphasis on certain subjects will vary with the nature of employment of those who are not ambulance personnel but who have a responsibility for delivery of health services, they should be equally trained so that minimum care can be assured,

The above may not have much meaning so early in your training. However, once you become an EMT, come back to this quotation. You will note that it is the framework on which your course is based. Also, keep in mind what emergency care must have been like in many areas of the country before direction, standards, and a national commitment were developed. With the preceding statement, the long-held concept of ambulance service as a means merely for transporting the sick and injured passed into oblivion. No longer could ambulance personnel be viewed as people with little more than the physical strength required to lift a victim in and out of an ambulance. Victims now became *patients*, receiving prehospital emergency care from highly trained professional personnel. Emergency care began to include treating both the sick and injured at the emergency scene and during transport, with the providers of this care being trained to consider the physical and emotional needs of the patient. The hospital emergency department was extended, through emergency medical services, to reach the sick and injured at the emergency scene and begin immediate care. The ambulance attendant was replaced by the **Emergency Medical Technician** (EMT).

The National Highway Safety Act of 1966 charged the United States Department of Transportation (DOT) with developing Emergency Medical Services (EMS) standards and assisting the states to upgrade the quality of their prehospital emergency care. The DOT created an 81-hour EMT course that is the basis for modern EMT training. In 1984, the DOT published a 110-hour course of instruction and clinical experience that served as a model for the development of most of today's EMT courses.

Added support for the emergency medical services came when the American Heart Association (AHA) began to produce training materials and programs for cardiopulmonary resuscitation (CPR) and basic life support in 1966. Their efforts were directed at the prehospital emergency care of patients who have suffered airway obstruction, the stoppage of breathing, and sudden death due to heart attack. A program for public education in basic cardiac life support came from the AHA and the National Academy of Sciences' National Research Council recommendations in 1973. By 1977, the AHA and the American Red Cross had trained over 12 million health care professionals and private citizens in basic life support. Their goal is to train 80 million persons, providing them with the skills that may save as many as 100,000 to 200,000 lives each year. Millions of citizens and EMS personnel are certified and recertified every year.

In 1970, the National Registry of Emergency Medical Technicians was founded. One of the goals of this organization was to establish professional standards for EMTs and to provide services for local EMS Systems wishing to upgrade their EMT training programs. Other national organizations were created to consider what could be done to improve prehospital emergency care (see p. 23).

In 1973, the National Emergency Medical Services Systems Act was passed at the national level. This legislation allowed the federal government to define 300 EMS regions in the United States and provide some of the initial funding for the development of specific emergency care services and facilities and the training of personnel for these units and facilities.

The National Health Planning and Resources Development Act of 1974 increased planning activities and services to help the states develop their EMS Systems. Today, most states have their own quality EMS System, offering basic, advanced, and continuing education programs to most providers of prehospital emergency care.

Members of the nation's EMS Systems are proud of their history and what they have been able to accomplish in the ongoing effort to improve prehospital emergency care.

Elements of the System

The EMS System is more than EMTs and emergency department personnel. It is a chain of human and physical resources brought together to provide total patient care. To better understand this chain of resources, consider an event in the life of Mr. Tom Henderson. Note how all the links of the chain of resources joined to carry Tom through an unfortunate experience (Figures 1–1 through 1–15).

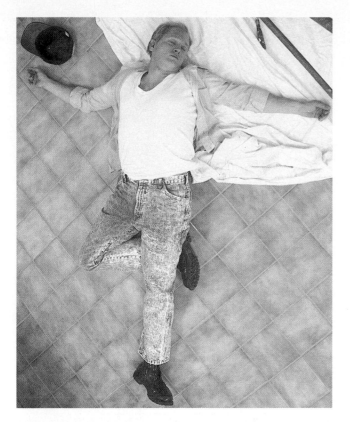

FIGURE 1–1. Wednesday, June 21, 11:50 A.M. Tom is working on scaffolding in the warehouse of the Acme Paper Products Company. While painting, he leans too far over the scaffold and falls nearly 8 feet to the floor. He lands on his right leg and falls backward, striking his upper back and shoulders on the floor.

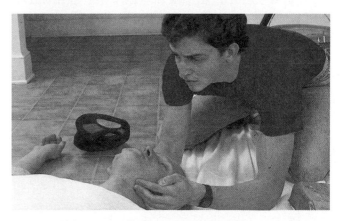

FIGURE 1–2. 11:51 A.M. A co-worker nearby sees Tom fall. Before going to Tom's assistance, he quickly calls out to the floor supervisor, who, in turn, notifies the nurse on duty in the plant infirmary. Before she leaves the infirmary, the nurse dials 911 and requests assistance from the local EMS System.

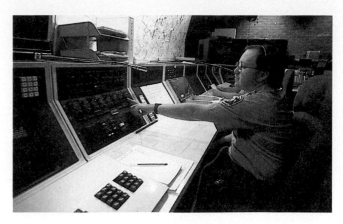

FIGURE 1–3. 11:51 A.M. The local emergency communications center dispatcher receives the call from the plant nurse. He gathers as much information about the accident as he can and passes this information on as he alerts the ambulance and rescue squad. In some areas of the country, if the caller had been a lay person without emergency care training or trained personnel at the scene, the dispatcher would have offered basic care instructions to be carried out until trained professionals arrived.

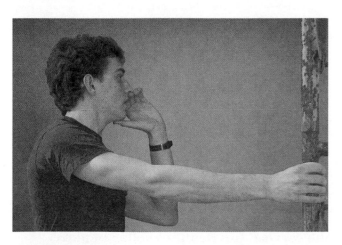

FIGURE 1–4. 11:52 A.M. The co-worker who witnessed the accident reaches Tom's side. It is obvious that Tom has been injured. A quick assessment shows him that Tom is unconscious and is having difficulty breathing. He quickly positions himself at Tom's head and opens Tom's airway by using a jaw-thrust maneuver that he learned in a plant-sponsored First Responder course. He is careful not to move Tom's head any more than absolutely necessary because of the possibility of spinal injuries. This simple maneuver reduces Tom's breathing problems. The co-worker does not move Tom; instead, he closely watches Tom's breathing efforts. He is ready to assist Tom in the event that respirations stop.

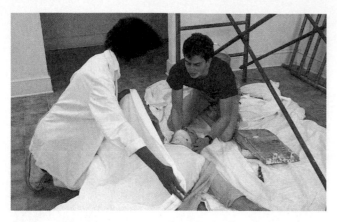

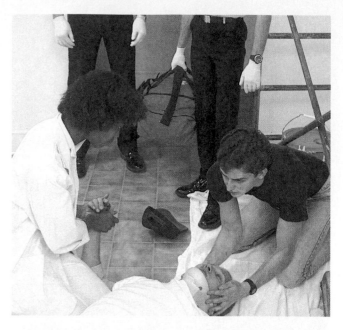

FIGURE 1–5.   11:56 A.M. The plant nurse arrives with a first aid kit and blankets. Tom's co-worker describes the breathing problem he noticed and the results of the jaw-thrust. The nurse determines that Tom is no longer having difficulty with his breathing. She makes a quick assessment and, based on her observation of the mechanism of injury, has the First Responder stabilize Tom's head and neck while she secures a rigid cervical collar (extrication collar) around Tom's neck. She has the co-worker continue to stabilize Tom's head after the collar is applied. Knowing that EMTs will soon arrive, she does not move Tom. However, she does cover him to help conserve body heat.

FIGURE 1–7.   12:03 P.M. The EMTs reach the site of Tom's accident. A quick survey shows that Tom is now alert, is breathing, has a full and regular pulse, and has no serious bleeding wounds. There are no indications that Tom is going into shock.

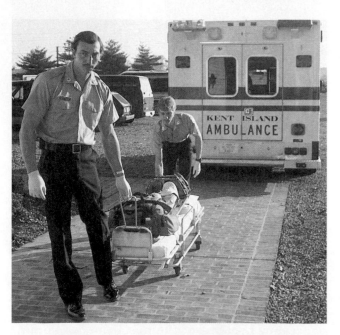

FIGURE 1–6.   12:01 P.M. The ambulance arrives on the scene. The EMTs enter the building, bringing with them a wheeled stretcher, a long spine board, a portable oxygen delivery system, and a trauma kit.

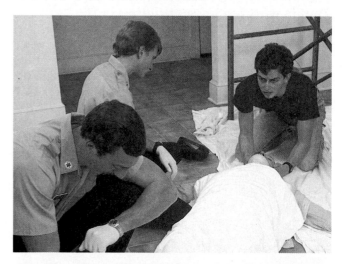

FIGURE 1–8.   The EMTs conduct a complete survey and find that Tom has a possible fracture of the right femur (thigh bone). He does not have any field-test indications of spinal injury. Nonetheless, they elect to leave the cervical (extrication) collar in place, knowing that spinal injuries are possible in this type of accident. To further protect Tom from additional injury, the EMTs plan to immobilize him on a long spine board after a traction splint is applied to the injured leg. Checking the pulse in the injured leg, the EMTs conduct a complete survey.

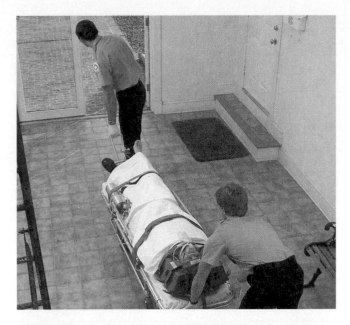

FIGURE 1–9.   12:09 P.M. The EMTs begin to administer oxygen to help lessen any complications should Tom develop shock. Properly splinted and immobilized, placed on a stretcher, covered, secured, and receiving oxygen, Tom is wheeled from the accident site.

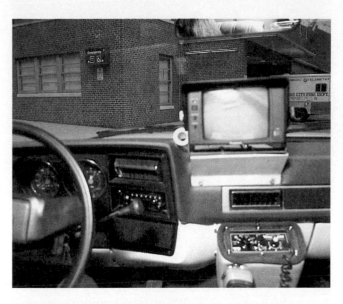

FIGURE 1–11.   12:30 P.M. The ambulance arrives at the medical facility. The EMTs transfer Tom to the emergency department and provide the staff with an oral and written report of the accident, patient assessment, and care rendered.

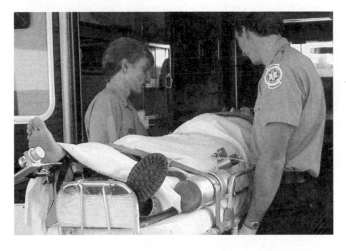

FIGURE 1–10.   12:13 P.M. Only ten minutes have passed since the EMTs reached the patient's side. Tom is loaded into the ambulance and transported to the hospital. He is attended by an EMT during transport in case additional emergency care is required. During transport, concise radio communications inform the emergency department staff of the circumstances of Tom's accident, the possible extent of his injuries, his condition, the care provided, and the estimated time of arrival. The emergency department staff will be alerted if there is any change in Tom's condition during transport.

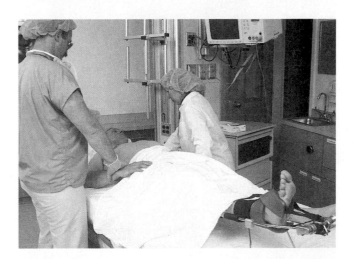

FIGURE 1–12.   Tom's immediate needs are cared for by the emergency department staff. Tests are performed and x-rays are taken. The emergency department physician finds that Tom does not have any spinal injuries. The required care for Tom's injuries is determined, and he is wheeled to an operating room where an orthopedic surgeon cares for Tom's fracture.

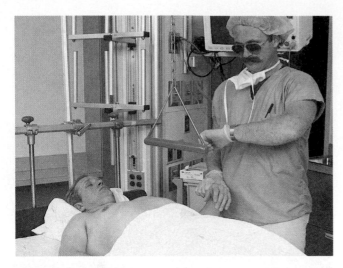

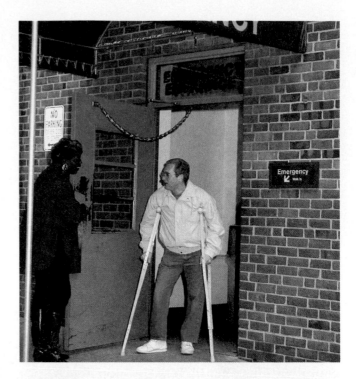

FIGURE 1–13.   Tom is moved to a recovery room and placed in traction. A nurse closely observes him until he is completely recovered from the anesthesia. When appropriate, he will be moved to a room in an area of the hospital where the staff specializes in the care of patients who have orthopedic injuries.

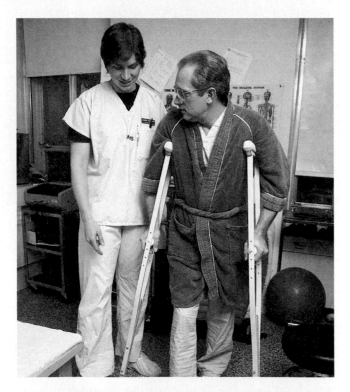

FIGURE 1–14.   Saturday, June 23. A physical therapist begins working with Tom, providing him with patient education and a program on exercises to prevent muscle wasting in his uninjured extremity. On Monday, August 14, Tom begins a program of rehabilitation for his injured leg under the supervision of a physical therapist.

FIGURE 1–15.   Sunday, August 20. Tom has received total patient care while he was in the hospital and has been discharged. He will be away from work for some time, and he will have to return to the hospital periodically for therapy. But . . . he is alive, and he can walk!

Having read of Tom's experience, consider how many different persons were involved with his care from accident through recovery. **AT ANY POINT, TOM COULD HAVE SUSTAINED IRREVERSIBLE INJURY IF ANY ONE OF THESE PERSONS FAILED TO ACT OR PROVIDED IMPROPER CARE.** The chain of human and physical resources, the EMS System in Tom's community, held together because none of the links in the chain failed. This chain of resources is reviewed in Figure 1–16.

Some parts of the EMS System were not visible in the preceding example. An advisory council and medical director for EMS decided how the system was to respond and what care procedures were to be used. Public information officers had provided the citizens with the knowledge of what the EMS System is, what it could do, and how to seek assistance. The EMS System trained instructors, who then trained the EMTs who responded to help Tom. Many other persons, including those involved with personnel, record keeping, and equipment and supplies were an important part of the EMS System being able to help Tom.

A person who has an accident, or a person who suddenly becomes ill, is called a *victim*. Once the

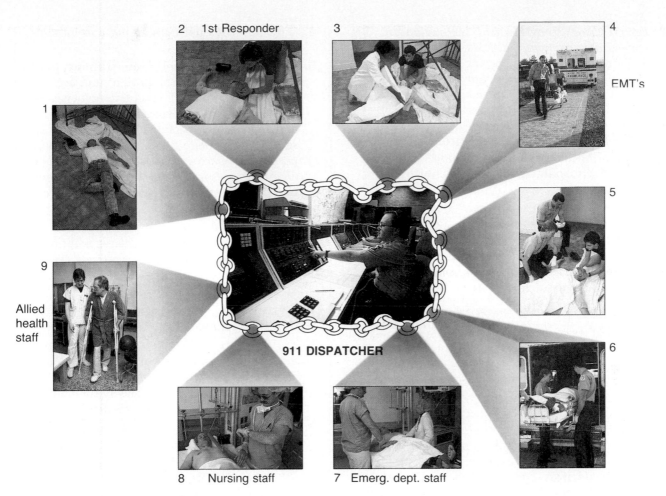

FIGURE 1–16. **The chain of human and physical resources of the EMS System.**

person enters into the EMS system, he becomes a *patient*.

As an EMT, you will be part of the EMS System. More specifically, you will carry out your duties as a part of a prehospital emergency care delivery subsystem. The components to this subsystem are:

- The EMT
- The ambulance
- The supplies and equipment carried on the ambulance

THE EMERGENCY MEDICAL TECHNICIAN

The EMT is a *professional* provider of emergency care. Both the volunteer and paid EMT are considered to be professional members of the EMS System.

The term *professional* does not imply payment for services. It refers to training, dedication, desire to perform to the best of one's abilities, and willingness to continue with formal training. Working within the EMS System, the EMT is a team member helping to provide total patient care. Trained and appropriately *certified*, the EMT is capable of providing emergency care at the scene and en route to the hospital.

There is more than one level of EMT. In this book, we will use the term to mean the *Basic EMT* unless otherwise stated. The levels of EMTs include:

1. *Basic EMT*: a person who has successfully completed the DOT EMT National Standard Training Program or its equivalent and has been certified as an EMT by a state emergency medical services board or other authorized agency. Some localities have the classification EMT-NA (Emergency Medical Technician–Nonambulance) for basic EMTs who are trained to provide care at the scene but not during transport.

2. *EMT-I* (*Emergency Medical Technician–Intermediate, pronounced EMT-eye*): a basic EMT who has passed specific training programs so that he may provide locally determined procedures in intermediate and advanced life support. In some states, this level includes those EMTs who are given the title of Cardiac Technician, Cardiac Rescue Technician, Shock-Trauma Technician, Critical Care Technician, and EMT-Defibrillator (EMT-D).

3. *EMT-P* (*Emergency Medical Technician–Paramedic*): a person who has successfully completed paramedic training including or equal to the DOT National Standard Paramedic Curriculum and has received the appropriate certification.

The EMT deals with both injury and illness and the emotional problems that result from such emergencies. You will have to provide basic life support for patients because they cannot breathe adequately, have stopped breathing, have developed cardiac arrest, or have developed shock. You will have to provide care for patients having cuts, bruises, fractures, burns, and internal injuries. You will be called on to deal with heart attacks, strokes, respiratory illnesses, seizures, diabetic coma, insulin shock, childbirth, poisoning, drug abuse, and problems due to excessive heat and cold. In addition, you will have to provide care for patients suffering emotional or psychiatric emergencies. Some problems will be simple, while others will be life threatening. All will require professional-level emergency care.

Roles and Responsibilities

At an emergency scene, the primary concern is the patient, but your primary responsibility will be one of personal safety. This responsibility requires you to make certain that you can safely reach the patient and remain safe during all aspects of care. You must never allow your desire to help the patient make you overlook the potential hazards at the scene.

In addition to hands-on care, each aspect of the activities carried out by EMTs is done to ensure efficient care, safety, and comfort to the patient.

As an EMT, you will have nine main duties:

1. Be prepared to respond.
2. Respond to the scene swiftly, but safely.
3. Make certain that the scene is safe, and when called on to do so, assist in the control of the activities at the scene (e.g., traffic).

4. Gain access to patients, using special tools when necessary.
5. Determine, to the level of your training, what may be wrong with the patient and provide the appropriate EMT-level emergency care. This would include recognizing the need for and requesting specialized personnel to be sent to the scene (e.g., advanced life support personnel). Care and assessments should be done with personal safety in mind. The scene must be safe and you must be protected from injury and disease.
6. Free, lift, and move the patient, when required, and do so without causing additional injury to the patient or to yourself. These procedures are also called disentanglement, extrication, and transfer.
7. Prepare and properly transfer the patient to the ambulance.
8. Transport the patient safely to the appropriate medical facility, providing the needed care and en route communications and transferring the patient and patient information to the staff at the medical facility.
9. Return safely from the run, complete records and reports, and prepare the ambulance, equipment, supplies, and yourself for the next response.

Depending on your training and where you will be working as an EMT, you may be called on to do any or all of the following as part of your duties:

- Function as a driver EMT, being familiar with emergency vehicle driving techniques; traffic regulations; how to select the best route depending on traffic conditions, weather, and other factors; and how to approach, park at, and leave the scene.
- Control an emergency scene in order to protect yourself and the patient and to prevent additional accidents. Hazard recognition is a key part of this activity. You must be able to use the appropriate protective clothing and apparatus required in your locality.
- Assess an emergency scene, determining and requesting any additional assistance from law enforcement, fire services, utility companies, or others that may be needed at the scene. Again, hazard recognition is critical in performing this function.
- Gain access to patients in special situations, such as motor vehicle accidents, water and ice accidents, cave-ins, and crime scenes.

SCAN 1–1   THE EMT—NINE MAIN DUTIES

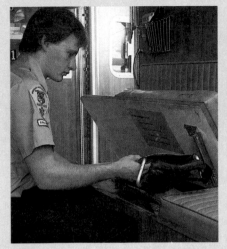

Preparation

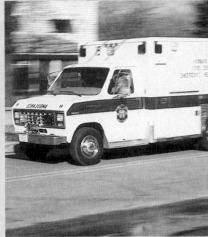

Response

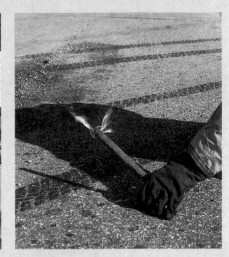

Scene control

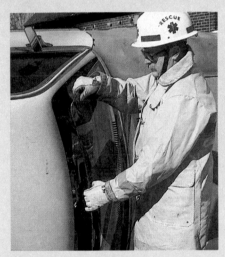

Gaining access

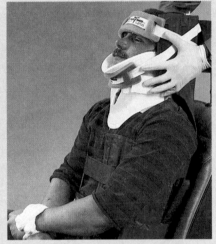

Assessment and emergency care

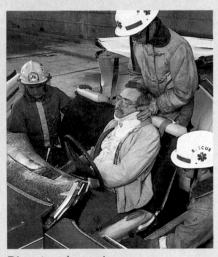

Disentanglement

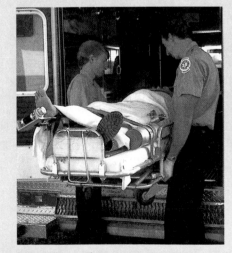

Transfer and transport

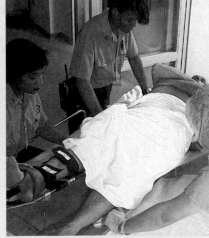

Transfer to medical facility

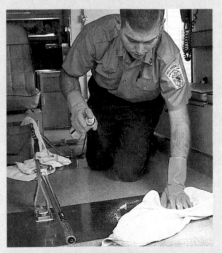

Termination of activities

- Determine what is probably wrong with the patient by gathering information from the scene, bystanders, and the patient and by examining the patient. This includes performing and/or directing the performance of triage. (See Chapter 20.)
- Provide EMT-level emergency care to the best of your ability and training.
- Reassure patients, relatives, and bystanders, providing emotional support as part of your care.
- Free trapped patients by using the techniques and tools of extrication.
- Properly prepare the patient for safe transfer to the ambulance and transport to the hospital (packaging the patient).
- Safely transport patients to the appropriate medical facility, monitoring the patient, providing needed emergency care, and communicating with the emergency department staff while en route.
- Transfer the patient, patient information, and personal effects to the emergency department staff, and on request, assist the emergency department staff.
- Complete all the necessary reports and forms that are required for the run.
- Make certain that everything necessary is done to be prepared for the next run.

These are only a few of the many things every EMT must be able to do. Some duties, such as basic life support, are dramatic. Report writing and taking inventory are far less glamorous. Remember, all duties are important to providing patient care.

You should now turn to page 26 at the end of this chapter. There you will find a list of all the skills and duties to be performed by an EMT. As you go through your training, check off the items that you believe you can accomplish at the professional level of the Emergency Medical Technician.

NOTE: Duties and skills may vary among localities. Within any given area, specific policies, laws, and regulations determine which member of an EMT team has what duties. Usually, all basic EMTs are equally trained in all duties and responsibilities so that they may function independently or interchangeably.

Background, Training, and Experience

Many areas of the nation use a job description for the EMT based on that which was prepared by the United States Department of Transportation and supported by the National Highway Traffic Safety Administration. In *most* localities, the minimum levels of training and experience required for the EMT include:

- Age of 18 years or older.
- Training to the level recognized as the DOT National Standard Curriculum for EMT–Ambulance personnel.
- Practical experience in the care and use of emergency care equipment commonly used by EMTs (e.g., suction devices, installed and portable oxygen delivery systems, anti-shock garments, splints and immobilization equipment, emergency medical kits, obstetric kits, patient transfer devices, and basic rescue tools).
- Practical experience in sanitizing and disinfecting procedures for all equipment, including the ambulance.
- Knowledge of safety and security procedures to allow for duties to be carried out in certain hostile environments.
- Knowledge of the territory within the EMT's service area.
- A valid driver's license, an acceptable driving record, and any professional certificate or license as required by law indicating that you know the motor vehicle codes and that you as a driver can skillfully and safely operate an ambulance. Many localities do not require all EMTs to be drivers.
- Ability to use communications equipment.
- Certification from your state or an appropriate agency that is responsible for EMT certification within a specific jurisdiction.

EMT Traits

There are certain physical traits and aspects of personality that are desirable for an EMT. Physically, you should be in good health, fit to carry out your duties. You have a responsibility to stay in shape so that you can carry out your duties. If you are unable to provide needed care because you cannot bend over or catch your breath, then all your training may be worthless to the patient who is in need of your help.

You should be able to lift and carry up to 100 pounds. Practice with other EMTs is essential so that you can learn how to carry your share of the combined weight of patient, stretcher, linens, blankets, and portable oxygen equipment. For such moves, coordination and dexterity are needed, as well as strength. You will have to perform basic rescue procedures, lower stretcher patients from upper levels, and negotiate fire escapes and stairways while carrying patients.

Your eyesight is very important in performing your EMT duties. Make certain that you can clearly see distant objects as well as those close at hand. Both types of vision are needed for patient assessment, driving tasks, and controlling emergency scenes. Should you have any eyesight problems, they must be corrected with prescription eye glasses or contact lenses.

Be aware of any problems you may have with color vision. Not only is this important to driving, but it could also be critical for patient assessment. Colors seen on the patient's skin, lips, nailbeds, ear lobes, and eyelids often provide valuable clues to a patient's condition.

You should be able to give and receive oral and written instructions. Eyesight, hearing, and speech are important to the EMT; thus all significant problems must be corrected if you are to be an EMT.

Good personality traits are very important to the EMT. You should be:

- Pleasant—to inspire confidence and help to calm the sick and injured.
- Sincere—able to convey an understanding of the situation and the patient's feelings.
- Cooperative—to allow for faster and better care, establish better coordination with other members of the EMS System, and bolster the confidence of patients and bystanders.
- Resourceful—able to adapt a tool or technique to fit an unusual situation.
- A self-starter—to show initiative and accomplish what must be done without having to depend on someone else to start procedures.
- Emotionally stable—to help overcome the unpleasant aspects of an emergency so that needed care may be rendered and any uneasy feelings that exist after care has been provided may be resolved.
- Able to lead—to take the steps necessary to control a scene, to organize bystanders, to deliver care, and, when necessary, to take complete charge of an emergency.
- Present a neat and clean appearance—to promote confidence in both patients and bystanders and to reduce the possibility of contamination.
- Of good moral character, having respect for others—to allow for trust in situations when the patient cannot protect his own body or valuables and so that all information relayed is considered to be truthful and reliable.

- In control of personal habits—to reduce the possibility of rendering improper care and to prevent discomfort to the patient. This would include not smoking when providing care (**REMEMBER:** smoking may contaminate wounds and is a danger around oxygen delivery systems) and never consuming alcohol within 8 hours of duty.
- Controlled in conversation—able to communicate properly, to inspire confidence, and to avoid inappropriate conversation that may upset or anger the patient or bystanders or violate patient confidentiality.
- Able to listen to others—to be accurate with interviews and to inspire confidence.

All of this leads to developing a CALM, PROFESSIONAL MANNER that will result in better patient care.

At first, some people do not see the importance of these personality traits. They believe that all that an EMT needs to worry about is how to efficiently provide the correct care procedure. Experience has shown that all of the traits listed are relevant to the complex world of emergency care.

For example, consider leadership ability. In many cases, others will be in charge at the scene. However, YOU may have to take control of an accident scene. YOU may have to initiate rescue efforts. YOU may have to direct the sorting and removal of multiple casualties from the scene. YOU may have to deal with distraught relatives. YOU may have to cope with spectators who are disrupting an otherwise smooth-running operation. YOU may have to make unpleasant decisions. In short, at one time or another, YOU will be in charge and there will be no one else to take over. In those instances you must be able to lead calmly, decisively, and firmly if you are to ensure cooperation, teamwork, and the best of patient care.

EMS Systems place a strong emphasis on a neat, clean appearance and good personal grooming (see Fig. 1–17). Put yourself in the place of an injured but conscious patient. If one EMT arrives in a clean uniform and another arrives in greasy overalls and if you know nothing of their capabilities, which one would you want to help you? You would probably pick the uniformed EMT, if for no other reason than he looks the part. The uniform indicates disciplined training, quality, and organization. Be it a full uniform, a jacket, or simply a cap with a badge, the recognition provided helps to put the patient at ease and to gain the cooperation of bystanders.

Neatness and good personal grooming not only inspire confidence, but they also serve to protect the patient from contamination that may come from

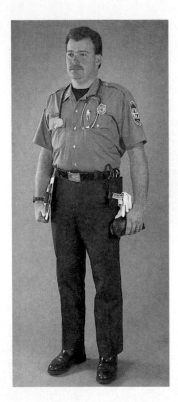

FIGURE 1–17. A professional appearance inspires confidence.

dirty clothing, hands, and fingernails and the unkempt hair of the rescuer.

One of the biggest mistakes made by new EMTs is *inappropriate conversation.* Saying the wrong thing or using the wrong words may upset a patient and worsen his condition. Inappropriate conversation also may upset relatives or bystanders, diminishing any chances you may have to gain their confidence and help. Remember, it is not only *what* you say but *how* you say it. Shouting only leads to confusion. A harsh voice may make others uncooperative or reluctant to accept your help. The tone of your voice may be the key that allows you to provide proper care.

People who are not trained to deal with emergencies often use phrases such as, "Don't worry, everything is all right" when dealing with the sick and injured. As an EMT, you must discipline yourself to avoid these types of statements. A patient knows that everything is not all right. An inappropriate statement, even if said in an effort to show concern, will not gain confidence or cooperation from the patient.

Learning to use appropriate, calm, **neutral** conversation is part of becoming a professional EMT. Conversation with a patient can help him to relax if you are calm and honest. Telling the patient that you are trained in emergency care and that you will help him eases his fear and inspires confidence. Telling the patient what you are going to do helps him to believe that you are competent.

As you can see, to provide emergency care, you must be able to do more than apply the correct procedures. You must do so in a professional manner, thus providing TOTAL PATIENT CARE.

THE EMT AND THE LAW

When it comes to the law, a textbook can only offer you general guidelines. Each state has its own laws in regard to emergency care provided by the nonphysician. This text covers some of the basics, using layperson's terms, but the legal advisors for your EMS System will have to provide you with the specifics that apply in your state. The information presented here is not intended as legal advice. When you are in doubt about the law and how it applies to your duties as an EMT, seek the advice of an attorney familiar with the EMS System in your state.

Most individuals involved in providing emergency care are concerned with the legal aspects of care. Often, they are concerned with being sued. No one will tell you to think lightly of this problem. You can be sued; however, you will probably be able to defend yourself if you provided proper care to the level of your training, within the laws of your state. You can be sued and held liable for many different acts, including (but not limited to):

- Not providing care—you have a duty to the patient to provide care to your level of training.
- Rendering *improper care* when what was needed should have been obvious to a trained EMT.
- Abusing or mistreating a patient—this includes assault (e.g., threatening to physically hurt someone), battery (e.g., touching someone who does not wish to be touched), or violating the patient's civil rights (e.g., denying care because of the patient's national origin).
- Providing care above the level of your certification, even if this act causes no injury or harm to the patient.
- Causing injury or mental anguish or allowing a correctable condition to worsen and cause damage.
- Forcing care on a competent adult who has refused your care—this may result in a charge of battery.
- Abandoning a patient before the completion of care or before being relieved by someone of equal or higher training.

- Irresponsible or reckless driving or violating other laws that apply to emergency driving.

There are other activities that can lead to your being sued. Your instructor can inform you of recent problems in your own state. Keep in mind that the laws have been written to help you carry out your duties and provide emergency care. If you know the law and you act as a professional EMT, you should have little to worry about in terms of successful lawsuits. Your worry should not be so great that it prevents you from caring for sick and injured patients.

NOTE: Learn to protect yourself by keeping accurate, detailed records on the "run sheets" provided by your EMS System.

Negligence

Negligence is the basis for the majority of lawsuits involving prehospital emergency care. To the layperson, negligence means that something that should have been done was not done or was done incorrectly. The legal concept of negligence in emergency care is not this simple. It requires that ALL of the following be proved to have occurred:

1. The EMT had a duty to the patient (duty to act).
2. The EMT did not provide the standard of care (breach of duty). This may include the failure to act, that is, not providing needed care as would be expected of an EMT in your locality.
3. The actions of the EMT in not providing the standard of care caused injury to the patient. This injury can be physical or psychological.

If the above are proved, the EMT may be required to pay damages if the harm to the patient is considered by the court to be a loss that requires *reimbursement* (compensable). The negligent EMT may be required to pay for medical expenses, lost wages (possibly including future earnings), pain and suffering, and various other factors as determined by the court.

Duty to Act

Laws vary from state to state as to the responsibility an individual has to attempt to help someone in an emergency. As an EMT, more is expected of you than of the general public, but these expectations may only apply to you when you are on duty. In your state you may be required to respond and to provide care. Usually, these laws have been written to take into consideration the level of your training and your emergency care skills. The safety of the rescuer may also be considered. Your instructor can inform you of the laws concerning the duty to act that apply to your locality. In most cases, if an agency is given the responsibility to provide care, and you are an EMT in that agency, you will have a responsibility to provide care at emergencies, perhaps even when off duty.*

If you have a duty to act and fail to do so, you can be held liable.

The Standard of Care

Each state has a **standard of care** that must be observed. This is the *minimum* accepted care based on sources such as state laws and judicial decisions, administrative orders, local protocols and locally accepted guidelines published by emergency care organizations and societies, and what has been found to be acceptable in the past (precedent). This standard of care allows you to be judged based on what is expected of someone with your training and experience acting in the same or a similar situation. A textbook is *not* the standard of care. Your course is based on the guidelines originally proposed by the DOT and other authorities who have studied what training, skills, and equipment are required for an EMT to provide the standard of care at the EMT level. You will be trained so you can provide this standard of care. Training and continuing education are your best ways to ensure that you will be able to provide the standard of care required in your state.

Abandonment

Once you stop to help someone having a medical emergency or someone who is injured, you have legally initiated care. If you leave this patient before completing care or if you transfer care to someone who has less training, then you have **abandoned** the patient and may be subject to legal action for negligence. This concept exists to ensure that required care is completed and to avoid situations in which someone else does not stop to provide care,

---

* Currently, Vermont is the only state to pass legislation requiring individuals with a certain level of training to provide needed care whenever they come upon an emergency. They do not have to be a member of the EMS System, or, if they are, they do not have to be on duty. Several other states are considering such legislation.

thinking that you are taking responsibility for the patient and will stay with him.

Some states view as abandonment a situation in which you leave a medical facility after bringing in a patient but have failed to turn over the information you had about the patient's problem and the care you provided. There are also states where abandonment may apply if you do not respond to a call or fail to complete a run. Abandonment may even apply if equipment failure or your own health prevents you from completing a response and you do not immediately report this failure.

Serious problems can occur when you decide that a patient does not need emergency care or transport. This may be viewed as abandonment if later it is shown that the patient did require care or transport. *Do not* make these decisions lightly. Interview all potential patients at the scene and conduct proper examinations. When in doubt, call the emergency department physician for assistance in care and transport decision making; otherwise, transport all patients.

Patient Rights—Consent

NOTE: Your state has specific laws as to when you can and cannot provide care. You must follow your local **protocols** (the accepted standard of care as defined by the local medical community). The following sections on consent are provided to inform you of some of the problems that exist in regard to consent and some of the solutions to these problems that have been created in various EMS Systems.

Adults, when conscious and mentally competent, have the RIGHT TO REFUSE CARE. Adults who are mentally and physically able to make judgments are assumed to be competent and cannot be forced by the EMT to accept emergency care.* This must be informed refusal, given after the persons know that assessment and care are recommended by a trained professional, the EMT (see informed consent in the next section). The reasons for refusal may be based on religious beliefs or a lack of trust. In some cases, you may believe their reasoning to be senseless. For whatever reasons, a competent adult can refuse care. You cannot treat such patients, nor can you restrain them.

The law recognizes *implied* refusal of care. If

---

* Persons who are intoxicated, under the influence of drugs, or suicidal are not considered to be able to make a rational decision concerning care. At times, it may be very difficult to determine if a patient belongs in one of these categories. Some states have laws that give the medical provider a margin of error in such decisions (e.g., an index of suspicion).

a patient pulls away from you, holds up his hand in a "universal" gesture to signal you to stop, or shakes his head to indicate "no," then you have received his refusal for care. The sign of refusal should be reasonably clear to the average individual.

If the patient is fearful or lacks confidence in your abilities, conversation may help you gain trust and approval for care. *Do not* argue with a patient, particularly if his reasons are based on religious belief. To do so will add stress that may intensify the patient's problem.

When a patient refuses your care, you should have this documented by having him sign a *release form*. In such cases, be certain to inform the patient of what may be wrong with him, what you think should be done, and why you believe such actions are necessary. Ask the patient to confirm that he has understood what you have told him. In rare cases a patient may refuse your care and also refuse to sign the form. You will have to rely on eyewitnesses to verify that the patient has refused care.

In all cases of refusal of care, have a witness to your offer of care, your explanations, the refusal, and the signing of any forms. Obtain the signatures and addresses of the witnesses, making certain that they have documentation to prove their identity.

NOTE: Law enforcement officers may make excellent witnesses to the refusal of care.

Report any refusal of care to the dispatcher, immediately. Be certain to fill out all necessary forms, including a description of the patient's problem, his condition, the number of times you asked for the patient's consent, how you stated this request for consent, and how the patient refused care (when possible, quote the patient's exact words).

Parents or legal guardians can refuse to let you treat their child. Once again, if fear or lack of confidence is the apparent reason, try to explain the situation to them using simple conversation. Do not try to make the adult feel guilty of wrongdoing, particularly if religious reasons are the basis for the decision. Obtain the necessary signatures and identifications. In some states you must immediately report any case in which a parent or legal guardian refuses emergency care for a minor. These states have special laws governing the welfare of children. The information you provide may be passed on quickly to the courts so that care may be ordered or to find out if the child received proper care or is still in need of care.

Actual Consent

An adult patient, when conscious and mentally competent, can give you **actual consent** to provide care. Oral consent is considered to be valid; however, a signed consent form provides you with more protection. Unfortunately, written consent is not practical for most emergency situations.

This consent must be **informed consent.** Most of the laws dealing with informed consent were created to cover surgical procedures being performed by physicians. These laws required that the physician must make known the risk of treatment and nontreatment and the alternatives to this treatment. These requirements cannot be applied to the EMT acting in an emergency situation. At best, you will be able to tell the patient who you are, the level of your training, and what you are going to do.

Actual consent for the adult patient can be *voluntary* as stated above, or it can be *involuntary*, as would occur with a court order.

The laws on actual consent for a minor vary widely from state to state. Usually, a parent, guardian, or a close adult relative (when the parents cannot be reached) can give you actual consent to care for the child. When this is done, actual consent exists, even if the child does not wish to be treated. In certain situations, the minor may be able to give you consent or refuse care. For example, a married minor may give you actual consent in your state. The same may hold true for a pregnant minor. In some states the minor who claims to be the victim of child abuse may be able to give you voluntary actual consent. You MUST follow the guidelines established in your state.

Involuntary consent for a *minor* may be issued by court order, a law enforcement officer who has arrested the minor or placed him in his custody, or a child welfare officer (in some states). A law enforcement officer may be able to place the minor in protective custody. This would make the minor a ward of the court and would allow for the officer to grant consent.

Implied Consent

In cases in which the adult is unconscious or for some other reason unable to give you his actual consent, and if he has what you believe to be a life-threatening illness or injury, the law assumes that the patient, if able to do so, would want to receive treatment. This is known as **implied consent.** Typically, the law requires an emergency in which there is a significant risk of death, but it also may recognize situations in which there is the possibility of the patient developing serious problems or a disability if care is not rendered immediately.

The law assumes that the parents or guardians would want care to be provided for their child. When they cannot be reached, and the child has a life-threatening condition, implied consent may be used to allow for care to begin.

The same may hold true in your state for patients who are mentally ill, emotionally disturbed, or developmentally disabled (e.g., mentally retarded) who have a life-threatening problem. If this is not the case in your state and if the patient will not or cannot give voluntary actual consent, you may have to seek involuntary consent. Since the EMT is not able to determine if a patient has any of these disorders, it is wise, when time allows, to seek advice from your medical director or emergency department physician and have a law enforcement officer place the patient in protective custody or seek a court order to begin care.

Patient Rights—Confidentiality

Many jurisdictions have yet to write specific laws about the confidentiality due a patient receiving emergency care from an EMT. Laws do exist that prevent the intentional invasion of a person's privacy. These may be applied to cases involving emergency care. In many states, the deliberate invasion of a patient's privacy by an EMT may lead to the loss of certification and could lead to legal actions being taken against you.

Individuals in emergency care usually feel very strongly about protecting the patient's right to privacy. You must not provide care for a patient and then speak to the press, your family, friends, or other members of the public about the details of the care. If you speak of the emergency, you must not relate specifics about what a patient may have said, who he was or was with, anything unusual about his behavior, or any descriptions of personal appearance. The same holds true if you receive this information from another member of the EMS System. Confidentiality applies not only to cases of physical injury, but also to cases involving possible infectious diseases, illnesses, and emotional and psychological emergencies.

Immunities

Each state has its own laws regarding the immunity granted to those who provide emergency care. Such laws spell out when you are *immune to liability* in cases in which you rendered care or were unable to render care. It is your responsibility to know the laws for your state. Note, too, that there is also governmental immunity provided to some government and military agencies.

Good Samaritan laws have been developed in most states to provide immunity to individuals trying to help people in emergencies. Most of these laws will grant immunity from liability if the rescuer acts in good faith to provide care to the level of his training, to the best of his ability. These laws do not prevent someone from initiating a lawsuit, nor will they protect the rescuer from being found liable for acts of gross negligence and other violations of the law. These laws are strongly tied to the standard of care laws.

You must familiarize yourself with the laws that govern your state. Good Samaritan laws may not apply to EMTs in your locality. In some states, the Good Samaritan laws only apply to volunteers. If you are a paid EMT, different laws and regulations may apply.

Some states have specific EMT statutes that authorize, regulate, and protect EMTs (also the physicians and other health care professionals who give instructions to these individuals by radio or telephone). To be protected by such laws, you must be recognized as an EMT in the state where care has been provided. Some states have specific licensing and certification requirements that must be met and obligate the holder to the standard of care recognized in the state.

Other Legal Aspects

Responsibility for Possessions

Some care procedures require you to remove articles of the patient's clothing and jewelry. When you do, you are legally responsible for these articles. Record what articles were removed from the patient and safeguard them until you transfer the patient at the medical facility. At such time, hand the possessions over to the emergency department staff and receive a signed receipt for the articles.

The trust given to you is an important part of being an EMT and carrying out your duties. The following is the EMT Oath that was formulated and adopted by The National Association of Emergency Medical Technicians in 1978. It is based on the traditional oaths of the medical professions. Note its strong emphasis on professionalism, the standard of care, ethics, and confidentiality.

Be it pledged as an Emergency Medical Technician, I will honor the physical and judicial laws of God and man. I will follow that regimen which, according to my ability and judgment, I consider for the benefit of patients and abstain from whatever is deleterious and mischievous, nor shall I suggest any such counsel. Into whatever homes I enter, I will go into them for the benefit of only the sick and injured, never revealing what I see or hear in the lives of men unless required by law.

I shall also share my medical knowledge with

those who may benefit from what I have learned. I will serve unselfishly and continuously in order to help make a better world for all mankind.

While I continue to keep this oath unviolated, may it be granted to me to enjoy life, and the practice of the art, respected by all men, in all times. Should I trespass or violate this oath, may the reverse be my lot. So help me God.

Records and Reporting Requirements

The information you gather when assessing and monitoring a patient is to be written down on standard forms. This form may become part of the patient's medical records. It is a legal document that must be complete and accurate.

There are situations that may require you to file a special report with the medical facility, the police, or a government agency. This varies from state to state. You may be required to report child abuse, rape, assault, drug-related injuries, injury received during the commission of a crime, all gunshot wounds, attempted suicide, communicable diseases, and animal bites. The failure to make such reports carries legal penalties in some states.

Legal Implications in Special Patient Situations

There are special patients and special care situations in which specific laws may apply. Some of these are described below.

Mentally Disturbed Patients Care is usually provided under the laws of implied consent. If the patient is violent and likely to hurt himself or others, then restraint may be necessary. The law does not expect an EMT to risk his own safety to care for any patient. Typically, local laws will not allow an EMT to apply restraints unless ordered to do so by a physician or by the police. In some cases, a court order may be required. The restraints must be applied so as not to harm the patient (police handcuffs may injure a person who is violent—wide strips of cloth or leather are usually recommended). Once restraints are in place, they must be kept in place until the patient is handed over to more highly trained personnel at a medical facility. See Chapter 19 for more information concerning these patients.

Alcohol and Substance Abuse Patients You must, when possible, carry out a complete patient assessment and provide needed care for patients who are under the influence of alcohol or drugs or who have been injured while under such influence. Since medical practice views both alcohol and drug abuse as illnesses and not crimes, you should know if your state requires you to report cases of alcohol and drug abuse to legal authorities. See Chapter 14, Section Two for more information on the care of these patients.

Attempted Suicide Patients   Specific care for such patients is covered in Chapter 19. You are not required to endanger yourself to reach and care for patients attempting suicide (unless your agency spells out such a responsibility). If you believe an injury or poisoning was due to an attempted suicide, your state may require you to report your suspicions to the emergency department staff or the police.

Felony-related Cases   If you have any reason to believe that the patient is the victim of a crime or was injured while committing a crime, then you may be required to report this suspicion to the police. This may hold true for possible cases of assault, rape, child abuse or neglect, gunshot wounds, knife wounds, and any other suspicious wound or injury. Your best course of action is to report to the emergency department staff and/or the police any cases in which you believe a possible crime is related to the patient's problem. EMT actions at the crime scene will be covered in Chapter 19.

Animal Bite Patients   Such cases are usually required to be reported to the hospital personnel or to the police. If the animal is dead, you should protect the carcass so that it can be examined by medical authorities. If the animal is at the scene, you should protect yourself first, then the patient and bystanders. *Do not* try to capture the animal unless you are specifically trained to do so and such action is part of your duties.

Care for the Deceased   In most states, an EMT does not have the authority to pronounce a patient dead. Therefore, if there is any chance of life still existing, you must provide basic life support measures (e.g., in cold water drowning, the patient may be successfully resuscitated 1 hour or more after he has stopped breathing). There are cases of obvious death, as when a person is decapitated, his body is severed, or he is virtually cremated. It is recommended and may be legally required that you do not move such bodies so as not to hinder possible police investigations.

In some states, you can phone the coroner or medical examiner and receive permission to declare a patient dead. There are even localities that allow EMTs to independently declare death. You will have to follow your local guidelines on this matter.

A major problem now exists because of home care programs for terminally ill patients. The patient may have requested and the physician may have ordered that no resuscitative measures be taken when the patient's lungs and heart cease to function.

Originally, this approach was designed to allow specific physician's orders to be on file at the patient's hospital or nursing home. Obtaining legal proof of this request and order may prove to be a difficult task, forcing you to initiate CPR as you would for any patient. Unless proof can be obtained and relayed to you immediately, resuscitative measures have to be initiated. Some localities have helped to solve this problem by having terminally ill patients registered at their local rescue squad or fire service. Such registrations let the EMTs know that they are not to initiate resuscitative procedures.

Malpractice Insurance

Having adequate malpractice insurance does not reduce your chances of being sued. The purpose of the insurance is to reduce your financial risk when providing care. Even though you believe that you will be the best EMT you can be, the unforeseen can occur. You cannot be certain how the courts will view your actions. Too many laws concerning emergency care are still in question.

As an EMT, you may be able to obtain malpractice insurance through a program offered to members of various EMT societies and organizations, from your own insurance company (most are highly selective if they offer such a service), or from your EMS System or employer. Legal advice as to how much coverage for each patient incident is desirable should be sought.

EQUIPMENT

It is doubtful that you will have time early in your course to go over all the equipment used by today's EMTs. The information provided in this section is presented to allow you to look over all the equipment you will be using and to cover only what your instructor wishes to introduce at this time.

The Ambulance

The **ambulance** is a vehicle for emergency care that provides a driver's compartment and a patient's compartment that usually can accommodate two EMTs and two litter patients. At least one of these patients must be able to be positioned so that intensive life-support measures can be provided during transport. The vehicle must be able to carry, at the same time, the equipment and supplies needed to provide optimum EMT-level emergency care at the scene and during transport. Equipment for light rescue procedures is recommended. Two-way radio communication with dispatch must be provided.

A good ambulance must be designed and constructed to provide maximum safety and comfort to patients and EMTs and to prevent aggravation of the patient's condition and exposure to any factors that may complicate the patient's condition or threaten his survival.

According to federal specifications for emergency care vehicles (KKK-A-1822C) there are *three* types of ambulances. These are shown and described in Figure 1–18. The vehicle that meets these specifications is identified by "the star of life." The word "AMBULANCE" should appear in mirror image on the front so that the drivers of other vehicles can identify the unit as seen in their rear-view mirrors. The vehicle is to have warning lights, including flashing roof lights in the upper corners of the vehicle body (this often varies according to local laws and regulations).

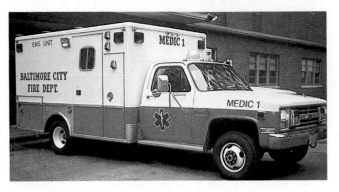

FIGURE 1–18a. A type-I ambulance has a conventional cab and chassis, on which is mounted a modular ambulance body. There is no passageway between the driver's and patient's compartments.

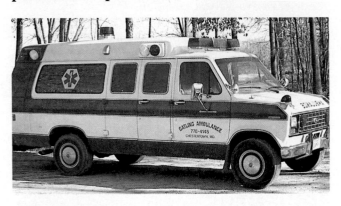

FIGURE 1–18b. A type-II ambulance is commonly called a van-type ambulance. The body and cab form an integral unit, and most models have a raised roof.

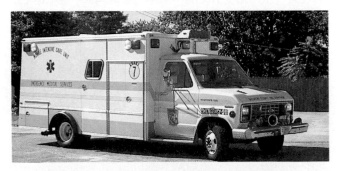

FIGURE 1–18c. A type-III ambulance is commonly called a specialty van ambulance. It has a forward cab and an integral body that is generally larger than that of a type-II ambulance. There is a walk-through compartment.

Equipment and Supplies

Federal specifications were set when federal funding was used in the purchasing of EMS System supplies. However, most ambulances and supplies are now purchased without federal funding. For this reason, the lists of equipment and supplies are presented as those items that *should* be carried and not those items that must be carried. Many systems base their equipment list on recommendations made in the American College of Surgeons' Essential Equipment List. A complete list is provided in Chapter 21. Your instructor will be able to tell you what is considered mandatory for your area.

The equipment and supplies carried may be categorized as follows:

1. Basic Supplies—those items carried to protect the patient (linens, pillows, blankets), to provide for patient needs (emesis bags, tissues, bedpans, towels), and to monitor the patient (stethoscope, penlight, and blood pressure measuring devices).
2. Equipment for Patient Transfer—including wheeled stretchers, folding stretchers and stair chairs, scoop-style stretchers, rigid cervical or extrication collars, and spine boards.
3. Equipment for Ventilation and Resuscitation—including airways, artificial ventilation devices, fixed and portable oxygen delivery systems, fixed and portable suction equipment, and spine or CPR boards for chest compression.
4. Supplies for Immobilizing Fractures—including lower extremity traction splints, padded board splints for upper and lower extremities, air-inflatable splints (where re-

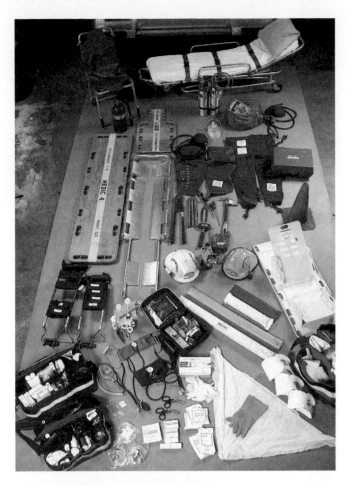

FIGURE 1–19. The well-equipped ambulance.

quired), anti-shock garments, and triangular bandages for slings and swathes.

5. Supplies for Wound Care—including sterile gauze pads, sterile universal or multitrauma dressings, self-adhering roller bandages, sterile nonporous occlusive dressings, and sterile burn sheets, as well as adhesive tape, safety pins, and bandage shears.

6. Supplies for Childbirth—a sterile childbirth (OB) kit, including all necessary gloves, towels, baby blankets, bags, sanitary napkins, gauze pads, surgical scissors, cord tape or clamps, and rubber bulb syringes.

7. Supplies for Poisonings and Substance Abuse—including syrup of ipecac (may be for advanced personnel use in some areas), activated charcoal, and drinking water.

8. Intermediate-level Care Supplies—mainly for the treatment of shock, including intravenous agents, sterile intravenous administration kits, and esophageal obturator airways (EOAs).

9. Physician and Paramedic Supplies (when carried)—including tracheal intubation kits, pleural decompression kits, drug administration kits, monitor/defibrillator (may also be for intermediate personnel in some areas), and a surgical kit (for some units).

10. Equipment for Gaining Access and Disentanglement—including hand tools, power tools, and required rope, blocks, wedges, chains, and straps.

11. Equipment for Safeguarding Ambulance Personnel—including disposable latex gloves, gowns, caps, masks, work gloves, safety goggles, helmets, reflective protective gear, and raingear.

12. Equipment for Warning and Signaling—including flares, battery-powered hand lights, and floodlights.

13. Equipment to Extinguish Fire—including the fire extinguishers required by local ordinance.

14. Communications Equipment—including fixed and portable two-way radios.

Remember that an EMT must be able to do more than carry out emergency care procedures. Gaining access, disentanglement and extrication, moving patients, and transferring patients are all part of the duties rendered.

NATIONAL ORGANIZATIONS

The National Registry of Emergency Medical Technicians (NREMT) exists to promote the improved delivery of emergency medical services by:

- Assisting in the development and evaluation of educational programs to train EMTs.
- Establishing qualifications for eligibility to apply for registration.
- Preparing and conducting examinations designed to ensure the competency of EMTs.
- Establishing a system for biennial registration.
- Establishing procedures for revocation of certificates of registration for just cause.
- Establishing continuing education requirements.
- Maintaining a centralized directory of registered EMTS.

Those applicants with the proper training must complete both written and practical examinations in order to be registered as EMT–Ambulance, EMT–Intermediate, or EMT–Paramedic. The identification devices for members of the National Registry are shown in Figure 1–20. For more information, write:

The National Registry of Emergency Medical Technicians
6610 Busch Boulevard
P.O. Box 29233
Columbus, OH 43229

The National Association of Emergency Medical Technicians (NAEMT) promotes the professional status of EMTs, encouraging the constant upgrading of skills, abilities, qualifications, and educational requirements of EMTs. The NAEMT provides support for the creation and upgrading of EMS Systems. The association is open to any state or nationally certified EMT. For more information, write:

National Association of Emergency Medical Technicians
9140 Ward Parkway
Kansas City, MO 64114

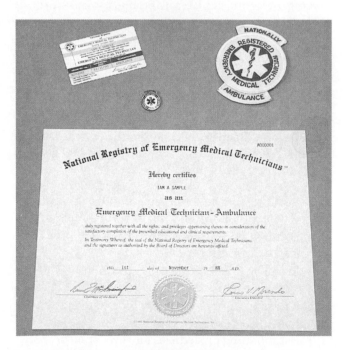

FIGURE 1–20. Identification devices for members of the National Registry of Emergency Medical Technicians.

The American Trauma Society is concerned with many aspects of emergency care, including educating the public as to the care of injured persons prior to the arrival of trained personnel. It is very involved with specialized burn and trauma units for the critically injured. For more information, write:

American Trauma Society
1400 Mercantile Lane
Suite 188
Landover, MD 20785

The National Association for Search and Rescue collects data, develops training programs, and participates in public education to help promote the implementation of a total, coordinated emergency response, rescue, and recovery system. For more information, write:

National Association for Search and Rescue
P.O. Box 3709
Fairfax, VA 22038

The American College of Emergency Physicians (ACEP) was established in 1968 with its goal set to improve the quality of emergency department care. Since 1979, it has had the medical specialty of emergency medicine recognized by the American Board of Medical Specialists. ACEP continues to set high standards for emergency department care and prehospital emergency care procedures.

American College of Emergency Physicians
P.O. Box 619911
Dallas, TX 75261

The American College of Surgeons (ACS), Committee on Trauma concerns itself with both prehospital and emergency department emergency care. The Committee on Trauma publishes lists of essential equipment, emergency department guidelines, emergency department posters, and new techniques for the management of trauma.

American College of Surgeons
Committee on Trauma
55 East Erie Street
Chicago, IL 60611

The National Council of State EMS Training Coordinators is involved with the national promotion of EMTs through standardization of courses, certification, reciprocity, and recertification. Concerned with more than training alone, the Council works with all activities required to upgrade the profession and to gain greater public recognition of the EMT and the EMS System. For more information, write:

National Council of State EMS Training Coordinators, Inc.
EMS Clearinghouse
P.O. Box 11910
Iron Works Pike
Lexington, KY 40578

SUMMARY

The Emergency Medical Services System is a chain of human and physical resources established to provide complete emergency care. The Emergency Medical Technician is trained and certified to provide professional-level emergency care at the scene and during transport to a medical facility.

The primary responsibility of the EMT is personal safety. To provide proper care, the EMT must carry out nine main duties. These duties include preparation to respond; responding; making certain that the scene is safe; gaining access to the patient; finding out what is wrong with the patient and providing emergency care; freeing and moving the patient; transferring the patient to the ambulance; transporting and handing over the patient and patient information; and returning to quarters and preparing for the next run.

As an EMT, you may be called on to drive an ambulance, control an accident scene, gain access in special situations, gather patient information, provide emergency care, provide emotional support, perform extrication, transport while monitoring the patient and communicating with the medical facility, transfer the patient over to the medical staff, and many other duties such as report writing and equipment inventory.

Basic EMT-level emergency care deals with both injury and illness, with care usually being provided at the emergency scene and during transport to a medical facility. Your duties are performed as part of an emergency care delivery subsystem consisting of EMTs, the ambulance, and equipment and supplies.

As an EMT, you are a health care professional, required to be pleasant, cooperative, resourceful, emotionally stable, and of good moral character. You must have leadership abilities and be a self-starter. You must be concerned with your personal appearance, your personal habits, and your conversation at the scene. All these traits help you to develop the calm, professional manner needed to provide proper emergency care.

When you begin to care for a patient, you have the responsibility to continue care until you are relieved by equally or more highly trained personnel or until you have transferred the patient and patient information to the staff of a medical facility. If you start care and then stop, or if you leave the scene, you may be charged with abandonment.

Some patients can refuse your care. You must have actual consent from a conscious, clear-thinking adult patient. It must be informed consent, with the patient knowing your level of training and what you are planning to do.

Actual consent may be voluntary or involuntary. A court order or the order of a law enforcement officer may be needed to assume involuntary consent.

There are cases in some states in which a minor can give actual consent (e.g., married minor). Usually, if voluntary consent is given it must come from a parent, legal guardian, or close adult relative (only when parents or guardians cannot be contacted). Involuntary consent requires a court order, an order from a law enforcement officer, or orders from a child welfare officer (in some states).

In cases in which the patient is unable to give consent, and has life-threatening problems, you may care for the patient under the law of implied consent.

In some localities, implied consent also may apply to children, to the mentally disturbed, and to developmentally disabled patients when their parents or legal guardians are not present.

Patients have a right to privacy. EMTs must respect and protect patient confidentiality.

In most states, specific laws have been written to allow you to provide emergency care. Good Samaritan laws may provide you with limited immmunity from civil liability. You may be protected if you act in good faith, providing the EMT standard of care, to your level of training and to the best of your abilities.

EMT SKILLS

As an EMT, you will be expected to perform your duties in a calm, professional manner. You must be able to apply the knowledge gained in your course to carry out the duties of a Basic EMT. You must be able to perform the activities of preparation, response, gaining access, patient assessment, basic EMT-level emergency care, disentanglement, moving and transfer, transport, termination of activities, and communications and reporting. You must be able to carry out all EMT-level patient assessment and emergency care procedures.

The following is a list of EMT skills. This is not a prioritized list. The major skills of an EMT include being able to:

- Perform assigned duties in accordance with the law
- Properly inform patients and gain informed actual consent
- Correctly apply implied consent
- File the proper reports for special patient situations
- Apply anatomical knowledge directly to patient assessment and care procedures
- Use correct medical terminology in communications and reports
- Present proper identification at the emergency scene
- Relate mechanisms of injury to accident patients in order to detect possible injuries
- Properly wear and use all assigned clothing and equipment supplied to help reduce the risk of exposure to infectious diseases
- Open and maintain an airway
- Determine adequate breathing
- Determine a carotid pulse
- Detect and control profuse bleeding
- Use direct pressure, pressure dressings, elevation, pressure points, the blood pressure cuff, and tourniquets to control bleeding
- Use pneumatic anti-shock garments for internal bleeding
- Complete a primary survey
- Gather information from bystanders
- Conduct a subjective patient interview
- Determine radial pulse rate, rhythm, and character
- Determine respiratory rate and character
- Determine blood pressure by auscultation
- Determine blood pressure by palpation
- Determine relative skin temperature
- Determine changes in skin color, including the indications of cyanosis
- Determine pupil size, equality, and reactivity
- Detect distal pulse and nerve activity during assessment of the upper and lower limbs
- Detect cervical and lower back point tenderness
- Use a stethoscope to determine equal air entry in the lungs
- Conduct an objective physical examination

- Complete a secondary survey
- Accurately record information gained during the patient assessment
- Detect and record changes in vital signs
- Detect and record changes in a patient's condition
- Clear partially and fully obstructed airways using back blows (infants only), manual thrusts, finger sweeps, and suction equipment for conscious patients, patients observed to have lost consciousness, and unconscious patients
- Establish respiratory arrest
- Provide safe pulmonary resuscitation
- Provide pulmonary resuscitation while in transport
- Establish cardiac arrest
- Locate the CPR compression site on infants, children, and adults
- Deliver external chest compressions at the proper rate and depth
- Provide proper ventilations, at the correct rate, for infants, children, and adults
- Provide one-rescuer CPR
- Provide two-rescuer CPR
- Carry out position changes during two-rescuer CPR
- Perform CPR while moving patients
- Provide CPR while in transport
- Deliver ventilations by bag-valve-mask, pocket face mask, and positive pressure resuscitator (in manual mode)
- Select and insert an oropharyngeal airway
- Select and insert a nasopharyngeal airway
- Take apart, clean, reassemble, and test fixed and portable suction devices
- Take apart, clean, reassemble, and test bag-valve-mask ventilators
- Provide ventilations with a bag-valve-mask ventilator, with and without supplemental oxygen
- Set up the equipment for oxygen therapy
- Provide supplemental oxygen to the breathing patient, selecting the proper delivery device and flow
- Provide supplemental oxygen to the breathing COPD patient, selecting the proper delivery device and flow
- Provide oxygen to nonbreathing patients by using the bag-valve-mask ventilator with supplemental oxygen, the pocket face mask with supplemental oxygen, and the positive pressure resuscitator
- Provide oxygen using the demand valve resuscitator in the patient demand mode
- Transfer patients receiving oxygen to the ambulance and from the ambulance to the emergency department
- Provide oxygen while in transport
- Determine when patients need supplemental oxygen based on symptoms and signs
- Detect external bleeding
- Control external bleeding
- Estimate external blood loss

FIGURE 1–21. EMT Skills.

EMT SKILLS CONT.

- Detect possible internal bleeding based on symptoms, signs, and mechanism of injury
- Estimate possible internal blood loss
- Detect shock based on symptoms and signs
- Detect anaphylactic shock based on symptoms and signs
- Care for shock
- Position patients to prevent fainting
- Detect soft tissue injuries and determine their type
- Expose, clear, dress, and bandage open wounds
- Use occlusive dressings for open chest wounds, open abdominal wounds, and bleeding from major neck veins
- Preserve and transport avulsed and amputated tissues
- Provide care for wounds to the scalp, face, eyes, nose, ears, mouth, and neck
- Provide care for an object impaled in the eye
- Provide care for an avulsed eye
- Provide care for an object impaled in the cheek
- Provide care for a nosebleed
- Provide care when there are clear or bloody fluids flowing from the nose and/or ears
- Wash debris from the eyes
- Provide care for acid and alkaline burns of the eyes
- Provide care for light burns of the eyes
- Provide care for heat burns of the eyes
- Remove contact lenses from a patient's eyes
- Provide care for unconscious patients' eyes
- Stabilize an impaled object
- Provide care for soft tissue wounds of the chest that do not puncture the thoracic cavity
- Detect possible internal abdominal injury
- Care for open and closed abdominal injury
- Place, apply, deflate, and remove pneumatic anti-shock garments for cases of abdominal injury as to local protocol
- Detect and care for injuries to the pelvis
- Detect and care for injuries to the groin
- Identify injuries to the extremities based upon symptoms and signs
- Provide soft tissue injury care to the extremities
- Straighten mildly angulated closed fractures of the humerus, radius, ulna, femur, tibia, and fibula
- Straighten angulations of the elbow, knee, and ankle in accordance with local protocol
- Utilize slings and swathes, upper extremity rigid board splints, lower extremity rigid board splints, air-inflated splints, pillow splints, and traction splints
- Provide care for fractures and dislocations of the pectoral girdle
- Provide care for fractures of the humerus
- Provide care for fractures and dislocations of the elbow
- Provide care for fractures of the forearm and wrist
- Provide care for fractures of the hand and fingers
- Provide care for pelvic fractures
- Provide care for anterior and posterior hip dislocations
- Provide care for fractures of the femur
- Provide care for fractures and dislocations of the knee
- Provide care for fractures of the leg and ankle
- Provide care for fractures of the foot
- Evaluate nerve and vascular function for the upper and lower extremities, before and after splinting
- Make and utilize noncommercial splints for emergency situations
- Transfer and transport splinted patients
- Apply patient assessment techniques to detect possible cranial fractures and facial fractures
- Apply patient assessment techniques to detect possible brain injury
- Apply patient assessment techniques to detect possible spinal injury
- Apply patient assessment techniques to detect possible blunt trauma to the chest and flail chest
- Detect and provide care for pneumothorax and spontaneous pneumothorax
- Detect and provide care for pneumothorax with tension pneumothorax
- Detect and provide basic life support for traumatic asphyxia (acute thoracic compression syndrome)
- Provide basic care for possible fractured skull and facial bones
- Provide basic care for possible brain injury
- Apply an extrication or rigid cervical collar
- Immobilize possible spinal injury patients to a long spine board
- Use the four-rescuer log roll or any approved alternate method when placing patients on a long spine board
- Position patients for drainage
- Apply a sling and swathe for possible rib fracture
- Correct paradoxical respirations in cases of flail chest
- Apply patient assessment techniques to detect possible angina pectoris, impending AMI, AMI, mechanical pump failure, and congestive heart failure
- Provide basic care for and transport patients with possible heart disorders
- Assess patients for stroke
- Provide proper care and positioning for possible stroke patients
- Assess patients for possible respiratory distress and for chronic obstructive pulmonary disease
- Care for patients in respiratory distress, including those with COPD
- Evaluate and care for hyperventilation as a condition and as a sign
- Distinguish between possible diabetic coma (diabetic ketoacidosis) and insulin shock (hypoglycemia)
- Provide proper care for patients having diabetic emergencies
- Use medical identification devices to collect patient information

- ☐ Care for patients having convulsive seizures
- ☐ Detect and provide basic care for possible acute abdomen
- ☐ Detect and provide safe basic care for patients with possible infectious diseases
- ☐ Provide care, protecting yourself from infectious disease
- ☐ Exercise proper personal hygiene after contact with patients who may have an infectious disease
- ☐ Ready the ambulance and its equipment and supplies after transporting patients who may have an infectious disease
- ☐ Detect possible cases of poisoning
- ☐ Call the poison control center, provide patient information, and carry out orders given by the staff at the center
- ☐ Administer syrup of ipecac and activated charcoal and water (follow local protocol)
- ☐ Collect vomitus at the scene and in transport
- ☐ Provide initial basic care for insect stings and snakebites
- ☐ Detect and care for possible alcohol abuse and withdrawal
- ☐ Detect and care for possible drug abuse and withdrawal
- ☐ Evaluate a woman in labor
- ☐ Use all items in the sterile emergency obstetric pack
- ☐ Prepare an expectant mother for delivery, including the use of sheets or towels to properly cover her
- ☐ Assist a woman in the delivery of her baby
- ☐ Provide postdelivery care for the newborn, including proper airway and umbilical cord care
- ☐ Provide resuscitative measures for newborns in respiratory and cardiac arrest
- ☐ Assist a woman in the delivery of the placenta
- ☐ Provide postdelivery care for the mother, including emotional support and care for postdelivery bleeding
- ☐ Collect and transport the afterbirth
- ☐ Provide basic care for predelivery, delivery, and postdelivery complications, including the proper administration of oxygen
- ☐ Provide basic care and needed life support procedures for abnormal deliveries, including breech and premature birth
- ☐ Administer oxygen properly for the newborn, when required, using the "tent method"
- ☐ Accurately record a birth
- ☐ Evaluate a woman for possible eclampsia, ectopic pregnancy, and abortion, and provide the appropriate care
- ☐ Assist a woman with a multiple delivery
- ☐ Provide emotional support in cases of stillborn infants
- ☐ Determine if a patient is an infant or a child
- ☐ Conduct a primary and secondary survey on infants and children
- ☐ Provide basic life support to infants and children
- ☐ Detect and care for head injury in infants and children
- ☐ Control your emotions during a pediatric emergency
- ☐ Interview child patients
- ☐ Provide emotional support in cases of possible sudden infant death syndrome
- ☐ Relate symptoms and signs to possible child abuse

- ☐ Properly report suspected child abuse
- ☐ Classify burns as first, second, or third degree
- ☐ Use the Rule of Nines (or Rule of Palm) to determine the severity of burns
- ☐ Provide care for thermal burns
- ☐ Provide care for chemical burns
- ☐ Provide care for electrical burns
- ☐ Provide care for radiation burns
- ☐ Provide care for cases of smoke inhalation
- ☐ Detect and care for heat cramps, heat exhaustion, and heatstroke
- ☐ Detect and care for incipient frostbite, superficial frostbite, and deep frostbite (freezing)
- ☐ Care for superficial and deep frostbite when transport is delayed
- ☐ Detect, classify as to severity, and provide proper care for hypothermia
- ☐ Provide care, to the level of your training, at special emergencies (electrical accidents, hazardous materials accidents, and radiation accidents)
- ☐ Follow local protocol to request the appropriate help when the scene involves electrical hazards, hazardous materials, and radioactivity
- ☐ Use appropriate patient assessment techniques at the scene of an accident involving an explosion
- ☐ Evaluate victims of swimming or diving accidents
- ☐ Solve basic problems faced in reaching patients in water- and ice-related accidents
- ☐ Apply resuscitative measures to near-drowning patients
- ☐ Work as a member of a team to turn patients in the water and place them on a long spine board (optional)
- ☐ Determine if patients may be having a possible stress reaction, emotional emergency, or psychiatric emergency
- ☐ Use personal interaction for cases of stress reaction, emotional emergency, and psychiatric emergency
- ☐ Initiate crisis management when appropriate
- ☐ Conduct efficient interviews with elderly patients
- ☐ Establish effective communications with deaf patients
- ☐ Provide care and comfort for blind patients
- ☐ Establish some form of communication with non-English-speaking patients
- ☐ Provide proper care for aggressive patients, when your own safety is ensured
- ☐ Provide proper care for patients attempting suicide, when your own safety is ensured
- ☐ Provide care at the controlled crime scene, helping to preserve the chain of evidence
- ☐ Provide care for rape victims, considering their emotional needs, privacy, comfort, and dignity, but preserving the chain of evidence
- ☐ Initiate and conduct triage
- ☐ Provide care when triage is in effect
- ☐ Apply basic assessment skills to triage
- ☐ Follow local protocol when providing care in a situation controlled by a disaster plan
- ☐ Reduce stress on rescuers during a disaster

EMT SKILLS CONT.

- □ Properly conduct a daily and postrun inspection of the ambulance and supplies
- □ Receive information from a dispatcher
- □ Drive an ambulance in accordance to the laws of your state
- □ Use emergency and defensive driving skills to avoid accidents while driving the ambulance
- □ Correctly use warning devices found on the ambulance
- □ Properly position an ambulance, taking into consideration the traffic, the roadway, and known hazards
- □ Control hazards at the emergency scene, doing only what you have been trained to do and using the required safety equipment
- □ Reach patients trapped in vehicles by gaining access through locked doors, through windows, and through the vehicle body (optional), doing only what you have been trained to do
- □ Effectively evaluate an emergency and summon the appropriate services to aid in scene control and gaining access
- □ Properly protect patients during disentanglement
- □ Make a pathway through the wreckage by helping to:
  - • Raise a crushed vehicle roof
  - • Remove the top of a vehicle
  - • Widen vehicle door openings
- □ Remove wreckage from the patient by helping to:
  - • Cut a seat belt
  - • Remove a steering wheel
  - • Displace a steering column
  - • Displace a vehicle floor pedal
  - • Displace a dash
  - • Displace a vehicle seat

- □ Decide when an emergency or nonemergency move is necessary
- □ Carry out one-, two-, and three-rescuer moves
- □ Package patients for transfer and transport
- □ Use the wheeled ambulance stretcher to transfer patients
- □ Use the stair chair, orthopedic (scoop-style) stretcher, and basket stretcher to transfer patients
- □ Apply a short spine board (or K.E.D. or other vest-type device) to patients found in a vehicle or confined space and move them to a long spine board
- □ Move patients to a long spine board by the four-rescuer straddle slide or other appropriate method
- □ Move patients to a long spine board when found under the dashboard or between the front and rear seat of an automobile
- □ Physically and mentally ready patients for transport
- □ Take vital signs and provide needed basic EMT-level care during transport
- □ Relay, by radio, patient information to the emergency department
- □ Conduct an orderly transfer of patients at a medical facility.
- □ Carry out all activities necessary at the medical facility, en route to quarters, and in quarters to ready the ambulance and crew for service
- □ Present oral reports in a calm, professional manner
- □ Conduct proper radio communications
- □ Complete all reports required by your system
- □ Take the appropriate steps to protect yourself from stress
- □ Carry out EMT-level steps in automated defibrillation if allowed in your state

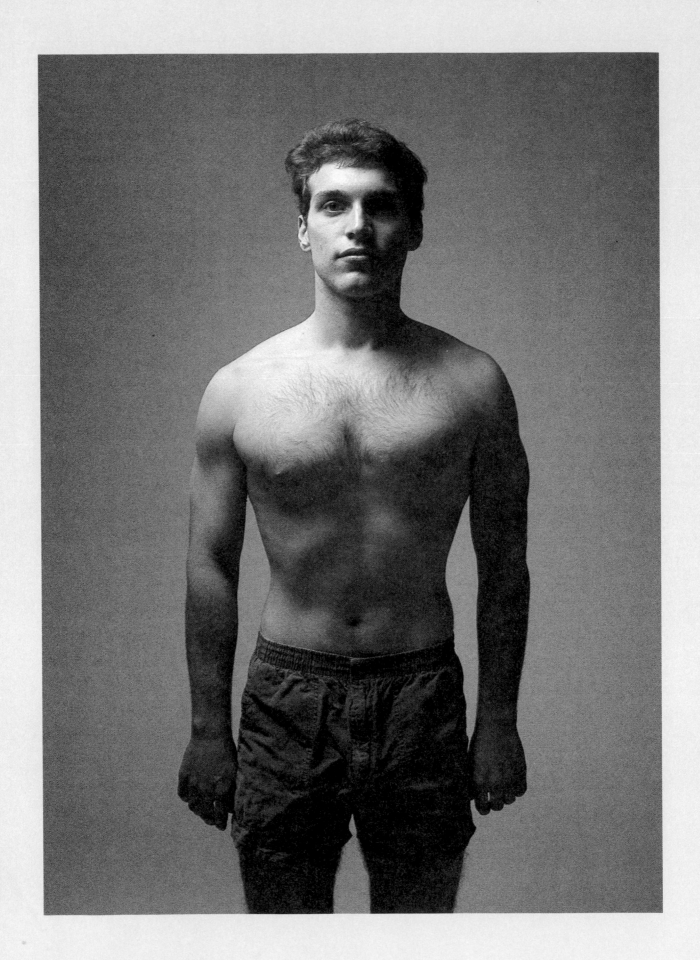

The Human Body

OBJECTIVES   As an EMT, you should be able to:

1. Describe the anatomical position. (p. 33)
2. Define and apply the terms *anterior*, *posterior*, *superior*, *inferior*, *midline*, *medial*, *lateral*, *proximal*, *distal*, *patient's left*, and *patient's right*. (pp. 33–34)
3. Identify FOUR anatomical postures. (p. 34)
4. Correctly use SIX terms that relate to direction of movement. (pp. 34 and 36)
5. List the FIVE major regions of the body and the subdivisions of each region. (p. 36)
6. Label the FIVE divisions of the spine. (pp. 36–37)
7. Name and locate the FOUR major body cavities. (p. 37)
8. Name and identify the FOUR abdominal quadrants. (pp. 37–38)
9. Match given body functions to specific body systems. (pp. 38–39)
10. Locate, on your own body, the position of the diaphragm, heart, lungs, stomach, liver, spleen, pancreas, gallbladder, small intestine, large intestine, kidneys, and urinary bladder. (p. 40)

SKILLS   As an EMT, you should be able to:

1. Apply the knowledge gained in this chapter so that you can look at a patient's body and mentally determine the positions of the major organs of the chest and abdomen.
2. Use correct terminology when communicating with other members of the patient care team.

TERMS   you may be using for the first time:

Abduction – movement away from the vertical midline of the body.

Abdominal Quadrants – the four zones of the abdominal wall used for quick reference.

Abdominopelvic (AB-dom-i-no-PEL-vik) **Cavity** – the anterior cavity below the diaphragm, made up of the abdominal portion and the pelvic portion.

Adduction – movement toward the vertical midline of the body.

Anatomical Position – the standard reference position for the body in the study of anatomy. The body is standing erect, facing the observer. The arms are down at the sides and the palms of the hands face forward.

Anterior – the front of the body or body part.

Cervical (SER-ve-kal) **Spine** – the section of the spine in the neck.

Coccyx (KOK-siks) – the lower end of the spine. It is sometimes referred to by the layperson as the tailbone.

Cranial (KRAY-ne-al) **Cavity** – the area within the skull that houses the brain.

Diaphragm (DI-ah-fram) – the dome-shaped muscle of respiration that separates the chest from the abdomen.

Distal – away from a point of reference or attachment (e.g., the shoulder or hip joint); used as a comparison with proximal.

Duodenum (du-o-DE-num or du-OD-e-num) – the first portion of the small intestine, beginning with its connection to the inferior (lower) portion of the stomach.

Erect – the upright position.

Extension – to straighten a joint.

Flexion – to bend at a joint.

Inferior – away from the head. Usually compared with another structure that is closer to the head (e.g., the lips are inferior when compared with the nose).

Lateral – to the side, away from the vertical midline of the body; used only in reference to another body part. Thus, there is a lateral side to the arm.

Lateral Recumbent – lying on the side.

Lateral Rotation – to turn the foot or hand outward away from the midline.

Lumbar (LUM-bar) **Spine** – the section of the spine that supports the small of the back.

Medial – toward the vertical midline of the body; used only in reference to another body part. Thus, you can have a medial side to the arm.

Medial Rotation – to turn the foot or hand inward toward the midline.

Midline – an imaginary line drawn down the center of the body, dividing it into right and left halves.

Posterior – the back of the body or body part.

Prone – lying face down.

Proximal – close to a point of reference or attachment (e.g., the shoulder or hip joint); used as a comparison with distal.

Sacrum (SA-krum) – the section of the spine in the lower back.

Spinal Cavity – the area within the spinal column that contains the spinal cord.

Sternum (STER-num) – the breastbone.

Superior – toward the head; often used in reference with inferior.

Supine – lying on the back.

Thoracic (tho-RAS-ik) **Cavity** – the anterior body cavity above the diaphragm, containing the heart and its great vessels, part of the trachea (windpipe), the lungs, and the esophagus (the tube connecting the throat and the stomach).

Thoracic (tho-RAS-ik) **Spine** – the section of the spine in the upper back, to which the ribs attach.

Thorax (THO-raks) – the chest.

Xiphoid (ZI-foyd) **Process** – the lower (inferior) extension of the sternum (breastbone).

OVERVIEW OF THE HUMAN BODY

The Language of Emergency Medical Care

To learn the materials presented in your EMT course, you will have to be able to understand what you hear and read. This chapter is an introduction to many of the terms that will be used in your training.

You need to be able to define these terms and apply them to your activities as an EMT.

Since you will be communicating with other medical professionals, you will have to use the vocabulary that is the language of your profession. Written and oral reports will require you to use this *medical terminology*. In addition, as an EMT, you will have many opportunities to read publications on emergency care and attend continuing education programs taught by physicians and other professionals in the EMS System. You will not be able to develop as a professional EMT unless you understand and correctly use the terminology that applies to emergency medical care.

There are a number of medical terms used in EMT–Basic training. You could try to memorize these terms; however, it is doubtful that you will remember them for very long unless you use them on a daily basis. You can keep a list and review it periodically, adding to the list each time you see or hear a new term. This is not very practical. It would be easier to learn the basic parts of medical terms that apply to EMT-level care and how these parts are put together to form terms. Once you know the parts and some basic rules for word formation you will be able to recall old terms and understand the meanings of new ones. If you wish to learn more medical terminology, Appendix 6 of this book contains a section on the formation of medical terms. You would do well to read through the introduction to this section early in your course. Each week, you should go through part of the list provided in this appendix to increase your knowledge of medical terminology.

The Study of Anatomy and Physiology

Two terms appear early and often in an EMT training program. They are anatomy and physiology. **Anatomy** is the study of body structure, while **physiology** is the study of body function. As an EMT, you will have to know the major body structures and systems and how these parts function. In general, you will need a working knowledge of the body in order to determine the nature of the patient's illness or injury (the patient assessment) and to provide the appropriate care.

It is impossible to learn all of basic anatomy in the standard EMT course. Nursing students average 180 classroom hours of study of anatomy and physiology. This is more time than you will have for the entire EMT course. However, you will learn enough to understand and be able to perform EMT activities and care. Also, your course will provide you with a strong foundation for your EMT continuing education.

This chapter will not attempt to cover all the anatomy that is included in your training. Instead, it is meant to serve as a foundation for your studies. At the end of the chapter, additional illustrations are provided as quick references for anatomical landmarks (points of reference seen or felt on the body surface) and the body systems. In later chapters, we will present entire body systems and important aspects of physiology and expand on anatomy. Throughout the text, anatomy and physiology will be related to patient assessment and specific care procedures.

First, learn to visualize where structures are located as you view a person who is fully clothed, since this is the way you will find most patients. Then, start looking for specific external body landmarks. These will help you locate structures within the body. Keep in mind that the patient's problem may be internal but all you will be able to see is the external body.

Directional Terms

The following is a set of very basic terms to use when referring to the human body (Figure 2–1):

Anatomical (AN-a-tom-i-kal) **Position**—Consider the human body, standing erect, facing you. The arms are down at the sides with the palms of the hands facing forward. Unless otherwise indicated, all references to body structures are made when the body is in the anatomical position. This is very important when considering anatomical structures.

Right and **Left**—As you face the patient, his left is on your right. When you assess the patient and note or report your findings, always make reference to the *patient's* right and *patient's* left.

Anterior and **Posterior**—Anterior is used to mean the front of the body, and posterior is used to indicate the back of the body. For the head, the face and top are considered anterior, while all of the remaining structures are posterior. The rest of the body can be easily divided into anterior and posterior by following the side seams of your clothing.

Midline—This is an imaginary vertical line that divides the body into right and left halves. Anything toward the midline is said to be **medial,** while anything away from the midline is said to be **lateral.** Remember the anatomical position, with the thumb on the lateral side of the hand and the little finger on the medial side of the hand.

Superior and **Inferior**—Superior means toward the top or toward the head, as in the eyes are superior to the nose. Inferior means toward the bottom or toward the feet, as in the mouth is inferior to the nose. (**NOTE:** you cannot correctly say something is superior or inferior unless you are comparing it with another structure or location. For example, the heart is not superior by itself, it is superior to the stomach.)

Proximal and **Distal**—Proximal means closer

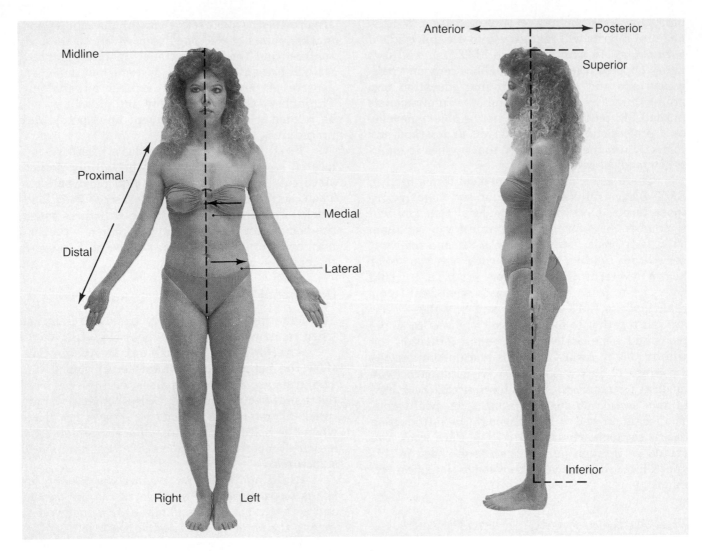

FIGURE 2–1. Directional terms.

to a point of reference, and distal means further away from a point of reference. These terms are used primarily for the upper and lower extremities, with the shoulder and the hip as the points of reference. The knee is proximal when compared with the ankle. The fingernails are on the distal ends of the fingers.

Anatomical Postures

The body is not always **erect** or in the upright position. When a person is lying on his back, he is in a **supine** position. Conversely, when he is lying face down, he is in the **prone** position. A person lying on one side is in a **lateral recumbent position.** To be more specific, if he is lying on his right side, he is in the right lateral recumbent position, and when on his left side, he is in the left lateral recumbent position. These terms are used frequently in communications between the hospital emergency department and EMTs en route and at the scene.

Direction of Movement

The term used to describe movement away from the midline of the body is **abduction** (to carry someone away is to ABduct). **Adduction** is movement toward the midline (think of ADDing to the body). Lateral rotation means to rotate outward or away from the midline. A lateral rotation of the leg twists the leg along its long axis so that the foot is turned outward. The opposite action is medial rotation, where twisting the leg along its long axis turns the foot inward.

Flexion is the act of bending at a joint, and **extension** is the act of straightening a joint. In the following sections on basic life support, you will learn that the airway can become obstructed when the head is flexed forward.

Variations of the terms **prone** and **supine** can be used when describing body movement. To rotate the forearm so that the palm of the hand is facing forward in the anatomical position is called a *supina-*

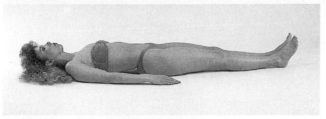
Supine

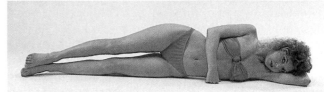
Prone

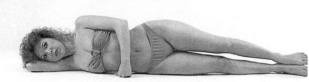
Right lateral recumbent

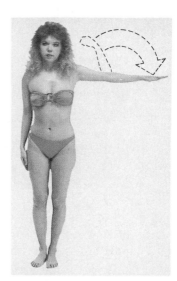
Left lateral recumbent

FIGURE 2–2. Anatomical postures.

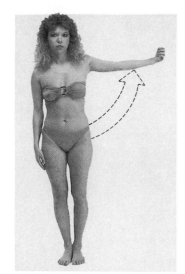
Abduction

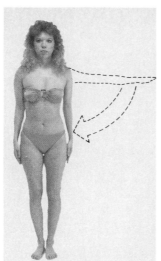
Adduction

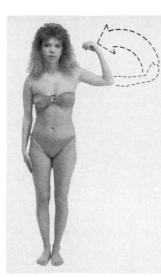
Flexion

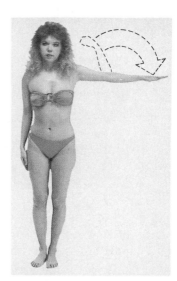
Extension

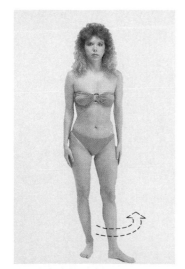
Lateral rotation

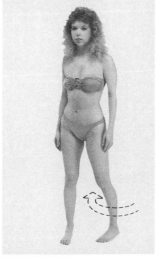
Medial rotation

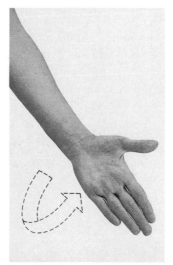
Supination

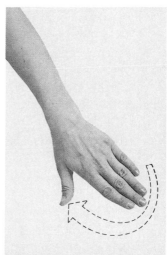
Pronation

FIGURE 2–3. Directions of movement.

tion. A rotation of the forearm that brings the back of the hand to a forward facing position is a *pronation.*

Body Regions

The human body can be divided into five regions: (1) the head, (2) neck, (3) trunk, (4) upper extremities (shoulders to tips of fingers), and (5) lower extremities (pelvis and hips to tips of toes). Later in this text you will study specific areas within each of these regions. You will find that each region has simple and complex subdivisions. We will start with the simplest to give you an opportunity to begin looking for these subdivisions as you consider illness, injury, and care. For now, you need to know the following:

1. **Head**
   - Cranium (KRAY-ne-um)—housing the brain. Many people use the term *skull* for cranium.
   - Face
   - Mandible (MAN-di-b'l)—the lower jaw, considered separately because its joints allow for movement
2. **Neck**
3. **Trunk**—from neck to the groin (anteriorly) and the buttocks (posteriorly)
   - Thorax (THO-raks)—the chest
   - Abdomen—extending from the lower ribs to the pelvis
   - Pelvis—formed and protected by the bones of the pelvic girdle (the pelvic bones are part of the lower extremities)
4. **Upper Extremities** (as found on each side)
   - Shoulder girdle and joint—composed of the scapula (SKAP-u-lah, shoulder blade) posteriorly, the clavicle (KLAV-i-kul, collarbone) anteriorly, and the joint formed by the head of the humerus (HU-mer-us, arm bone) and the scapula
   - Arm—sometimes referred to as the upper arm
   - Elbow
   - Forearm—sometimes referred to as the lower arm
   - Wrist
   - Hand
   - Fingers
5. **Lower Extremities**
   - Pelvic girdle and joint—composed of the fused bones of the pelvis and lower spine and the joint made with the femur (FE-mur, thigh bone)

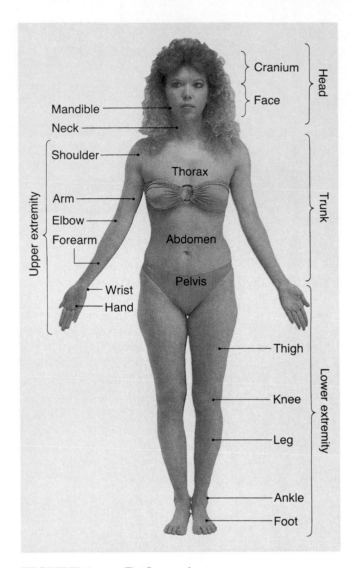

FIGURE 2–4. Body regions.

   - Thigh—extends from the hip to the knee. Sometimes it is referred to as the upper leg.
   - Knee
   - Leg—also called the lower leg or shin and calf
   - Ankle
   - Foot
   - Toes

The Spine

In Chapter 11 you will study the spinal column in detail. For now, you need to know that the spine is divided into five regions (levels) and that each of these regions can be used as points of reference to locate other structures and injuries. The five divisions of the spine are as follows:

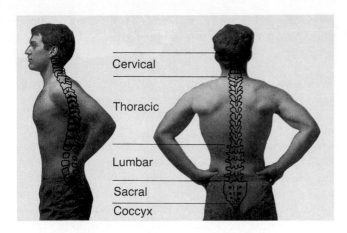

FIGURE 2–5. The divisions of the spine.

- Cervical (SER-ve-kal)—the neck
- Thoracic (tho-RAS-ik)—the upper back. The ribs attach to the bones (vertebrae) of the thoracic spine.
- Lumbar (LUM-bar)—the midback
- Sacral (SA-kral)—the lower back. When referring to all the bones of the sacral region, use the term *sacrum* (SA-krum).
- Coccygeal (KOK-si-JE-al)—the inferior end of the spine. Some laypersons call this the tailbone. It is easiest to remember this as the region of the *coccyx* (KOK-siks).

A puncture wound to the back just above the waist would be reported as a wound to the lumbar region of the back.

Body Cavities

There are four major body cavities, two anterior and two posterior. Housed in these cavities are the vital organs, glands, blood vessels, and nerves.

Anterior Cavities

- **Thoracic** (tho-RAS-ik) **Cavity**—the entire chest cavity, enclosed by the rib cage, protecting the lungs, heart, great blood vessels, part of the **trachea** (windpipe), and most of the **esophagus** (the tube connecting the throat and the stomach). The lower border of the thoracic cavity is the **diaphragm,** a dome-shaped muscle used in breathing. The diaphragm separates the thoracic cavity from the lower anterior cavity.
- **Abdominopelvic** (ab-DOM-i-no-PEL-vik) **Cavity**—the anterior body cavity below the diaphragm. There are two portions of the abdominopelvic cavity: abdominal and pelvic.
- **Abdominal Cavity**—extending between the diaphragm and the pelvis, containing all the abdominal organs, including the liver, stomach, gallbladder, pancreas, spleen, small intestine, and most of the large intestine are found in this cavity. Most of the abdominal cavity, unlike the other body cavities, is not surrounded by bones. Only the upper portion of the cavity is protected by the lower ribs. If you consider all the organs in this cavity and the lack of bony protection, it is easy to see why blows to the abdomen can be so potentially harmful.
- **Pelvic Cavity**—protects a portion of the lower anterior cavity with bones of the pelvic girdle. This cavity contains the urinary bladder, portions of the large intestine, and the internal reproductive organs.

Posterior Cavities

- **Cranial Cavity**—This is the portion of the skull housing the brain and its specialized membranes.
- **Spinal Cavity**—This cavity runs through the center of the backbone, protecting the spinal cord and its specialized membranes.

Abdominal Quadrants

The abdomen is a large body region, and the abdominal cavity contains many vital organs. In other body regions, bones may be used for reference, such as counting the ribs or feeling a bump or notch on a bone. This is not the case when trying to be specific

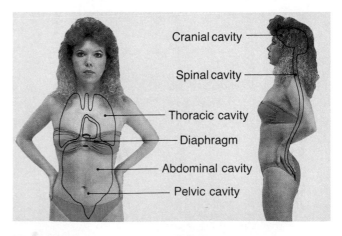

FIGURE 2–6. Body cavities.

about references to the areas of the abdomen. The navel or **umbilicus** (um-BIL-i-kus) is the only quick point of reference available for the beginning student. To improve this situation, the abdominal wall is divided into four quadrants (Figure 2–7):

1. **Right Upper Quadrant** (RUQ)—containing most of the liver, the gallbladder, and part of the large intestine.
2. **Left Upper Quadrant** (LUQ)—containing most of the stomach, the spleen, the pancreas, and part of the large intestine.
3. **Right Lower Quadrant** (RLQ)—containing the appendix and part of the large intestine.
4. **Left Lower Quadrant** (LLQ)—containing part of the large intestine.

Some organs and glands are located in more than one quadrant. As you can see from the previous list, the large intestine is found, in part, in all four quadrants. The same is true for the small intestine. Most of the stomach is in the left upper quadrant, but part of it can be found in the right upper quadrant. The bulk of the liver is found in the right upper quadrant; however, the left lobe of the liver extends into the left upper quadrant.

These quadrants also are used to help locate the pelvic organs. For example, the right ovary is located in the right lower quadrant and the left ovary is in the left lower quadrant. The uterus (womb) and the urinary bladder are assigned to both lower quadrants.

The kidneys are a special case.* They are not within the abdominal cavity but located behind the cavity's membrane lining, the peritoneum (per-i-to-NE-um). Consider one kidney to be in the right upper quadrant and the other to be in the left upper quadrant. However, do not let this abdominal classification make you forget that the kidneys are behind the abdominal cavity and subject to injury from blows to the mid-back. Any pain or ache in the back may be caused by problems with the kidneys.

You now have four ways to locate body structures or the sites of injuries. You can make reference to body regions, the divisions of the spine, body cavities, and the abdominal quadrants. As you continue your studies, you will learn how to make use of body landmarks as points of reference. These are specific structures, notches, joints, and "bumps" on bones. Some are obvious (navel, nipples); some you know by other names but will have to learn the medical terms (Adam's apple = thyroid cartilage); and some will probably be new to you (xiphoid process). Figures are included at the end of this chapter to help you review these points of reference as they are studied in your course.

Body Systems

A body system is a group of organs that carry out specific body functions. Learning as much as you can about the body systems and their functions will prove to be of great value when you begin to provide emergency care. Remembering the different body functions can be useful when trying to determine the extent of injury or the nature of a medical emergency. The following is a list of the major body systems and their primary functions:

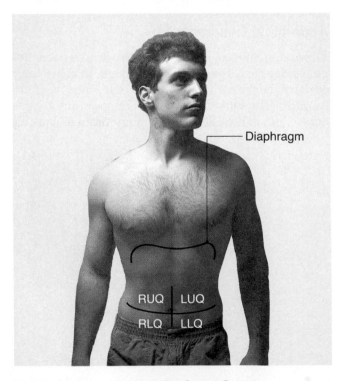
- *Circulatory System*—the heart and vessels that move blood, carrying oxygen and food to the body's cells and removing wastes and carbon dioxide from these cells.
- *Respiratory System*—exchanges air to bring in oxygen and expel carbon dioxide. This oxygen is placed into the bloodstream as carbon dioxide is being removed to be expelled into the atmosphere.
- *Digestive System*—enables us to eat, digest, and absorb foods and provides for the removal of wastes.

FIGURE 2–7. Abdominal quadrants.

* The pancreas also is located behind the peritoneum (retroperitoneal); however, most general anatomy textbooks classify it along with the abdominal organs.

- *Urinary System*—involved in the removal of chemical wastes from the blood and helps balance water and salt levels of the blood.
- *Reproductive System*—the structures of the body involved with sexual reproduction. Sometimes this is classified with the urinary system as the genitourinary (jen-E-to-U-re-NER-e) system.
- *Nervous System*—controls movement, interprets sensations, regulates and coordinates body activities, and generates memory and thought.
- *Special Senses*—various organs that link with the nervous system to provide sight, hearing, taste, smell, and the sensations of pain, cold, heat, and tactile (touch) responses.
- *Endocrine* (EN-do-krin) *System*—produces chemicals called hormones that help regulate most body activities and functions (e.g., growth).
- *Musculoskeletal System*—bones provide protection and support, and skeletal muscles act with the bones to permit body movement. Skeletal muscles are voluntary muscles. This means that we can consciously direct these muscles to contract and relax. (Not all the body's muscles are part of the musculoskeletal system. The heart is made of cardiac muscle that keeps the heart functioning automatically. The walls of organs are made up of smooth, involuntary muscles that contract and relax without our conscious control.)
- *Integumentary* (in-TEG-u-MEN-ta-re) *System*—the skin and its accessories (hair, oil glands, sweat glands, and nails).
- *Immune System*—a network of specialized cells found in the bloodstream, lymphatic system, liver, spleen, thyroid, and throughout the body's connective tissues. These cells function mainly to kill, or otherwise render harmless, microorganisms (germs).*

RELATING STRUCTURES TO THE BODY

In this section we will use a series of illustrations to show what you, as an EMT, should know about

* Detailed references to this system often are found in medical textbooks under the heading of the reticuloendothelial (re-TIK-u-lo-EN-do-THE-li-al) system.

the general anatomy of the human body. Your task as you study this section is a complex one that requires much thought and practice before you will be comfortable with the new knowlege gained in your training. Basically, you will be asked to consider your own body and the bodies of others so that you may visualize where structures are located within the body. As stated earlier, your job is to learn the general location of these structures as you view the external body. On many of the following illustrations, you will see a line representing the diaphragm. Being able to visualize the position of the diaphragm will give you a point of reference that will greatly help you understand how the various organs and glands fit into the body.

In Scan 2–1, we see the position of the heart in the thoracic cavity. As a quick point of reference, use your fingers to find a small hard spot just below your sternum (breastbone). This is the **xiphoid** (ZI-foyd) **process,** a major body landmark. You can find a point directly over the heart by measuring two to three finger widths up from this point. Look at yourself in a mirror and find this point. Each time you look in the mirror during your training, try to visualize where your heart is located.

Scan 2–1 shows you the position of the lungs in the chest cavity. Notice that the lungs do not extend downward as far as the bottom of the rib cage. The diaphragm forms the inferior border of the lungs. By studying SCAN 2–1, you will have a very good idea of the size, shape, and position of the lungs.

As you study Scan 2–1, keep in mind that the abdomen is rich in blood vessels, nerves, and membranes. Punctures and blunt trauma can rupture blood vessels and hollow organs. Blood loss may quickly prove to be life threatening. The blood and body fluids released may cause the rapid inflammation of membranes and other body tissues, causing intense pain and adding to the patient's decline.

Scan 2–1 shows the positioning of the *stomach*, *liver*, and the first portion of the *small intestine* called the **duodenum** (du-o-DE-num). Note how the lower ribs partially protect the stomach, spleen, pancreas, duodenum, and liver. The point at which the esophagus enters the stomach, immediately after passing through the diaphragm, is at the level of the xiphoid process.

The duodenum is held in a more rigid position than the rest of the small intestine. Forceful blows to the abdomen, such as those often received in motor vehicle accidents, may damage the duodenum without causing any immediate significant damage to the rest of the intestine.

Before leaving this region of the abdomen, you can quickly learn the positions of three other struc-

SCAN 2–1 MAJOR BODY ORGANS

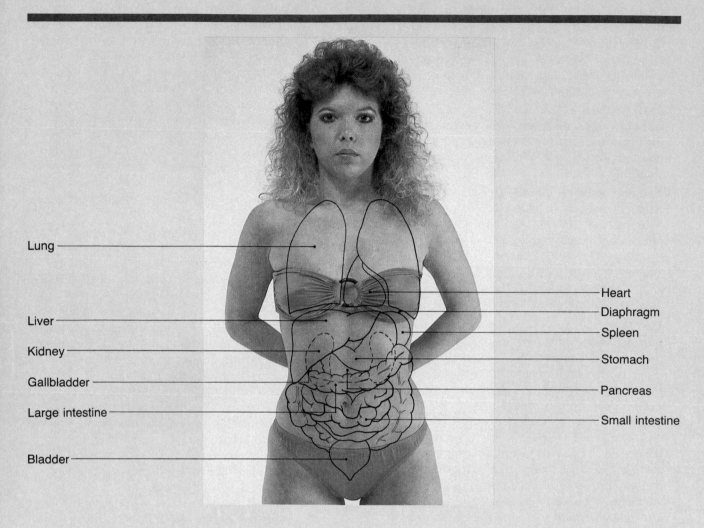

Lung

Liver

Kidney

Gallbladder

Large intestine

Bladder

Heart

Diaphragm

Spleen

Stomach

Pancreas

Small intestine

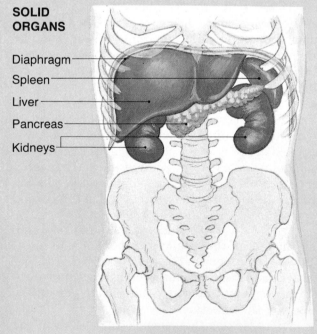

SOLID ORGANS

Diaphragm
Spleen
Liver
Pancreas
Kidneys

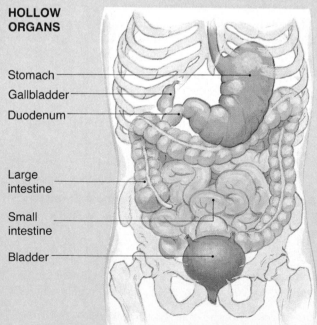

HOLLOW ORGANS

Stomach
Gallbladder
Duodenum

Large intestine

Small intestine

Bladder

tures based on what you have already learned. The *gallbladder* is below the liver, the *pancreas* is behind the lower part of the stomach, and the *spleen* is lateral to the left side of the stomach (Scansheet 2–1).

Scan 2–1 shows the space occupied by the *small intestine*. As you can see, most of the abdominal cavity is filled with this structure. The illustration shows the space occupied by the *large intestine*. Note how it passes through each of the four abdominal quadrants.

The *kidneys* and the *urinary bladder* are shown in Scan 2–1. Remember, the kidneys are behind the abdominal cavity and the bladder is in the pelvic cavity.

SUMMARY

All references made to body structures consider the body to be in the anatomical position. Always use *patient right* and *patient left*. Remember that *medial* is toward the midline, while *lateral* is away from the midline.

- Anterior = front
- Posterior = back
- Superior = top, higher, or toward the head
- Inferior = bottom, lower, or away from the head

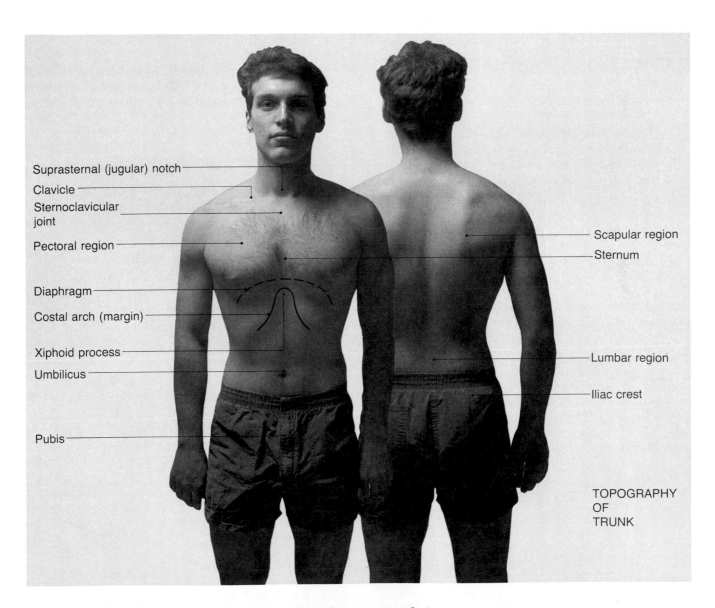

FIGURE 2–8. **The chest, abdomen, and back (topography).**

- Proximal = closest to the point of origin or reference
- Distal = farthest from the point of origin or reference

There are two anterior body cavities: thoracic and abdominopelvic (abdominal and pelvic). The posterior body cavities are the cranial and the spinal.

Divide the spine into five regions: cervix (neck), thorax (upper back), lumbar (mid back), sacrum (lower back), and coccygeal (inferior tip).

Divide the abdomen into abdominal quadrants: right and left upper (RUQ, LUQ) and right and left lower (RLQ, LLQ).

Before returning to the list of objectives for Chapter 2, use your own body as a reference and:

- Apply the terms *anterior*, *posterior*, *medial*, and *lateral*.
- Apply the terms *superior*, *inferior*, *proximal*, and *distal*.
- Outline your own major body cavities. Trace the anterior position of your diaphragm. Can you name the organs found in each cavity?
- Point to each of your abdominal quadrants. Can you name the organs found in each quadrant?

- Look in a mirror. Where are your heart, lungs, xiphoid process, liver, stomach, gallbladder, spleen, pancreas, small intestine, and large intestine? Can you locate your kidneys and your urinary bladder?

Go back to the Chapter Objectives and be sure that you can meet every one. Throughout the rest of your course, practice locating the positions of the body's organs, glands, and other major structures. Refer to Scan 2–1. Add new structures to your list as they are presented, and remember to add more details to what you now know as these details appear in the text.

In this chapter you will find 12 color anatomical inserts. They are designed to help you learn the anatomy and physiology of the major body systems as you progress through your EMT course. They are not grouped together to indicate that they should be learned all at once. Use these inserts throughout your course to aid you in learning various structures and systems as they are covered and needed in your training.

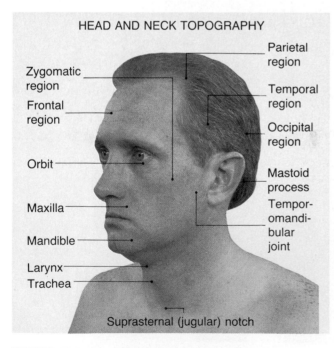

FIGURE 2–9. The head and neck (topography).

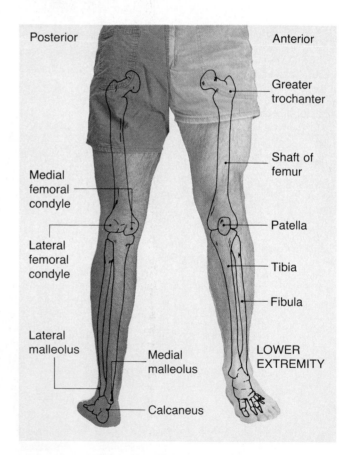

FIGURE 2–10. The lower extremity (topography and skeletal).

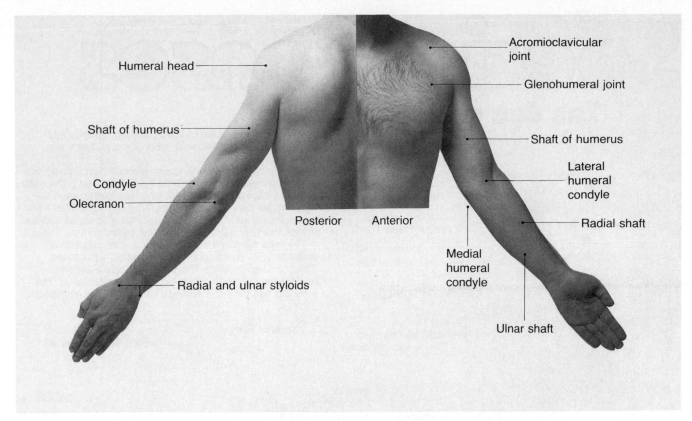

FIGURE 2–11. **The upper extremity (topography and skeletal).**

ANATOMY AND PHYSIOLOGY PLATES AND ATLAS OF INJURIES PHOTOGRAPHS

The anatomical plates are designed to help you learn the anatomy and physiology of the major body systems as you progress through your EMT course. The plates are not grouped together to indicate that they should be learned all at once. You may wish to refer to them throughout your course as aids in learning the various body structures and systems as they are covered and needed in your training.

The injuries photographs that follow show major types of bodily injuries.

Anatomy Plates

- Special Senses, p. 44
- Membranes, p. 45

Special Senses
The Eye and Ear

The body has the sense of vision, hearing, balance and equilibrium, touch, pain, heat, cold, pressure, taste, and smell.

The eye can receive and focus light and then convert this energy into nerve impulses to be sent to the brain. The nerve impulses originate from the retina. Visual receptors in the retina called rods can work in low intensity light. They have no color function. The visual receptors called cones operate in high intensity light and do receive colors.

The ear's functions include hearing, static equilibrium (balance while standing still), and dynamic equilibrium (balance when moving). The outer and middle ear are responsible for sound gathering and its transmission. The inner ear has the nerve endings for hearing and equilibrium.

The Eye

The Ear

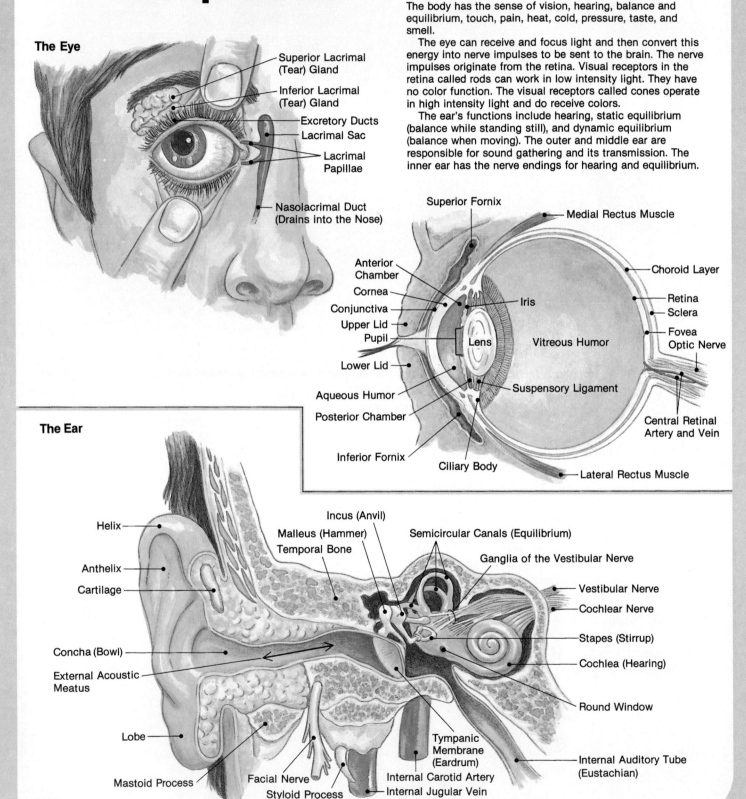

Superior Lacrimal (Tear) Gland
Inferior Lacrimal (Tear) Gland
Excretory Ducts
Lacrimal Sac
Lacrimal Papillae
Nasolacrimal Duct (Drains into the Nose)

Superior Fornix
Medial Rectus Muscle
Anterior Chamber
Cornea
Conjunctiva
Upper Lid
Pupil
Lower Lid
Aqueous Humor
Posterior Chamber
Inferior Fornix
Ciliary Body
Iris
Lens
Vitreous Humor
Suspensory Ligament
Choroid Layer
Retina
Sclera
Fovea
Optic Nerve
Central Retinal Artery and Vein
Lateral Rectus Muscle

Helix
Anthelix
Cartilage
Concha (Bowl)
External Acoustic Meatus
Lobe
Mastoid Process
Facial Nerve
Styloid Process
Incus (Anvil)
Malleus (Hammer)
Temporal Bone
Semicircular Canals (Equilibrium)
Ganglia of the Vestibular Nerve
Vestibular Nerve
Cochlear Nerve
Stapes (Stirrup)
Cochlea (Hearing)
Round Window
Tympanic Membrane (Eardrum)
Internal Carotid Artery
Internal Jugular Vein
Internal Auditory Tube (Eustachian)

44

Membranes

The Skin

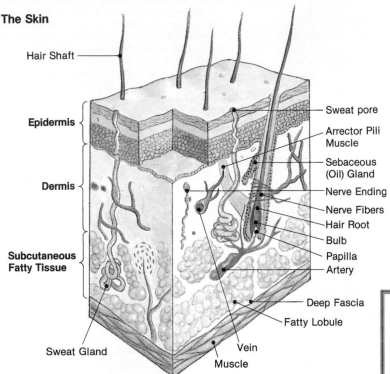

Hair Shaft

Epidermis

Dermis

Subcutaneous
Fatty Tissue

Sweat Gland

Sweat pore
Arrector Pili Muscle
Sebaceous (Oil) Gland
Nerve Ending
Nerve Fibers
Hair Root
Bulb
Papilla
Artery
Deep Fascia
Fatty Lobule
Vein
Muscle

The skin is the largest organ of the body. In the adult the skin covers about 3000 square inches (1.75 square meters) and weighs about 6 pounds. It is involved with protection, insulation, thermal regulation, excretion, and the production of vitamin D.

Membranes

Membranes cover or line body structures to provide protection from injury and infection. There are four major classes of membranes. Mucous membranes line those structures that open to the outside world (for example, the mouth, the airway, digestive tract, urinary tract, and vagina). Serous membranes line the closed body cavities and cover the outsides of organs. The cutaneous membrane is the skin. Synovial membranes line joints to reduce friction during movement.

A serous membrane that covers an organ is called a visceral layer. The term parietal layer is used for the part of the serous membrane that lines a cavity. The serous membrane in the thoracic cavity is called pleura (for example, the parietal pleura lines the chest cavity). In the abdominal cavity, it is called peritoneum (for example, the parietal peritoneum). A double layer of peritoneum is called mesentery. The membrane that lines the sac surrounding the heart is pericardium.

Synovial Joint

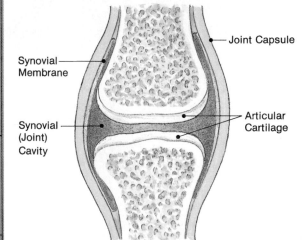

Synovial Membrane

Synovial (Joint) Cavity

Joint Capsule

Articular Cartilage

The Peritoneum

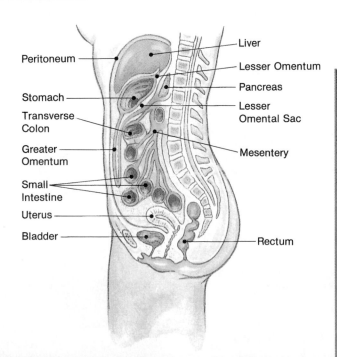

Peritoneum
Stomach
Transverse Colon
Greater Omentum
Small Intestine
Uterus
Bladder

Liver
Lesser Omentum
Pancreas
Lesser Omental Sac
Mesentery
Rectum

The Pleura

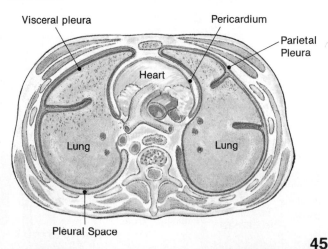

Visceral pleura
Pericardium
Parietal Pleura
Heart
Lung
Lung
Pleural Space

45

Skeleton

The skeleton is a living framework made by the joining of bones. It serves to provide support, body movement powered by muscular contractions, protection for the vital organs and other soft structures, blood cell production, and storage for essential minerals. There are 206 bones in the adult body, forming the two divisions of the skeletal system. The axial skeleton is comprised of skull, vertebrae, rib cage, and sternum. The upper and lower extremities and the shoulder and pelvic girdles form the appendicular skeleton.

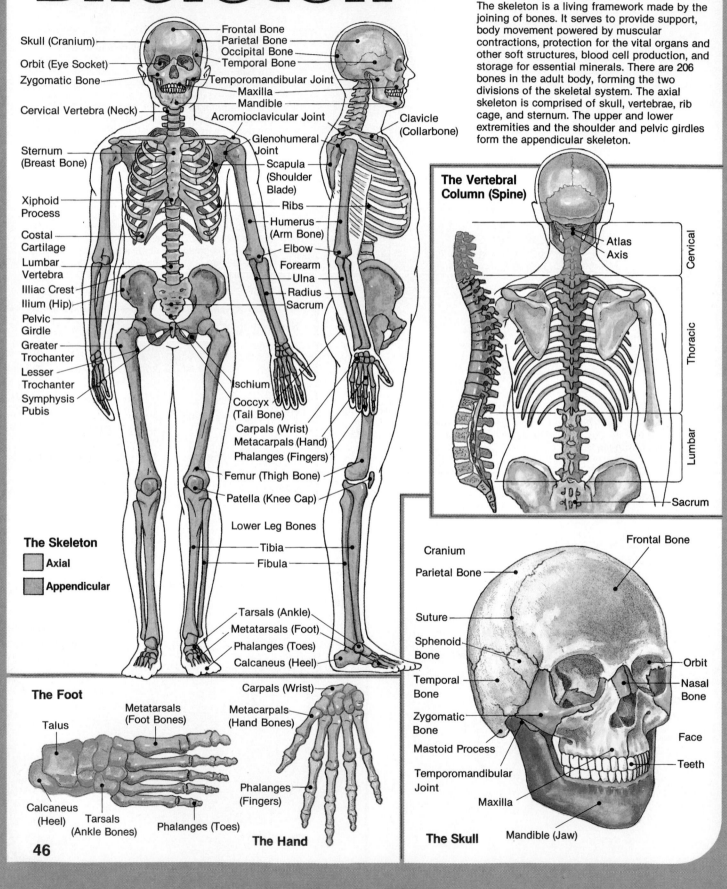

Skull (Cranium)
Orbit (Eye Socket)
Zygomatic Bone
Cervical Vertebra (Neck)
Sternum (Breast Bone)
Xiphoid Process
Costal Cartilage
Lumbar Vertebra
Illiac Crest
Ilium (Hip)
Pelvic Girdle
Greater Trochanter
Lesser Trochanter
Symphysis Pubis

Frontal Bone
Parietal Bone
Occipital Bone
Temporal Bone
Temporomandibular Joint
Maxilla
Mandible
Acromioclavicular Joint
Glenohumeral Joint
Scapula (Shoulder Blade)
Ribs
Humerus (Arm Bone)
Elbow
Forearm
Ulna
Radius
Sacrum

Clavicle (Collarbone)

Ischium
Coccyx (Tail Bone)
Carpals (Wrist)
Metacarpals (Hand)
Phalanges (Fingers)
Femur (Thigh Bone)
Patella (Knee Cap)
Lower Leg Bones
Tibia
Fibula

Tarsals (Ankle)
Metatarsals (Foot)
Phalanges (Toes)
Calcaneus (Heel)

The Skeleton
Axial
Appendicular

The Vertebral Column (Spine)
Atlas
Axis
Cervical
Thoracic
Lumbar
Sacrum

The Foot
Metatarsals (Foot Bones)
Talus
Calcaneus (Heel)
Tarsals (Ankle Bones)
Phalanges (Toes)

The Hand
Carpals (Wrist)
Metacarpals (Hand Bones)
Phalanges (Fingers)
Phalanges (Toes)

The Skull
Cranium
Parietal Bone
Suture
Sphenoid Bone
Temporal Bone
Zygomatic Bone
Mastoid Process
Temporomandibular Joint
Maxilla
Mandible (Jaw)
Frontal Bone
Orbit
Nasal Bone
Face
Teeth

46

Muscles
The Muscular System

The tissues of the muscular system comprise 40 to 50% of the body's weight. The skeletal muscles of the body are voluntary muscles, subject to conscious control. They exhibit the properties of excitability; that is, they will react to nerve stimulus. Once stimulated, skeleton muscles are quick to contract and can relax and very quickly be ready for another contraction. There are 501 separate skeletal muscles that provide contractions for movement, coordinated support for posture, and heat production. Muscles connect to bones by way of tendons.

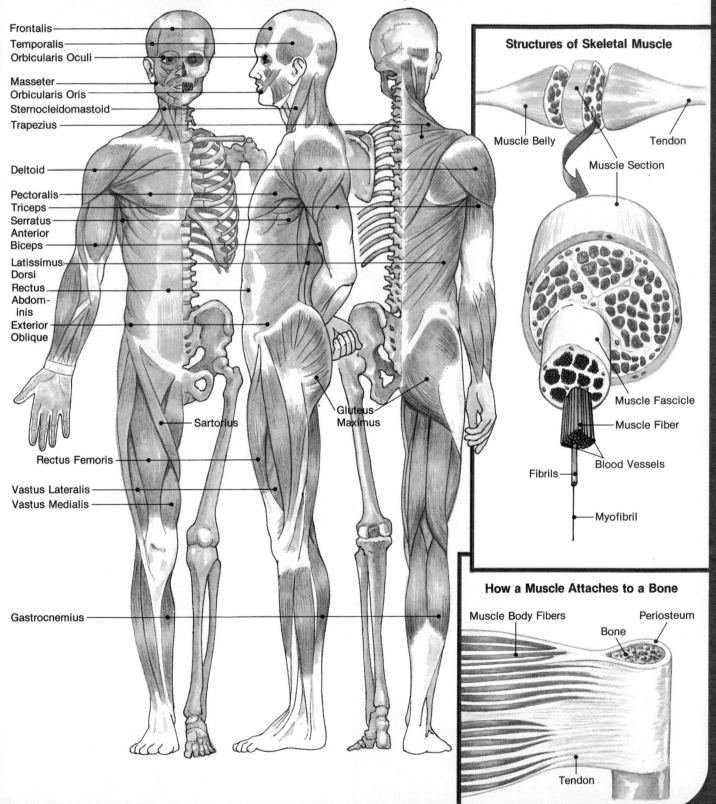

Frontalis
Temporalis
Orbicularis Oculi
Masseter
Orbicularis Oris
Sternocleidomastoid
Trapezius
Deltoid
Pectoralis
Triceps
Serratus Anterior
Biceps
Latissimus Dorsi
Rectus Abdominis
Exterior Oblique
Sartorius
Gluteus Maximus
Rectus Femoris
Vastus Lateralis
Vastus Medialis
Gastrocnemius

Structures of Skeletal Muscle

Muscle Belly
Tendon
Muscle Section
Muscle Fascicle
Muscle Fiber
Blood Vessels
Fibrils
Myofibril

How a Muscle Attaches to a Bone

Muscle Body Fibers
Periosteum
Bone
Tendon

The Heart
The Cardiovascular System

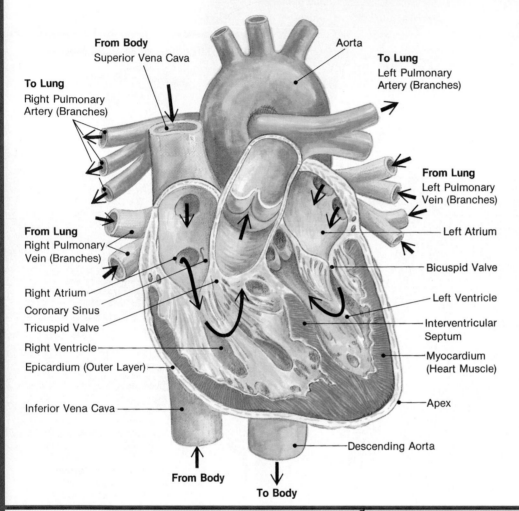

From Body
Superior Vena Cava

To Lung
Right Pulmonary
Artery (Branches)

Aorta

To Lung
Left Pulmonary
Artery (Branches)

From Lung
Left Pulmonary
Vein (Branches)

From Lung
Right Pulmonary
Vein (Branches)

Left Atrium

Bicuspid Valve

Right Atrium

Coronary Sinus

Tricuspid Valve

Right Ventricle

Epicardium (Outer Layer)

Left Ventricle

Interventricular
Septum

Myocardium
(Heart Muscle)

Inferior Vena Cava

Apex

Descending Aorta

From Body

To Body

The heart is a hollow, muscular organ that pumps 450 million pints of blood in the average lifetime. Its superior chambers, the atria, receive blood. Both atria fill and then contract at the same time. The inferior chambers are the ventricles. They pump blood out of the heart. Both ventricles fill and then contract at the same time. When the atria are relaxing, the ventricles are contracting.

The right side of the heart receives blood from the body and sends it to the lungs (pulmonic circulation). The heart's left side receives oxygenated blood from the lungs and sends it out to the body (systemic circulation).

The heartbeat originates at the sinoatrial node (pacemaker) and spreads across the atria to stimulate contraction. After a slight delay, the impulse is sent from the atrioventricular node, down the bundles of His, and out across the ventricles. This stimulates the ventricles to contract while the atria are relaxing.

The heart muscle (myocardium) receives its blood supply by way of the right and left coronary arteries. These vessels are the first branches of the aorta.

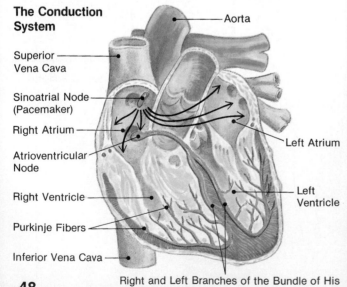

The Conduction System

Aorta

Superior
Vena Cava

Sinoatrial Node
(Pacemaker)

Right Atrium

Atrioventricular
Node

Right Ventricle

Purkinje Fibers

Inferior Vena Cava

Left Atrium

Left
Ventricle

Right and Left Branches of the Bundle of His

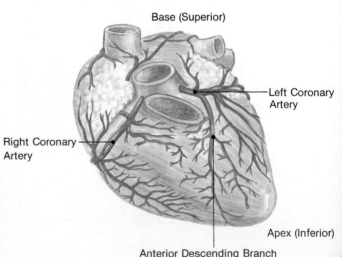

The Coronary Arteries

Base (Superior)

Left Coronary
Artery

Right Coronary
Artery

Apex (Inferior)

Anterior Descending Branch

48

Blood Vessels

The Circulatory System

Major Arteries

Internal Carotid
External Carotid
Common Carotid

Subclavian
Innominate
Axillary
Pulmonary
Aorta
Brachial

Radial
Ulnar
Common Iliac

Palmar Arches
Digital

Deep Femoral
Femoral

Popliteal

Anterior Tibial
Peroneal

Posterior Tibial

Dorsal Pedis
Arcuate

Major Veins

External Jugular
Internal Jugular
Innominate

Brachial
Cephalic   Antecubital

Axillary
Subclavian
Basilic

Venae Cavae

Volar Digital

Right Gastric Artery and Vein
Hepatic Artery and Vein
Splenic Artery and Vein
Renal Artery and Vein
Mesenteric Arteries and Veins

Common Iliac

Great Saphenous

Femoral

Popliteal

Peroneal

Posterior Tibial

Anterior Tibial

Dorsal Venous Arch

Any blood vessel that carries blood away from the heart is an artery. Arteries have strong muscular walls and are very elastic, changing their diameter as the heart contracts to force blood into circulation. They decrease in diameter to become arterioles. These structures join with capillary beds. A capillary is thin-walled, being no thicker than the lining of an arteriole. Blood moves through the capillaries in a constant flow know as **perfusion.** During perfusion, oxygen and nutrients are given up to the body's tissues and cellular carbon dioxide and wastes are picked up.

Any blood vessel that carries blood back to the heart is a vein. The small diameter veins that leave capillary beds are called venules. These join with larger veins. The walls of veins are not as thick or elastic as those of arteries. Some veins have valves to prevent the backward flow of blood.

Nervous System

The Brain

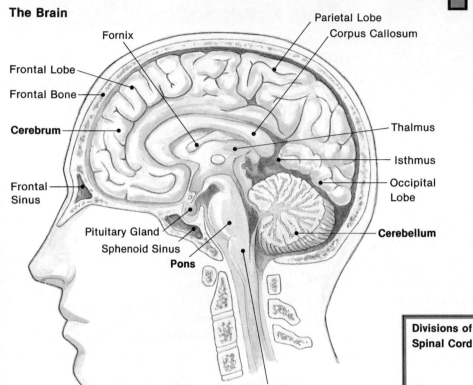

- Parietal Lobe
- Corpus Callosum
- Fornix
- Frontal Lobe
- Frontal Bone
- **Cerebrum**
- Frontal Sinus
- Pituitary Gland
- Sphenoid Sinus
- **Pons**
- Thalmus
- Isthmus
- Occipital Lobe
- **Cerebellum**
- **Medulla Oblongata**

The nervous system includes the brain, spinal cord, and nerves. Structures within the system may be classified according to divisions: central, peripheral, and autonomic divisions of the nervous system. The central nervous system includes the brain and spinal cord. The sensory (incoming) and motor (outgoing) nerves make up the peripheral nervous system. The autonomic nervous system has structures that parallel the spinal cord and then share the same pathways as the peripheral nerves. This division is involved with motor impulses (outgoing commands) that travel from the central nervous system to the heart muscle, blood vessels, secreting cells of glands, and the smooth muscles of organs. The impulses will stimulate or inhibit certain activities.

The Spinal Cord

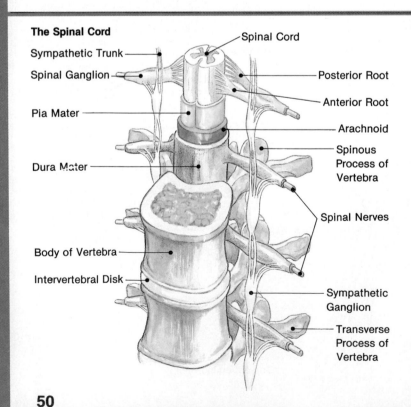

- Spinal Cord
- Sympathetic Trunk
- Spinal Ganglion
- Pia Mater
- Dura Mater
- Body of Vertebra
- Intervertebral Disk
- Posterior Root
- Anterior Root
- Arachnoid
- Spinous Process of Vertebra
- Spinal Nerves
- Sympathetic Ganglion
- Transverse Process of Vertebra

Divisions of the Spinal Cord

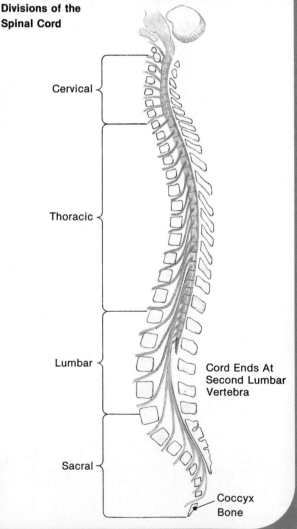

- Cervical
- Thoracic
- Lumbar
- Sacral
- Cord Ends At Second Lumbar Vertebra
- Coccyx Bone

Nervous System Continued

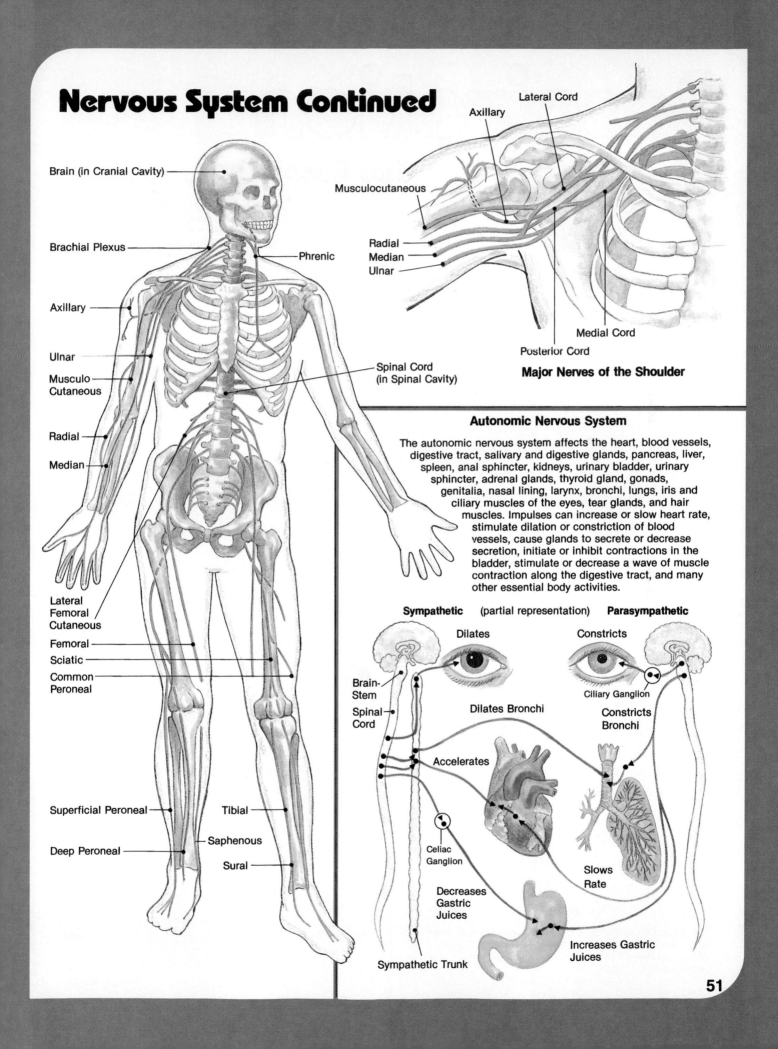

Brain (in Cranial Cavity)

Brachial Plexus

Axillary

Ulnar

Musculo Cutaneous

Radial

Median

Phrenic

Spinal Cord (in Spinal Cavity)

Lateral Femoral Cutaneous

Femoral

Sciatic

Common Peroneal

Superficial Peroneal

Deep Peroneal

Tibial

Saphenous

Sural

Major Nerves of the Shoulder

Axillary

Lateral Cord

Musculocutaneous

Radial

Median

Ulnar

Medial Cord

Posterior Cord

Autonomic Nervous System

The autonomic nervous system affects the heart, blood vessels, digestive tract, salivary and digestive glands, pancreas, liver, spleen, anal sphincter, kidneys, urinary bladder, urinary sphincter, adrenal glands, thyroid gland, gonads, genitalia, nasal lining, larynx, bronchi, lungs, iris and ciliary muscles of the eyes, tear glands, and hair muscles. Impulses can increase or slow heart rate, stimulate dilation or constriction of blood vessels, cause glands to secrete or decrease secretion, initiate or inhibit contractions in the bladder, stimulate or decrease a wave of muscle contraction along the digestive tract, and many other essential body activities.

Sympathetic (partial representation) **Parasympathetic**

Dilates

Constricts

Brain-Stem

Spinal Cord

Ciliary Ganglion

Dilates Bronchi

Constricts Bronchi

Accelerates

Celiac Ganglion

Slows Rate

Decreases Gastric Juices

Increases Gastric Juices

Sympathetic Trunk

Respiration

The Respiratory System

The airway consists of structures involved with the conduction and exchange of air. Conduction is the movement of air to and from the exchange levels of the lungs. Air enters through the nose (primary) and mouth (secondary) and travels down the pharynx to enter the larynx. After passing through the larynx, air enters the trachea. At its distal end, the trachea branches into the right and left primary bronchi. These bronchi branch into secondary bronchi, which then branch into the bronchioles. Some of the bronchioles end as closed tubes. Air movement in them helps the lungs expand. The rest of the bronchioles carry the air to the exchange levels of the lungs.

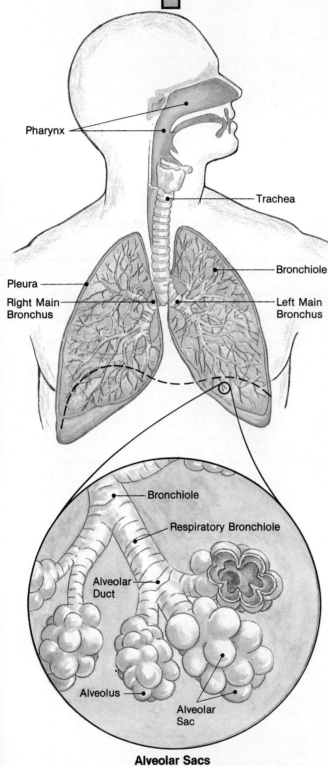

Pharynx

Trachea

Bronchiole

Pleura

Right Main Bronchus

Left Main Bronchus

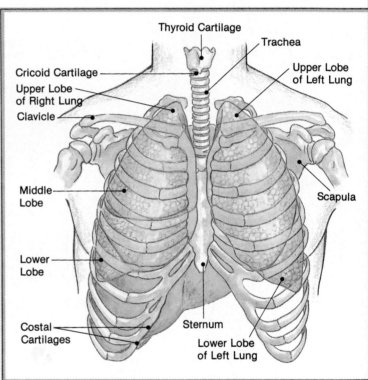

Thyroid Cartilage

Trachea

Cricoid Cartilage

Upper Lobe of Right Lung

Clavicle

Upper Lobe of Left Lung

Middle Lobe

Scapula

Lower Lobe

Costal Cartilages

Sternum

Lower Lobe of Left Lung

Alveolar Sacs

Bronchiole

Respiratory Bronchiole

Alveolar Duct

Alveolus

Alveolar Sac

The respiratory bronchioles turn into alveolar ducts. These form alveolar sacs that are made up of the alveoli. Gas exchange takes place between the alveoli and the capillaries in the lungs.

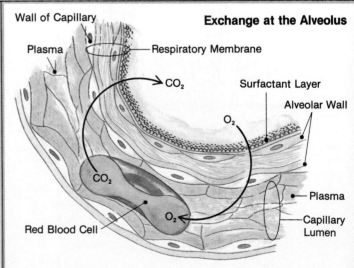

Exchange at the Alveolus

Wall of Capillary

Plasma

Respiratory Membrane

CO_2

Surfactant Layer

Alveolar Wall

O_2

CO_2

O_2

Plasma

Red Blood Cell

Capillary Lumen

Digestion

The Digestive System

The digestive system includes the digestive tract and various supportive structures and accessory glands. The tract begins at the oral cavity with the teeth and tongue. The salivary glands release saliva into the mouth to moisten food for swallowing. The tract continues down the throat to the esophagus, through the cardiac sphincter, and into the stomach. Acid and digestive enzymes are added to the food to produce chyme. The chyme passes through the pyloric sphincter to enter the small intestine. Digestive enzymes from the pancreas and bile from the liver are added to the chyme. The process of digestion and absorption are completed in the small intestine. Wastes are carried through the ileoceccal valve into the large intestine. The wastes are moved to the rectum, from where they can be expelled through the anus.

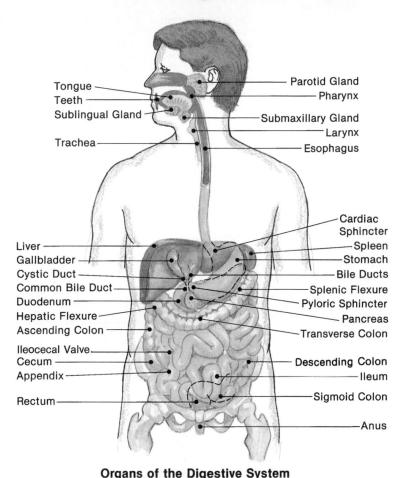

Tongue
Teeth
Sublingual Gland
Trachea

Parotid Gland
Pharynx
Submaxillary Gland
Larynx
Esophagus

Liver
Gallbladder
Cystic Duct
Common Bile Duct
Duodenum
Hepatic Flexure
Ascending Colon
Ileocecal Valve
Cecum
Appendix
Rectum

Cardiac Sphincter
Spleen
Stomach
Bile Ducts
Splenic Flexure
Pyloric Sphincter
Pancreas
Transverse Colon
Descending Colon
Ileum
Sigmoid Colon
Anus

Organs of the Digestive System

Liver, Stomach, and Pancreas

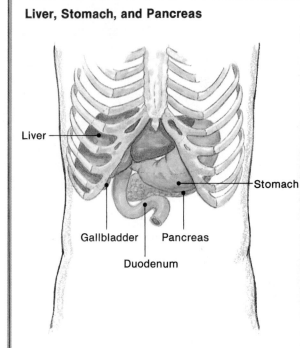

Liver

Stomach

Gallbladder   Pancreas

Duodenum

Large Intestine

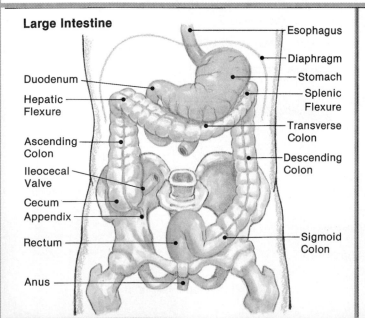

Duodenum
Hepatic Flexure
Ascending Colon
Ileocecal Valve
Cecum
Appendix
Rectum
Anus

Esophagus
Diaphragm
Stomach
Splenic Flexure
Transverse Colon
Descending Colon
Sigmoid Colon

Small Intestine

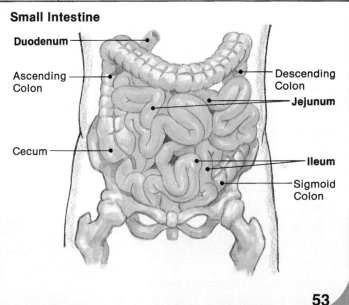

Duodenum
Ascending Colon
Cecum

Descending Colon
Jejunum
Ileum
Sigmoid Colon

Excretion The Urinary System

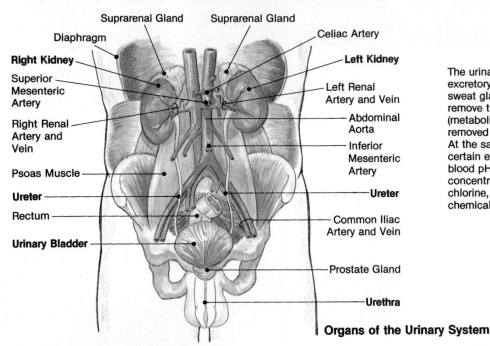

Suprarenal Gland
Suprarenal Gland
Diaphragm
Celiac Artery
Right Kidney
Left Kidney
Superior Mesenteric Artery
Left Renal Artery and Vein
Right Renal Artery and Vein
Abdominal Aorta
Inferior Mesenteric Artery
Psoas Muscle
Ureter
Ureter
Rectum
Common Iliac Artery and Vein
Urinary Bladder
Prostate Gland
Urethra

Organs of the Urinary System

The urinary system is part of the body's excretory structures (urinary system, lungs, sweat glands, and intestine). The kidneys remove the wastes of chemical activities (metabolism) in the body. These wastes are removed from the blood to produce urine. At the same time, the kidneys remove certain excess compounds, regulate the blood pH (acid-base balance), and the concentration of sodium, potassium, chlorine, glucose and other important chemicals.

The Nephron

Each kidney is made up of microscopic nephrons. Both wastes and needed chemicals are filtered from the blood. As these materials are passed through the nephron, the needed compounds (including water) are sent back into the blood. Wastes are collected as urine.

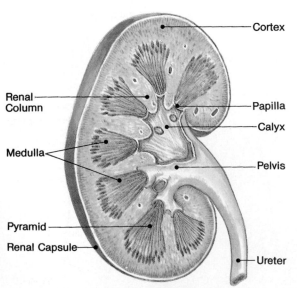

Cortex
Renal Column
Papilla
Calyx
Medulla
Pelvis
Pyramid
Renal Capsule
Ureter

Sectioned Kidney

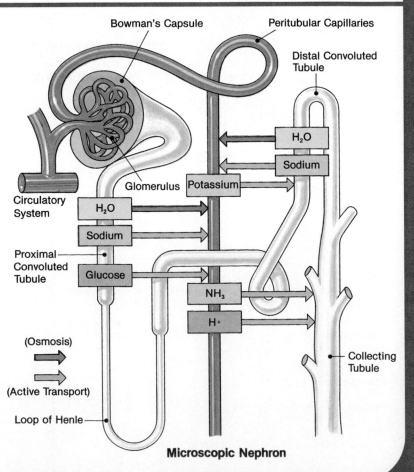

Bowman's Capsule
Peritubular Capillaries
Distal Convoluted Tubule
H_2O
Sodium
Glomerulus
Potassium
Circulatory System
H_2O
Sodium
Proximal Convoluted Tubule
Glucose
NH_3
H^+
(Osmosis)
(Active Transport)
Collecting Tubule
Loop of Henle

Microscopic Nephron

54

Reproduction
The Reproductive System

The reproductive system consists of the organs, glands, and supportive structures that are involved with human sexuality and procreation. In the male, spermatozoa and the hormone testosterone are produced in the testes. The female produces ova (eggs) and the hormones estrogen and progesterone in her ovaries. The union of ovum and sperm produce a single cell called a zygote. Through growth, cell division, and cellular differentiation (the formation of specialized cells) the new individual develops and matures.

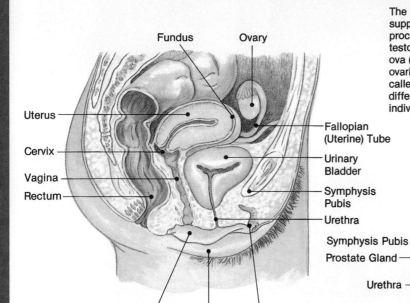

Female

Fundus
Ovary
Uterus
Cervix
Vagina
Rectum
Fallopian (Uterine) Tube
Urinary Bladder
Symphysis Pubis
Urethra
Labium Minus
Clitoris
Labium Majus

Labium Minus (singular), Labia Minora (plural)
Lablum Majus (singular), Labia Majora (plural)

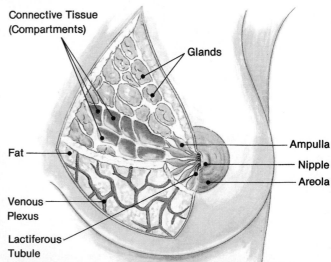

Male

Ductus Deferens
Urinary Bladder
Seminal Vesicle
Rectum
Ejaculatory Duct
Bulb of Urethra
Symphysis Pubis
Prostate Gland
Urethra
Corpus Cavernosum
Corpus Spongiosum
Testis
Epididymis
Duct of Bulbourethral Gland

The Ovary

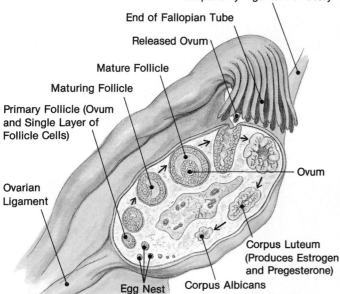

Suspensory Ligament of Ovary
End of Fallopian Tube
Released Ovum
Mature Follicle
Maturing Follicle
Primary Follicle (Ovum and Single Layer of Follicle Cells)
Ovarian Ligament
Ovum
Corpus Luteum (Produces Estrogen and Pregesterone)
Corpus Albicans
Egg Nest

The developing ovum and its supportive cells are called a follicle. Each month, follicle stimulating hormone (FSH) from the pituitary gland starts the growth of several follicles. Usually, only one will mature and release an ovum (ovulation). During its growth, the follicle produces estrogen. After ovulation, the remaining cells of the follicle form a specialized structure that produces both estrogen and progesterone.

The Breast

Connective Tissue (Compartments)
Glands
Fat
Ampulla
Nipple
Areola
Venous Plexus
Lactiferous Tubule

The breasts contain the mammary glands that produce milk (lactation). A mammary gland is a highly modified form of sweat gland. Estrogen stimulates the growth of the ducts, while progesterone stimulates the development of the secreting (milk-producing) cells. Lactic hormone from the pituitary stimulates milk production. Another pituitary hormone, oxytocin, stimulates the milk-producing cells to eject their milk into the ducts.

ATLAS OF INJURIES

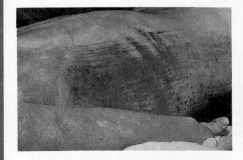

ABRASION (Gravel Roadway)

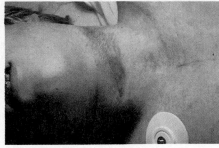

ABRASION (Rope or Cord)

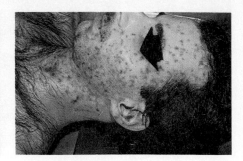

PITTED ABRASION

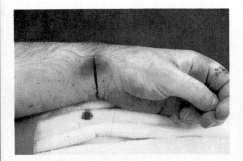

INCISION

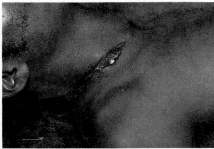

INCISION

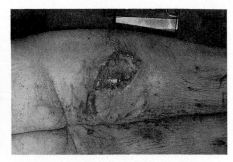

LACERATION (Jagged Margins)

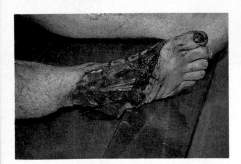

LACERATION (Tendons Still Intact)

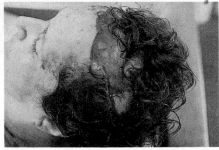

SCALP LACERATION (With Skin Separation)

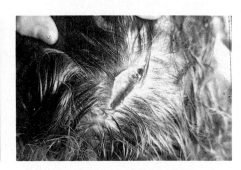

SCALP LACERATION (Minor)

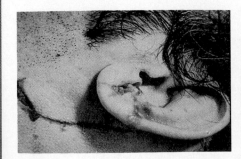

PUNCTURE WOUNDS (Stab Wounds)

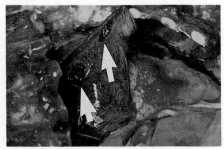

PUNCTURED LUNGS — FROM STAB WOUNDS (Autopsy)

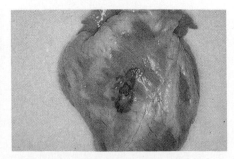

PERFORATED HEART (Bullet Wound)

ALL PHOTOGRAPHS ON THIS PAGE ARE FROM:
Dr. Lee J. Abbott, PO Box 1285, Laxahatchee, FL 33470

ATLAS OF INJURIES

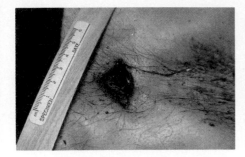

ENTRANCE WOUND (Bullet)

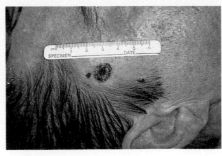

ENTRANCE WOUND (Bullet — Close Range)

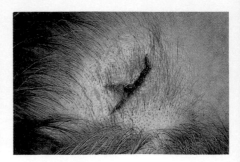

EXIT WOUND (Bullet)

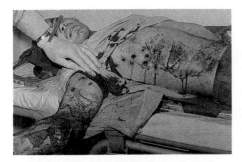

SHOTGUN WOUND

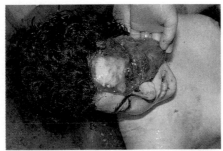

FACIAL AVULSION

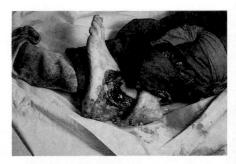

SKIN AVULSION (All Layers)

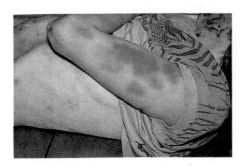

CONTUSIONS

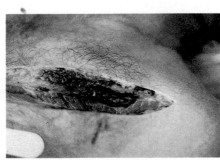

CONTUSION (Opened to Show Blood Accumulation)

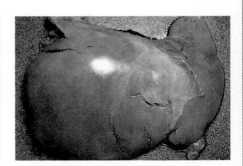

LACERATED LIVER (Abdominal Trauma)

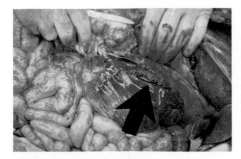

LACERATED SPLEEN

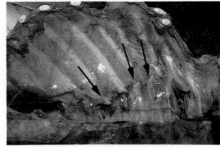

FRACTURED RIBS (Death due to Blood Loss from Lacerated Lungs)

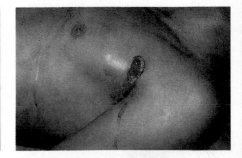

PERFORATED CHEST (Sucking Chest Wound)

ALL PHOTOGRAPHS ON THIS PAGE ARE FROM:
Dr. Lee J. Abbott, PO Box 1285, Laxahatchee, FL 33470

ATLAS OF INJURIES

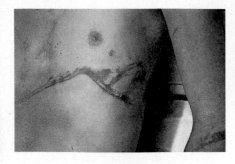

BLUNT TRAUMA TO CHEST

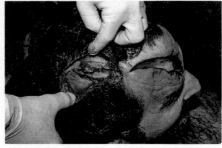

OPEN HEAD WOUND — SKULL FRACTURE

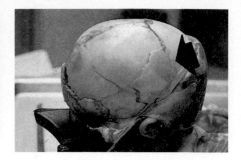

RADIATING SKULL FRACTURE (Blunt Trauma)

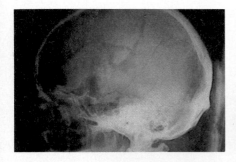

MULTIPLE SKULL FRACTURES (X-ray)

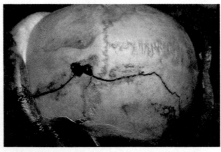

DEPRESSED SKULL FRACTURE (Force from Small Object)

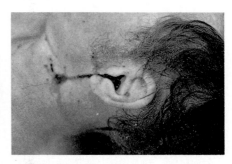

BLEEDING FROM EAR (Possible Skull Fracture)

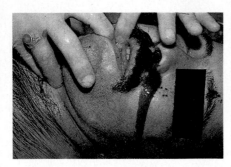

BLEEDING FROM NOSE (Possible Skull Fracture)

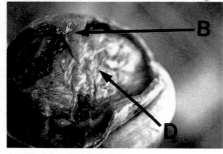

EPIDURAL HEMATOMA (D = Dura, B = Bone Fragment)

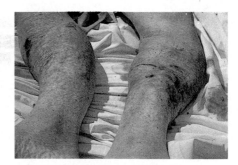

EXTENSIVE BILATERAL INJURY — LOWER EXTREMITIES (Impact with Car)

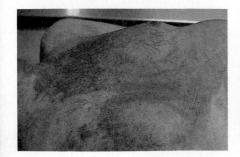

FIRST-DEGREE BURN

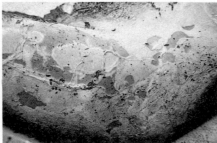

SECOND-DEGREE BURN

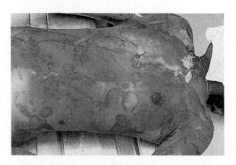

THIRD-DEGREE BURN

ALL PHOTOGRAPHS ON THIS PAGE ARE FROM:
Dr. Lee J. Abbott, PO Box 1285, Laxahatchee, FL 33470

ATLAS OF INJURIES

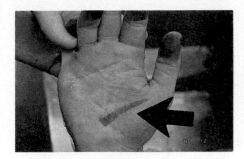

ELECTRICAL BURN
(Contact with Source) LJA

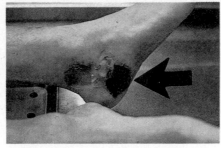

ELECTRICAL BURN (Exit)
LJA

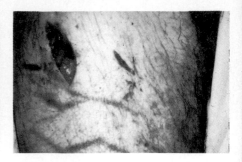

OPEN FRACTURE (Femur)
UT

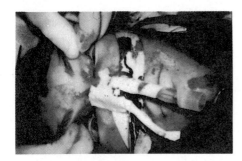

FROSTBITE

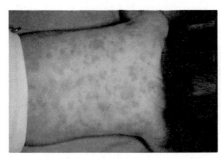

SNAKEBITE
UT

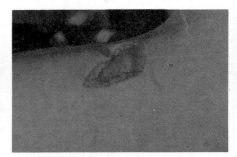

BOWEL EVISCERATION

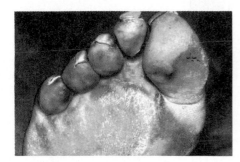

ORBITAL EDEMA

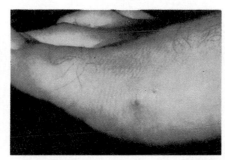

HIVES
AFIP Neg. No. 65-6982-4

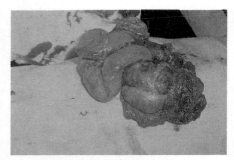

DOG BITE (Leg)
AFIP Neg. No. 62-12291

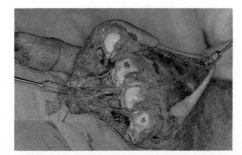

AMPUTATION (Fingers)
AFIP Neg. No. 75-20914

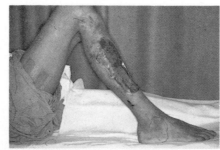

LACERATED LEG
AFIP Neg. No. 68-15269

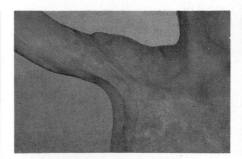

BURN (Hot Water)
AFIP Neg. No. 64-8320

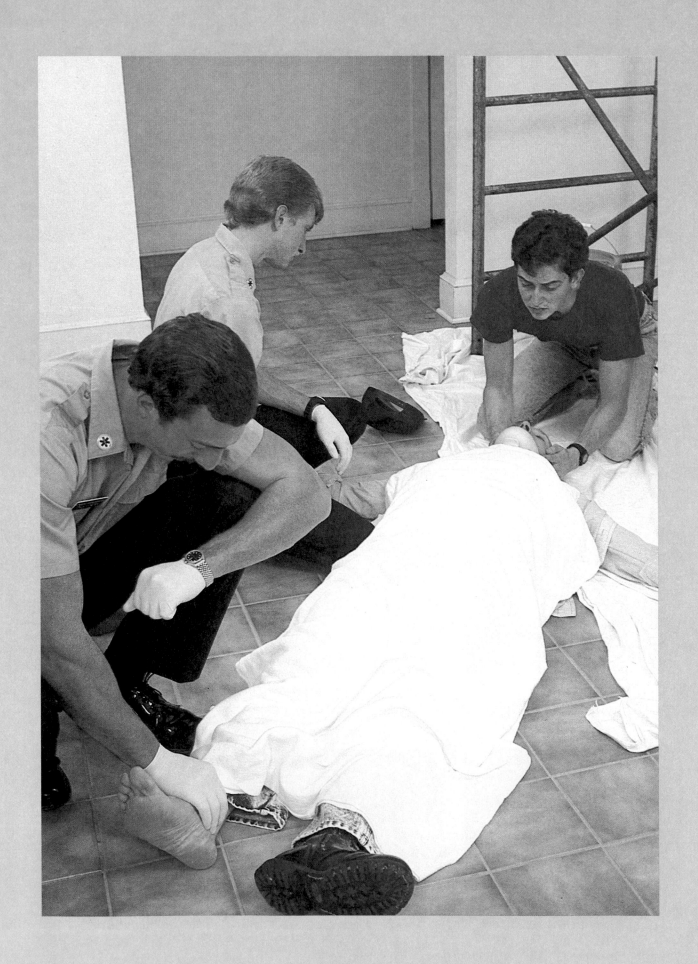

Patient Assessment

WARNING: The procedures of patient assessment may bring you into contact with patient blood and body fluids. Be certain to wear protective latex gloves and follow all local guidelines established to help prevent the spread of infectious diseases.

OBJECTIVES   As an EMT, you should be able to:

1. List the THREE major concerns you have as an EMT in gathering information. (pp. 63–64)

2. List at least FIVE problems at the emergency scene that can complicate the information gathering process. (p. 64)

3. State how you should identify yourself on arrival at the emergency scene. (p. 64)

4. List at least SIX quick sources of patient information. (p. 65)

5. Define *mechanism of injury* and relate types of accidents to types of injuries. (pp 66–67, 69)

6. Define *primary survey,* stating its purpose and indicating when it is done during the patient assessment. (p. 70)

7. Describe how to determine patient responsiveness and indicate how you can tell if a patient is alert and oriented. (p. 71)

8. Describe how to ensure an open airway and check a patient for adequate breathing. (p. 72)

9. Describe how to detect a carotid pulse. (pp. 72–73)

10. Define *secondary survey*, stating its purpose and when it is done during the patient assessment. (p. 75)

11. List the equipment an EMT should have to perform the secondary survey. (p. 75)

12. Define *subjective interview* and *objective examination*. (p. 75)

13. Define *symptom*, *sign*, and *vital sign*. (p. 82)

14. List the types of information that should be sought during your interviews of patients and bystanders. (pp. 79–82)

15. Describe the procedures used by an EMT in the gathering of vital signs. (pp. 84–90)

16. List, in the correct order, the steps of the head-to-toe survey. (pp. 91–105)

17. State the TEN examination rules you must consider when conducting the patient assessment. (pp. 105 and 107)

SKILLS   As an EMT, you must be able to:

1. Determine level of consciousness.
2. Ensure an open airway.

3. Take a carotid pulse, radial pulse, and distal lower extremity pulse (both dorsalis pedis and

posterior tibialis) and determine rate, rhythm, and character of a radial pulse.

4. Determine respiratory rate and character.
5. Measure blood pressure by auscultation and palpation.
6. Determine relative skin temperature.
7. Gather information and conduct a primary survey and a secondary survey at an emergency scene.

8. Record and communicate the information gained from the patient assessment.
9. Use the Glasgow Coma Scale (or other similar scales) if required in your EMS System.
10. Use a stethoscope to assess breathing sounds (if this is required in your EMS System).

NOTE: In this chapter you will be learning patient assessment, including the physical examination of patients. We have presented the assessment in detail. Read through the chapter once, then use the scan sheets and the summary to study each aspect of assessment. Once you can list all the steps, go back and reread the detailed description, adding the additional information to your basic list of procedures. After you are certain that you understand the various elements of patient assessment, begin to practice the skills required for all the procedures that are part of this assessment.

TERMS you may be using for the first time:

Airway – the pathway from nose and mouth that carries air to the gas exchange levels of the lungs.

Auscultation (os-skul-TAY-shun) – the process of listening to sounds that occur within the body. An example is the procedure that uses a blood pressure cuff and a stethoscope to determine blood pressure. This method requires you to listen for certain sounds and changes in sound that correspond to systolic and diastolic blood pressures.

Brachial (BRAY-key-al) **Artery** – the major artery supplying blood to the arm.

Carotid (kah-ROT-id) **Pulse** – the pulse that can be felt on each side of the patient's neck, over top of the carotid arteries.

Cerebrospinal (ser-e-bro-SPI-nal) **Fluid** – the clear, watery fluid that surrounds and protects the brain and spinal cord.

Cervical (SER-ve-kal) – in reference to the neck. The cervical spine is that portion of the spine that passes through the neck.

Clavicle (KLAV-i-kal) – collarbone.

Diastolic (di-as-TOL-ik) **Blood Pressure** – the pressure in the arteries when the lower left chamber of the heart (left ventricle) is refilling.

Mechanisms of Injury – what forces caused the injury, allowing you to relate types of accidents to certain types of injuries. You must consider the kind of force, its intensity and direction, and the area of the body that is affected.

Objective Examination – a part of the secondary survey. This is a hands-on survey of the patient in which you determine vital signs and perform a head-to-toe examination.

Palpate, Palpation – to feel any part of the body, as to palpate the radial pulse; also, to use the blood pressure cuff and the feeling of the radial pulse to determine approximate patient systolic blood pressure.

Patient Assessment – the systematic gathering of information in order to determine the nature of a patient's illness or injury.

Pedal (PEED-al) **Pulse** – a foot pulse. There are two locations used in field emergency care: the dorsalis pedis and the posterior tibial.

Primary Survey – a patient assessment process carried out to detect life-threatening problems. Basic life support is provided as needed during the primary survey.

Radial Pulse – a pulse found in the lateral wrist.

Secondary Survey – a patient assessment process that includes the subjective interview, the head-to-toe survey of the patient, and the taking of vital signs.

Sign – what you see, hear, feel, and smell in relation to a patient's problem.

Sphygmomanometer (SFIG-mo-mah-NOM-e-ter) – the cuff and gauge used in blood pressure determination.

Sternum (STER-num) – breastbone.

Stoma (STO-mah) – a permanent opening surgically made in the body. A "neck breather" breathes through a stoma in the anterior neck.

Subjective Interview – a part of the secondary survey that uses the patient and bystanders as sources of information by having them answer specific questions.

Symptom – what the patient tells you about his problem.

Systolic (sis-TOL-ik) **Blood Pressure** – the pressure created in the arteries when the lower left chamber of the heart (left ventricle) contracts and forces blood out into circulation.

Trauma – a physical injury caused by an external force (e.g., a fracture) or a medical problem (e.g., heart tissue that has been damaged by a heart attack). The term also may be applied to the emotional stress suffered by a specific event.

Vital Signs – the patient's pulse rate, rhythm and character, respiratory rate and character, blood pressure, and temperature. Some approaches consider level of consciousness and appearance of the pupils of the eyes to be part of the vital signs.

Tracheostomy (TRA-ke-OS-to-me) – a surgical opening made through the anterior neck entering into the windpipe (trachea).

OBTAINING INFORMATION

Patient Assessment

Patient assessment is the gathering of the information needed to help determine what is wrong with the patient. During this process, the first concern is to identify and correct any life-threatening problems. Always keep this in mind. It is foolish to be gathering information from bystanders while the patient is in cardiac arrest (his heart has stopped beating) or has some other life-threatening problem.

The patient assessment is a *systematic* procedure, but it is not always done in the same step-by-step order. Different types of patients will require different types of assessment. A patient who has been injured in an accident will need to be assessed differently than one who is having breathing problems related to a known illness. A serious injury to a patient's chest may require care that cannot wait until a complete survey is performed.

As an EMT, you will have to assess:

- Medical Patients—those who have problems related to infections, the failure of a body organ or system, a psychological problem, certain environmental factors (e.g., excessive cold), drugs or other chemical substances, or childbirth.
- Trauma Patients—those who have suffered trauma, that is, they have been injured or have a problem that has developed as a result of injury.*

* The word *trauma* is often used in prehospital emergency care to refer to injury brought about by an accident or act of aggression. Note that the word also may be used to refer to psychological injury or the injury to tissues brought about by disease (e.g., traumatized heart muscle).

You *must* always do as complete a survey as possible. Medical patients who are clearly free of injury can be assessed to obtain information relating directly to their medical problem. However, some medical patients suffer falls or other types of accidents and will require assessments that consider possible injury. Trauma patients will need to be assessed so that you may determine the nature and extent of their injuries and, when possible, any medical problems. This is done because trauma patients may have preexisting medical problems that need attention, may have caused an accident to take place because of medical problems, or may have medical problems surface because of an accident (e.g., a heart attack).

A patient's condition must be considered as a *dynamic process*. Basically, something may change, requiring you to stop in the middle of an assessment and repeat a procedure you completed only seconds after you arrived. Also, the gathering of information does not end after the initial assessment. You will have to keep reassessing the patient, gathering new information. This is called *monitoring* the patient.

No matter where you are in the information gathering process, you must remember:

- Your First Concern is to identify and attempt to correct life-threatening problems.
- Your Second Concern is to identify any injuries or medical problems and to provide basic EMT-level care in an effort to stabilize the patient and, when possible, to reduce the severity of his problem.

> • Your Third Concern is to try to keep the patient stable and continue reassessing the patient in case his condition worsens or improves.

Throughout the entire process of patient assessment, your goal is to **DO NO HARM,** protecting the patient from additional injury and stress as you gather the information needed to allow for proper and efficient care.

Problems with Assessment

As an EMT, you may face all the problems that interfere with patient assessment. You will have to overcome other problems that may be unique to the emergency scene. Problems with assessment can include:

- Dangerous scenes (e.g., fires, collapsing buildings, hazardous materials)
- Harsh environments (including unfavorable weather conditions)
- Unfavorable conditions (e.g., too much noise, darkness, no privacy for the patient)
- Unfavorable location (e.g., the bottom of a hill, around a blind curve, in water)
- Uncooperative bystanders and motorists
- Uncooperative patients
- Special patients (children, elderly, blind, deaf, non-English speaking, chronically ill, handicapped, and those affected by drugs, including alcohol)
- More than one patient
- Severe injury (especially spinal or head injury)
- Patients with more than one serious injury (multitrauma)
- Grotesque injuries that tax your emotional stability

Each of these problems will be considered at various points throughout this text. Many are covered in Chapters 19, 20, 22, and 27. For now, we will skip the special problems at the scene of an accident or medical emergency, focusing attention instead on the actual processes used in patient assessment. As part of your complete training you will study traffic, crowd control, fire, toxic gases, possible falling objects, and other dangers and problems at the scene. Some special problems (e.g., spinal injury) will be mentioned in this chapter, but we will delay in-depth studies of these problems until later.

Assessment and care are meant to be done without risk to the rescuer. Keep in mind that direct contact with the patient's blood and body fluids may expose you to a dangerous infectious disease. Make certain that you wear the assigned protective equipment needed for assessment and care of trauma patients and some medical patients. The minimum is the wearing of latex gloves. Eye protection (goggles or faceshield), gowns, and masks should be worn as needed. Follow all local protocols.

Arrival at the Scene

Again, let us assume that the only problems at the scene will be injuries or medical emergencies. If you receive your calls from an efficient dispatching center, you may learn something of a person's illness or injury before leaving quarters. Even though this information may later prove to be erroneous, you can at least be thinking of what equipment you will have to remove from the ambulance and what special procedures may be required immediately on arrival.

When you arrive at the scene, stay alert and begin to gather information. Do not allow the dispatcher's report or information given to you by untrained bystanders to be the basis of a quick conclusion. You will have to consider many factors before you will know what is wrong with a patient and what course of action you will take in order to provide emergency care.

On arrival, you must:

> 1. State your name (and rank or classification and the organization you represent).
> 2. Identify yourself as an Emergency Medical Technician (not everyone knows what "EMT" means).
> 3. Ask the patient if you may help.

While doing the above, remember to be looking for any obvious life-threatening problems.

Identifying yourself is very important, even if you believe the patient is unconscious. If you are in uniform, most patients and bystanders will respond to the uniform and let you take charge. When out of uniform, identifying yourself may be the only way you will be allowed to provide care. State your name and the name of your organization, and then the following: "I am an Emergency Medical Technician. I have been trained to provide emergency care." Even if you believe the patient to be unconscious, your next statement should be, "May I help you?" Keep in mind that some patients who appear to be unconscious may respond to your voice. Many patients maintain a functional sense of hearing, even when near death.

Surprisingly, some patients will say "no" to your offer of help. Usually, their fear is so great that they are confused. Simple conversation works best in gaining confidence. Even if the patient says "no" to your offer of help, continue to talk to him quietly, offering reassurance. His first refusal may be due to an initial lack of trust, denial that anything is wrong, confusion, or fear. In the vast majority of cases, the patient will allow you to help.

Quick Sources of Information

In a few seconds, you can gain valuable information as to what may be wrong with a patient. Now is not the time to ask a lot of questions or to look over the entire scene trying to detect all possible causes of injury. Instead, you must observe and listen as you quickly, but safely, reach the patient as soon as possible. *You must not delay the detection of life-threatening problems.* At this time in the assessment, clues to the patient's problem must be obvious or quickly provided to you by others. Some immediate sources of information may come from the following:

- The Scene—Is it safe or hazardous? Does the patient have to be moved? Are conditions harsh?
- The Patient—Is he alert, trying to tell you something or pointing to a part of his body?
- Bystanders—Are they trying to tell you something? Listen, they might be saying, "He's had a bad heart for years," "He was having chest pains before he fell," "He fell off that ladder."
- Mechanisms of Injury—Has something fallen on the patient? Is this a burn injury? Has the patient been thrown against the steering column? Is the steering wheel bent, the dashboard dented, or the windshield broken?
- Deformities or Injuries—Does the patient's body appear to be lying in a strange position? Is there blood around the patient? Are there burns, crushed limbs, or any other obvious wounds?
- Signs—What do you quickly see, hear, or smell when approaching the patient? Is there blood around the patient? Has he vomited? Is the patient having convulsions? Is there obvious pain?

You must be highly observant as you approach the patient. What you see before touching the patient may indicate that there are life-threatening problems or that the patient's condition will probably

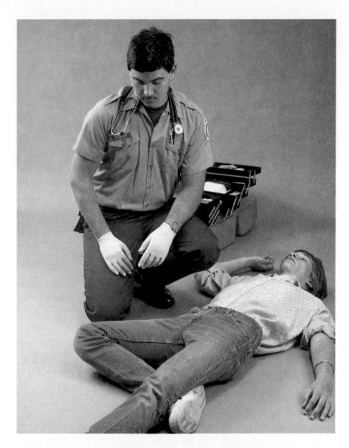

FIGURE 3–1. **Obvious deformities and injuries may provide clues as to the extent of a patient's problem.**

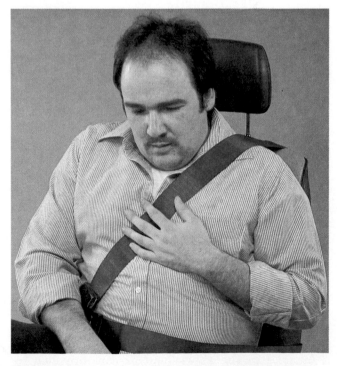

FIGURE 3–2. **Begin to gather information when you first observe the patient.**

worsen rapidly. At the scene of a motor vehicle accident, these observations are part of what is sometimes called the "windshield survey," that is, what you see walking up to and looking in the vehicle. These early observations can be critical factors in how soon you can initiate care.

First Responders

There will be times when the first person on the scene is someone with formal training in first aid, basic life support, or elementary emergency care. This person may be a police officer, a firefighter, or an industrial health officer. In some cases, this person may have advanced training, such as nursing. These individuals have traditionally been called first responders.

As an EMT, you will interact with first responders who have had American Red Cross training, American Heart Association basic cardiac life support training, or special industrial first responder training. Today, many police officers, firefighters, and industrial health personnel are trained to Department of Transportation guidelines and are certified First Responders. As a member of the EMS System, you should respect the work done by all of these individuals as they attempt to help the patient and you at the emergency scene.

First responders can provide valuable information about how the emergency came about, how the patient was acting when they arrived, what they found to be wrong with the patient, and what care procedures have been started. True, you will still have to do a patient assessment and you must evaluate the care already provided, but you should appreciate what the first responders have done before you arrived. Their assessment and care may often make a difference, improving or stabilizing the patient's condition. The information they give you, along with your own assessment may alert you to the fact that the patient is improving or deteriorating.

When you arrive at an emergency scene and find first responders providing care for a patient, tactfully assume responsibility for the patient. Remember to thank the first responders and to give them credit for any prompt and efficient care they provided for the patient. Allow first responders to help when you need assistance.

Most emergency scenes will not provide you with the time or privacy necessary to give on-the-scene training to the first responders. When practical, point out any errors made by first responders, but do so tactfully and in private. Should you notice a mistake in the assessment or care provided by the first responders, and they are members of the police department, fire department, or industrial

squads, alert the appropriate training officer as soon after the run as possible. Do not act as though the training officer is at fault or the first responders lacked ability. Be a professional helping another professional to improve the quality of care.

Mechanisms of Injury

What caused the injury? If you know this, you can suspect certain types of injuries and be able to decide the possible extent of them. The **mechanism of injury** is the force that caused the injury and how it was applied to the body (e.g., a direct blow to the head caused by a heavy falling object). Knowing this helps direct you to look for certain types of injuries. Certain injuries must be considered "common" to particular accident situations. Fractured bones are usually associated with falls and motor vehicle accidents; burns are common to fires and explosions; soft tissue injuries can be associated with gunshot wounds, and so on.

Knowing the mechanism of injury allows you to assume that a particular injury has occurred simply because it is often associated with the forces generated and the way they are applied to the body.

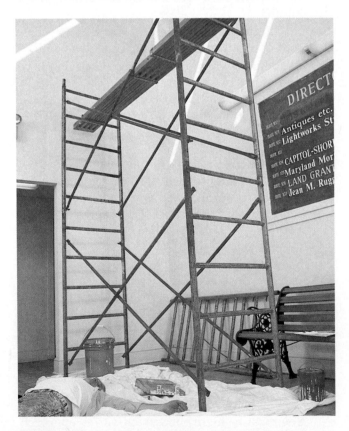

FIGURE 3–3. **Mechanisms of injury may provide valuable clues to the nature of a patient's injury.**

For example, if an automobile traveling at 30 miles per hour hits a utility pole and the driver's head strikes the windshield, the head injury may be obvious. However, even though possible spinal injury may not be apparent, the forces produced during this type of injury are usually enough to cause some kind of damage to the spine. In such a case, you must assume there is spinal injury.

There are many ways in which injuries can be classified into different categories. One system

Table 3–1. EXAMPLES OF MECHANISM OF INJURIES—FRACTURES

Upper Extremities		Lower Extremities	
Structure	*Mechanism*	*Structure*	*Mechanism*
SHOULDER		PELVIS	Fall (landing on the buttocks), fall (more common with elderly), forceful direct blow, crush injury, strenuous activity (young patients)
• Clavicle (collarbone)	Fall on lateral shoulder direct blow, blow to upper back and posterior shoulder, downward blow striking the bone		
• Scapula (shoulder blade)	Direct blow, severe downward blow to the shoulder (e.g., falling objects), fall on the lateral shoulder	HIP	Direct blow to knees (e.g., striking dashboard), direct blow (e.g., vehicle strikes pedestrian's hip), posterior dislocation
• Proximal humerus (arm bone near shoulder)	Direct blow to the lateral arm (falls or striking vehicle compartment wall in crash)	FEMUR (thigh bone)	
		• Femoral head	Direct blow, anterior dislocation
HUMERUS (arm bone)— shaft	Direct blow from striking an object (motor vehicle accidents), direct blow from a fall, fall on the elbow, fall on the hand of an outstretched arm	• Proximal shaft	Fall on hip, fall on hip with twisting forces
		• Shaft	Severe blow to thigh, severe blow to knees
ELBOW		KNEE	
• Distal humerus	Direct blow to flexed elbow, indirect force of landing on outstretched arm, forceful hyperextension of elbow	• Distal femur	Direct blow (usually motor vehicle accidents or falls), hyperextension or severe twist of the knee
• Proximal forearm bones	Direct blow to elbow, indirect force from fall on outstretched arm, elbow dislocation	• Proximal leg (lower leg bones)	Direct force from a fall, transfer of force from falling and landing on the feet, object strikes leg (e.g., vehicle strikes pedestrian)
FOREARM BONES		• Patella (kneecap)	Direct blow (e.g., falls, knee strikes dashboard), severe muscle contractions (e.g., from the force of a fall)
• Shaft	Direct blow (often to forearm while raised to protect face), compression occurring from a fall (usually to children)		
		LEG (lower leg bones)	Direct blow, twisting forces, blow to the side of the knee
• Distal forearm	Fall on hand, forced flexion or extension of hand	ANKLE	Twisting forces, crush injury, falls (landing on the feet)
WRIST	Forced flexion or hyperextension, direct blow, indirect force from falling on an outstretched hand, crush injury, force of thumb being driven back into its joint with the wrist	FOOT	Heel strikes ground during fall, forced extreme flexion or hyperextension of foot, severe ankle twist, direct blow to the toes (falling objects or kicking an object)
HAND	Direct blows (falls), objects striking the distal fingers, falling objects striking the hand, forced flexion or hyperextension of fingers, twisting force to the fingers, impact to the fist		

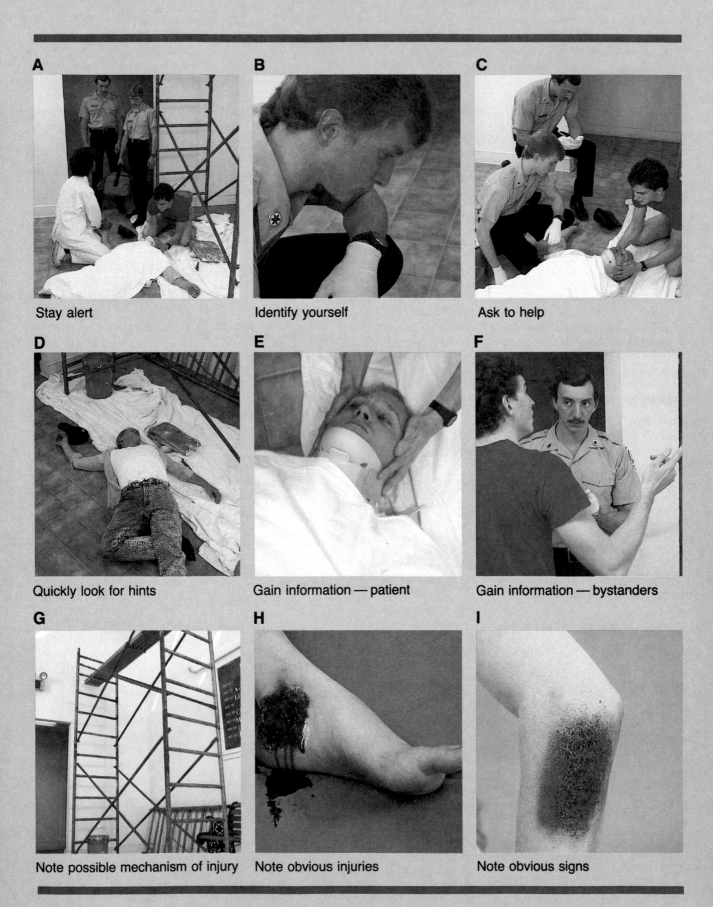

A Stay alert

B Identify yourself

C Ask to help

D Quickly look for hints

E Gain information — patient

F Gain information — bystanders

G Note possible mechanism of injury

H Note obvious injuries

I Note obvious signs

considers the type of tissue or structure injured, as in soft tissue injuries, fractures, dislocations, and internal organ injuries. Another system uses the force causing the damage, such as blunt trauma, penetrating trauma, deceleration injury, and thermal injury. The accidents that produce these injuries can also be categorized. According to the National Safety Council, people usually are injured in:

- Motor vehicle accidents
- Falls
- Fires and explosions
- Assaults (e.g., beatings, knife wounds, gunshot wounds)
- Swimming and boating accidents
- Firearms accidents
- Poisonings by solids, liquids, and gases
- Machinery accidents
- Accidents involving electricity (including lightning)

If you study the types of accidents, forces produced and applied, types of injuries produced, and tissues involved, you will be able to predict certain types of injury associated with given types of accidents.

Such an approach can be helpful if your study considers more than the most commonly occurring injury. Otherwise, you may develop "tunnel vision." Do not become so busy looking for the one thing in common to an accident that you forget to consider all of the major possibilities. Instead, learn that a variety of injuries can be produced in any accident situation. For example, a patient who was in a fire may have burns, but he may also have lung damage from smoke and hot gases. Perhaps he fell trying to escape and fractured his leg. Appreciate what an accident can do to the human body, then you will not be easily led into missing an obvious injury or overlooking other injuries.

Knowing the mechanism of injury is very important when dealing with motor vehicle accidents. A collapsed or bent steering column suggests that the driver has suffered a chest wall injury, with possible lung damage and perhaps damage to the heart and its great blood vessels. A bent steering wheel tells of the possibility of fractured ribs. A shattered, blood-spattered windshield may point to the likelihood of a forehead or scalp laceration (cut) and possibly a severe blow to the head that may have caused brain damage and spinal injury.

REMEMBER: For every obvious injury, there may be a number of hidden ones. Knowing what an accident can do and being able to recognize the mecha-

nisms of injury are important to the patient assessment procedure.

THE FIELD ASSESSMENT

The quick sources of information stated earlier provide you with a starting point to begin your field assessment of the patient. This assessment must:

- Be appropriate for both medical and trauma emergencies.
- Allow for the quick detection of life-threatening problems.
- Enable you to detect problems that are not immediately life-threatening but may be if they are allowed to remain uncorrected.
- Detect non-life-threatening problems that should receive care.
- Be organized to allow for effective communications with the emergency department.
- Include questioning of the conscious patient as well as a hands-on physical examination.
- Take only a few minutes to complete carefully.

The field assessment will call on you to evaluate and use the information you have gained from the dispatcher, observations of the scene, interviews with the patient and bystanders, and the physical examination of the patient.

As noted earlier, not every person requiring emergency care will have to be surveyed to the same depth. Some examples of assessment approaches are shown in Table 3–2. Every unconscious patient should be thoroughly examined, regardless of whether the emergency is due to illness or injury. Of course, if a life-threatening problem is found, it is to be cared for immediately. *Never* delay basic life support in order to conduct a complete hands-on examination.

The field assessment detects problems and helps to establish a priority of care. This priority changes somewhat depending on the stability of the patient, what other injuries are present, how many patients and rescuers there are, how long it will take to transport the patient, and factors that may be unique to a particular emergency. Each EMS System has established a definite order of care, stating what you should do first for any particular patient. There is also an order of care for situations having more than one patient. In Chapter 20, we will recon-

Table 3-2. **EXAMPLES OF APPROACHES TO PATIENT ASSESSMENT**

Medical Problem (No Injuries)

Conscious Patient	Unconscious Patient
• Begin an interview, continuing to maintain verbal contact through the rest of assessment and care. Assess airway and if breathing is adequate during interview.	• Make certain that the patient has an open airway, adequate breathing, and a carotid pulse. Look for and control profuse bleeding. Care for any life-threatening problems as they are detected.
• Determine vital signs (pulse, respirations, blood pressure, and relative skin temperature) and continue to determine level of consciousness.	• Determine vital signs.
• Examine the patient as required, directed by the information obtained during the interview.	• Examine the patient, but at the same time
	• Begin to formally interview bystanders.

Trauma

Conscious Patient	Unconscious Patient
• Look for mechanism of injury	• Look for mechanism of injury
• Begin to interview the patient and check for adequate breathing and profuse bleeding. Stop the interview and care for any life-threatening problems as they are found.	• Assess the patient for airway, adequate breathing, carotid pulse, and profuse bleeding. Correct any life-threatening problems as they are found.
• Determine vital signs if the patient appears to be unstable.	• Take vital signs.
• Do a complete examination of the patient.	• Conduct a complete examination of the patient, but at the same time
• Determine the patient's vital signs.	• Begin to formally interview bystanders.
	• Determine the patient's vital signs.

sider patient assessment and the order of care if there is more than one patient.

An example of an order of care is provided in Table 3-3. As you learn about a specific type of injury or illness, check to see where the care fits into this list. Modify the list as necessary to comply with your EMS System's order of care. Do not try to memorize this table. If you keep track of each procedure, you will have the order memorized by the end of your course.

The field examination consists of the primary and secondary survey.

REMEMBER: Learning the steps of the field examination is a simple matter, but you must know more than how to conduct a primary and secondary survey. Unless you understand the significance of the information gathered during a patient assessment, you may not be able to provide the proper care for the patient.

The Primary Survey

The **primary survey** is a process carried out to detect life-threatening problems. As these problems are detected, lifesaving measures are taken. Many conditions can become life threatening if they remain uncorrected; however, certain problems require immediate attention. An obstructed airway may quickly lead to respiratory arrest. Cardiac arrest will occur shortly after respiratory arrest. If a patient's heart is not beating, irreversible changes will begin to occur in the brain in 4 to 6 minutes. Brain cell death will usually begin within 10 minutes of cardiac arrest. Profuse bleeding is another problem requiring immediate attention. Such bleeding will quickly produce severe shock, leading to death within a few minutes.

Conducting the primary survey does not require any special instruments or equipment. During this survey, you are concerned with the ABCs of emergency care:

> • **A = Airway:** You must assess responsiveness, and open the airway.
> • **B = Breathing:** Assess breathing. When necessary, you must provide rescue breathing (pulmonary resuscitation).
> • **C = Circulation:** Assess circulation. When necessary, you must provide cardiopulmonary resuscitation (CPR).

NOTE: Your course and local requirements may state that you should check the patient's pupils and look for medical identification devices during the primary survey. Your instructor is the authority on such matters. It is understood, however, that you are not to delay lifesaving care.

As an EMT, the primary survey procedures you should follow are:

Table 3–3. PRIORITY OF CARE EXAMPLE—ONE PATIENT INCIDENT

The following example is meant to serve as a guide as you learn your EMS System's order of care. Note that some of these problems overlap and that care for one often provides partial care for another. Note, too, that the care for *shock* is a part of the required treatment for most illness and injury.

1. Determine responsiveness (LOC)*
2. Maintain an open airway, protecting spine.
3. Make certain the patient is breathing or receiving rescue breathing (artificial ventilations).
4. Make certain there is circulation or CPR is provided.
5. Control severe, life-threatening bleeding.
6. Treat chest wounds that have opened the thoracic cavity and flail chest that compromises breathing.
7. Provide care for severe to moderate breathing distress.
8. Care for spinal injuries (cervical collar, etc).
9. Treat severe, life-threatening shock.
10. Treat possible heart attack (patient unstable).
11. Determine severe head injuries and expedite transport.
12. Care for severe injuries of the chest, abdomen, and pelvis.
13. Treat severe medical problems or drug overdose.
14. Provide care for severe burns.
15. Control moderate bleeding.
16. Care for moderate medical problems.
17. Splint fractures.
18. Care for minor burns.
19. Care for minor cuts and bruises.

* LOC, level of consciousness.

1. Check for RESPONSIVENESS (LOC). A conscious patient indicates breathing and circulation. Breathing may not be adequate and you may have to clear the airway, but the patient is breathing. Keep in mind that consciousness may be lost quickly, breathing may change, and circulation may stop. To check for responsiveness, *gently* tap the patient's shoulder and say: "Are you okay?"

2. Reposition the patient if necessary. You will find it difficult to determine if an unconscious patient in the prone position has an open airway and adequate breathing. Even though you have not surveyed the patient for possible spinal and other serious injuries, you will have to place him in a supine position (Figure 3–5; see also Chapter 4). If the patient is not breathing, or you cannot tell if he is breathing, use a simple **log-roll maneuver** to move the patient from a prone to a supine position. Kneel at his side, leaving enough room so that the patient will not roll

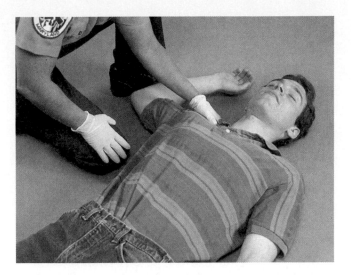

FIGURE 3–4. Establish unresponsiveness.

into your lap. Gently straighten his legs and position the arm that is closest to you above his head. Place one of your hands so that it cradles the head and neck from behind. Place your other hand under the patient's distant shoulder, at the armpit. Move the patient as a unit onto his side and then onto his back. You must move his head, neck, and torso as a unit to reduce the chances of aggravation to spinal injuries.

NOTE: This log roll is best done by two or more rescuers. One rescuer must be responsible for stabilizing the head and neck. This person directs the actual repositioning of the patient. The one-rescuer log roll is to be used only when basic life support may be needed and adequate personnel are not immediately on hand to assist.

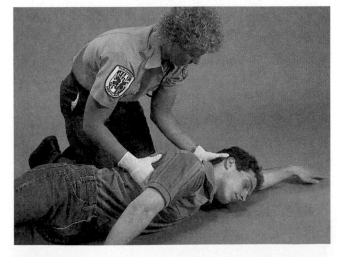

FIGURE 3–5. Placing a patient in the supine position.

3. If the patient is unresponsive, always ensure an open airway (Figure 3–6) and determine if there is adequate breathing.

• Open Airway—For cases in which you do not suspect spinal injury, position yourself at the patient's side. Perform a **head-tilt, chin-lift maneuver** (see Ch. 4). Use the fingers of your hand that is closest to the patient's chest to support the lower jaw. Place these fingers under the jaw at the chin. Your fingers should rest on the bony part of the jaw, avoiding the soft tissue that is found under the chin. Lift to move the jaw forward.

   For patients with possible spinal injury, you should use the **jaw-thrust** (see Ch. 4). Manage all unconscious trauma patients as if they have spinal injuries.

• Adequate Breathing—You must check to ensure that there is sufficient air exchange. Position the side of your head close to the patient's face, then Look, Listen, and Feel (Figure 3–7).

   LOOK—for chest movements that are associated with breathing. (**NOTE**: Males often show the most pronounced respiratory movement at the level of the dia-

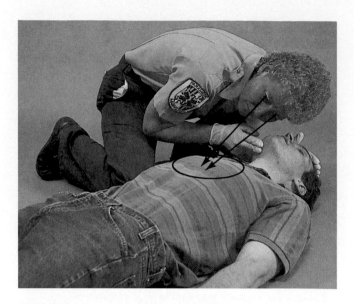

FIGURE 3–7. **LOOK, LISTEN, and FEEL for adequate breathing.**

phragm; females tend to show more pronounced movement at the clavicles.)

   LISTEN—for air moving at the patient's mouth and nose.

   FEEL—for air being expired through the patient's nose and mouth.

   Take 5 seconds to establish breathlessness.

   If the patient is not breathing, or if there is an airway obstruction, YOU MUST TAKE IMMEDIATE ACTION. Also, some patients with very erratic chest movements may not be exchanging air and may develop cardiac arrest. The procedures to follow are covered in Chapter 4. If the patient is breathing adequately through an open airway, continue the primary survey.

4. Check for CIRCULATION. If the patient has been in respiratory arrest for a few minutes, he may have developed cardiac arrest as well. Determine if there is heart action and blood circulation by palpating (feeling for) a **carotid** (kah-ROT-id) **pulse** (Figure 3–8).

   While stabilizing the patient's head and maintaining the proper head-tilt by keeping one hand on the patient's forehead, use your hand that is closest to the patient's neck to locate his "Adam's apple" (the most prominent part of the thyroid cartilage). Place the tips of your index and middle fingers directly over the midline of this structure. (Do not use your thumb. It has a pulse that you may feel instead of the patient's carotid pulse.) Slide your fingertips to the side of the pa-

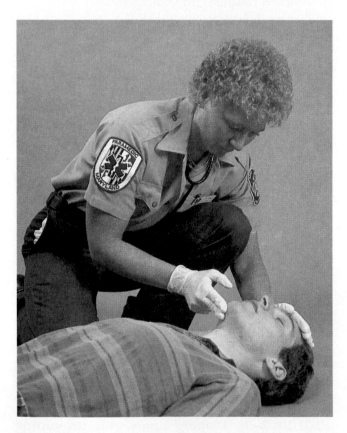

FIGURE 3–6. **Ensure an open airway.**

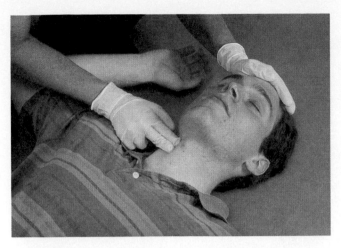

FIGURE 3–8. A quick check of the carotid pulse confirms circulation.

tient's neck closest to you. Keep the palm side of your fingertips against the patient's neck. *Do not* slide your fingertips to the opposite side of the patient's neck.* Feel for a groove between the Adam's apple (larynx) and the muscles located along the side of the neck.

Very little pressure need be applied to the neck to feel the carotid pulse. Precise pulse rate is not important; however, you should note the strength and regularity of the pulse. You should take no less than 5 and no more than 10 seconds to establish pulselessness.†

If there is no carotid pulse, basic life support measures in the form of **cardiopulmonary resuscitation** (KAR-de-o-PUL-mo-ner-e re-SUS-ci-TA-shun) or CPR will have to be initiated (see Chapter 5). If there is a pulse, but no breathing, continue your efforts at artificial ventilation with periodic checking for a carotid pulse. If the patient is breathing and has a carotid pulse, then continue with the primary survey.

5. Check for PROFUSE BLEEDING. Only *profuse* bleeding is considered during the primary survey. Look and feel for this bleeding,

---

* To do so may place your fingers on the patient's windpipe, reducing your ability to palpate the pulse and possibly causing you to apply incorrect pressure that may interfere with the patient's airway or reduce the proper head-tilt. Also, this will keep you from having your thumb on one side of the neck and your fingers on the other side. You should never try to feel for a pulse on both sides of the neck at the same time. To do so may cause you to interrupt circulation to the brain.

† Up to 1 minute is recommended for cases of hypothermia (see Chapter 18).

but do so with extreme care. Keep in mind that the patient may have spinal injuries and other serious injuries requiring him to be kept still.

Bleeding wounds are not always as severe as they may first appear, so be certain that you are dealing with bleeding that requires immediate action. Look for wounds from which blood is *spurting* or *flowing freely*. Methods to control such bleeding will be covered in Chapter 7.

On completing the primary survey, having ensured that the patient has an open airway, adequate breathing, a carotid pulse and that any profuse bleeding is controlled, you should proceed to the next phase of patient assessment.

Special Considerations

There are special cases in which you find a patient who has been bleeding slowly for a long period of time, having lost a significant amount of blood. Such cases may require you to consider any additional bleeding as life threatening. Taking care not to aggravate spinal and other serious injuries, control bleeding and begin to treat for shock immediately following the primary survey.

In situations in which you immediately notice profuse bleeding, you may have to begin to control it while, at the same time, you begin to check for respiration. Keep in mind that severe bleeding, with blood spurting from a wound, indicates some heart action (circulation). Remember, even though bleeding is occurring, assessment of respiration cannot be ignored.

During the primary survey, if you notice breath-

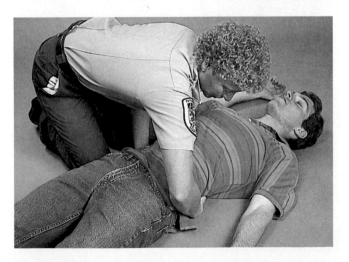

FIGURE 3–9. Locate and control all profuse bleeding.

1

Responsiveness

2

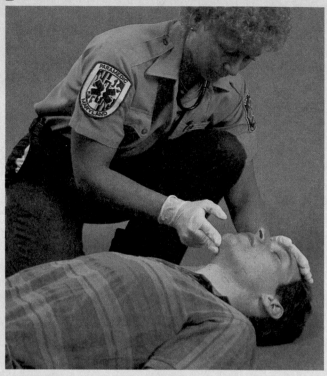

Open Airway

3

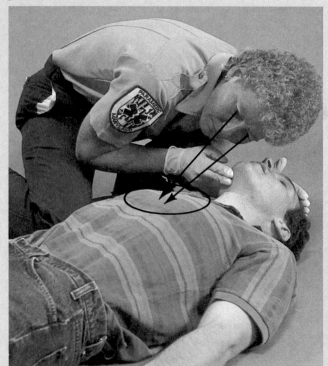

Breathing

4

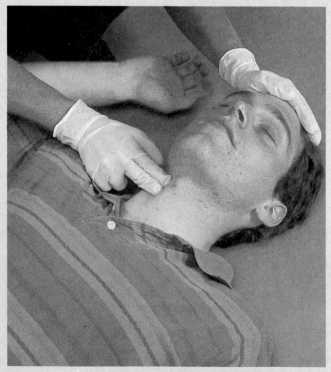

Circulation: Pulse, Profuse Bleeding

ing problems, you should quickly check to see if the patient has a chest wound that has opened the thoracic cavity. This type of injury will need immediate care (see p. 352). The same holds true if you notice a section of ribs or the sternum has broken free from the rib cage.

If the patient shows indications of severe shock or is likely to develop shock, you should carefully begin your care for shock before moving on to the next step of the assessment (see p. 205). Remember that the best treatment for shock is prevention.

> It is very important to protect the patient's spine throughout the patient assessment. In cases in which the trauma patient is unconscious, or the mechanism of injury indicates possible spinal injury, you should stabilize the head and neck before moving to the next step in the assessment.

When you have determined if the patient was responsive, you have completed the first step in assessing the patient's level of consciousness. Completion of this process flows into the next steps of the patient assessment.

The Secondary Survey

The objective of the secondary survey is to discover medical and injury-related problems that do not pose an immediate threat to survival but may do so if allowed to go untreated. There are two parts to the secondary survey: the subjective interview and the objective examination. NOTE: If the patient has a life-threatening illness or injury, it may not be possible to complete the secondary survey before starting to transport the patient.

The **subjective interview** is not unlike that conducted by a physician prior to a complete physical examination. During the interview, whenever possible use the patient as a source of information. Relatives and bystanders also may serve as sources of information; however, do not interrupt interviewing the patient to gather information from a bystander.

The **objective examination** is a comprehensive hands-on, head-to-toe survey of the patient, during which you check the patient's body for less than obvious injuries or the effects of illness. The findings from the interview and the examination are combined and related to allow you to make an assessment of your patient's condition and form a plan of emergency care.

You must be realistic when conducting a secondary survey. If you are too systematic, you may find yourself asking the patient a lot of questions while he becomes upset simply because he wants you to look at his leg. In such cases, you may find yourself doing two things at once during the survey. Your activities must fit the situation.

Keep in mind that you will have to reconsider and reevaluate some of the things you did on arrival at the scene. Since the primary survey has to begin as soon as possible, you may have missed something or something may have changed. Before starting the secondary survey, always:

- Look over the scene—Is it still safe? Did you overlook a mechanism of injury? Are there any other patients in need of attention?
- Look over your patient—Are there obvious injuries or indications of illness? Is his condition deteriorating? Is the patient wearing a medical identification necklace or bracelet you can read without moving him?

Examination Equipment

Unlike the primary survey, which required no special equipment or instruments, the secondary survey requires some basic items:

- A **sphygmomanometer** (SFIG-mo-mah-NOM-e-ter), commonly called a blood pressure cuff—used to measure and monitor blood pressure.
- A stethoscope—used in conjunction with a blood pressure cuff in the determination of blood pressure. A stethoscope can also be used for listening to the sounds of air entering and leaving the lungs.
- A penlight—used for examining the patient's mouth, nose, ears, and pupils. It is also useful in poorly lighted situations.
- Heavy-duty bandage scissors—to cut away clothing and footwear that may obscure an injury site or prevent access to a pulse or blood pressure site.
- A pocket notebook and a pen, clipboard and paper, and patient survey form—to record the results of the survey and to list actions taken.
- A watch with either a sweep second hand or digital seconds counter—to measure pulse and respiration rates.
- Protective equipment—latex gloves, goggles, face mask, devices for artificial respirations.

Several examination instruments can be carried in a belt holster.

The Survey Form

A standard survey form provides a quick, positive means of recording information obtained during the interview and examination. In your system, this may be an individual form or it may be part of a prehospital care report (trip sheet). This form may become a legal document and made part of the patient's medical records. If practical to do so, findings should be recorded as they are found. The survey procedure can be speeded up if one EMT conducts the survey while another records the findings.

Many EMS Systems are now including a trauma score that includes a coma scale as part of the survey form. An example of one such form in common use is shown in Figure 3–12. Table 3–4 shows the coded values for the revised trauma score that is used in some EMS Systems. More will be said about using the coma scale in Chapter 11.

Table 3–4. REVISED TRAUMA SCORE BREAKPOINTS. (> means greater than)

Glasgow Coma Scale	Systolic Blood Pressure	Respiratory Rate	Coded Value
13–15	>89	10–29	4
9–12	76–89	>29	3
6–8	50–75	6–9	2
4–5	1–49	1–5	1
3	0	0	0

The Subjective Interview

Time is to be used wisely at the emergency scene. As you become an experienced EMT, you will find that it is possible to begin the physical examination of a patient while you are conducting the subjective interview.

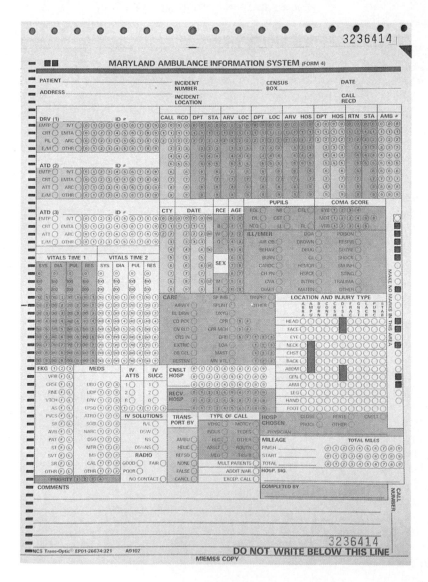

FIGURE 3–10. A typical survey form.

The subjective interview is a conversational, information-gathering effort (Figure 3–11). When a patient is unconscious, you may gain some of this same type of information from bystanders and medical identification devices while the physical examination is taking place. With a conscious patient, you should conduct an interview. Not only will you gain needed information, but you will also reduce the patient's fear and promote cooperation.

When conducting a patient interview, you should:

1. *Position yourself close to the patient.* Depending on the patient's situation, kneel or stand close to him. If possible, position yourself so that the sun or bright lights are not at your back. When practical, allow the patient to see your face.

2. *Identify yourself and reassure the patient.* It is important that the patient know he is in competent hands. Maintain eye contact with the patient and state your name, that you are an Emergency Medical Technician, and the organization you represent.

   Speak in your normal voice. If you ask a question, wait for a reply. Remember, at first the patient may not want you to help. Work to gain his confidence through calm conversation. Avoid inappropriate remarks like "Don't worry," and "Everything is all right."

   If you believe it to be appropriate, gently touch the patient's shoulder or rest your hand over his. A simple touch is comforting to most people. Keep in mind that a sign of caring for the sick and injured is to place

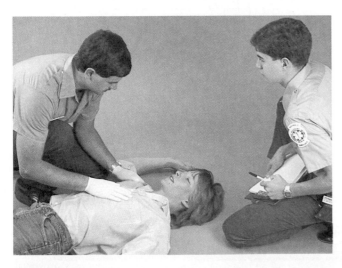

FIGURE 3–11. A carefully conducted interview can be as important as the physical examination.

the back of your hand on a person's forehead. Not only will you help reassure the patient, but you will also gain some information about his skin temperature.

3. *Learn your patient's name.* Once you know it, use it in the rest of your conversations. Children will expect you to use their first names. For adults, use the appropriate "Mr.," "Mrs.," "Miss," or "Ms."

   You need the patient's name for completion of your evaluation forms and to give a personal touch that is often very reassuring to the patient. Having the patient's name could prove to be of great importance should he become unconscious and not be carrying any identification.

4. *Learn your patient's age.* This may not be required in your locality, but some areas need this for reports and transmissions to the medical facility. If you cannot judge your patient as to a general age (early adulthood, middle adulthood, late adulthood) always ask his age.

   Children expect to be asked their age. To do so will help keep a "normal" tone to the conversation. You should ask adolescents their age to be certain that you are dealing with a minor.

   It is a good idea at this time to ask minors how you can contact their parents. Sometimes, this question upsets children because it intensifies the fear they are having about being sick or hurt without their parents being there to help. Be prepared to offer comfort and assure the child that someone will contact the parents.

5. *Seek out what is wrong.* This is the patient's primary (chief) complaint. Be certain to record this complaint even if you suspect several more significant problems. Ask the patient what is wrong. If he tells you several things, ask what is bothering him the most. Find out if the patient is in pain and where he hurts. Unless the pain of one injury or medical problem masks that of another, or unless a spinal injury has interrupted nerve pathways, most injured people will be able to tell you of painful areas. A sick person will be able to tell you of pain or discomfort.

   When your patient has been injured in an accident, try to ask open-ended questions, that is, questions that do not limit the response because they are too specific. Start by asking if anything feels wrong. Then, if necessary, become more specific to direct the patient's responses. For example, if the pa-

THE CHAMPION SACCO TRAUMA SCORE

The Trauma Score is used to give each injured patient a numerical score that can be used to estimate the severity of injury. The patient is graded in terms of cardiopulmonary and neurologic functions. Each category receives a numerical score. A high number indicates normal function, while a low number signifies impaired function. The numbers are totaled to give a Trauma Score. The lowest possible score is 1 (severe impairment). The highest possible score is 16 (normal for all categories).

The use of the Trauma Score can help to determine the order of care and transport, the level of care required, and if transport to a special facility is needed.

Each patient should be scored during the initial assessment and each time that vital signs are taken.

The following is based on the Trauma Score developed by Champion and Sacco. For additional information, see: Champion HR, Sacco WJ, Carnazzo AJ, et al: Trauma Score. *Critical Care Medicine* 9 (9): 672-676, 1981. Note that variations of this procedure have been adopted by some EMS Systems.

WARNING: Follow local guidelines if you are allowed to apply painful stimuli to a patient. Your local protocol should include what actions you may take when the mechanism of injury or state of consciousness indicates possible spinal injury.

TRAUMA SCORE

Respiratory Rate	10-24/min	4	
	24-35/min	3	
	36/min or greater	2	
	1-9/min	1	
	None	0	
Respiratory Expansion	Normal	1	
	Retractive	0	
Systolic Blood Pressure	90 mmHg or greater	4	
	70-89 mmHg	3	
	50-69 mmHg	2	
	0-49 mmHg	1	
	No Pulse	0	
Capillary Refill	Normal	2	
	Delayed	1	
	None	0	
Cardiopulmonary Assessment			

GLASGOW COMA SCALE

Eye Opening	Spontaneous	4	
	To Voice	3	
	To Pain	2	
	None	1	
Verbal Response	Oriented	5	
	Confused	4	
	Inappropriate Words	3	
	Incomprehensible Words	2	
	None	1	
Motor Response	Obeys Command	6	
	Localizes Pain	5	
	Withdraw (pain)	4	
	Flexion (pain)	3	
	Extension (pain)	2	
	None	1	
Glasgow Coma Score Total			

TOTAL GLASGOW COMA SCALE POINTS

14 – 15 = 5	CONVERSION =
11 – 13 = 4	APPROXIMATELY
8 – 10 = 3	ONE-THIRD
5 – 7 = 2	TOTAL VALUE
3 – 4 = 1	

Neurologic Assessment

Total Trauma Score = Cardiopulmonary + Neurologic ➡

FIGURE 3–12. The Champion Sacco Trauma Score.

SCORING THE PATIENT

There are four elements to the cardiopulmonary assessment. The numerical values are added together to produce a cardiopulmonary score.

There are three elements to the neurological assessment. These are derived from the Glasgow Coma Score. Each category of the Glasgow Coma Score is given a numerical value. These numerical values are added together to produce a subtotal. This number is then reduced by approximately one-third its value to produce the neurologic assessment score.

The cardiopulmonary assessment and the neurologic assessment scores are added together to give the Trauma Score.

For example, a patient has a respiratory rate of 30 breaths per minute (3), retractive chest movements (0), a systolic blood pressure of 80 mmHg (3), and delayed capillary refill (1). The total score for cardiopulmonary function is 3+0+3+1=7.

This same patient shows no eye opening (1), no verbal response (1), and an extension reaction to pain (2). Added together, the total is 4. Approximately one-third of this number is 1. The cardiopulmonary and neurologic scores are added together (7+1) to give a Trauma Score of 8.

TRAUMA SCORE DEFINITIONS

RESPIRATION RATE
The number of respirations (1 inspiration and 1 expiration) in 30 seconds, multiplied by two.

RESPIRATION EXPANSION
NORMAL — clearly visible chest wall movements that are associated with breathing.
RETRACTIVE — the use of accessory muscles (neck and abdominal muscles) to assist with breathing.

SYSTOLIC BLOOD PRESSURE
The systolic pressure recorded by auscultation or palpation (see pages 60-61).

CAPILLARY REFILL
This is determined by pressing a nail bed, the skin on the forehead, or the lining of the mouth (oral mucosa) until there is a loss of normal color (blanching or turning white). The pressure is released and the time for color return is measured. Normal return of color will take place in approximately two seconds (about the time it takes to say to yourself, "capillary refill").
NORMAL REFILL — the color returns within two seconds.
DELAYED REFILL — the color returns sometime after two seconds.
NONE — there is no indication of capillary refill.

GLASGOW COMA SCALE DEFINITIONS

EYE OPENING
This test is valid only if there is no injury or swelling that prevents the patient from opening the eyes.
SPONTANEOUS — the patient opens his or her eyes without any stimulation.
TO VOICE — the patient will open his or her eyes in response to your request. Say, "Open your eyes." If the patient's eyes remain unopened, shout the command.
TO PAIN — if the patient does not open his or her eyes in response to your voice command, pinch the back of his or her hand or the skin at the ankles (apply the stimulus to an uninjured limb).

VERBAL RESPONSE
ORIENTED — an aroused patient should be able to tell you his or her name, where he or she is, and the date in terms of the year and month.
CONFUSED — the patient cannot give accurate responses, but he or she is able to say phrases or sentences and perhaps take part in a conversation.
INAPPROPRIATE WORDS — the patient says one or several inappropriate words, usually in response to a physical stimulus. Often, the patient will curse or call for a specific person. This may happen without any stimulus.
INCOMPREHENSIBLE SOUNDS — the patient mumbles, groans, or moans in response to stimuli.
NO VERBAL RESPONSE — repeated stimulation will not cause the patient to make any sounds.

MOTOR RESPONSE
OBEYS COMMANDS — this is limited by the apparent nature of the patient's injuries and the injuries that can be associated with the mechanism of injury. The patient is asked to perform a simple task such as moving a specific finger or holding up two fingers.

If the patient does not carry out the command, painful stimuli can be utilized by applying firm pressure to an uninjured nail bed for five seconds or pinching the skin on the back of an uninjured hand or at an uninjured ankle.

LOCALIZES PAIN — the patient reaches to the source of the pain. Often, the patient will try to remove your hand from the pain site.
WITHDRAWS — the patient moves the limb rapidly away from the source of the pain. The arm may be moved away from the trunk.
FLEXION — the patient slowly bends the joint (elbow or knee) in an attempt to move away from the pain. The forearm and hand may be held against the trunk.
EXTENSION — the patient will straighten a limb in an effort to escape the pain. The movement appears slow and "stiff." There may be an internal rotation of the shoulder and forearm.
NONE — the patient does not respond to the repeated application of the stimulus.

NOTE: A special thanks is given to the people at Emergency Health Services, Department of Health, Commonwealth of Pennsylvania for their help in supplying information for this figure.

tient says that everything feels fine or if he appears to be confused by your broad questions, you could ask if his arms and legs feel OK. If he says that there is a problem and does not offer a description of that problem, you may have to ask more specific questions. You may have to ask if there is numbness, tingling, burning, or any other unusual sensations in his arms or legs. Such sensations in the extremities suggest damage to the spinal cord and warn you against moving the patient any more than necessary during the remainder of the survey.

As you learn more about various illnesses and injuries, you will see what additional questions can be asked to develop specific responses.

6. *In cases of injury—ask how it happened.* You are trying to learn the circumstances of the complaint. In an accident, try to determine exactly how the injury was sustained. Knowing how the patient was injured will help direct you to problems that may not be noticeable to you or the patient. Any time you come on a patient who is lying down, always find out if he lay down, was knocked down, fell, or was thrown into that position. Do this even if the patient's primary complaint appears to be medical. The knowledge gained could help direct you to possible spinal injuries and internal bleeding.

In accidents involving two parties, such as motor vehicle accidents, word your questions with great care. If you say, "What happened?" you may find yourself listening to a story of how the other person was wrong. Some bystanders wait for the question to be asked so they can tell their stories. Start with a general question such as, "How were you hurt?" Then ask more specific questions such as, "Did you hit the dash (windshield, steering wheel)?" "Were you thrown from the car?" and "Do you know if you lost consciousness?" to provide you with needed information.

In cases of illness—find out how long the patient has felt ill. You will need to know if the problem occurred suddenly, has been developing over the past few days, or has taken some time to develop.

7. *Learn if the problem has happened before or if the patient has ever felt this way before.* You are seeking any previous *relevant* experience. Injuries and illnesses alike can sometimes be attributed to a past medical condition. Certain accidents, such as falling from a ladder, may keep happening to a patient, indicating a possible medical problem. If the patient complains of shortness of breath, dizziness, chills, chest pains, or some other medical problem, then you need to know if this is the first time or if it is a recurring problem.

8. *Determine current medical status.* Find out if the patient has been having any medical problems. Has he been feeling ill? Has he been seeing a doctor? If so, then ask the patient for the name of his physician. You may need to transmit this information to the emergency department staff so they can contact the doctor and possibly learn what may be critical in helping the patient.

9. *Find out if any medications are being taken.* Again, such information could prove to be critical to the emergency department staff. If you fail to ask and the patient becomes unconscious, this information may take hours, if not days, to determine. Use the word "medications." The word "drugs" implies illicit use. If the patient is on medications that are at the scene, gather all the containers and transport them with the patient. Ask if the patient knows the dosage (how many and how many times a day) and when he last took the medication.

10. *Ask if the patient has any known allergies or reactions to medications.* Any medical problem or injury may prove to be enough for a patient to handle without adding the additional stress of an allergy. The health care team needs to know if a patient is allergic to a medication or some other substances or foods so that these can be kept away from the patient.

You may question the need for the subjective interview and even argue the merit of asking questions that appear to have no direct bearing on emergency care measures. It takes only a few minutes to conduct the interview, however, and the brief history obtained may gain information that is essential to patient care. This is especially true if the patient loses consciousness before he can be interviewed by the emergency department staff.

Remember, stay in control by conducting the interview in a calm, professional manner. Avoid inappropriate conversation. Record information as it is gathered. A typical interview might be as follows:

EMT: Good morning, I'm Mark Bennett. I'm an Emergency Medical Technician with the Glen Echo Fire Department. May I help you?

PT: Please!

EMT: Sir, would you tell me your name?

PT: I'm Tom Henderson.

EMT: Mr. Henderson, I'd like to ask you a few questions. Would that be all right with you?

PT: Sure. (If the patient were to say, "Look! I'm in pain!", then skip to his primary complaint.)

EMT: Would you tell me how old you are?

PT: I'm 34.

EMT: Mr. Henderson, can you tell me where you hurt?

PT: My right leg hurts, and I have an awful headache.

EMT: Which is bothering you the most?

PT: My leg.

EMT: Does anything else feel wrong with your leg?

PT: I don't think so . . . ah, what do you mean?

EMT: Do you have any numbness, or is there any tingling or burning in your arms or legs?

PT: No.

EMT: Do you remember what happened, Mr. Henderson?

PT: I was up on the ladder working on the light. I don't remember whether I leaned over too far, or whether I got dizzy and slipped.

EMT: Did you become unconscious?

PT: What?

EMT: Did you pass out?

PT: I don't think so.

EMT: You said you may have had a dizzy spell, Mr. Henderson. Have you ever had a dizzy spell before?

PT: I get lightheaded every once in a while, but the spell usually passes quickly.

EMT: Mr. Henderson, are you under a doctor's care at this time?

PT: Yes, Dr. Johnson.

EMT: What is Dr. Johnson treating you for?

PT: High blood pressure.

EMT: Are you taking any medications?

PT: Water pills. I think they're called Lasix.

EMT: How many do you take and when do you take them?

PT: One in the morning.

EMT: Are you allergic to anything, Mr. Henderson?

PT: Not that I know of.

The above interview went well and information was gathered by the EMT. However, what if the patient had been unconscious? In such cases, you will have to depend on first responders, bystanders, medical identification devices, and your own suspicions based on the mechanism of injury.

When interviewing bystanders, determine if any are relatives or friends of the patient. They usually have more information to provide about past problems. See which of the bystanders saw what happened. When questioning bystanders, you should ask:

1. *The patient's name*. If the patient is obviously a minor, you should ask if the parents are present or if they have been contacted.
2. *What happened*? You may be told that the patient fell off a ladder, appeared to faint, was hit on the head by a falling object, or any other possible clues.
3. *Did they see anything else*? For example, was the patient clutching his chest or head before he fell?
4. *Did the patient complain of anything before this happened*? You may learn of chest pains, nausea, concern about odors where he was working, or other clues to the problem.
5. *Did the patient have any known illnesses or problems*? This may provide you with information about heart problems, alcohol abuse, or other problems that could cause a change in the patient's condition.
6. *Do they know if the patient was taking any medications*? Be sure to use the words "medications" or "medicines." If you say "drugs" or some other term, bystanders may not answer you, thinking that you are asking questions as part of a criminal investigation. In rare cases, you may feel that the bystanders are holding back information because the patient was abusing drugs. Remind them that you are an EMT and you need all the information they can give you so proper care can begin.

If your patient is the victim of a motor vehicle accident and was taken from the wreckage prior to your arrival, ask if he was the driver or a passenger and if he was wearing a seat belt. You can often associate the mechanism of injury with where a person was sitting in a vehicle. Also ask if the person was alert when he was extricated and if he has lost consciousness, even for a brief moment. Document the removal of the patient before your arrival at the scene.

Do not ask these questions as an isolated part of the secondary survey. You can be active, beginning the examination while you ask questions and listen to bystanders' answers.

Medical identification devices can provide needed information. One of the most commonly used medical-alerting devices is the Medic Alert emblem shown in Figure 3–13. Over one million people wear a medical identification device in the form of a necklace or wrist or ankle bracelet. One side of the device has a star of life emblem. The patient's medical problem is engraved on the reverse side, along with a telephone number to call for additional information. Look for necklaces and bracelets. Never assume you know the form of every medical identification device. Check carefully any necklace or bracelet, taking usual care when moving the patient or any of his extremities. You should alert the emergency department staff (usually by radio transmission) that the patient is wearing a medical identification device. Give the staff the wearer's identification number, the nature of the problem, and the telephone number they are to call. See page 208 for information on the "Vial of Life."

Do not move the patient to reach for his wallet in order to find a medical alert card. You should not check his wallet unless you are directed to do so on the bracelet or necklace. If there is any chance

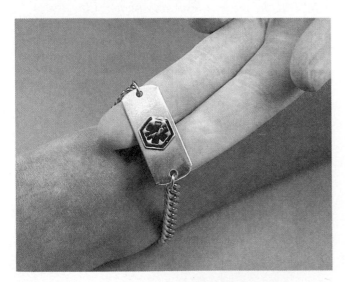

FIGURE 3–13. A medical identification device.

of spinal injury, you should not move the patient to gain access to his wallet. To do so may cause severe injury to the patient.

The Objective Examination

The objective examination begins the search for very specific signs and symptoms. Before going on, make certain you understand the following terms:

- SYMPTOMS—What the patient tells you is wrong. Such things as chest pains, dizziness, and nausea are considered symptoms. Many of these may have been gathered through the interview with the patient. Others can be gained by continuing to ask questions during the examination.
- SIGNS—What you see, hear, feel, and smell when examining the patient. Since you will use these signs to try to determine what is wrong with the patient, they are sometimes called diagnostic signs.
- VITAL SIGNS—Pulse, respiration, blood pressure, and skin temperature. Some localities also use pupils, skin color, and level of consciousness. They are not vital signs but they are very important and can be gathered at the same time.

The objective examination of your patient may begin with a head-to-toe examination and conclude with the taking of vital signs. However, if your patient has a medical problem and does not have injuries, he is unconscious, he has apparent serious injuries, or he appears unstable (he appears to be growing worse), you may start with vital signs, do the examination, and take vital signs again.

When the patient is alert, be certain to obtain actual consent before starting to determine vital signs or conducting the examination. Before you begin, TAKE A GOOD LOOK AT YOUR PATIENT. Note whatever you can that is obvious about his condition (Figure 3–14).

Examination Rule No. 1

If you should notice anything unusual about a patient's awareness or behavior, consider that something may be seriously wrong with the patient. Stay alert for changes.

First, continue with the determination of the patient's **level of consciousness** and orientation. Determining if the patient is conscious or unconscious is usually no problem; it is the level of con-

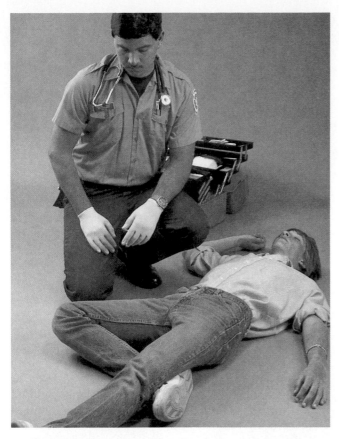

FIGURE 3–14. Briefly observe the patient before beginning the objective examination.

sciousness that requires special skills. Many terms are used to describe a person's level of consciousness: semiconscious, incoherent, hysterical, stuporous, and so on. These terms often have different meanings, even in the same locality. *Do not* depend on these terms to give you a quick "classification" of the patient. Instead, as you ask questions and ask the patient to do specific things, note simply whether he is alert and oriented to what you are doing, or if he is confused and disoriented. An alert person is aware of what is going on around him. He is oriented if he knows who he is, where he is, and the day of the week and can respond quickly to both vocal and physical stimuli. A confused, disoriented person usually has trouble answering questions and responding to specific instructions. Experience will soon allow you to determine easily a person's level of consciousness.

If the coma scale is part of your EMS System's patient assessment, use it to determine the patient's level of consciousness. Some systems use a simple form for level of consciousness. This form uses the "AVPU" method, which stands for:

- *Alert and oriented*—the patient is aware of what is happening around him.
- *Verbal*—the patient responds to your voice.
- *Painful stimuli*—the patient will not obey your commands or may not respond at all to your voice. He does withdraw from painful stimuli (e.g., being pinched).
- *Unconscious*—the patient is unresponsive.

You should stay aware of the patient's level of consciousness until he is turned over to the emergency department staff. More specifics on measuring the level of consciousness will be presented in Chapter 11.

Examination Rule No. 2

Even patients who appear to be stable may worsen rapidly. An EMT must always be aware of changes in a patient's condition. Constant monitoring of patients is an essential part of emergency care.

Look for change as you continue the survey. Be on the alert for loss of awareness, failing respiration, distress due to pain, new bleeding, and indications of the onset of shock, such as restlessness, anxiety, and profuse sweating. Remember that patient improvement is also a change to be noted.

Examination Rule No. 3

You must watch the patient's skin for color changes. Observe your patient's skin color and condition. A great deal of emphasis is often placed on the significance of a sick or injured person's skin color. Skin color suggests a variety of medical problems and is a good indicator of heart and lung function (Table 3–5).

You need to note any odd colorations of the patient's skin and stay alert for changes. When a person has deeply pigmented or dark skin it may be necessary to look for color changes in his lips, nailbeds, palms, ear lobes, whites of the eye, inner surface of lower eyelid, gums, or tongue.

Table 3–5. MEDICAL SIGNIFICANCE OF CHANGES IN SKIN COLOR

Skin Color	Possible Cause of Abnormality
Red	High blood pressure, stroke, heart attack, alcohol abuse, sunburn, infectious disease, simple blushing
White	Shock, heart attack, fright, anemia, simple fainting, emotional distress
Blue	Asphyxia (suffocation), hypoxia (lack of oxygen), heart attack, poisoning
Yellow	Liver disease
Black and blue	Seepage of blood under skin surface

Examination Rule No. 4

You must look over the patient and note *anything* that looks wrong. Quickly look for obvious wound sites, burns, fractures and any obvious deformities, swellings and puffiness, ulcers and blotches on the skin, and any blood-soaked areas.

Examination Rule No. 5

Unless you are certain that you are dealing with a patient free from spinal injury (e.g., medical patient, no trauma), *assume* the patient has such injuries. Always assume that the unconscious trauma patient has a spinal injury.

Spinal injuries can occur even in apparently minor accidents. Keep in mind that a patient with a medical emergency may have fallen and hurt his spine. You must conduct the physical examination without aggravating spinal injuries.

Examination Rule No. 6

Fully explain what you will be doing during the examination. Tell the patient what you are going to do. Let him know if there may be pain or discomfort. Always let the patient know if you must lift, rearrange, or remove any article of his clothing. Do all you can to ensure privacy for the patient. Stress the importance of the examination and work to build the patient's confidence. Ask the patient if he understands what you are doing, seeking his response. Try to maintain eye contact whenever possible, and never turn away while you are talking or while the patient is answering your questions.

Vital Signs

Vital signs include pulse, respiration, blood pressure, and temperature. In basic EMT-level emergency care, *relative skin temperature* is usually measured. In some localities, level of consciousness and pupil size and reactivity are recorded with vital signs. Even though they are not technically vital signs, they can be conveniently observed when vital signs are being taken. It is also very convenient to determine other skin characteristics (e.g., color, dry, moist) when assessing skin temperature.

Your EMS System may have you take vital signs after the physical examination, thus having an assessment protocol of primary survey, interview, examination, and vital signs. In some areas of the country, vital signs are taken for conscious patients after the subjective interview and for unconscious patients after the physical examination. This is done to reduce the risk of aggravating spinal injuries and fractures and dislocations of the extremities. Most EMS Systems use variations in the approach to patient assessment described earlier. These variations are based on consciousness or unconsciousness and trauma or medical emergency.

Examination Rule No. 7

Determine vital signs. The process will take you a little over 1 minute. The information gained could save a patient's life.

As an EMT, you should follow a simple procedure in determining vital signs. This procedure allows you to gather quickly the needed measurements in an uninterrupted manner. You will have to develop a smooth, efficient method of determining vital signs. Most patients will have to have their vital signs taken more than once. In some cases, when the patient is unstable and the transport is short, you may find yourself completing the determination of vital signs only to begin the next determination.

First, place the stethoscope around your neck, with the earpieces pointing forward. Position yourself at the patient's side and place the blood pressure cuff on his arm. Be certain that there are no suspected or obvious injuries to this arm. There must be no clothing under the cuff. If you can expose the arm sufficiently by rolling the sleeve up, do so, but make sure that this roll of clothing does not become a constricting band.

Wrap the cuff around the patient's upper arm so that the lower edge of the cuff is about one inch above the anterior crease of the elbow. Know the equipment that you are using. The center of the bladder must be placed over the brachial (BRAY-key-al) artery. The marker on the cuff (if provided) should indicate where you place the cuff in relation to the artery, but many cuffs do not have markers in the correct location. Tubes entering the bladder are not always in the right location either. The Amer-

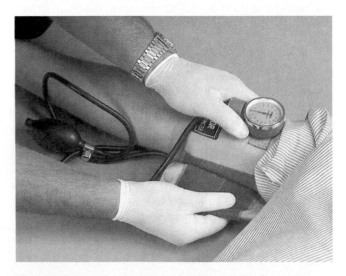

FIGURE 3–15. Positioning the blood pressure cuff.

ican Heart Association states that the only accurate method is finding the bladder center. If you know your equipment, then you will know if the markers are correct, if you can use the tubes entering the bladder, or if you will have to find the center of the bladder. Always apply the cuff securely but not overly tight. You should be able to place one finger easily under the bottom edge of the cuff.

You are now ready to begin your determination of the patient's vital signs.

Determination of Pulse Rate and Character The pumping action of the heart is normally rhythmic, causing blood to move through the arteries in waves, not smoothly and continuously at the same pressure like water flowing through a pipe. A fingertip held over an artery where it lies close to the body's surface and crosses over a bone can easily feel characteristic "beats" as the surging blood causes the artery to expand. What you feel is called the *pulse.*

When "taking a patient's pulse," you are concerned with two factors: rate and character. For **pulse rate,** you will have to determine the number of beats per minute. This will allow you to decide if the patient's pulse rate is *normal, rapid,* or *slow.* The rhythm and force of the pulse are considered for **pulse character.** You will have to judge the patient's pulse as *regular* or *irregular* in regard to rhythm and *full* (strong) or *thready* (weak) in regard to force.

Pulse rate varies among individuals. Factors such as age, sex, physical condition, degree of exercise just completed, medications or substances being taken, blood loss, and stress all have an influence on the rate. The normal rate for an *adult at rest* is between 60 and 80 beats per minute. Any pulse rate above 100 beats per minute is **rapid** (tachycardia), while a rate below 60 beats per minute is **slow** (bradycardia). An athlete may have a normal at-rest pulse rate between 40 and 50 beats per minute. This is a slow pulse rate, but it is certainly not an indication of poor health. As an EMT, you are concerned with the typical adult having a pulse rate that stays above 100 or below 60 beats per minute.

In an emergency it is not unusual for this rate to be between 100 and 150 beats per minute. An adult patient must see a physician as soon as possible whenever the pulse rate stays above 150 beats per minute. If you take a patient's pulse several times during care at the scene and find him holding a pulse rate above 120 beats or below 50 beats per minute, you must consider this to be a sign that something may be seriously wrong with the patient and that he should be transported as soon as possible.

The normal pulse rate for children from 1 to 5 years of age is between 80 and 150 beats per minute; this rate gradually slows as the child grows older. Some newborns may reach as high as 150 to 180 beats per minute. Rates above or below the 80 to 150 range are considered to be serious, with the patient needing to see a physician as soon as possible. For children from 5 to 12 years of age, the rate is usually between 60 and 120 beats per minute. Again, rates above or below this range require immediate medical care rendered by a physician.

Pulse rhythm relates to regularity. A pulse is said to be regular when the intervals between beats are constant. When the intervals are not constant, the pulse is irregular. You should report irregular pulse rhythm and if you felt what seemed to be a skipping of a beat or beats.

Pulse force refers to the pressure of the pulse wave as it expands the artery. Normally, the pulse should feel as if a strong wave has passed under your fingertips. This is a full pulse. When the pulse feels weak and thin, the patient has a thready pulse.

Many disorders can be related to variations in pulse rate, rhythm, and force (Table 3–6).

Table 3–6. PULSE VARIATIONS AND MEDICAL CONDITIONS

Pulse	*Possible Cause of Abnormality*
Rapid, regular and full	May be caused by nothing more than exertion; may also be caused by fright, fever, hypertension (high blood pressure), or first stage of blood loss
Rapid, regular and thready	Reliable sign of shock; often evident in later stage of blood loss
Slow	Head injury, drug use (barbiturates and narcotics), some poisons, certain cardiac (heart) problems
No pulse	Cardiac arrest leading to death

Pulse Rates *(beats per minute, at rest)*		
Adult	60 to 80	Normal
	100+	Rapid
	Below 60	Slow
Infant	120 to 150	Normal
	Above 150	Rapid
	Below 120	Slow
Child (1 to 5 yrs)	80 to 150	Normal
	Above 150	Rapid
	Below 80	Slow
Child (5 to 12 yrs)	60 to 120	Normal
	Above 120	Rapid
	Below 60	Slow

Note: For more information on children, see Table 15–1.

Pulse rate and character can be determined at a number of points throughout the body. During the determination of vital signs, a **radial pulse** is measured. This is the wrist pulse, named for the radial artery found in the lateral portion of the forearm (remember the anatomical position). If you cannot measure one radial pulse, try the radial pulse of the other arm. When you cannot measure either radial pulse, use the carotid pulse, as described earlier on pp. 72–73.

In order to measure a radial pulse, find the pulse site by placing your first three fingers on the middle of the patient's wrist (Figure 3–16), just above the crease (toward the proximal end). Do not use your thumb. It has its own pulse that may cause you to measure your own pulse rate. Slide your fingertips toward the lateral (thumb) side of the patient's wrist, keeping one finger over the crease. Apply moderate pressure to feel the pulse beats. A weak pulse may require applying greater pressure, but take care. If you experience difficulty, try the patient's other arm. Count the pulsations for 30 seconds and multiply by 2 to determine the beats per minute. While you are counting, judge the rhythm and force. Record the information: for example, "Pulse 72, regular and full," and the time of determination. It is best to wait until you also have determined respiratory rate and character before recording pulse information (see below). When recording the pulse rate and character, also record the time of the determination.

If the pulse rate, rhythm, or character is not normal, continue with your count and observations for a full 60 seconds. The number counted is the rate in beats per minute.

Determination of Respiratory Rate and Character
For the determination of vital signs, you also are concerned with the rate and character of breathing. **Respiration** is the act of breathing in and out; therefore, a single breath is the complete process of breathing in, followed by breathing out.

Respiratory rate is the number of breaths a patient takes in one minute. The rate of respiration is classified as normal, rapid, or slow. Respiratory character includes rhythm, depth, sounds, and ease of breathing.

The normal respiration rate for an adult at rest is between 12 and 20 breaths per minute. Keep in mind that age, sex, size, physical conditioning, and emotional state can influence breathing rates. Fear and other emotions experienced during an emer-

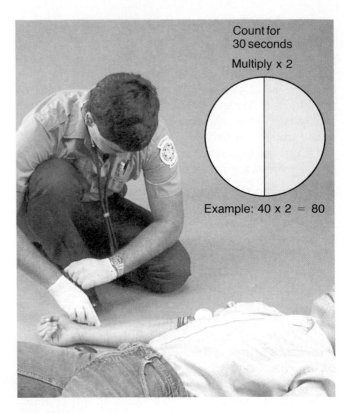

FIGURE 3–16. Pulse rate and character are vital signs.

gency can cause an increase in respiratory rate. However, if you have an adult patient maintaining a rate above 28 breaths per minute, you must consider this to be a serious emergency in need of a physician's care as soon as possible. The same holds true for rates that stay below 10 breaths per minute.

Children breathe more quickly than adults. The rate for infants can range from 35 to 60 breaths per minute. For children from 1 to 5 years old, a respiratory rate above 44 breaths per minute is considered serious. Children from 5 to 12 years of age are considered in immediate need of a physician's care when their respiratory rate exceeds 36 breaths per minute.

Rhythm refers to the manner in which a person breathes. Breathing is considered *regular* when the interval between breaths is constant and *irregular* when the interval varies.

Depth relates to the amount of air moved with each breath. Normal is something you will have to judge for yourself by watching people breathe when at rest. Then you will be able to differentiate between *deep* and *shallow* respirations. While judging depth, also note the ease of respirations. Does the patient exhibit *labored* breathing, *difficult* breathing, or *painful* breathing? If the patient shows pronounced movement of his shoulder and neck and/or abdominal muscles while breathing, report this as the use of accessory muscles.

Listen for any sounds of respiration such as *snoring, wheezing, crowing,* and *gurgling* (Table 3–7). More will be said about these sounds in Chapter 4.

NOTE: If you are to use a stethoscope for the assessment of breathing sounds, see page 107. Usually, this assessment is done during the head-to-toe survey.

Table 3–7. VARIATIONS IN RESPIRATION AND MEDICAL CONDITIONS

Respirations	Possible Cause of Abnormality
Deep, gasping, labored	Airway obstruction, heart failure, asthma
Rapid, deep	Diabetic coma, hyperventilation, destructive lung disease
Rapid, shallow	Shock, cardiac problems, chest injury
Painful, difficult, labored	Respiratory distress, lung disease, heart problems
Difficulty in breathing while lying down	Heart failure, lung infection, asthma
Stertorous (snoring)	Stroke, fractured skull, drug influence and alcohol intoxication
Wheezing	Asthma
Gurgling (as though the breaths are passing through water)	Foreign matter in throat, pulmonary edema (accumulation of fluid in lungs)
Crowing (birdlike sounds)	Spasms of the larynx
Temporary cessation of respirations	Hypoxia (lack of oxygen), congestive heart failure, head injuries
Slowed breathing	Stroke, head injury, chest injury, certain drugs (e.g., narcotics)
No respirations	Respiratory arrest, airway obstruction

Respiration Rates
(breaths per minute, at rest)

Adult	12 to 20	Normal
	Above 30	Very serious
	Below 10	Very serious
Infant	30 to 70	Normal (above
30 to 70 at birth		60 is rapid,
30 at 6 months		below 35 is slow)
	Above 70	Very serious
	Below 30	Very serious
Child (1 to 5 yrs.)	25 to 28	Normal
	Above 44	Very serious
	Below 20	Very serious
Child (5 to 12 yrs.)	20 to 24	Normal
	Above 36	Very serious
	Below 16	Very serious

Note: For more information on children, see Table 15–1.

As soon as you have determined pulse rate, start counting respirations. Many individuals change their breathing rate if they know someone is watching them breathe. For this reason, do not move your hand from the patient's wrist. After you have counted pulse beats, immediately begin to watch the patient's chest for breathing movements. Count the number of breaths taken by the patient during 30 seconds and multiply by 2 to obtain the breaths per minute. While counting, note rhythm, depth, ease, and sounds of respiration. Record your results. For example. "Respirations are 16, regular and normal." Record the time of the assessment.

Determination of Blood Pressure   Since the blood pressure cuff is already in place, you can begin to measure blood pressure as soon as you complete the determination of pulse and respirations. Keep in

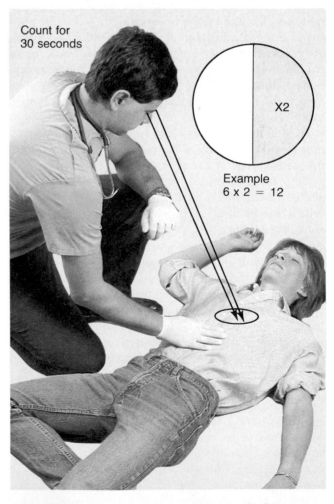

FIGURE 3–17. Breathing rate and character are vital signs.

mind that you have no way of knowing the patient's *normal* blood pressure unless the patient is alert and knows this information (his information must be current). For this reason, one reading of blood pressure may not be very meaningful. You will have to make several readings over a period of time while care is provided at the scene and during transport. Remember that changes in blood pressure are very significant. The patient's blood pressure may be normal in the early stages of some very serious problems, only to change rapidly in a matter of minutes.

Each time the lower chamber of the left side of the heart contracts it forces blood out into circulation. The pressure created in the arteries by this blood is called the **systolic** (sis-TOL-ik) blood pressure. When the lower left chamber of the heart is relaxed and refilling, the pressure remaining in the arteries is called the **diastolic** (di-as-TOL-ik) blood pressure. The systolic pressure is reported first, as in 120 over 80.

Just as pulse and respiratory rates vary among individuals so does blood pressure. There is a generally accepted rule for estimating blood pressure of adults up to the age of 40. For an adult male at rest, add his age to 100 to estimate his systolic pressure. For an adult female at rest, add her age to 90 to estimate her systolic pressure. Thus, using this formula, a 36-year-old man would have an estimated normal systolic blood pressure of 136 millimeters of mercury (mmHg). **Millimeters of mercury** refers to the units of the blood pressure gauge. A 36-year-old woman would have an estimated normal systolic pressure of 126 mmHg. Normal diastolic pressures usually range from 60 to 90 mmHg.

Serious low blood pressure (hypotension) is generally considered to exist when the systolic pressure falls below 90 mmHg. High blood pressure (hypertension) exists once the pressure rises above 140/90. Keep in mind that many individuals in emergency situations will exhibit a temporary rise in blood pressure. More than one reading will be necessary to decide if a high or low reading is only temporary. If your patient's blood pressure drops, the patient may be developing shock (other signs are usually more important early indicators of shock). Report any major changes in blood pressure to emergency department personnel without delay.

In adults, consider any systolic reading above 180 or below 90 mmHg to be very serious. A diastolic reading above 104 or below 60 mmHg must also be considered to be very serious. For children from 1 to 5, any systolic reading above 120 or below 70 mmHg means that the child should be seen by a physician as soon as possible. In this age group, diastolic readings above 76 or below 50 mmHg must be considered as indications of serious problems.

Table 3–8. BLOOD PRESSURE—INDICATIONS OF VERY SERIOUS PROBLEMS

Patient	Systolic (mmHg)	Diastolic (mmHg)
Adult	Above 180	Above 104
	Below 90	Below 60
Child (1 to 5 yrs.)	Above 120	Above 76
	Below 70	Below 50
Child (5 to 12 yrs.)	Above 150	Above 86
	Below 90	Below 60

Note: For more information on children, see Table 15–1.

Children 5 to 12 are classified as needing to see a physician as soon as possible when their systolic pressure is above 150 or below 90 mmHg. The same is true in cases where the diastolic pressure is above 86 or below 60 mmHg (see Table 3–8).

There are two common techniques used to measure blood pressure with a sphygmomanometer: (1) **auscultation** (os-skul-TAY-shun), when a stethoscope is used to listen for characteristic sounds; and (2) **palpation,** when the radial pulse is palpated (felt) with the fingertips.

Determining Blood Pressure by Auscultation. Begin by placing the tips of the stethoscope arms in your ears (the earpieces should be pointing forward). The patient should be seated or lying down. If the patient has not been injured, support his arm at the level of his heart. With your fingertips, palpate the brachial artery at the crease of the elbow. Position the diaphragm of the stethoscope directly over the brachial pulse site or over the medial anterior elbow if no brachial pulse site can be determined. Do not touch the cuff with the diaphragm, since this will give you false readings. With the bulb valve (thumb valve) closed, inflate the cuff. As you do so, you soon will be able to hear pulse sounds. Inflate the cuff, watching the gauge. At a certain point, you will no longer hear the brachial pulse. Continue to inflate the cuff until the gauge reads 30 mmHg higher than the point where the pulse sound disappeared.

Slowly release air from the cuff by opening the bulb valve, allowing the pressure to fall smoothly at the rate of approximately 2 mmHg per second.

Listen for the start of clicking or tapping sounds. When you hear the beginning of these sounds, note the reading on the gauge. This is the systolic pressure. Continue to deflate the cuff, listening for the point at which these distinctive sounds fade (not when they disappear*). When the sounds turn to dull, muffled thuds, the reading on the gauge is the diastolic pressure. After obtaining the diastolic pressure, let the cuff deflate rapidly. If you are not certain of a reading, repeat the procedure. You should use the other arm or wait one minute before reinflating the cuff. Otherwise, you will tend to obtain an erroneously high reading.

Record the measurements and the time of determination. For example, "B.P. is 140/90." Blood pressure is reported in even numbers. If a reading falls between two lines on the gauge, use the higher number.

Sometimes you will have difficulty hearing the pulse sound in patients with hypovolemia or inside a moving ambulance. If this is the case, use your fingertips to find the patient's radial pulse at the wrist of the arm to which the cuff has been applied. Make certain that the adjustable valve on the rubber bulb assembly is closed; then inflate the cuff. Note the point at which the radial pulse disappears. Continue inflating the cuff until the needle (or column) shows 30 mmHg higher than the point of radial pulse cutoff. The rest of the procedure remains the same.

REMEMBER: Blood pressure must be measured when a person is seated or lying down. Use usual caution when moving a patient or extremity to determine blood pressure. To do so may aggravate existing injuries. Always try to keep the cuff at heart level. If the patient is sitting up, support his arm (e.g., on the arm of a chair) or hold the patient's arm during the entire procedure.

Some patients who have high systolic blood pressures will have the pulse sounds *disappear* as you deflate the cuff, only to have these sounds *reappear* as you continue with the deflation. When this happens, *false* systolic and diastolic readings may be obtained. If you determine a high diastolic reading, wait from 1 to 2 minutes and take another reading. As you inflate the cuff, feel for the disappearance of the radial pulse to ensure that you are not measuring a false diastolic pressure. Listen as you deflate the cuff down into the normal range. The diastolic pressure is the reading at which the last fade of sound takes place.

Determination of Blood Pressure by Palpation. This method is not as accurate as the auscultation method, since only an *approximate* systolic pressure can be determined. The technique is used

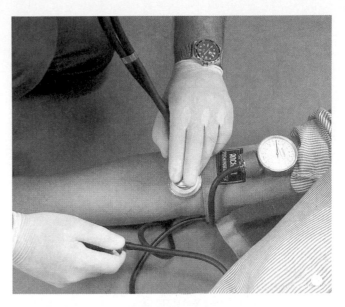

FIGURE 3–18. **Measuring blood pressure by auscultation.**

when there is too much noise around a patient to allow the use of the stethoscope or when the situation involves many patients and too few persons to deliver care.

Begin by finding the radial pulse site on the limb to which the blood pressure cuff has been applied. Make certain that the adjustable valve is closed on the bulb and inflate the cuff to a point where you can no longer feel the radial pulse. Note this point on the gauge and continue to inflate the cuff 30 mmHg beyond this point.

Slowly deflate the cuff, noting the reading at which the radial pulse returns. This reading is the patient's systolic pressure. Record your findings as, for example, "Blood pressure 140 by palpation," and the time of the determination.

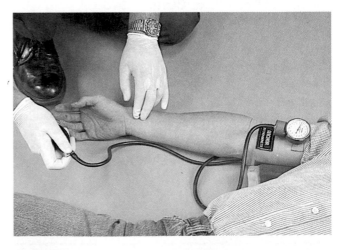

FIGURE 3–19. **Measuring blood pressure by palpation.**

Determination of Skin Temperature

Some areas have EMTs measure oral, axillary (armpit), or rectal temperatures for a determination of body temperature for certain patients. However, most area guidelines for basic EMT-level care call for a measurement of relative skin temperature. This is not a true vital sign in higher levels of care, but in the field it is useful to find abnormally high and low temperatures.

NOTE: While determining relative skin temperature you also should note skin color and condition.

To determine skin temperature and condition, feel the patient's forehead with the back of your hand. Note if his skin feels *normal*, *warm*, *hot*, *cool*, or *cold*. At the same time, notice if his skin is *dry*, *moist*, or *clammy*. Look for "goose pimples," which are often associated with chills. Many patient problems are exhibited by changes in skin temperature and condition. As you continue with the assessment and care of the patient, be alert for major *temperature differences* on various parts of the body. For example, you may note that the patient's trunk is warm but his left arm feels cold. Such a finding can direct you to detecting problems with circulation. A relatively hot area on the abdomen may indicate inflammation or infection within the cavity (Table 3–9).

The Head-to-Toe Survey

The head-to-toe procedure may cause the patient some pain and discomfort. Warn the patient of these possibilities. Ask the patient to let you know when anything that you do causes pain. The more systematic you are in your approach and the better you know how to conduct each aspect of the examination,

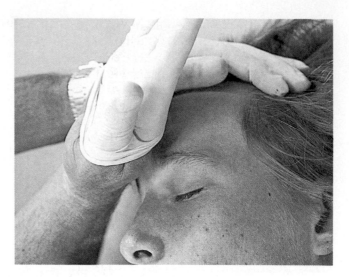

FIGURE 3–20. Determining relative skin temperature.

the less likely you are to cause pain and discomfort. As an EMT, you MUST know the head-to-toe procedures and be able to perform each move without any hesitation.

All the survey does not have to be performed on every patient. The survey is geared to the patient's chief complaint, the nature of the accident or illness, and the seriousness of his condition. A commonsense approach should be taken.

Take care not to contaminate wounds and aggravate injuries. If bleeding has obviously stopped, *do not* pull the clothing or skin around the site. *Do not* probe into the site.

Readjust, remove, or cut away only those articles of patient clothing that interfere with your ability to examine the patient. *Do not* try to pull clothing off the limbs of a patient. Such procedures could increase bleeding and worsen existing injuries.

Be certain to tell the patient that you have to rearrange his clothing and explain why this must be done. Do all you can to ensure the patient's privacy, even if it means asking bystanders to face away from the patient or to hold up a blanket to serve as a shield. Some authorities recommend having a woman EMT present during the examination of a female patient by a male EMT. However, no one recommends delaying the examination or care of a patient of the opposite sex. As a professional EMT, your intentions should be respected.

During the head-to-toe survey:

- LOOK—for discolorations, deformities, penetrations, wounds, openings in the neck, and any unusual chest movements.

Table 3–9. TEMPERATURE VARIATIONS AND RELEVANT MEDICAL CONDITIONS

Skin Temperature	Possible Cause of Abnormality
Cool, clammy	Usual sign of shock, anxiety
Cold, moist	Body is losing heat
Cold, dry	Body has been exposed to cold and has lost considerable heat
Hot, dry	Excessive body heat (as in heatstroke and high fever)
Hot, moist	High fever
"Goose pimples" accompanied by shivering, chattering teeth, blue lips and pale skin	Chills, communicable disease, exposure to cold, pain, or fear

- FEEL—for deformities, tenderness, pulsations, abnormal hardness or softness, spasms, and skin temperature.
- LISTEN—for changes in breathing patterns, unusual breathing sounds, and any grating noises made by the ends of broken bones (do not ask the patient to move or move his limbs so that you can confirm grating sounds).
- SMELL—for any unusual odors coming from the patient's body, breath, or clothing.

Examination Rule No. 8

Conduct a head-to-toe examination, wearing all necessary protective equipment. If anything looks, feels, sounds, or smells strange to you, assume that there is something seriously wrong with the patient.

There may be some variation in the head-to-toe survey depending on local guidelines. Traditionally, the examination started with the head. However, most medical authorities now recommend that the neck be examined first in an effort to detect possible spinal injuries and any serious injury to the trachea (windpipe) that may lead to airway obstruction. When such injuries are detected, the head and neck can be immobilized to reduce chances of aggravating spinal or airway injury during the rest of the survey.

Begin your head-to-toe survey by placing yourself in a full kneeling position at the side of the patient's head. Take a quick overview of the patient's body. You should then perform the following:

PATIENT ASSESSMENT

Head-to-Toe Survey

1. CHECK THE CERVICAL SPINE FOR POINT TENDERNESS AND DEFORMITY.

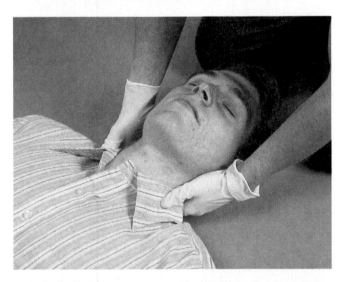

PROCEDURE: The portion of the spinal column that runs through the neck is called the **cervical** (SER-ve-kal) **spine.** Prepare the patient for possible pain. With the palms up, *gently* slide your hands under the sides of the patient's neck, moving your fingertips toward the cervical midline. Check the back of the neck from the shoulders to the base of the skull. Apply gentle finger pressure. A painful response to this pressure is **point tenderness.**

POSSIBLE FINDINGS: Midline deformities, point tenderness, or muscle spasms indicate possible cervical spinal injury. You cannot rule out cervical spine injury if there is no point tenderness.

NOTE: If there are signs of possible spinal injury, *stop the survey* and provide temporary immobilization of the head and neck. This can be done manually by another EMT with a blanket roll or by two EMTs applying a rigid cervical or extrication collar (see Ch. 11). Another rescuer will have to stabilize the head and neck during application of the device and after it has been applied. If the patient is unconscious, assume that there is spinal injury.

WARNING: If the patient is seated or in an unusual position, stabilize the head with one hand on his chin while you inspect with your other hand. If possible, have another EMT stabilize the head. If a rigid collar is to be applied, make certain that you have examined the anterior neck and the sides of the neck before its application.

2. INSPECT THE ANTERIOR NECK FOR INDICATIONS OF INJURY AND NECK BREATHING.

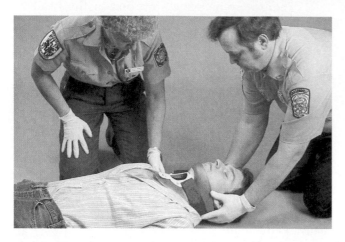

PROCEDURE: The anterior neck must be exposed so that you can check for surgical openings or a metal or plastic tube that indicates the patient is a "neck breather." Look for signs of injury. Does the larynx (voice box) or trachea (windpipe) appear to be deviated from the midline of the neck? Are there bruises or deformities? If so, the patient may have an obstructed airway, a cervical spine injury, damage to the trachea, or a serious chest injury.

See if the patient has a **stoma** (STO-mah) (permanent surgical opening) in the neck through which he breathes. He may have a **tracheostomy** (TRA-ke-OS-to-me). This is a surgical incision held open by a metal or plastic tube or tubes. In either case, the patient will breath through the opening.

Look for a medical identification necklace. Note the information provided, but *do not* remove the necklace.

POSSIBLE FINDINGS: Cuts, bruises, discolorations, deformities, or signs of airway deviation may be seen. Bruises or deformities directly over the trachea may indicate a serious airway obstruction exists or will soon occur owing to tissue swelling or a ruptured trachea (immediate care is needed). The patient may have a stoma. There may be a medical identification necklace.

3. INSPECT THE SCALP FOR WOUNDS.

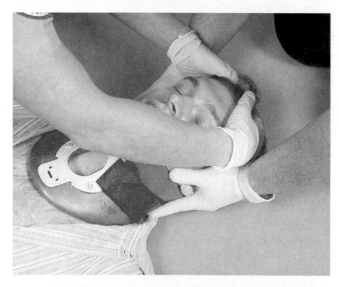

PROCEDURE: Extreme care must be exercised so as not to move the patient's head, aggravating possible spinal injuries. Move to the top of the patient's head and run your fingers gently through the patient's hair, feeling the scalp. If you believe you have found an injury site, *do not* separate strands of hair matted over the site. To do so may restart bleeding. When the patient is found lying on his back, check the hidden part of his scalp by placing your fingers behind his neck. Slide them upward toward the top of his head. Check your fingers for blood. If you have any reason to believe there are spinal or neck injuries, *delay* this procedure until the head and neck are immobilized.

POSSIBLE FINDINGS: Blood, cuts, puncture wounds, swellings or "goose eggs," deformities, and any other indications of injury may be found.

NOTE: You may find the patient is wearing a hairpiece or wig. If so, you will feel the netting of the hairpiece or the border where the piece or wig joins the patient's natural hairline. *Do not* try to remove the hairpiece. It may be held in place by adhesive, tape, or permanent glue. To attempt removal may aggravate injuries or restart bleeding. Some wigs remove easily; others may have to be cut away. This may prove to be a difficult procedure, forcing you to combine cutting and sliding to remove the wig, which may cause undesired movement of the head and neck. Proper immobilization of the head and neck must be done before attempting wig removal. Unless you suspect profuse bleeding, it is best to leave the wig in place. It is probably acting as an effective dressing. If the patient is wearing a hairpiece, gently feel through the netting for bleeding or deformity. *Do not* reach under a wig to inspect the scalp.

WARNING: Take great care not to drive bone fragments or force dirt into any scalp wound.

4. CHECK THE SKULL AND FACE FOR DEFORMITIES AND DEPRESSIONS.

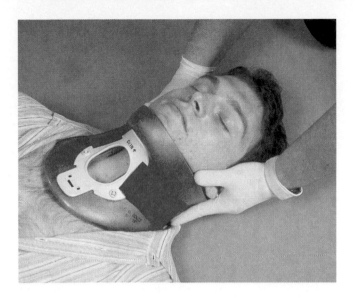

PROCEDURE: While feeling the scalp, note any depressions or bony projections that would indicate possible injury to the skull. Visually check the facial bones for any signs of fractures. Gently palpate the cheekbones, forehead, and lower jaw unless there are obvious signs of injury.

POSSIBLE FINDINGS: Depressions, bony projections, obvious breaks in the bones, swellings, heavy discolorations, or the obvious crushing of bones.

5. EXAMINE THE PATIENT'S EYES.

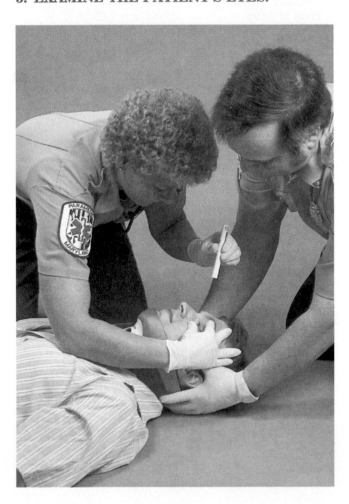

PROCEDURE: Return to a side position. Begin by looking at the patient's eyelids. Have the patient open his eyes. With unresponsive patients, gently open their eyes by sliding back the upper eyelids. Visually check the globe of each eye. Do not apply pressure on the eyeballs.

POSSIBLE FINDINGS: Cuts, foreign objects, impaled objects, and signs of burns may be noted.

WARNING: Do not attempt to open the eyelids of a patient with burns, cuts, or other injuries to the eyelids. Assume there is damage to the eye and treat accordingly.

6. CHECK THE PUPILS FOR SIZE, EQUALITY, AND REACTIVITY.

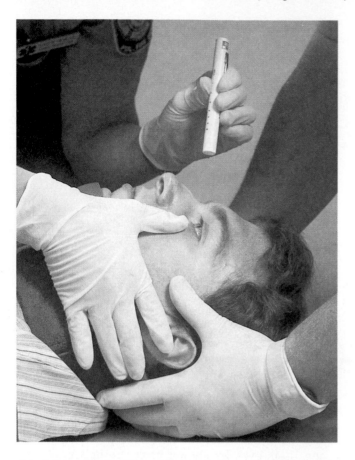

PROCEDURE: Use your penlight to examine both eyes. Note pupil size and if both pupils are equal in size. See if the pupils react to the beam of light.

Note if the pupils are slow to react. Note any eye movements. Both eyes should move as a pair when they *track* persons or objects.

POSSIBLE FINDINGS: Pupils are *normal, constricted* (small), or *dilated* (large). Pupils are either *equal* or *unequal* in size. Pupils *react* to the beam of light, or one or both are *fixed*. The eyes may appear *lackluster* (dull). Tracking may be *normal* or *abnormal*.

Pupil Size	*Possible Cause of Abnormality*
Dilated, unresponsive	Cardiac arrest, influence of drugs such as LSD and amphetamines, unconsciousness from numerous causes
Constricted, unresponsive	Central nervous system disease or disorder, influence of narcotic such as heroin, morphine, or codeine
Unequal	Stroke, head injury
Lackluster, pupils do not appear to focus	Shock, coma

NOTE: Check the unconscious patient for contact lenses. Many EMS Systems' guidelines recommend prompt removal of these lenses to help prevent damage to the patient's eyes. Contact lens removal procedures are described in Chapter 12.

7. INSPECT THE INNER SURFACES OF THE EYELIDS.

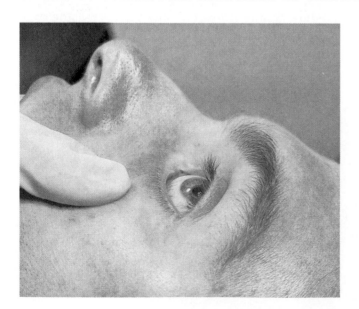

PROCEDURE: Gently pull down either lower eyelid and check the color of the inner surface.

POSSIBLE FINDINGS: Normally these surfaces should be pink. However, with blood loss they become pale or with jaundice, they become yellow.

WARNING: *Do not* attempt to open the eyelid of a patient with obvious eye injury.

8. INSPECT THE EARS AND NOSE FOR INJURY AND BLOOD OR CLEAR FLUIDS.

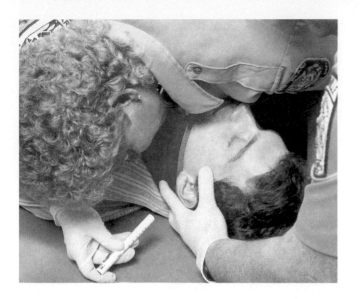

PROCEDURE: Observe the ears and nose for cuts, tears, and burns. Look carefully in the ears and nose for blood, clear fluids, or bloody fluids. Carefully look for bruises behind the ears.

POSSIBLE FINDINGS: Blood in the nose may be the result of simple nasal tissue injury (a bloody nose). It could also indicate a skull fracture. Blood in the ears and clear fluids in the ears or nose are strong indicators of skull fracture. This clear fluid may be **cerebrospinal** (ser-e-bro-SPI-nal) **fluid,** a watery substance that surrounds the brain and spinal cord. Bruises behind the ears are strong indicators of possible skull and cervical spine injury. Burned or singed nasal hairs indicate possible burns to the airway.

WARNING: *Do not* rotate the patient's head to inspect the ears.

9. INSPECT THE MOUTH.

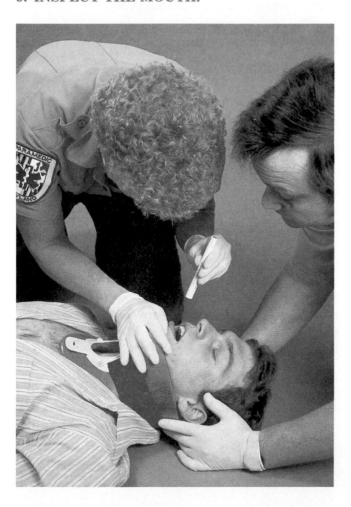

PROCEDURE: Look for anything that may have been missed during the primary survey that may be causing or could become an AIRWAY OBSTRUCTION. Take care not to move the patient's head during this inspection. Look for chemical burns around the mouth.

POSSIBLE FINDINGS: Foreign objects, broken teeth, broken dentures, blood, or vomitus may be found. The tongue may be swollen, discolored, injured, or obstructing the airway. Chemical burns suggest that the patient may have ingested a poison.

10. SNIFF FOR AN ODD BREATH ODOR.

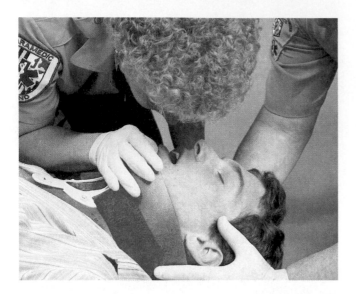

PROCEDURE: Position your face close to the patient's mouth and nose and note any unusual odors.

POSSIBLE FINDINGS: A fruity smell (diabetic coma or prolonged vomiting and diarrhea), petroleum odor (ingested poisoning), or alcohol (alcohol intoxication) may be noted.

NOTE: You will need to expose the examination areas. The lower chest and abdomen must be exposed to observe chest movements, listen for equal air entry, check for penetrations, and palpate the abdomen for tenderness. Be certain to protect the patient from the stares of onlookers. Remember, clothing that cannot be easily rearranged should be cut away.

11. INSPECT THE CHEST FOR WOUNDS.

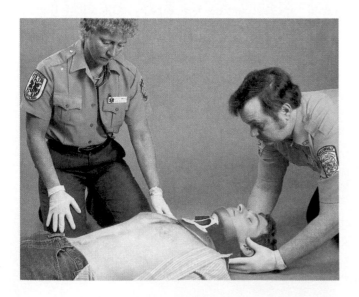

PROCEDURE: Look for obvious injuries. Follow local protocol in regard to baring the patient's chest. It is best to bare the chest of an unconscious patient or trauma patient. If there are any indications of chest injury or the patient has breathing problems, completely bare the patient's chest.

POSSIBLE FINDINGS: Cuts, bruises, penetrations, impaled objects, deformities, burns, or rashes. If puncture wounds are found, they may indicate that an object has passed through the chest. You will have to feel or look for exit wounds when inspecting the back.

12. EXAMINE THE CHEST FOR POSSIBLE FRACTURES.

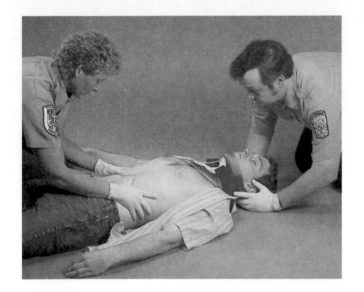

PROCEDURE: Warn the patient of possible pain and gently feel the **clavicles** (KLAV-i-kuls). These are the collarbones. Next, gently feel the **sternum** (STER-num). This is the breastbone. Use your hands to apply gentle pressure to the sides of the rib cage. This process, known as **compression,** usually produces pain in cases of fractured ribs. When applying compression, position your forearms as shown to the left. Finally, gently slide your hands under the patient's **scapulae** (SKAP-u-le). These are the shoulder blades. Feel for deformity and tenderness.

POSSIBLE FINDINGS: Point tenderness, painful reaction to compression, deformity, or grating sounds may occur. If air is felt or heard (crackling sounds) under the skin, this indicates that at least one rib has been fractured or that there is a pneumothorax. (punctured lung). Air is escaping into the chest cavity and the wound.

13. CHECK FOR EQUAL EXPANSION OF THE CHEST.

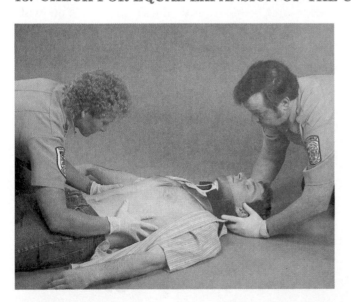

PROCEDURE: Look for chest movements and feel for equal expansion. Be on the alert for sections of the chest that seem to be "floating" or moving in opposite directions to the rest of the chest during respirations.

POSSIBLE FINDINGS: Deformed chest, loss of chest symmetry, or floating (flail) sections may be found.

14. LISTEN FOR SOUNDS OF EQUAL AIR ENTRY.

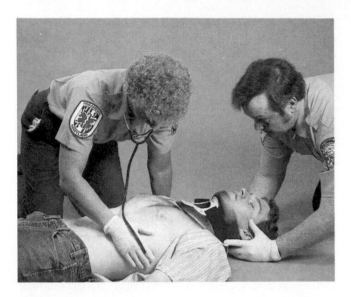

PROCEDURE: Use your stethoscope to listen to both sides of the chest. The sounds of air entry will usually be clearly present or clearly absent. See page 106 for more details.

POSSIBLE FINDINGS: The absence of air movement indicates injury or illness to the internal chest or lungs.

15. INSPECT THE ABDOMEN FOR WOUNDS.

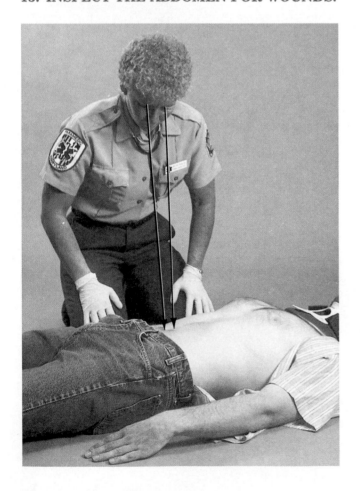

PROCEDURE: Look for obvious signs of injury.

POSSIBLE FINDINGS: Cuts, bruises, penetrations, impaled objects, open wounds with protruding organs (evisceration), rashes, or burns may be seen. The patient may have his legs drawn up to help guard his abdomen.

NOTE: The patient may have had a colostomy (ko-LOS-to-me) or ileostomy (il-e-OS-to-me). You will see a surgical opening in the abdominal wall and a bag in place to receive excretions from the digestive tract. *Do not* remove the bag. Having this bag exposed may be embarrassing to the patient. If you note this bag when rearranging or cutting away clothing, make every effort to keep it covered by clothing or other suitable materials.

16. PALPATE THE ABDOMEN FOR TENDERNESS.

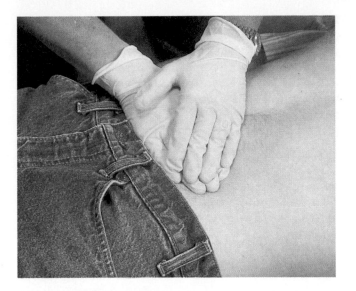

PROCEDURE: Look for any attempts by the patient to protect the abdomen (e.g., knees pulled up). Prepare the patient for possible pain and then *gently* palpate his entire abdomen (all four quadrants). If the patient tells you he has pain limited to a specific area of the abdomen, palpate this site last. When practical, make sure your hands are warm. Press in on the abdomen with the palm side of your fingers, depressing the surface about one inch. Many rescuer's prefer to use two hands, one on top of the other at the fingertips. Do not palpate over an obvious injury site or where the patient is having severe pain. Always start away from an area of pain. Note any painful response. Ask the conscious patient. "Does this hurt?" "Can you feel this?" The patient may show tensing of the abdominal muscles. While palpating the abdomen for tenderness, note any tight (rigid) or swollen (distended) areas. Stay alert for any lumps (masses) that may be felt through the abdominal wall.

POSSIBLE FINDINGS: If the pain is confined to one spot, it is said to be **localized.** Should it be spread over the entire abdomen, it is classified as **general** or **diffuse.** Relate painful responses to the abdominal quadrants. Specifically note guarding, rigidity, distention, masses, tenderness, spasms, or pulsations.

17. FEEL THE LOWER BACK FOR POINT TENDERNESS AND DEFORMITY.

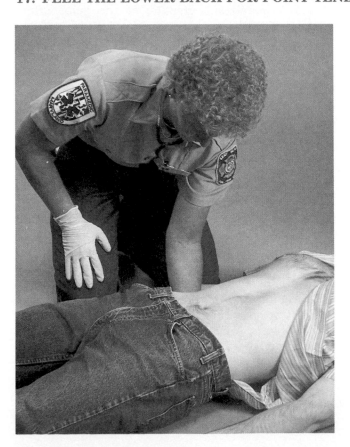

PROCEDURE: Prepare the patient for possible pain and gently slide your hand under the void (space) created by the curve of the spine. Apply gentle finger pressure to detect both point tenderness and deformity.

POSSIBLE FINDINGS: Point tenderness or deformity suggests possible spinal injury and may require you to immobilize the patient's spine before continuing the survey.

WARNING: *Do not* attempt to inspect the upper back of the patient at this time. To do so will require you to lift the patient slightly. You have yet to rule out spinal damage and damage to the upper extremities that could be aggravated by such a procedure.

18. EXAMINE THE PELVIS FOR INJURIES AND POSSIBLE FRACTURES.

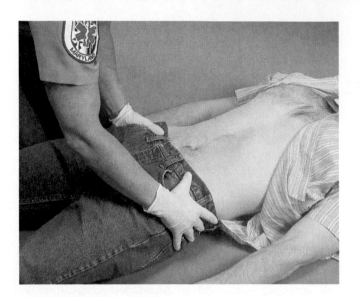

PROCEDURE: Evaluate the pelvic area for obvious injuries. Next, gently slide your hands from the small of the patient's back to the lateral wings of the pelvis and gently apply compression toward the mid-line. Again, warn the patient of possible pain, then lightly apply compression to the pelvis, noting any painful response and pelvic deformities. *Do not* place your hands over any obvious injury site.

POSSIBLE FINDINGS: Penetrating wounds, impaled objects, deformity, and compression pain or pain upon the release of compression may be found. There may be grating sounds if the injury also involves the hip joint or if the pelvis is fractured.

19. NOTE ANY OBVIOUS INJURY TO THE GENITAL (GROIN) REGION.

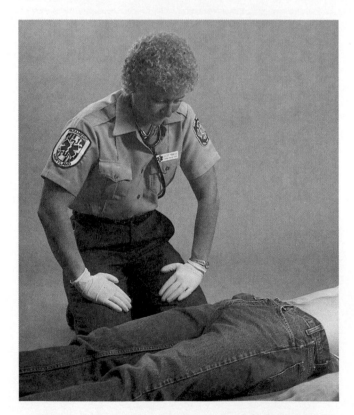

PROCEDURE: Look for bleeding and impaled objects, but *do not* expose the area unless you are reasonably sure that an injury has been sustained.

Look for **priapism** (PRI-a-pizm) in male patients. This is a persistent erection of the penis often brought about by spinal injury or certain medical problems (e.g., sickle cell crisis). Usually, there are other signs of spinal injury or the mechanism of injury requires you to assume that there is spinal injury. Noting this sign by touching the patient will not provide you with any information that will change the care to be rendered.

POSSIBLE FINDINGS: Bleeding wounds and impaled objects, burns, and the spinal injury sign of priapism.

NOTE: When examining the lower limbs and feet, it may be necessary to rearrange or cut away clothing. Injury to the lower limb is best observed with little additional aggravation if pants legs are cut away from the site. Cutting is best done along the seams. If there is a painful response when you feel the patient's foot, or there is no sign of injury, you may not need to remove the patient's shoes (follow local protocol). A pulse can be taken without removing low-cut shoes. If the patient is wearing gym shoes, high-top dress shoes, or boots, it may be necessary to cut the laces or to cut away the footwear if unlacing and removal might aggravate an injury. *Do not* attempt to remove ski boots unless you are specifically trained in the procedure.

20. EXAMINE THE LOWER LIMBS AND FEET.

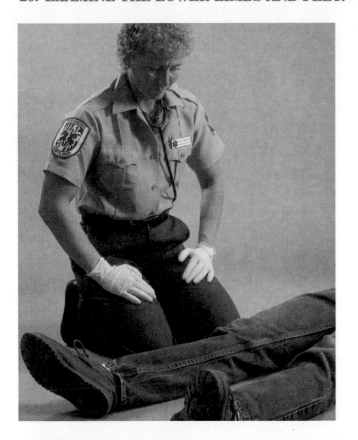

PROCEDURE: Inspect each limb, one at a time, from hip to foot, looking for signs of injury. Look for any abnormal inward or outward rotation of the lower limbs. Gently feel along the front and sides of each limb. Unless the injury is obvious, carefully palpate any suspected fracture site for point tenderness, warning the patient beforehand.

POSSIBLE FINDINGS: Deformities, bleeding, bone protrusions, swellings, and discolorations may occur. One or both limbs may be rotated inward or outward.

WARNING: *Do not* move or lift the patient's lower limbs. *Do not* change the positions of the limbs or feet from the position they were in at the beginning of the examination.

21. CHECK FOR A DISTAL PULSE.

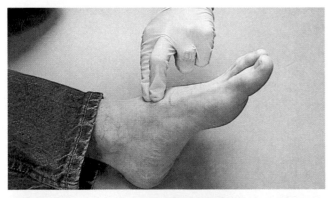

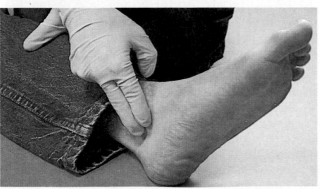

PROCEDURE: You need to know if circulation to both feet is impaired or interrupted. Palpate the distal pulse of each foot either behind the medial ankle (**posterior tibial pulse**) or on the anterior surface of the foot, lateral to the large tendon of the great toe (**dorsalis pedis pulse**). You must bare the patient's foot to palpate the dorsalis pedis pulse. The posterior tibial pulse is not as reliable as the dorsalis pedis pulse because in many healthy, uninjured people this pulse cannot be felt.

Compare the quality of the pulses in each lower limb.

POSSIBLE FINDINGS: Presence of a pulse indicates that circulation is intact, while no pulse suggests that a major artery supplying the limb has been pinched or severed, usually by a broken or displaced bone end or a blood clot.

NOTE: if you are unable to feel a pulse, check for skin color and capillary refill. (See page 205.)

22. CHECK FOR NERVE FUNCTION AND POSSIBLE PARALYSIS OF THE LOWER EXTREMITIES—CONSCIOUS PATIENT.

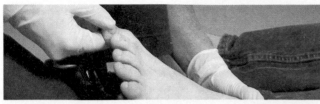

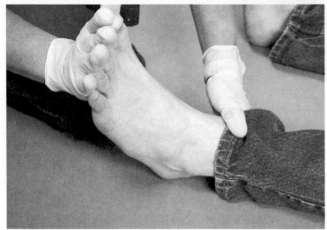

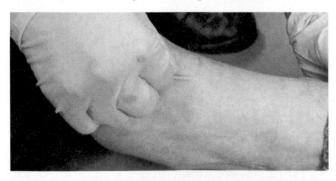

PROCEDURE: Touch a toe and ask the patient to identify which toe you touched. Do this for each foot. If the patient cannot feel your touch or the touch sensations for each foot are not the same, assume nerve damage in the limb or spinal damage (it is best to assume spinal damage). If sensation appears normal, have the patient wave his feet. Finally, ask the patient to press the sole of his foot gently against the palm of your hand. Do this for each foot if there are no signs of injury to the limbs.

POSSIBLE FINDINGS: Failure by the patient to accomplish any of these tasks or any difference in sensations for either limb indicates the possibility of injury to nerve pathways. At this point, ASSUME SPINAL INJURY.

CHECK FOR NERVE FUNCTION AND POSSIBLE PARALYSIS OF THE LOWER EXTREMITIES— UNCONSCIOUS PATIENT. (This may be optional since other signs and the mechanism of injury are more useful. Follow your local protocol.)

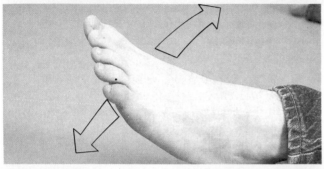

NOTE: Most EMS guidelines now recommend that an unconscious patient be treated as if he has spinal injuries. The field test for nerve action in the unconscious patient is not very reliable. If you have reason to believe that spinal injury has occurred, or if dam-

age to the pelvis, limbs, or feet is severe, do not try this test. Instead, ASSUME THERE IS SPINAL INJURY and treat accordingly.

PROCEDURE: To test the unconscious patient for nerve function, grasp the patient's limb at or near the ankle and pinch an accessible distal area that appears free of injury.

POSSIBLE FINDINGS: The patient, even though unconscious, may show a reflex action by pulling the leg away or by making a pronounced upward or downward toe movement. There should be a reaction to pain. Failure to do so MUST be assumed to be the result of spinal injury; however, movement by the patient does not allow you to rule out possible spinal injury.

23. EXAMINE THE UPPER EXTREMITIES FOR INJURY.

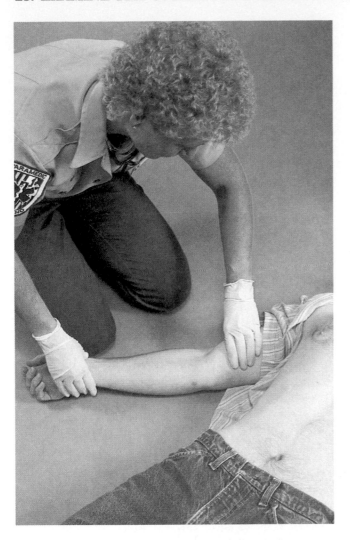

PROCEDURE: Check the patient from clavicles (collarbones) to the fingertips. Look for signs of injury. Check for point tenderness at the site of possible fractures. Look for a medical identification bracelet.

POSSIBLE FINDINGS: Note any deformities, bleeding, bone protrusions, swellings, discolorations, rashes, or burns. Assume point tenderness to mean possible fracture. A medical identification bracelet may be found.

24. CHECK FOR A DISTAL PULSE.

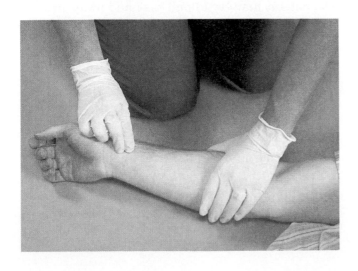

PROCEDURE: Confirm a radial pulse for each limb (see p. 86). *Do not* measure pulse rate. Compare the quality of each pulse. If the pulse is not palpable, check skin color and capillary return.

NOTE: Some EMS systems have the EMT check for capillary refilling. See page 205 for more information.

POSSIBLE FINDINGS: Presence of a pulse indicates circulation is intact. The absence of a pulse suggests shock or that a major artery has been pinched, severed, or blocked by a clot. Most often, this is the result of a fracture to a bone in the limb.

25. CHECK FOR NERVE FUNCTION AND POSSIBLE PARALYSIS OF THE UPPER EXTREMITIES—CONSCIOUS PATIENT.

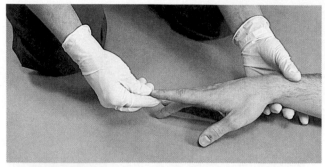

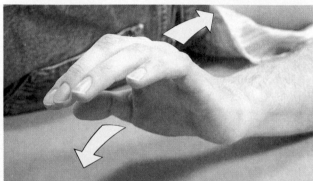

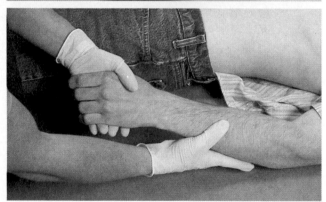

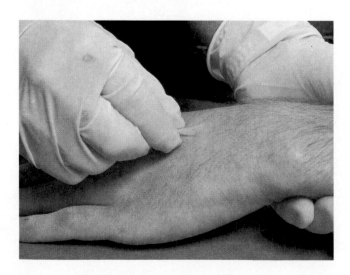

PROCEDURE: Have the conscious, responsive patient identify the finger you touch, wave his hand, and grasp your hand. Do this for each upper limb, only if the extremity is apparently uninjured.

POSSIBLE FINDINGS: If the patient fails to accomplish any of these tasks, there is possible injury to the nerve pathways. At this point, ASSUME SPINAL INJURY.

WARNING: If an awake, alert patient cannot move his hands or arms, be on the alert for the rapid onset of difficult breathing or respiratory arrest. The patient's breathing will have to be constantly monitored.

CHECK FOR NERVE FUNCTION AND POSSIBLE PARALYSIS OF THE UPPER EXTREMITIES—UNCONSCIOUS PATIENT

(optional: other signs and the mechanism of injury are more useful).

PROCEDURE: If the patient is unconscious or unresponsive, grasp his limb at or near the wrist and pinch an accessible distal area. Do this for each limb. The patient may try to pull his hand away or show some other reaction to the pain. If the patient is deeply unconscious, he will not move his hand. This test must be considered to be fairly unreliable under field conditions.

POSSIBLE FINDINGS: Failure of the patient to react to the pain stimulus must be considered to be a sign of possible spinal injury. You would do well to assume that all unconscious trauma patients have possible spinal injury.

Examination Rule No. 9

If a patient fails to respond properly on any test for upper or lower extremity nerve function, you *must* consider this to be a sign of spinal injury.

26. INSPECT THE BACK SURFACES FOR INJURY.

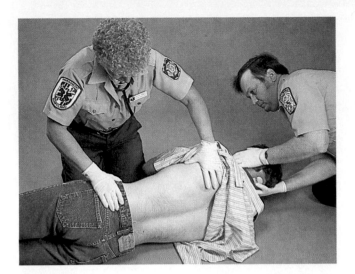

PROCEDURE: Provided there are no indications of injuries to the skull, neck, spine, or extremities, and you have no evidence of severe injury to the chest or abdomen, gently roll the conscious patient as a nit toward your knees and inspect the back surfaces for bleeding and obvious injuries.

The back surface can be inspected prior to positioning the patient for transport or delayed until the patient is transferred to a spine board or other immobilizing device.

POSSIBLE FINDINGS: Cuts, puncture wounds, impaled objects, and burns may be noted.

NOTE: Since possible neck and spinal injuries are difficult to detect in some unconscious patients, your local guidelines may state that this procedure should not be done unless you need to control profuse bleeding or it can be done while repositioning or immobilizing the patient.

The head-to-toe survey appears to be a long process, but as you practice the procedure you will find that it can be done in a few minutes.

After completing the patient examination you will have to consider all the signs recorded and the combinations of these signs that may point the way to specific illness or injury. A *lack* of certain findings may also prove to be important. For example, if the patient has a severe obvious injury, but shows no reactions to indicate pain, you will have to consider problems such as spinal injury, brain damage, shock, or drug abuse. Later in this text, you will learn what care should be provided based on your findings obtained during the patient assessment procedures.

The patient assessment is the most critical professional function of an EMT. It must be done smoothly, efficiently, and as accurately as possible under field conditions. With training and field experience, you will find that this assessment works to gather the information you will need to provide appropriate care.

In this chapter, we listed nine examination rules and mentioned two others. Follow these rules closely to ensure a proper assessment. These rules are:

- Do no harm.
- If the patient's condition warrants, it may be necessary to start transport before the head-to-toe survey can be completed.
- If you notice anything unusual about a patient's awareness or behavior, consider that something may be seriously wrong with the patient.
- Even patients who appear to be stable may worsen rapidly. An EMT must always be aware of changes in a patient's condition. Constant monitoring of patients is an essential part of emergency care.
- You must watch a patient's skin for color changes.

SCAN 3–3 ASSESSING BREATHING SOUNDS

BREATHING SOUNDS:

- Rales—Heard during inspiration. Air is passing through secretions or fluids in lower airway. Sounds range from crackling or powdery to gravelly or gurgling.
- Rhonchi—Coarse "popping" or snoring noises heard during expiration (exception: asthma—also may be heard during inspira-tion). Sounds indicate a narrowing of larger lower airways.
- Wheezing—Heard on expiration. A high-pitched, whistling sound associated with a narrowing of or an obstruction in the lower airways.

SIMPLE ASSESSMENT

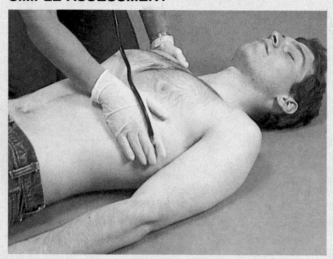

Listen for equal air entry. This can be done for all patients who are breathing.

MIDCLAVICULAR

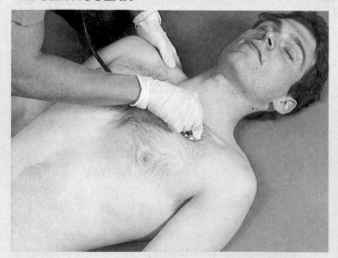

Listen for entry and sounds. For medical patients, assess supine and seated.

MIDAXILLARY

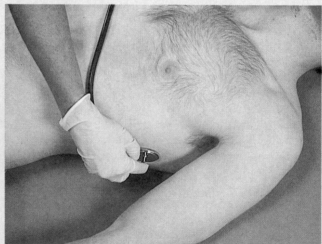

Listen for entry and sounds. For medical patients, assess supine and seated.

- You must look over the patient and note anything that appears to be wrong.
- Unless you are certain that you are dealing with a patient free from serious spinal injury, assume the patient has such injuries. Always assume the unconscious trauma patient has spinal injury.
- Fully explain what you will be doing during the examination.
- Take vital signs. The process will take you a little over one minute. The information gained could save a patient's life.
- Conduct a head-to-toe examination. If *anything* looks, feels, sounds, or smells strange to you, assume there is something seriously wrong with the patient.
- If a patient fails to respond properly on any test for upper or lower extremity nerve function, you *must* consider this to be a sign of spinal injury.

Assessing Breathing Sounds

Most EMS Systems have their EMTs perform breathing sound assessment using a stethoscope. Most EMTs are trained to assess equal entry and breathing sounds for the supine and the seated patient (anterior and lateral assessment). The majority of EMS Systems have been training their EMTs to increase their level of skills in this assessment. See SCAN 3–3.

SUMMARY

Patient assessment is one of the most important things you will learn in your EMT training. Before going back to the chapter objectives, you should review the following:

1. ARRIVAL—Use the information gained from the dispatcher. Gain information quickly from the scene, patient, bystanders, mechanisms of injury, and obvious deformities and signs of injury or illness.
2. PRIMARY SURVEY—This involves assessment of the airway, breathing, circulation, and profuse bleeding. Determine the level of consciousness of the patient. You must make certain that there is an open airway and adequate breathing. You have to confirm a carotid pulse. You must detect and stop all life-threatening bleeding. Attempt to correct all life-threatening problems as they are found.
3. SECONDARY SURVEY—Interview: Look over the scene, look over the patient, and look for medical identification devices. Gather information by asking specific questions and listening to the patient's and bystanders' responses. The more organized you are in the interview, the better are your chances of accurately gaining needed information in a quick and efficient manner.
4. SECONDARY SURVEY—Vital Signs: As part of the examination phase of the secondary survey, you must take vital signs. You have to determine radial pulse rate and character. You must measure respiratory rate and note the character of respirations. You will have to measure blood pressure by auscultation or palpation. You will have to determine relative skin temperature. At this time also note skin color and the general condition of the skin.
5. SECONDARY SURVEY—Head-to-Toe Survey:
   - NECK—Gently examine for cervical point tenderness, midline deformity, and muscle spasms. Check to see if the patient is a neck breather: Examine for neck injury. Look for a medical identification necklace.
   - HEAD—Check scalp for cuts, bruises, swellings, and other signs of injury. Examine the skull for deformities, depressions, and other signs of injury. Include the facial bones. Inspect the eyelids for injury and do the same for the eyes. Determine pupil size, equality, and reactivity. Check for abnormal eye tracking. Note any discoloration on the inner eyelid. Look for blood, clear fluids, or bloody fluids in the ears and nose. Examine the mouth for obstructions, bleeding, and any odd odors.
   - CHEST—Examine for injury (cuts, bruises, penetrations, impaled objects, and fractures). Use compression as a test for fractures. Check for equal expansion and watch for unusual chest movements. Listen for equal air entry (and assess breathing sounds).
   - ABDOMEN—Examine for injuries (cuts, bruises, penetrations, and impaled objects). Check for local and general pain as you examine the abdomen for tenderness, distention, masses, and rigid areas.
   - LOWER BACK—Feel for deformity and point tenderness.
   - PELVIS—Use compression to check for fractures and look for signs of injury.

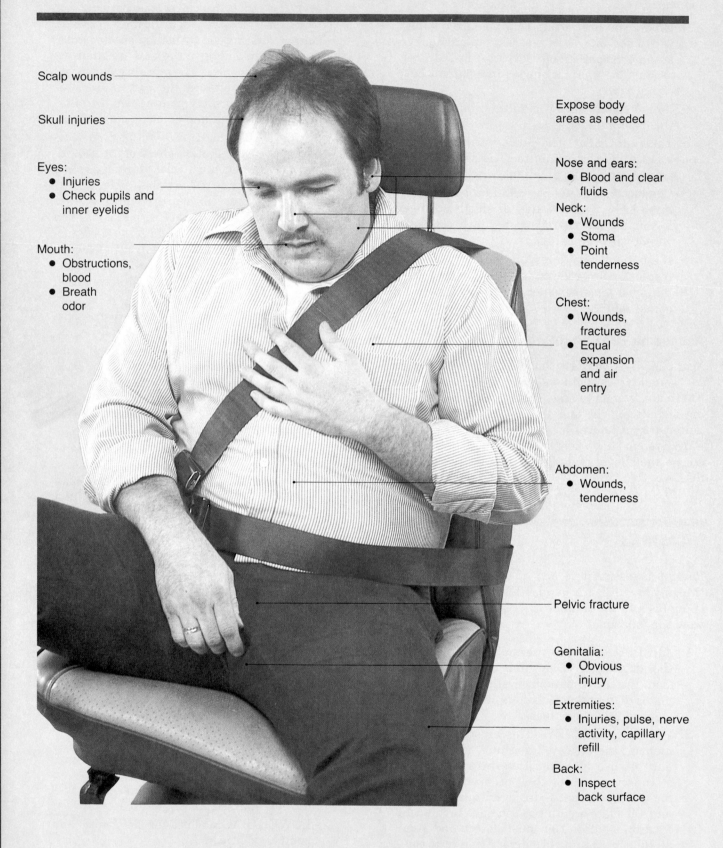

Scalp wounds

Skull injuries

Eyes:
- Injuries
- Check pupils and inner eyelids

Mouth:
- Obstructions, blood
- Breath odor

Expose body areas as needed

Nose and ears:
- Blood and clear fluids

Neck:
- Wounds
- Stoma
- Point tenderness

Chest:
- Wounds, fractures
- Equal expansion and air entry

Abdomen:
- Wounds, tenderness

Pelvic fracture

Genitalia:
- Obvious injury

Extremities:
- Injuries, pulse, nerve activity, capillary refill

Back:
- Inspect back surface

- GENITAL REGION—Note any obvious injury. Look for priapism when assessing male patients suspected of having spinal injuries.
- LOWER EXTREMITIES—Examine for injury (deformities, swellings, discolorations, bone protrusions, and fractures). Run point tenderness tests on suspect fracture sites. Confirm a distal pulse in each limb, and check each lower limb for nerve function. Capillary refill may be checked at this time.
- UPPER EXTREMITIES—Examine for injury (deformities, swellings, discolorations, bone protrusions, and fractures). Run point tenderness tests on suspected fracture sites. Confirm a radial pulse for each wrist and check for nerve function. Check for a medical identification bracelet. Capillary refill may be checked at this time.
- BACK SURFACES—Examine for bleeding and obvious injury, if indicated.

Remember to explain to the patient what you are going to do before you perform the head-to-toe survey. Be certain to warn the patient when there is the possibility of pain. At all times, be reassuring.

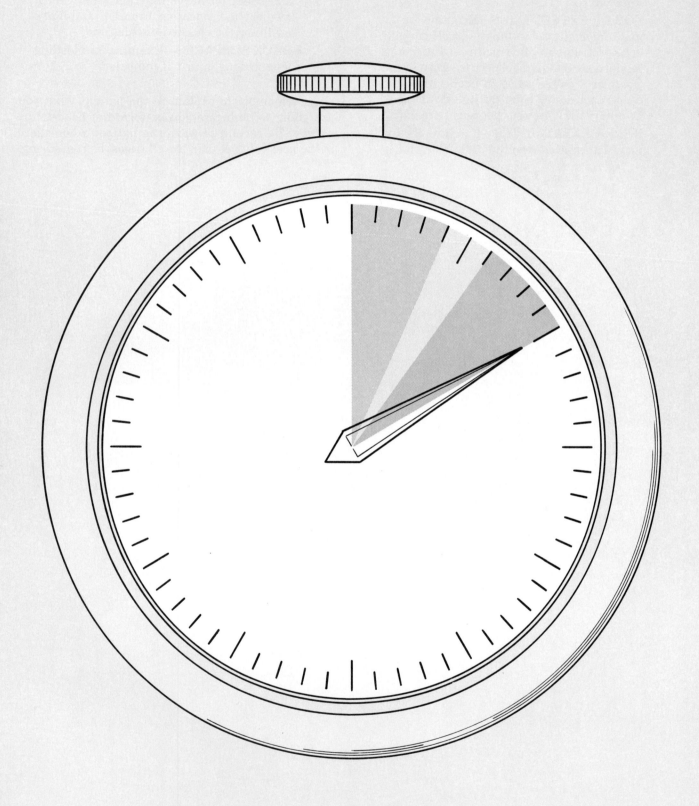

CHAPTER 4

Basic Life Support I
The airway and pulmonary resuscitation

WARNING: It is recommended that prehospital emergency health care personnel reduce the risk of contracting infectious diseases by employing pocket face masks with one-way valves or bag-valve-mask units when ventilating patients (see Chapter 6). Gloves should be worn when clearing a patient's mouth or suctioning the airway.

OBJECTIVES   As an EMT, you should be able to:

1. State three reasons why breathing is essential to life. (p. 113)
2. Define and compare *clinical death* and *biological death*. (p. 114)
3. Name and label the major structures of the respiratory system. (p. 114)
4. Name the major muscles used in breathing. (p. 115)
5. Relate, in general terms, changes in volume and pressure to the process of breathing, (p. 115)
6. List FIVE signs of adequate breathing. (p. 116)
7. List the major signs of inadequate breathing. (p. 116)
8. Describe, step by step, the head-tilt, chin-lift maneuver and the jaw-thrust. (pp. 117 and 119)
9. List, step by step, the actions taken when providing mouth-to-mouth ventilation. (pp. 120–121)
10. Compare and contrast mouth-to-nose ventilation and mouth-to-stoma ventilation with the mouth-to-mouth techniques. (p. 122)

11. List, step by step, the actions taken when providing rescue breathing to an infant or a small child. (p. 122)
12. State what the EMT can do to correct problems of gastric distention caused by artificial ventilation. (pp. 124–125)
13. List FOUR factors that may cause partial or full airway obstruction. (p. 125)
14. List THREE major signs of partial airway obstruction. (p. 126)
15. State when you must treat a partial airway obstruction as if it were a full airway obstruction. (p. 126)
16. Describe TWO signs displayed by a conscious patient with a full (total) airway obstruction. (p. 126)
17. Describe, step by step, the procedures used in correcting airway obstructions, including:
   • Manual thrusts
   • Back blows (infants only)
   • Finger sweeps (pp. 127–130)

18. State the sequence of procedures used for correcting an airway obstruction in a conscious patient. (pp. 131 and 132)
19. List the procedure used for correcting an airway obstruction when the patient being cared for suffers a loss of consciousness. (page 131 through page 133)
20. List the procedures used for correcting an airway obstruction in an unconscious patient. (pp. 131–133)

SKILLS   As an EMT, you should be able to:

1. Determine if a patient has an airway obstruction and if there is adequate breathing.
2. Recognize upper airway obstruction and apply the proper techniques in the correct sequence necessary to correct such an airway obstruction.
3. Properly employ the head-tilt, chin-lift maneuver and the jaw-thrust.
4. Determine respiratory arrest.
5. Correctly perform mouth-to-mouth, mouth-to-nose, and mouth-to-stoma ventilations.
6. Correctly perform pulmonary resuscitation techniques on infants and small children.
7. Correct gastric distention brought about by artificial ventilations.
8. Provide airway care and resuscitation for patients with possible neck and spinal injuries.

TERMS   you may be using for the first time:

Alveoli (al-VE-o-li) – the microscopic air sacs of the lungs where gas exchange with the bloodstream takes place.

Biological Death – when the brain cells begin to die.

Bronchiole (BRONG-key-ol) – the smaller branches of the airway that connect the bronchi to the air sacs of the lungs. The plural of this structure is bronchioles.

Bronchus (BRONG-kus) – one of the first of two large sets of branches that come off the trachea and enter the lungs. There are right and left primary (main-stem) bronchi.

Clinical Death – when breathing and heart action stop.

Cyanosis (sigh-ah-NO-sis) – when the skin, lips, ear lobes, or nailbeds turn blue or gray owing to a lack of oxygen in circulation. The patient is said to be cyanotic (sigh-ah-NOT-ik).

Edema (e-DE-mah) – swelling due to the accumulation of excess fluid in the tissues.

Intercostal (in-ter-KOS-tal) **Muscles** – the muscles found between the ribs. When they contract during an inspiration, the ribs are lifted and spread apart to increase the volume of the thoracic cavity.

Laryngectomee (LAR-in-JEK-to-me) – a "neck breather." The patient has had a surgical opening into or removal of the larynx.

Larynx (LAR-inks) – that portion of the airway connecting the pharynx and the trachea. It contains the voicebox and the vocal cords.

Pharynx (FAR-inks) – the throat.

Pleura (PLOOR-ah) – a double-layered membranous sac. The outer layer lines the thoracic cavity. The inner layer clings to the outside of the lungs. Between the two layers lies the pleural space. Under normal conditions, the inner and outer layers of pleura are in contact, making this a potential space.

Pleural Cavities – the right and left portions of the thoracic cavity, containing the lungs.

Pulmonary (PUL-mo-ner-e) **Resuscitation** – providing ventilations (rescue breathing) to the patient in an attempt to artificially restore normal lung function.

Respiratory Arrest – when a patient stops breathing.

Resuscitation (re-SUS-si-TAY-shun) – any efforts used to artificially restore normal lung or lung and heart function.

Thyroid (THY-roid) **Cartilage** – the Adam's apple.

Trachea (TRAY-ke-ah) – the windpipe.

THE RESPIRATORY SYSTEM

Basic Life Support

There are several conditions that can rapidly cause death, including the cessation of breathing, the absence of breathing and circulation, severe bleeding, and shock. You must be able to detect these problems quickly and take prompt and efficient action.

The techniques used in an attempt to keep a patient alive when he has a life-threatening problem are known as **basic life support.** The procedures used in basic life support use no drugs, intravenous (IV) fluids, or electrical stimulus as would be applied during advanced life support. As an EMT, you must know how to provide basic life support using a minimum of equipment. In some cases, you will have to sustain life with no more than your hands, your breath, a great deal of common sense, and a few basic supplies.

There is more gained by the application of basic life support measures than just keeping a patient alive until he reaches the hospital. It may help stabilize the patient or even allow him to improve during care and transport.

Studies have shown that there is a critical hour called the "golden hour" in caring for trauma patients. If advanced care is not started and the patient stabilized (including Emergency Department and/or Operating Room care) during the first hour after a severe injury, the chances for survival decline drastically.

Basic life support can keep the cardiac arrest patient alive and perhaps stable until definitive care can begin. As an EMT, you will usually be initiating and providing care during the critical minutes of cardiac arrest. You must know all the procedures of basic life support and you must be efficient in performing these procedures.

The Importance of Breathing

The ensurance of breathing takes precedence over all other emergency care measures. The reason is stated simply: if a person cannot breathe, he cannot survive.

The body's cells must be provided with oxygen and have carbon dioxide removed by means of circulating blood. The act of breathing, or **respiration,** is the process that carries oxygen from the atmosphere to the gas exchange levels of the lungs, where it moves into the bloodstream. Also during the process of respiration, carbon dioxide moves from the blood into the lungs, and is carried out into the atmosphere.

A series of chemical processes continually convert food into the energy that is needed for life. These processes are collectively called **metabolism.** Oxygen is required for many of the metabolic processes occurring within the body's cells. An adequate and continuing supply of oxygen is needed to make energy-rich compounds. When these compounds are broken down, the cells again need oxygen for the process. The energy released is used to contract muscles, send nerve impulses, build new tissues, digest foods, and carry out all other life processes.

Carbon dioxide is a waste product produced as a result of certain metabolic processes. If allowed to accumulate in the body, carbon dioxide can become a deadly poison. As the concentration of carbon dioxide increases, a person will start panting, trying to rid the body of the carbon dioxide. Heart rate and blood pressure increase. Soon, brain cells will start to malfunction. The person may become restless or combative. As more carbon dioxide builds up in the body, the person may start to hallucinate owing to the narcotic effects of the excess carbon dioxide. Unconsciousness becomes a strong possibility. Unless corrected, many body functions, including respiration, will fail, causing the person to die.

The process of respiration does more than supply oxygen and remove carbon dioxide. It is difficult for things to stay in balance when there is constant change. Many chemical reactions take place in our bodies, causing such change. Some of these reactions make the blood too acidic, while others make it too basic (alkaline). The respiratory system plays a key role in preventing this by regulating the amount of carbon dioxide that is in circulation. The carbon dioxide is involved in a complex series of reactions that produce chemicals that help to regulate acid–base balance. These compounds are known as buffers. Should breathing become inadequate, the acid–base balance of the blood will become upset, causing cells to die. Some of the cells most sensitive to this imbalance are those in the brain.

The brain and the other structures of the nervous system are very sensitive to a lack of oxygen, an increase in carbon dioxide, or an acid–base imbalance. The brain uses approximately 20% of the oxygen that is in the circulatory system. Even a slight decrease in available oxygen can affect brain function. A marked decrease can lead to drastic changes and, eventually to death.

REMEMBER: Breathing provides needed oxygen for the cells, removes potentially dangerous carbon dioxide, and helps to maintain the acid–base balance of the blood.

Biological Death

The process of respiration cannot be separated from circulation. It is not enough to receive oxygen at the exchange level of the lungs. This oxygen must be transported by the blood to the cells. Likewise, carbon dioxide must be carried to the lungs for removal from the body. You must always relate breathing to circulation, making sure that both processes are taking place. In Chapter 5 we will consider heart action and circulation.

As an EMT, you must know the difference between *clinical death* and *biological death*.

> • **CLINICAL DEATH**—a patient is clinically dead the moment breathing stops and the heart stops beating.
> • **BIOLOGICAL DEATH**—if a patient is not breathing and the heart is not circulating oxygenated blood, potentially lethal changes begin to take place in the brain within *4 to 6 minutes*. Biological death occurs when the patient's brain cells die. *Usually,* brain cell death begins within *10 minutes* after the heart stops beating (this can be delayed by cold temperatures, see p. 489). You may be able to reverse clinical death, but biological death is irreversible.

Respiratory System Anatomy

The major structures of the airway include:

- NOSE—the primary pathway for air to enter and leave the system.
- MOUTH—the secondary pathway for air.
- PHARYNX (FAR-inks)—the throat. The common passageway for air and food.
- LARYNX (LAR-inks)—the neck structure that connects the pharynx and the trachea.

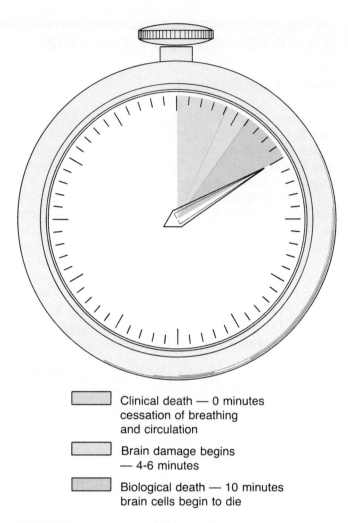

Clinical death — 0 minutes
cessation of breathing
and circulation

Brain damage begins
— 4-6 minutes

Biological death — 10 minutes
brain cells begin to die

FIGURE 4–1. Clinical and biological death.

The voicebox is contained in the larynx. When viewed externally, the most prominent feature is the **thyroid** (THY-roid) **cartilage,** or Adam's apple. A trap-door-like structure, the **epiglottis** (EP-i-GLOT-is), normally prevents food, liquids, and foreign objects from entering the airway as it passes through the larynx.

- TRACHEA (TRAY-ke-ah)—the windpipe.
- BRONCHIAL TREE—branching from the trachea to the microscopic air sacs of the lungs. The first branches are the right and left main stem (primary) **bronchi** (BRONG-ki). These branch into secondary bronchi. The smaller branches coming off the secondary bronchi are called the **bronchioles** (BRONG-key-ols).
- LUNGS—the spongy, elastic organs containing **alveoli** (al-VE-o-li), the microscopic air sacs where oxygen and carbon dioxide exchange takes place. (See page 52.)

Those structures found superior to the larynx are called the *upper airway*. The *lower airway* comprises all the structures from the larynx to the alveoli. The structures of the airway do more than provide a passageway for air to and from the lungs. As air passes through the upper airway, it is filtered, adjusted to body temperature, and humidified. Hairs in the nose start the filtration process, trapping large particles. The mucus on the surface of the airway lining picks up most of the smaller particles. The blood vessels in the airway lining can either provide heat to air that is below body temperature or absorb heat from air that is too warm. The tissues of the lining add water to the air so that it is nearly saturated with moisture. These processes combine to condition the air to help prevent lung damage.

The Thoracic Cavity

Most of the trachea and all of the lungs are situated in the thoracic cavity (see Chapter 2). A double-layered membrane sac, the **pleura** (PLOOR-ah), is found inside this cavity. One layer lines the cavity, while the other layer coats the outside of the lungs.

The portion of the thoracic cavity containing the lungs is called the **pleural portion** of the thoracic cavity.

The thoracic cavity is separated from the abdominal cavity by the **diaphragm.** This is a major muscle used in normal breathing.

Respiratory Function

The physical process of respiration is so constant in a healthy person that he is seldom aware of his own breathing. The act of breathing is an *automatic function*. We can, for short periods, control the rate and depth of our breathing. However, most of the time breathing is *involuntary*, controlled by respiratory centers in the brain that are sensitive to the carbon dioxide level in the blood. The amount of carbon dioxide in our blood is constantly being monitored. If this level becomes too high, we automatically begin to breathe faster and deeper. A low level of oxygen can also be detected, setting off a faster and deeper breathing rate. The structures responsible for this oxygen detection (carotid bodies) are located in the carotid arteries.

If you try to hold your breath, the respiratory centers in your brain will urge you to breathe. Should you try to run, taking very slow, shallow breaths, these centers would automatically adjust the rate, depth, and rhythm of breathing to suit the needs of your cells. If you are asleep, or even unconscious, and if there is no damage to the respiratory centers

and the heart continues circulating oxygenated blood to the brain, your breathing will remain an involuntary, automatic function.

Breathing takes place because of changes in volume and pressure brought about as a result of the combined actions of the muscles attached to the rib cage, the **intercostal** (in-ter-KOS-tal) **muscles,** and the diaphragm. An **inspiration** (the process of breathing in) takes place when these muscles contract. When the diaphragm and the intercostal muscles relax, an **expiration** (the process of breathing out) takes place. An inspiration is an active process, requiring the body to do work (contract muscles). An expiration is a passive process since the muscles involved are relaxing.

A basic law of physics governs breathing: AS VOLUME INCREASES, PRESSURE DECREASES. Consider the moment just before you begin an inspiration. The thoracic cavity has a certain volume and internal pressure. The lungs also have a certain volume and internal pressure. If the volume of the cavity is increased, the pressure within the cavity will decrease. If the volume of the lungs increases, the pressure within the lungs decreases. For an inspiration to take place, there must be a pressure decrease in the lungs to a point where it is less than the pressure of the atmosphere. Once this occurs, air will move from a place of high pressure (atmosphere) to one of low pressure (lungs).

Inspiration and Expiration

You begin an inspiration by increasing the volume of the thoracic cavity. The intercostal muscles attached to the ribs contract and the ribs are pulled outward. The diaphragm flattens downward as it contracts, further increasing the volume in the chest cavity above its position. During this process the pressure on the outside of the lungs decreases and the lungs start to expand. These two events cause the volume of the lungs to increase. AS THE VOLUME OF THE LUNGS INCREASES, THE PRESSURE INSIDE THE LUNGS DECREASES (Figure 4–2). At a certain point, the pressure inside the lungs becomes less than atmospheric pressure. Air begins to flow from an area of high to one of low pressure, or from the atmosphere into the lungs. The air flowing into the lungs helps the lungs to expand.

In the expiration phase, the diaphragm and the intercostal muscles relax. The chest cavity and the lungs are reduced in volume. As the volume is decreased, the pressure increases. At a certain point, the pressure within the lungs becomes greater than the pressure in the atmosphere. Air then moves from an area of high pressure (lungs) to one of low pressure (atmosphere) until the two pressures are equal.

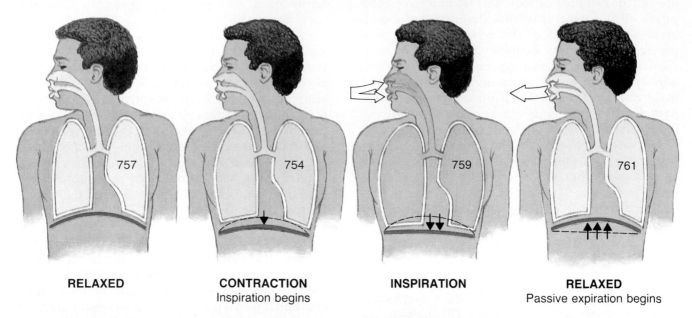

| RELAXED | CONTRACTION Inspiration begins | INSPIRATION | RELAXED Passive expiration begins |

FIGURE 4–2. Changes in volume and pressure produce inspirations and expirations (mmHg = millimeters of mercury pressure).

> The process of breathing is repeated 12 to 20 times each minute in the average adult male at rest, with each breath moving about one-half liter (500 cc or 1 pint) of air.

RESPIRATORY FAILURE

Simply stated, **respiratory failure** is either the cessation of normal breathing or the reduction of breathing to the point where oxygen intake is not sufficient to support life. When breathing stops completely, the patient is in **respiratory arrest.**

Respiratory arrest can develop during heart attack, stroke, airway obstruction, drowning, electrocution, drug overdose, poisoning, brain injury, severe chest injury, suffocation, and prolonged respiratory failure.

Diagnostic Signs

To determine the SIGNS OF NORMAL BREATHING, you should:

- LOOK for the even (bilateral) rise and fall of the chest associated with breathing.
- LISTEN for air entering and leaving the nose or mouth. The sounds should be typical, free of gurgling, gasping, crowing, and wheezing.
- FEEL for air moving out of the nose or mouth.
- CHECK for typical skin coloration. There should be no blue or gray colorations.
- NOTE that the rate and depth of breathing should be typical for a person at rest (see p. 86).

SIGNS OF INADEQUATE BREATHING include:

- Chest movements are absent, minimal, or uneven.
- Movements associated with breathing are limited to the abdomen (abdominal breathing).
- The use of neck muscles during respirations.
- No air can be felt or heard at the nose or mouth, or exchange is evaluated as below normal.
- Breathing is noisy.
- The breathing rate is too rapid or too slow (see p. 87).
- Breathing is very shallow or very deep and labored.
- The patient's skin is blue or gray. This is called **cyanosis** (sigh-ah-NO-sis).

- Inspirations are prolonged (possible upper airway obstruction) or expirations are prolonged (possible lower airway obstruction).
- The patient is unable to speak or cannot speak in a normal fashion.

PULMONARY RESUSCITATION

The procedures for airway evaluation and rescue breathing are best carried out with the patient lying flat on his back. Any movement of a trauma patient before the patient assessment and necessary immobilization of spinal injuries and fractures is complete can produce serious injury to the patient; however, breathing *must* be ensured as quickly as possible. If the patient must be moved, every effort must be made to protect the patient's neck and spine during any repositioning procedure. In Chapter 3, a method was discussed for repositioning the patient. SCAN 4–1 reviews this procedure.

Opening the Airway

As an EMT, you are to ensure an open airway during the primary survey. You may have to open a patient's airway to correct a partial or full upper airway obstruction or to provide rescue breathing for respiratory or cardiac arrest.

Most airway problems are caused by the tongue. As the head flexes forward the tongue may slide into the airway, causing an obstruction. If the patient is unconscious, the muscles of the lower jaw relax. Since the tongue is attached to the lower jaw, the risk of airway obstruction by the tongue is even greater during unconsciousness. The basic procedures for opening the airway help to correct the position of the tongue.

There are several methods recommended for opening the airway.

Head-Tilt Maneuver

WARNING: This procedure is not recommended for use on any patient with possible injuries to the head, neck, or spine. The trauma patient should be conscious. The procedure can be used on unconscious nontrauma patients.

The head-tilt procedure is a simple repositioning of the head (Figure 4–4). For cases in which the patient is conscious and in a seated position, reposition the head so that it does not flex forward on the chest. When the conscious patient is lying

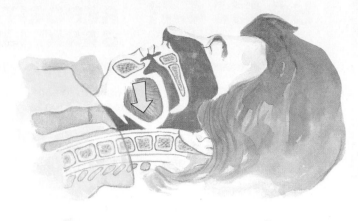
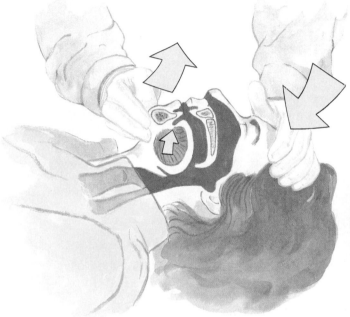

FIGURE 4–3. Procedures for opening the airway help reposition the tongue.

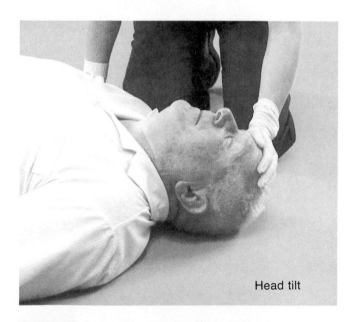

Head tilt

FIGURE 4–4. The head-tilt maneuver.

SCAN 4–1 REPOSITIONING THE PATIENT FOR BASIC LIFE SUPPORT

WARNING: This maneuver is used to initiate basic cardiac life support when you must act alone. For all other repositionings, use the four-rescuer log roll (Chapter 11).

1

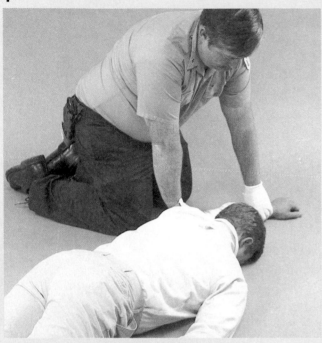

Straighten the legs and position the closest arm above the head.

2

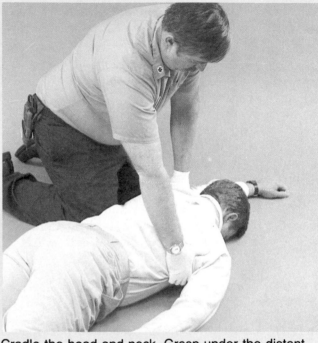

Cradle the head and neck. Grasp under the distant armpit.

3

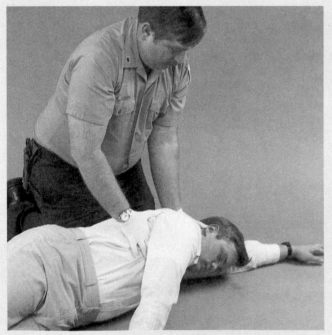

Move the patient as a unit onto his side.

4

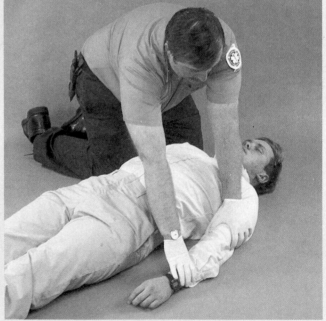

Move the patient onto his back and reposition the extended arm.

down, place one of your hands on the forehead and apply gentle, firm, backward pressure using the palm of your hand. This will tilt the patient's head backward.

In some cases you will find a patient lying down with his head on several pillows or with his head against some object. Repositioning of the head or removal of the object will prevent his head from flexing too far forward.

Head-Tilt, Chin-Lift Maneuver

WARNING: This procedure is not recommended for use on any patient with possible neck or spinal injuries.

This technique provides for the *maximum* opening of the airway. It is useful on both conscious and unconscious patients in need of assistance in breathing, providing one of the best methods for correcting obstruction caused by the tongue. Many rescuers have found that it works well for patients with loose dentures.

One hand is placed on the patient's forehead while the fingertips of the other hand are placed under the chin. The fingertips are used to bring the patient's chin forward and to support the lower jaw. This movement also will help to tilt the head. Most of the head-tilt is provided by gentle pressure applied to the patient's forehead (do not push down on his forehead). During the entire procedure, it is important that you do not compress the soft tissues under the lower jaw and that you lift the chin and move it to a point where the lower teeth are almost touching the upper teeth. The patient's mouth is *not* to

be closed. To provide an adequate opening at the mouth, you may find it necessary to use your thumb to pull back the patient's lower lip. *Do not* insert your thumb into the patient's mouth.

Jaw-Thrust Maneuver

NOTE: This is the *only* widely recommended procedure for use on unconscious patients with possible neck or spinal injuries.

The patient should be lying on his back. Kneel at the top of his head, resting your elbows on the same surface on which the patient is lying. Carefully reach forward and gently place one hand on each side of the patient's chin, at the lateral angles of the lower jaw. Stabilize the patient's head with your forearms, then push his jaw forward, applying most of the pressure with your index fingers (Figure 4–6). *Do not* tilt or rotate the patient's head. For some patients, it may be necessary to retract the lower lip with your thumb.

Rescue Breathing

NOTE: You will be instructed in the basic procedures of mouth-to-mouth and mouth-to-nose ventilations as per AHA guidelines. It is *recommended* that you provide breaths to patients using a pocket face mask with one-way valve, bag-valve-mask, or other acceptable device that protects you from infectious diseases. The use of these devices is covered in Chapter 6. Follow your local protocols in regard to how rescue breathing is to be done in your EMS system.

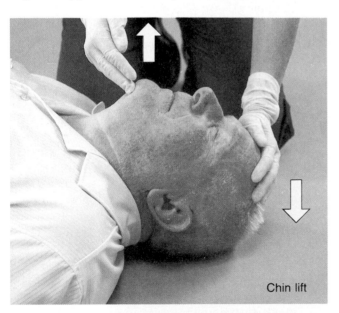

Chin lift

FIGURE 4–5. The head-tilt, chin-lift maneuver.

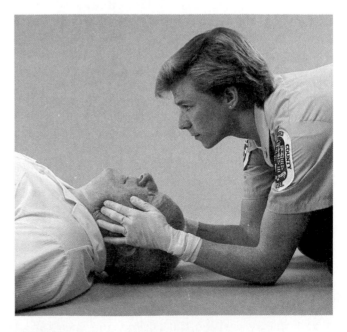

FIGURE 4–6. The jaw-thrust.

Rescue breathing, or artificial ventilation, is called **pulmonary resuscitation** (PUL-mo-ner-e re-SUS-si-TAY-shun). When you perform pulmonary resuscitation, you are providing artificial ventilations to the patient in an effort to maintain normal lung function. The patient may not start *breathing on his own* (spontaneous breathing), but the procedure will help to keep the patient alive by allowing oxygen to enter the bloodstream and carbon dioxide to be removed.

Many students wonder how artificial ventilations provide enough oxygen to the patient, since the air has already been in the rescuer's lungs. Atmospheric air contains 21% oxygen. The air you exhale contains 16% oxygen. This means that the air you provide for the nonbreathing patient still contains about three times the amount of oxygen that is normally removed by the lungs.

NOTE: As an EMT, you must know how to provide artificial ventilations without the use of supplemental oxygen; however, pulmonary resuscitation is much more effective when a high concentration of supplemental oxygen is provided. While on duty, you may start pulmonary resuscitation without using supplemental oxygen, but you must provide this oxygen as soon as possible to render more efficient care and to improve the patient's chances of survival. See Chapter 6 for more information on the use of supplemental oxygen when providing care for the nonbreathing patient.

Mouth-to-Mouth Ventilation

This technique can be performed by one person, with no special equipment (see SCAN 4–2). It is the most expedient of the basic resuscitative techniques, and it is easy for the rescuer to tell if his efforts are effective; however, when performed without a pocket face mask or other adjunct device, the rescuer may be exposed to infectious diseases. Primarily, this procedure is used when the patient is in **respiratory arrest,** that is, when he is no longer breathing. The procedure may be used when a patient's respiratory rate or depth is not sufficient to sustain life.

Keep in mind that you may use the head-tilt, chin-lift maneuver, or if there is a possibility of spinal injuries, the jaw-thrust should be used.

When providing mouth-to-mouth ventilations, you should:

1. Establish if the patient is unresponsive. If you are working alone, call out for help if the patient is unresponsive.
2. Properly position the patient and open the airway. If necessary, remove any vomitus,

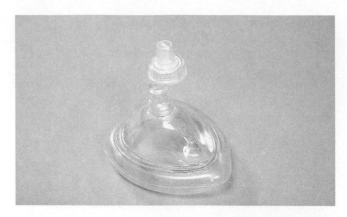

FIGURE 4–7A.   Pocket face mask with one-way valve.

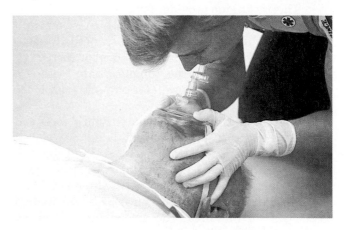

FIGURE 4–7B.   Providing breaths with a pocket face mask.

bloody fluids, or foreign objects obstructing the airway (see pages 129–130).
3. Determine if the patient is breathing and if the breathing is adequate.
   - LOOK for chest movements.
   - LISTEN for air flow (note any unusual sounds).
   - FEEL for air exchange (against your cheek).
   - NOTE anything that appears wrong, such as blue coloration of the skin or abnormal chest movements.
      Take 3 TO 5 SECONDS to determine if the patient is breathing.
4. Maintain the patient in the optimum head-tilt position and pinch the nose closed with the thumb and forefinger of the hand you are using to hold the patient's forehead. You will be safer if you employ a pocket face mask with one-way valve.
5. Open your mouth wide and take a deep breath.

6. Place your mouth on the mask's chimney or around the patient's mouth and make a tight seal with your lips against the patient's face over the top of his mouth.

7. Exhale into the patient's mouth until you see his chest rise and feel the resistance offered by his expanding lungs. Stop when you see the chest rise so that you do not overventilate the patient.*

8. Break contact with the patient's mouth to allow him to exhale passively or allow time for the patient to exhale through the mask's one-way valve. Take in another deep breath and exhale this air into the patient's airway. Each ventilation should take 1 to 1.5 seconds. Allow for deflation between breaths.

9. If the patient does not begin spontaneous breathing after two breaths, check for a carotid pulse (see Chapter 5). If there is a pulse, but no breathing, continue with the following cycle:
   • Take a deep breath and pinch the patient's nostrils closed.
   • Form a seal with the patient's mouth and exhale air into the patient's airway.
   • Break contact with the patient's mouth and allow his nostrils to open. Air should be passively released from his lungs while you . . .
   • Turn your head to watch the patient's chest fall and listen and feel for the return of air.
   • Take another deep breath, close the patient's nostrils, and begin the cycle again.

IMPORTANT: For artificial respirations provided to the adult patient, you must deliver breaths to the patient at **one every 5 seconds** to give a rate of **12 breaths per minute.** To help establish this rate, count, "One, one thousand; two, one thousand; three, one thousand; four, one thousand; five, one thousand."

If you are working alone, make certain that someone alerts EMS dispatch, informing the dispatcher that pulmonary resuscitation or CPR has been initiated.

Once you are breathing for the patient, you must continue to do so until he starts to breathe on his own (spontaneous breathing) or until you transfer the responsibility to another trained person.

* If this initial attempt to ventilate fails, reposition the patient's head and try again.

If you detect cardiac arrest, you must begin CPR, continuing to breathe for the patient as part of this procedure.

You will know that you are *adequately ventilating* the patient if you:

• SEE the chest rise and fall.
• HEAR and FEEL air leaving the patient's lungs.
• FEEL resistance to your ventilations as the patient's lungs expand.

You also may note that his skin color improves or remains normal. In some cases, another rescuer may note that the pupils of the patient's eyes react to light.

The most common *problems* with the mouth-to-mouth technique include:

• Failure to form a tight seal over the patient's mouth (often caused by pushing too hard in an effort to form a tight seal).
• Failure to pinch the nose completely closed in mouth-to-mouth procedures.
• Failure to establish an open airway because of inadequate head-tilt or head positioning.
• Failure to have the patient's mouth open wide enough to receive ventilations.
• Failure to clear the upper airway of obstructions.

Many students wonder how big the rescue breath should be. There is no set answer for this question. That is why it is so important to watch the patient's chest rise and feel for resistance to your breaths. As stated earlier, the average breath of an adult at rest moves 500 cc of air. More air is needed for an effective artificial ventilation. The size should be somewhere between a normal breath and a double-sized breath. You are trying to deliver at least 800 to 1,200 cc* of air to the adult patient. Often, each of these initial breaths turns out to be around 500 cc if you try to deliver the breaths too quickly.

REMEMBER: If there is a possibility of spinal injury, employ the jaw-thrust maneuver to open the airway. Use your cheek to seal the nose. This technique is difficult, even when practiced on a regular basis. The procedure is very tiring for the rescuer. If the jaw-thrust is used, the mouth-to-nose technique is preferred. This is not a consideration if a pocket face mask or bag-valve-mask is used.

* For this size of volume, a cubic centimeter and a milliliter can be considered to be the same thing.

Mouth-To-Nose-Ventilation

Occasionally, you will not be able to ventilate a non-breathing patient by the mouth-to-mouth technique. An accident victim may have severe injuries to the mouth and lower jaw. A patient lacking teeth or dentures may have a pronounced receding chin. For this patient, you may have to use the mouth-to-nose technique. Most of the procedure is very similar to the mouth-to-mouth technique. The airway must be opened, and two breaths are delivered. As with the mouth-to-mouth procedure, breaths are delivered **one every 5 seconds** to equal **12 breaths per minute.** The differences in the mouth-to-nose procedure include:

- You must keep one hand on the patient's forehead to maintain an open airway and use your other hand to close the patient's mouth.
- The patient's nose is left open.
- To provide breaths, you must seal your mouth around and deliver ventilations through the patient's nose. The patient's mouth must be kept shut during delivery of the ventilation.
- When allowing the patient to exhale passively, you must break contact with his nose and slightly open his mouth. You keep your hand on the patient's forehead to help keep his airway open as he exhales.

REMEMBER: The jaw-thrust should be used if there is a possibility of spinal injury. For the mouth-to-nose technique, do not allow the lower lip to retract as you push with your thumbs. Use your cheek to seal the patient's mouth.

Ventilating Infants and Children

NOTE: In basic life support, an infant is any patient from birth to one year of age and a child is any patient from one to eight years of age.

To provide ventilations to the infant or child, you should:

1. Establish whether the patient is responsive. If you are working alone, call out for help if the patient is unresponsive.
2. Lay a child on a hard surface. Cradle an infant in your arms.
3. Open the airway and determine if the patient is breathing. Take 3 TO 5 SECONDS to determine breathlessness.

WARNING: A slight head-tilt is all that is required to open the airway of infants and children. Too great a tilt might actually obstruct the airway of a young infant. If the patient's chest does not rise when you provide a breath, it may be due to an improper head-tilt. Some rescuers are too cautious with the head-tilt. Make certain that you do not underventilate the patient because of a failure to maintain an open airway.

4. Take a breath and cover both the mouth and nose of the infant or small child patient (mouth-to-mouth and nose technique). If a pocket face mask is used, it must be the correct size for the patient.
5. Use SLOWLY DELIVERED BREATHS. Only small breaths are required to ventilate infants. Ventilate TWO times, taking 1 to 1.5 seconds per ventilation, pausing between each to take a breath.

WARNING: You must stay alert for resistance to your ventilations and for chest movements. If you are too forceful with your ventilations, air will be forced into the patient's stomach. Provide a breath that is just large enough to make the patient's chest rise. If your efforts are met with resistance, there may be an upper airway obstruction. Do not use excessive pressure to force air into the lungs.

6. When allowing the patient to exhale, uncover both mouth and nose. Allow for deflation between breaths.
7. Determine pulselessness if the patient is not breathing (Ch. 5). When working alone, have someone phone EMS dispatch to report that pulmonary resuscitation or CPR has been started. If the patient has a pulse, start pulmonary resuscitation and . . .
8. Provide ventilations to the infant as one gentle breath every 3 SECONDS in order to deliver 20 breaths per minute. For the child, provide one gentle breath every 4 SECONDS to provide 15 breaths per minute.

Ventilating Neck Breathers

Although such occasions are rare, you may have to ventilate a neck breather, or **laryngectomy** (LAR-in-JEK-to-me) **patient.** This is someone who has had a surgical procedure in which part or all of the larynx has been removed. The trachea is shortened and is usually brought to the front of the neck as a

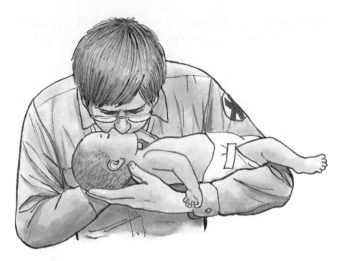

FIGURE 4–8. **Ventilating infants and small children. Deliver one slow breath every 3 seconds for the infant and every 4 seconds for the child. *Do not* hyperextend the neck, but do establish an adequate airway.**

permanent opening called a stoma (Figure 4–9). The patient is called a laryngectomee (LAR-in-JEK-to-me). At present, there are approximately 30,000 laryngectomees in the United States.

A laryngectomy requires the construction of a permanent stoma. A **tracheostomy** (TRAY-ke-OS-to-me), the creation of an artificial opening into the trachea through the neck, may be temporary or permanent, depending on the reason for the surgery (Figure 4–9). The opening of a tracheostomy is round and usually no more than several millimeters in

diameter. This opening often contains two concentric metal tubes, although some patients may have only one tube made of metal or plastic. When two tubes are used, there is an outer tube and an inner one passing from outside the skin to the trachea. In the laryngectomy, the opening is large and round and the edge of the tracheal lining can be seen attached to the skin. There is no metal tube. The method of ventilation is the same for both types of patients.

When you examine a patient's stoma, you may find that there is a breathing tube (or tubes) in the opening. This tube may become clogged and need cleaning. Do not remove the tube. The tube should be cleaned while in place. Quickly clean the neck opening of encrusted mucus and foreign matter using a gauze pad or handkerchief (*do not* use tissue). Pass a sterile suction catheter tube through the stoma and into the trachea. *Do not* insert the catheter more

LARYNGECTOMY   **TRACHEOSTOMY**

Larynx removed
Stoma

Temporary opening

FIGURE 4–9. **Differences between the laryngectomy and the tracheostomy.**

INSERT 3 TO 5 INCHES

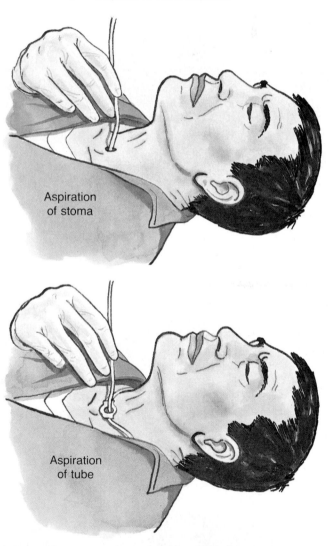

Aspiration of stoma

Aspiration of tube

FIGURE 4–10. **Suctioning techniques for the laryngectomy and tracheostomy patient.**

than 3 to 5 inches into the trachea. Allow suctioning to take place for a few seconds while withdrawing the catheter (see p. 168). *Do not* waste time by attempting to do a complete suctioning. Once the airway is partially open, start mouth-to-stoma ventilations. If approved in your EMS system, protect yourself by using a pediatric pocket face mask over the top of the stoma.

Since the patient's airway from throat to trachea has been interrupted, you will have to use the **mouth-to-stoma** technique on neck breathers (Figure 4–11). Use the same basic technique as for mouth-to-mouth ventilation, but *do not* tilt the head. Best results come from keeping the patient's head straight and his shoulders slightly elevated. Place your mouth directly over the patient's stoma rather than his mouth (mouth-to-stoma ventilation is bacteriologically cleaner than mouth-to-mouth ventilation). Use the same size breaths you normally would during mouth-to-mouth resuscitation, and provide ventilations at the rate of **one every 5 seconds.** Make certain that you watch for the patient's chest to rise and fall as you provide ventilations.

If the patient's chest does not rise, it may mean that the patient is a *partial neck breather.* This type of patient does take in and expel some air through the mouth and nose. In such cases, you will have to pinch closed the nose and seal the mouth with the palm of your hand.

NOTE: Other special patients, including the elderly, near-drowning victims, and accident victims, will be covered in this text. The special problems of airway obstruction and artificial ventilation will be discussed when these cases are presented.

WARNING: You may be exposed to infectious diseases when using the mouth-to-stoma technique. Follow local protocols in regard to the use of a pediatric-sized pocket face mask or other suitable shield.

Gastric Distention

The mouth-to-mouth and the mouth-to-nose procedures can force some air into the patient's stomach. The stomach becomes **distended** (bulges), often indicating that the airway is blocked. This may indicate improper head position or that the ventilations being provided are excessive. This problem is seen most frequently in infants and children but can occur with any patient. A slight bulge is of little worry, but a major distention can cause two serious problems. First, the air-filled stomach reduces lung volume by forcing up the diaphragm. Second, *regurgitation* (the slow expulsion of fluids and partially digested foods from the stomach into the throat) or *vomiting* (the forceful expulsion of the stomach's contents) are strong possibilities. This could lead to additional airway obstruction or the **aspiration** (breathing in) of vomitus into the patient's lungs. When this happens, lung damage can occur and a lethal form of pneumonia may develop.

The best way to avoid gastric distention is to position the patient's head properly, avoid too forceful and too quickly delivered ventilations, and to limit the volume of ventilations delivered. This is one reason why it is so important to watch the patient's chest rise as each ventilation is delivered. The volume delivered should be limited to the size breath that causes the chest to rise.

WARNING: The American Heart Association states that no attempt should be made to force air from the stomach unless suction equipment is on hand for immediate use.

Once gastric distention begins, try to reposition the patient's head to provide a better airway. Be

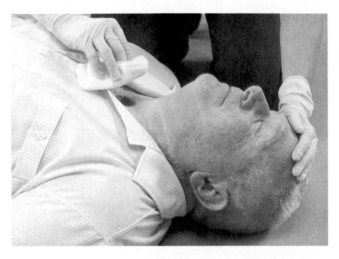

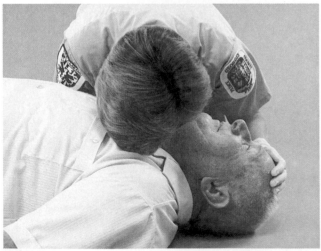

FIGURE 4–11. **Mouth-to-stoma ventilations. If allowed, use a pediatric-sized pocket face mask.**

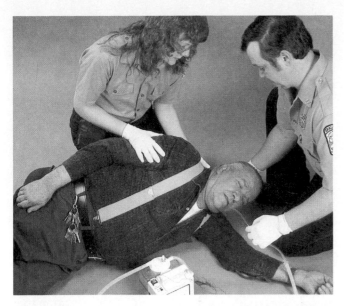

FIGURE 4–12. Be prepared for vomiting when attempting to relieve gastric distention.

prepared for vomiting, and turn the patient to the side should it occur. You have to turn the entire patient, protecting his head and neck. *Do not* simply turn the patient's head. If suction equipment is on hand and the patient has marked distention, you can turn him on his side, facing away from you. Support the patient's head with one hand and use the palm of your other hand to apply moderate pressure to the abdomen between the rib cage and the navel. Be prepared to use suction to clear the patient's mouth and throat of vomitus. Finger sweeps with gloved hands (see pp. 129–130) may also be necessary.

AIRWAY OBSTRUCTION

Causes of Airway Obstruction

Every year in the United States, as many as 3,000 people die of airway obstruction. As noted in Chapter 3, in the ABCs of basic life support, establishing an open airway may be critical. As an EMT, you must be able to quickly detect and, when possible, correct airway obstructions.

Many factors can cause the patient's airway to become partially or completely obstructed, including:

- *Obstruction by the Tongue*—as noted earlier, the tongue can fall back and block off the pharynx (throat). This often occurs when a patient's head flexes forward and is allowed to remain in that position. This problem is most commonly seen with unconscious patients and patients who have abused alcohol or some other drug.

- *Obstruction by the Epiglottis*—attempts by the patient to force inspirations may create a negative pressure that forces the epiglottis (and tongue) to block the airway.

- *Foreign Objects* (mechanical obstruction)— these can include pieces of food, ice, toys, dentures, broken teeth, vomitus, and liquids pooling in the back of the throat. This problem is most commonly seen with children and patients who have abused alcohol or drugs.

- *Tissue Damage*—these accident-related tissue problems can be caused by puncture wounds to the neck, crushing wounds to the face, breathing hot air (as in fires), poisons, and severe injury due to blows to the neck or chest. Swelling (edema, e-DE-mah) of the pharynx and tracheal tissues presents a major problem in providing emergency care.

- *Diseases*—respiratory infection, allergic reactions, and certain chronic illnesses such as asthma can cause edema or bronchial spasms that will obstruct the airway.

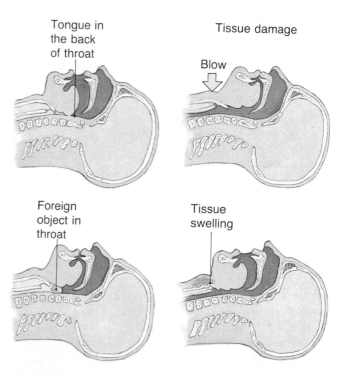

FIGURE 4–13. Four possible causes of airway obstruction.

There is little that the EMT can do to clear obstructions from the lower airway. Most of the time, such obstructions are due to respiratory disease. Upper airway obstruction caused by the tongue or by foreign objects may be cleared using a few simple techniques. These procedures are very important to know. In 1984, the National Safety Council reported 3,100 deaths due to foreign object airway obstruction.

Signs of Partial Airway Obstruction

Keep in mind the mechanisms of injury. Look over the scene. Together, such knowledge will tell you when to be alert for airway problems. Something as simple as noticing a half-eaten sandwich may make a difference.

Be on the alert for partial airway obstruction if you note:

- Unusual breathing sounds. Listen for:
  Snoring—probably caused by the tongue obstructing the pharynx.
  Gurgling—often due to a foreign object or blood and other fluids in the trachea.
  Crowing—probably caused by spasms in the larynx.
  Wheezing—this may not indicate any major problems along the airway. However, wheezing should not be treated lightly since it may be due to serious edema or spasms along the airway.
- Skin discoloration. The patient is breathing, but there is a noticeable blue or blue-gray color to the skin, lips, tongue, fingernail beds, or ear lobes. This is recorded as cyanosis, and the patient is said to be cyanotic.
- Changes in breathing. The patient's breathing may keep changing from near normal to very labored and back again.

A conscious patient will usually point to his mouth or hold his neck trying to indicate an airway problem. Many do this even when a partial obstruction does not prevent speech. Ask the patient if he is choking. Then, ask the patient if he can speak or cough. If he can, then the obstruction is partial. For the conscious patient with an apparent partial airway obstruction, have him cough. A strong and forceful cough indicates he is exchanging enough air. Continue to encourage the patient to cough in the hope that such action will dislodge and expel the foreign object. *Do not* interfere with the patient's efforts to clear the partial obstruction by means of forceful coughing.

WARNING: In cases where the patient *has* an apparent partial airway obstruction but he cannot cough or has a very weak cough, begin to treat the patient AS IF THERE IS A COMPLETE AIRWAY OBSTRUCTION. This rule also applies to the patient who is cyanotic or shows other indications of poor air exchange.

Signs of Complete Airway Obstruction

The *conscious* patient will try to speak, but he will not be able to do so, nor will he be able to cough. Usually, he will display the distress signal for choking, by clutching the neck between thumb and fingers. It will soon become apparent that he cannot breathe. The *unconscious* patient with a complete airway obstruction exhibits none of the usual signs of breathing, namely rhythmic chest movements and air exchange at the nose and mouth. We will study shock in Chapter 7. For now, keep in mind that the typical signs of shock can be seen in unconscious patients with full airway obstruction.

Correcting Airway Obstructions

The conscious patient will usually be able to indicate that he is having problems with his airway. This will allow you to act swiftly to provide an adequate

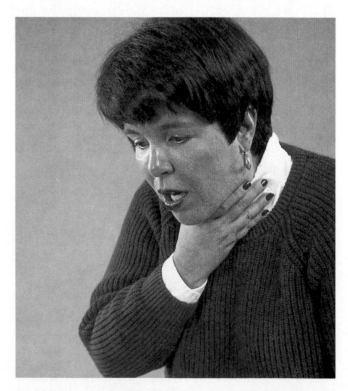

FIGURE 4–14. The distress signal for choking.

airway. However, if the patient is not able to communicate or is unconscious, you must be able to determine quickly that the airway is obstructed and take appropriate measures to clear it. Since so many obstructions are caused by the tongue, you must always make certain the airway is open. Once this is done, two maneuvers are recommended for removal of foreign materials. These are manual thrusts and finger sweeps. On any given patient you may have to use both methods.

When providing care for the unconscious patient, you should not delay opening the airway and checking for adequate breathing. If the patient is not breathing, *do not* waste time looking for an airway obstruction; attempt to provide the initial ventilations that are part of pulmonary resuscitation. If there is an obstruction, it will become evident once you try to ventilate.

The techniques used in clearing the airway vary depending on whether the patient is conscious, loses consciousness while being treated, or is unconscious. We will begin by describing the techniques used to clear the airway, then we will apply specific procedures to each type of patient.

NOTE: If the cause of airway obstruction is blood, liquids, or vomitus pooling in the throat, you should consider the use of sunctioning to clear the airway (see Chapter 6). However, *do not* delay efforts to clear the airway in order to locate and set up suctioning equipment.

Manual Thrusts—Abdominal

Abdominal thrusts are used to force a burst of air from the lungs that will be sufficient to dislodge an obstructing object.

WARNING: Do not use abdominal thrusts on pregnant patients or infants and very small children.

With the conscious patient standing or sitting:

1. Stand behind him and slide your arms under his armpits, wrapping both of your arms around his waist.

2. Make a fist and place the thumb side of this fist against the midline of the patient's abdomen, between the waist and rib cage. Avoid touching the patient's chest, especially the area immediately below the sternum (the region of the xiphoid process).

3. Grasp your properly positioned fist with your other hand and apply pressure inward and up toward the patient's diaphragm in one smooth movement. This will cause your fist to press into the patient's abdomen. Deliver SIX TO TEN RAPID INWARD THRUSTS up toward the diaphragm.

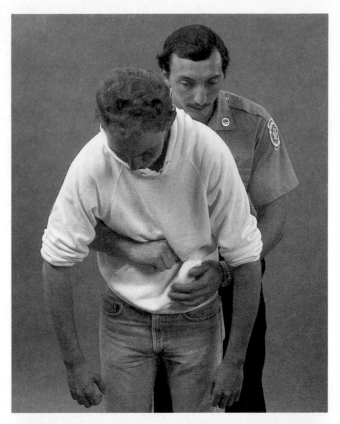

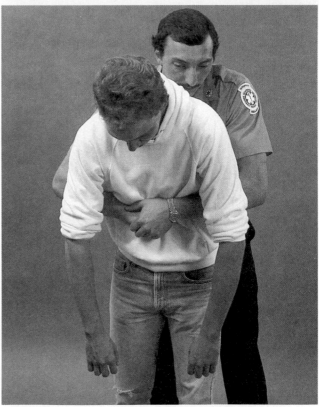

FIGURE 4–15. **Abdominal thrusts. Place your fist on the patient's midline, between the waist and rib cage. Grasp this fist and rapidly deliver six to ten inward and upward thrusts.**

Abdominal thrusts are best delivered to the unconscious patient when he is in a supine position. The same technique can be used for a conscious patient who cannot sit up or be seated with your assistance. When the patient is lying down:

1. Move the patient into a supine position.
2. Kneel and straddle the patient at the level of the hips, facing his chest.
3. Place the heel of your hand on the midline of his abdomen, slightly above the navel and below the xiphoid process.
4. Now place your free hand over the positioned hand and lock your arms at the shoulders and elbows. Your shoulders should be directly over the patient's abdomen.
5. Deliver compressions by pressing your hands inward and upward toward the patient's diaphragm. Deliver SIX TO TEN RAPID ABDOMINAL THRUSTS.

If the patient is very large or if you are a small individual, you can deliver more effective thrusts if you straddle one leg of the patient.

Manual Thrusts—Chest

The chest thrust is used in place of abdominal thrusts when the patient is pregnant, when a patient is too large for you to wrap your arms around his waist, or for infants and very small children.

When the conscious adult patient is standing or sitting:

1. Position yourself behind the patient and slide your arms under his armpits, so that you encircle his chest.

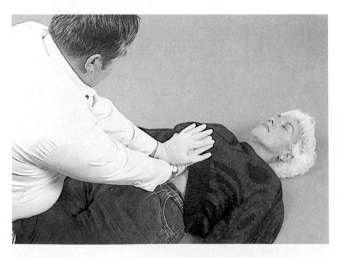

FIGURE 4–16. Abdominal thrust technique used on a patient who is supine.

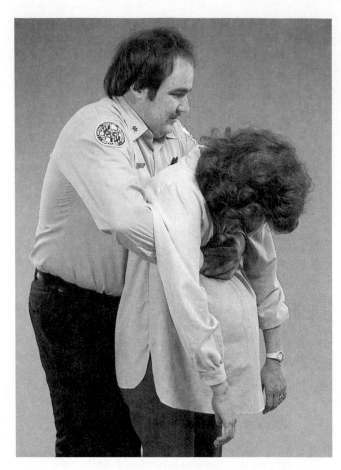

FIGURE 4–17.   The chest thrust applied to a pregnant patient.

2. Form a fist with one hand and place the thumb side of this fist on the patient's sternum. You should make contact with the midline of the sternum, about two to three finger widths above the xiphoid process.
3. Grasp the fist with your other hand and rapidly deliver thrusts directly backward until the object is expelled or the patient loses consciousness (p. 131). Do not exert this force in an upward or downward direction or off to one side.

Again, the best procedure for an unconscious adult patient is carried out when the patient is in a supine position. Once the patient is properly positioned, you should:

1. Kneel alongside the patient at the level of the chest. Have both of your knees facing the patient's chest.
2. Position the heel of one hand on the midline of the sternum, two to three finger widths from the lower tip (your fingers should be perpendicular to the sternum). Lift and

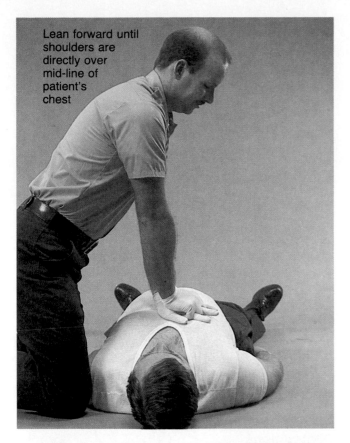

Lean forward until shoulders are directly over mid-line of patient's chest

FIGURE 4–18. The chest thrust method can be used when the patient is lying on his back.

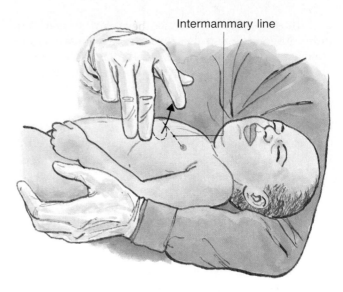

Intermammary line

FIGURE 4–19. For infants, chest thrusts are applied to the middle of the sternum, one finger width below the intermammary line.

spread your fingers to avoid applying too much pressure to the ribs.

3. Place your other hand on top of the first, interlocking your fingers. Lock your elbows and lean forward until your shoulders are directly over the midline of the patient's chest.

4. Deliver DISTINCT THRUSTS in a downward direction, applying enough force to compress the chest cavity. Continue until the object is expelled.

If you find it necessary to use the chest thrust procedure on an infant or small child, you should:

1. Place the patient in a face-up position on your thigh, making certain that you provide adequate support for the head throughout the turn.

2. Reposition the patient so that the head is lower than the trunk.

3. Deliver FOUR SLOW DISTINCT CHEST THRUSTS, using the tips of two or three fingers, applying pressure along the midline of the sternum, with the index finger placed

just below (one finger width) an imaginary line drawn directly between the nipples.

If your patient is a very small child but is too large to hold, support the child's head and back and place him face up on the floor or ground. Apply FOUR CHEST THRUSTS to the sternum, between the nipples, using the heel of one hand.

Finger Sweeps

Manual removal of an object can be tried if the object is dislodged or partially dislodged. Wear gloves to protect yourself from infectious agents. Always take great care not to force the object farther down the patient's throat. This is especially true in infants and small children. *Do not use "blind" finger sweeps and probes in infants and children.* You *must* see the object before trying to grasp it with your fingers. For infants and small children, use your little finger.

You can open an unconscious patient's mouth and airway by using the **tongue-jaw lift** procedure. This requires you to grasp both tongue and lower jaw between your gloved thumb and fingers and lift to move the tongue away from the back of the pharynx. This movement will also move the tongue away from any foreign object that might be lodged in the back of the throat. The procedure may partially solve the problem of obstruction. However, it will be necessary to keep the patient's face up and insert the index finger of your free gloved hand into the patient's mouth and move this finger along the inside of the cheek to the base of the tongue. Using your finger as a hook, attempt to dislodge the object and sweep it into the mouth so it can be removed.

In some cases, it may be necessary to use your index finger to push the foreign object against the opposite side of the patient's throat in order to dislodge and lift the object. During such a procedure, you must take extra care not to push the object farther down the patient's throat.

WARNING: A conscious patient has a gag reflex that can induce vomiting. This vomitus can be aspirated into the lungs. This is why EMS Systems do not sanction the use of finger sweeps on conscious patients. Some localities believe that there are situations in which aggressive actions must be taken during basic life support. If an obstructing object becomes visible, the EMT can use a finger sweep to dislodge and remove the object. If you are using a finger sweep method on a conscious patient, or you are trying to grasp a dislodged object, take great care not to induce vomiting or force the object farther down the patient's airway. Stay alert to avoid being bitten by the patient.

You can use the crossed-finger technique to open the mouth of an unconscious patient (Figure 4–20). Use one gloved hand to steady the patient's forehead. Take your free gloved hand and cross the thumb under the index finger. Place your thumb against the patient's lower lip and your index finger against his upper teeth. Crossing the thumb and finger will force open the patient's mouth. Once the mouth is open, hold the lower jaw so that it cannot close.

Once you have opened the patient's mouth, release the the patient's forehead and use the index finger of this hand as you would in the tongue-jaw lift procedure.

NOTE: When using the finger sweep technique, remember: If the object comes within reach, grasp the

object and remove it. Be careful not to push it down the patient's airway. Be prepared for the patient to vomit.

Back Blows

Back blows can be used when providing care for infants and very small young children. An **infant** is any patient between birth and one year of age. (A **child** is any patient between the ages of one and eight.) When the patient is an infant or small child, cradle the patient face down on your forearm, with the head lower than the trunk. Best results can be obtained if you are seated and rest this forearm on one of your thighs. You MUST support the patient's head by placing a hand around the lower jaw and chest. Use the heel of your free hand to rapidly deliver FOUR SHARP BLOWS to the spinal area between the shoulder blades.

NOTE: Do NOT place infants or small children into this head-down position if they have a partial obstruction and can breathe adequately in an upright position. Keep in mind that forceful coughing is a good sign in cases of partial airway obstruction.

Procedures for Correcting Airway Obstructions

A procedure or combination of procedures used to clear the airway is considered to be effective if any of the following happen:

- The patient reestablishes good air exchange or spontaneous breathing.
- The foreign object is expelled from the mouth.
- The foreign object is expelled into the mouth where it can be removed by the rescuer.

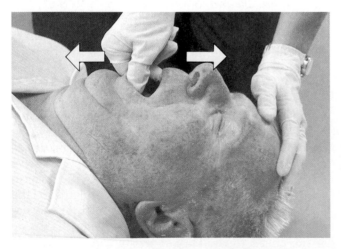 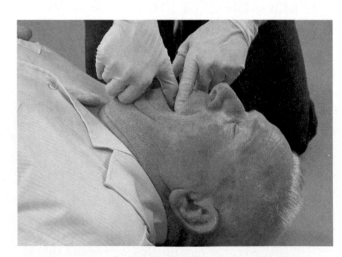

FIGURE 4–20.   Open the patient's mouth using the crossed-fingers technique. Use finger sweeps to remove foreign objects from the airway and mouth.

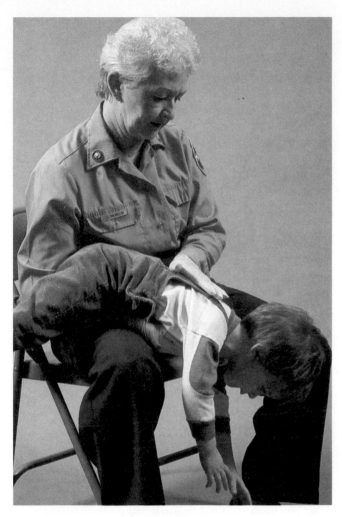

FIGURE 4–21. **Cradle the *infant* face down on your forearm. (Child model used for demonstration purposes only.)**

- The patient regains consciousness.
- The patient's skin color improves.

When an obstruction is not easily corrected, you will have to combine procedures in an attempt to open the airway.

The use of manual thrusts requires a little common sense. Even though six to ten abdominal thrusts are called for, if the first one works, the remaining thrusts are not needed. You must stay aware of what is happening to the patient when applying the procedure. The thrusts are to be delivered rapidly, but some restraint is needed. Too forceful and too rapid a blow may injure the patient. An improperly delivered thrust may cause damage in the thoracic or abdominal cavity. Trying to do the thrusts as quickly as you can move will probably cause you to lose your balance and deliver an improper and possibly harmful thrust. You must practice these techniques on the manikins provided in your course and keep your skills up to date.

If a person has only a partial airway obstruction and is still able to speak and cough forcefully, *do not* interfere with his attempts to expel the foreign body. Carefully watch him, however, so that you can immediately provide help if this partial obstruction becomes a complete one.

An unconscious patient or a conscious patient with total airway obstruction will present the greatest problems.

Conscious Adult Patient If the adult patient is conscious, you should:

1. Determine if there is a COMPLETE OBSTRUCTION or poor air exchange. Look, listen, and feel for the signs of complete obstruction. Be certain to ask, "Are you choking?" or "Can you speak?" If the patient can speak, see if he can produce a forceful cough. If the patient has a complete obstruction or poor air exchange . . .
2. Provide SIX TO TEN ABDOMINAL THRUSTS in rapid succession. If the manual thrusts have not expelled the obstruction . . .
3. Repeat the thrusts until you are successful or the patient loses consciousness.

REMEMBER: Chest thrusts must be used for infants and small children, for very obese patients, and for pregnant patients.

Adult Patient Loses Consciousness If the patient loses consciousness, you should:

1. Protect the patient who suffers a loss of consciousness from possible injury due to falling. Establish unresponsiveness. If you are working alone, call out for help.
2. Use the tongue-jaw lift to open the mouth. Perform finger sweeps.
3. Open the airway and attempt to ventilate. If this fails . . .
4. Deliver SIX TO TEN ABDOMINAL THRUSTS.
5. Repeat the tongue-jaw lift and finger sweeps.
6. Open the airway and repeat your attempt to ventilate the patient. If this fails . . .
7. Continue with the following cycle until you are successful:
   - Abdominal thrusts
   - Finger sweeps
   - Attempt to ventilate

Unconscious Adult Patient If the patient is unconscious when you arrive:

1. Establish unresponsiveness. If you are working alone, call out for help.
2. Position the patient on his back with the arms at his side.
3. Attempt to open the patient's airway by the head-tilt, chin-lift (no possible trauma), or jaw-thrust maneuver. Remember to look, listen, and feel for breathing.
4. Provide mouth-to-mask ventilations or pinch the patient's nostrils closed. Typically, this is done with the hand used to hold the patient's forehead. Try to give TWO VENTILATIONS as described in the section on mouth-to-mouth ventilation (see pp. 120–121). You can usually tell if ventilation will be successful after the first attempt. When working alone, have someone alert the EMS dispatch. If your attempts to ventilate the patient fail, you should . . .
5. Reposition the patient's head, attempt to create an open airway, and try to ventilate. If this fails . . .
6. Provide SIX TO TEN abdominal thrusts in rapid succession. If this fails . . .
7. Use the tongue-jaw lift and attempt finger sweeps. After removing the object, or if you cannot find and remove the obstruction, you should . . .
8. Open the airway and attempt to ventilate. If attempts to ventilate fail . . .
9. Continue with the cycle of abdominal thrusts, finger sweeps, and attempts to ventilate until successful.

If you are unable to dislodge the obstruction, you have a critical emergency, requiring transport to a medical facility without delay. You must continue efforts to clear the obstruction, even if you can do no more than partially dislodge the object. The chances of at least partially dislodging the object will improve with time as the muscles of the patient's jaw and upper airway relax. Once the object is partially dislodged, you should be able to keep the patient alive by artificial ventilations. Keep in mind that cardiopulmonary resuscitation may be necessary.

REMEMBER: You must persist in your efforts until the airway is clear or until you have dislodged the object enough to allow for you to provide artificial ventilations. If the patient's brain cells do not receive oxygen, they will begin to die within 10 minutes.

Keep in mind that procedures used to clear the airway may at first fail, only to be successful later as muscles in the patient's body relax.

Conscious Child Start by determining if there is an airway obstruction. Ask the child, "Are you choking?" "Can you speak?" "Can you cough?" If the child cannot cough or has an ineffective cough, or if the child's breathing problems continue to worsen, deliver SIX TO TEN abdominal thrusts. Continue with the thrusts until the object is expelled or the child loses consciousness.

Child Loses Consciousness If the child who has an airway obstruction loses consciousness while you are providing care, provide the same care as you would for an adult, but DO NOT ATTEMPT BLIND FINGER SWEEPS (look for and remove any visible foreign objects). Abdominal thrusts are best delivered if you kneel at the child's feet. You may place the child on a table and stand at his feet.

If your attempts to clear the airway fail, continue the cycle of abdominal thrusts, finger sweeps, and attempts to ventilate until you are successful.

Unconscious Child If the child is unconscious when you arrive, carry out the same procedures as you would for an adult patient. The abdominal thrusts are best delivered if you kneel at the child's feet. You may place the child on a table and stand at his feet.

DO NOT attempt to provide blind finger sweeps. Look for and remove any visible foreign objects.

If you fail at your attempts to clear the airway, repeat the cycle of abdominal thrusts, visible foreign object removal, and attempts to ventilate until you are successful.

Conscious Infant If the patient is a conscious infant who requires your assistance to clear an airway obstruction, you should:

1. Determine that there is an airway obstruction by assessing breathing difficulties.
2. Support the infant's head with one hand and straddle him face down on your forearm. Support your forearm on your thigh. Keep the infant's head lower than his trunk.
3. Deliver FOUR BACK BLOWS in 3 to 5 seconds. If this fails . . .
4. Support the infant's head and sandwich him between your hands. Turn the patient over on the back, keeping the head lower than the trunk.
5. Deliver FOUR CHEST THRUSTS, using the tips of two or three fingers, applying pressure

along the midline of the sternum, with the index finger placed just below (one finger width) an imaginary line drawn directly between the nipples. Deliver the compressions more slowly than you would during CPR (see page 156).

6. Continue with the sequence of back blows and chest thrusts until the object is expelled or the infant loses consciousness.

NOTE: The above procedures are recommended only in cases where the infant's problem is a known or strongly suspected obstruction due to a foreign object, vomitus, or blood. If the problem is caused by tissue swelling related to an allergy or infection, transport the infant and follow the care protocol for epiglottitis as explained on p. 429.

Infant Loses Consciousness   If the infant suffers a loss of consciousness while you are attempting to clear the airway, you should:

1. Establish unresponsiveness. If working alone, call out for help.
2. Position the patient and use the tongue-jaw lift. Look for and remove any visible foreign objects. DO NOT use blind finger sweeps.
3. Attempt to ventilate. If this fails . . .
4. Deliver FOUR back blows. If this fails . . .
5. Deliver FOUR chest thrusts.
6. Employ the tongue-jaw lift and look for and remove any foreign objects. DO NOT use blind finger sweeps.
7. Reattempt to ventilate. If this fails . . .
8. Continue with the sequence of back blows, chest thrusts, foreign object removal (not "blind"), and attempts to ventilate until you are successful.

Unconscious Infant   If the infant is found unconscious:

1. Establish unresponsiveness. When alone, call out for help.
2. Place the infant on his back, supporting the head and neck.
3. Open the airway and establish breathlessness.
4. Attempt to ventilate, using the mouth-to-mouth and nose technique (see p. 122) or appropriate mouth-to-mask technique or other approved delivery device. Should this fail . . .
5. Reposition the patient's head and attempt to ventilate. If this fails . . .

6. Support the infant's head with one hand and straddle him face down over your forearm. Support your forearm with your thigh. Keep the infant's head lower than his trunk and deliver FOUR back blows in 3 to 5 seconds. If this fails . . .
7. Sandwich the infant between your arms and place the patient in a face-up position on your thigh (protect the head). Deliver four chest thrusts, keeping the head lower than the trunk. Deliver the FOUR thrusts in 3 to 5 seconds. If this fails . . .
8. Insert your gloved thumb into the mouth, over the tongue. Wrap your fingers around the lower jaw and lift the tongue and jaw forward, opening the patient's mouth. Look for any objects causing the obstruction. If you can see the object, remove it using your little finger, but *do not* attempt "blind" finger sweeps. If you cannot see and remove an object . . .
9. Open the airway and attempt to ventilate using the mouth-to-mouth and nose or appropriate mouth-to-mask technique.
10. Repeat the sequence of:
    • Back blows
    • FOUR chest thrusts
    • Looking for and removing visible objects
    • Attempts to ventilate until you are successful.

Should the patient develop respiratory arrest and you have cleared enough of the obstruction to provide adequate ventilation, provide two breaths and check for heart action to see if CPR must be initiated (see Chapter 5).

SUMMARY

We breathe to bring in oxygen, to remove carbon dioxide, and to help regulate the acid–base balance of our blood. The major muscle of respiration, the diaphragm, and the intercostal muscles contract to increase the volume in the thoracic cavity. The lungs expand, thus becoming greater in volume. As the volume increases, the pressure decreases. When the pressure in the lungs decreases to less than the atmosphere, air rushes into the lungs (an inspiration). When the diaphragm and the intercostal muscles relax, the volume in the lungs decreases, causing the pressure to increase. Once the pressure becomes

SCAN 4-2 CLEARING THE AIRWAY— UNCONSCIOUS INFANT

1

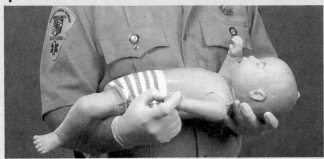

Establish unresponsiveness. Position the infant.

2

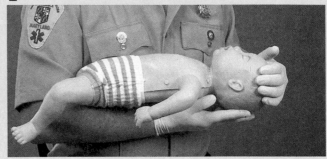

Open airway. Establish breathlessness.

3

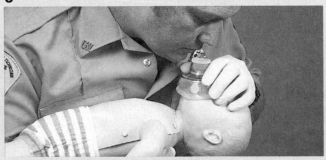

Attempt to ventilate. If this fails, reposition head and try again.

4

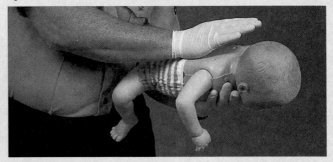

Deliver 4 back blows.

5

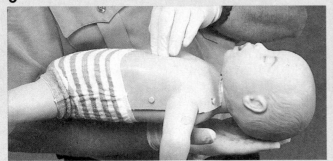

Deliver 4 chest thrusts.

6

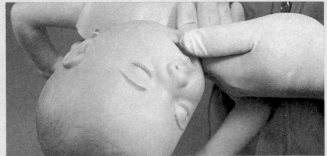

Remove visible objects.

7

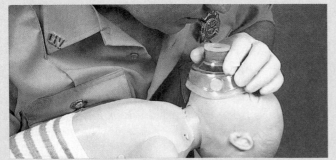

Reattempt to ventilate.

8

Repeat the sequence of:

- Back blows
- Chest thrusts
- Removing visible objects
- Reattempting ventilations.

greater than that of the atmosphere, air rushes out of the lungs (an expiration). All of this is an involuntary, automatic process, controlled mainly by respiratory centers in the brain.

Clinical death occurs when an individual stops breathing and the heart stops beating. Biological death occurs when the brain cells start to die. This takes place when the brain cells are without oxygen for approximately 10 minutes.

In addition to the respiratory centers in the brain, the diaphragm, and the muscles between the ribs, the respiratory system includes the nose and mouth, the pharynx (throat), the larynx (including the voicebox and the epiglottis), the trachea (windpipe), the bronchial tree (from bronchi through the bronchioles), and the lungs with their microscopic alveoli.

When evaluating a patient for adequate breathing, look for the chest movements associated with breathing, listen and feel for air exchange, and note anything that may indicate problems with breathing (unusual rate, depth, and skin color changes).

The most common cause of airway obstruction is the tongue. Opening the airway can sometimes be done by simply repositioning the patient's head or performing a head-tilt maneuver.

If the patient does not have spinal injuries, the head-tilt, chin-lift maneuver can be employed. If there is any possibility of spinal injury, the jaw-thrust should be used. Do not hyperextend the neck of an infant or small child, but make certain that the airway is open to allow for adequate ventilation.

Mouth-to-mouth ventilation is the most immediate form of pulmonary resuscitation. There are no shortcuts to this procedure. Learn all the steps in this chapter, including the mouth-to-nose, mouth-to-stoma (for neck breathers), and mouth-to-mouth and nose (for infants and small children) techniques.

It is recommended that EMTs utilize a pocket face mask with one-way valve, a bag-valve-mask unit, or another approved device to avoid direct contact with the patient's body fluids.

Remember that artificial ventilations for the adult are provided at the rate of 1 BREATH EVERY 5 SECONDS to equal 12 BREATHS PER MINUTE. This is true for mouth-to-mouth, mouth-to-nose, and mouth-to-stoma techniques.

Infants receive a gentle but adequate breath every three seconds (20 breaths per minute), while children receive a gentle but adequate breath every four seconds (15 breaths per minute).

Be on the alert for gastric distention, when air is forced into the patient's stomach. Reposition the patient's head and be on the guard for vomiting. Watch the patient's chest rise to adjust your ventilations. *Do not* attempt to force air from the patient's stomach unless you have suction equipment on hand for immediate use.

A variety of problems can cause partial or full airway obstruction. These include the tongue, foreign objects, tissue damage, and disease. Listen for snoring, crowing, gurgling, and wheezing sounds that may indicate partial obstruction. In cases of total obstruction there will be no chest movements typical of normal breathing, no sounds of respiration, and no air exchange felt at the nose and mouth. The conscious patient will not be able to speak.

Encourage patients with partial airway obstructions to cough. If they cannot cough, or their coughing is very weak, *treat as if they had a complete airway obstruction.*

Conscious patients with airway obstructions will often grasp the neck, trying to communicate the problem. Be sure to ask patients, "Can you speak?" If they can, then the obstruction is partial.

Correcting airway obstruction may be accomplished by manual thrusts and finger sweeps. It is sometimes necessary to use combined procedures:

- Opening the airway and attempt TWO ventilations
- SIX TO TEN abdominal thrusts
- Finger sweeps

Remember that abdominal thrusts are not recommended for infants and pregnant patients. Use chest thrusts for these patients. Back blows are not to be used except for foreign object airway obstruction in the infant.

These various procedures are used in a very specific pattern. Before completing this chapter, make certain that you can list the combined procedure steps for the conscious patient, the patient who becomes unconscious after care is started, and the unconscious patient. You should be able to do this for adult, child, and infant.

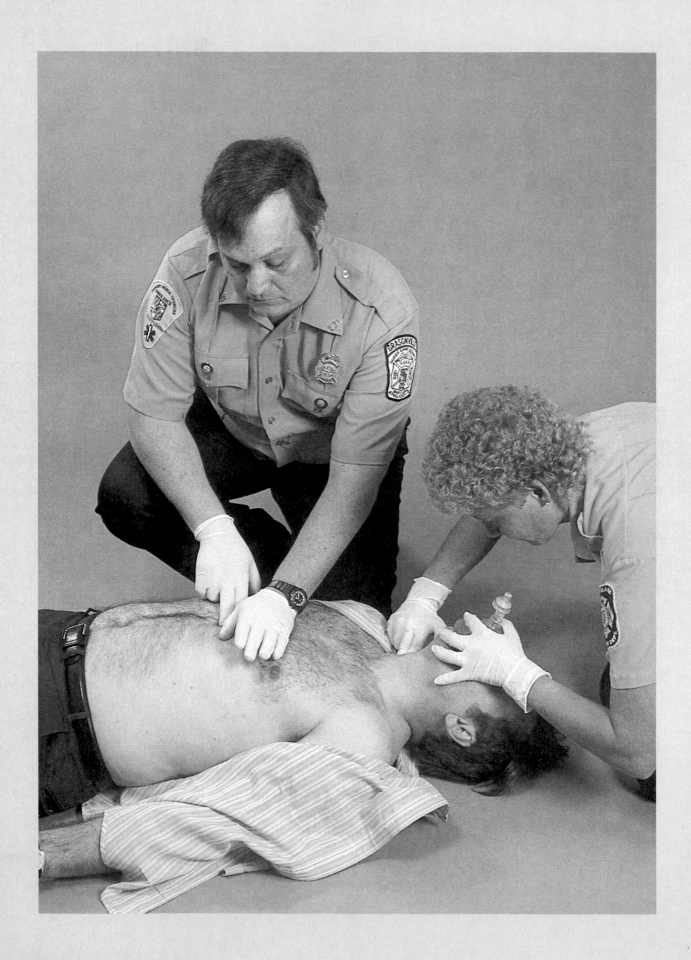

CHAPTER 5

Basic Life Support II
CPR—cardiopulmonary resuscitation

WARNING: It is recommended that prehospital emergency health care personnel protect themselves from infectious diseases by using pocket face masks with one-way valves or bag-valve-mask units (if appropriate) when ventilating patients. Wear protective gloves to avoid contact with the patient's blood and body fluids.

OBJECTIVES   As an EMT, you should be able to:

1. List and define the FIVE main components of the circulatory system. (p. 139)
2. Locate the anatomical position of the heart. (p. 139)
3. Describe the relationship of heart, lung, and brain activity. (pp. 140–141)
4. Define *CPR*. (p. 141)
5. Describe, in terms of oxygen and circulation, how CPR keeps a patient alive. (pp. 141–142)
6. Explain how CPR works. (pp. 141–142)
7. List the signs of cardiac arrest. (p. 143)
8. Relate starting CPR to the results of the primary survey. (p. 143)
9. Define *CPR compression site* and describe how to find this site on the adult patient. (p. 144)
10. Describe how to deliver external chest compressions and interposed (CPR) ventilations. (pp. 144–146)
11. List the rates and ratios of compressions and ventilations used during CPR on adults, children, and infants. (p. 145, pp. 155–156)
12. State how the EMT can determine that CPR is effective. (p. 146)
13. State at least FIVE causes of ineffective CPR. (p. 146)
14. List, step by step, the procedures for performing CPR on adults, children, and infants. (pp. 150–151, pp. 155–156)
15. Cite at least THREE complications that can occur during CPR. (p. 147)
16. State when an EMT can stop CPR. (pp. 147–148)
17. List at least THREE advantages of two-rescuer CPR over one-rescuer CPR. (p. 149)
18. Compare one-rescuer CPR and two-rescuer CPR in terms of rates of compression and rates of ventilations. (p. 157)
19. List, step by step, the procedures for two-rescuer CPR. (p. 153)
20. State how often you should check for a spontaneous carotid pulse and breathing when performing two-rescuer CPR. (p. 152)
21. State for how long compressions may be

interrupted when checking for breathing and carotid pulse when performing two-rescuer CPR. (p. 152)

22. List, step by step, the sequence of procedures for changing positions during two-rescuer CPR. (pp. 152–154)

23. State what the ventilator should do if he misses an interposed ventilation during two-rescuer CPR. (p. 152)

24. Describe, step by step, how to provide CPR when moving a patient. (pp. 156–158)

SKILLS As an EMT, you should be able to:

1. Correctly evaluate a patient to detect cardiac arrest.
2. Perform one-rescuer CPR on adult patients, children, and infants.

3. Perform two-rescuer CPR, including the proper change of positions.
4. Perform CPR on a patient while he is being moved.

TERMS you may be using for the first time:

Aorta (a-OR-tah) – the largest artery in the body. It transports blood from the left ventricle to begin systemic circulation.

Atrium (A-tree-um) – an upper chamber of the heart. There is a right atrium (which receives unoxygenated blood returning from the body) and a left atrium (which receives oxygenated blood returning from the lungs). The plural of atrium is atria.

Brachial (BRAY-key-al) **Pulse** – the pulse measured by palpating the major artery (brachial artery) of the arm. This pulse is used to detect heart action and circulation in infants.

Cardiac Arrest – when the heart stops circulating blood or stops beating entirely. The term *cardiac standstill* is sometimes used interchangeably with the term *cardiac arrest*.

Cardiopulmonary Resuscitation (KAR-de-o PUL-mo-ner-e re-SUS-ci-TA-shun), **CPR** – Heart–lung resuscitation. A combined effort is made to restore or maintain respiration and circulation, artificially.

Clavicle (KLAV-i-kul) – the collarbone. There are two, with one attached to the right side of the superior sternum and one attached to the left side.

Conduction System – modified heart muscle that acts as nervous tissue to initiate heart contraction.

CPR Compression Site – for the adult and child, this is the sternal point placement of the hands approximately one finger width superior to the substernal notch. For infants it is the point on the midline of the sternum that is one finger width lower than an imaginary line drawn through the nipples.

CPR Ventilation – the artificial ventilations provided during CPR. The ventilations are provided

between a set of compressions. Today, "rescue breathing" is the more popular term.

Mediastinum (me-de-as-TI-num or me-de-ah-STI-num) – the central portion of the thoracic cavity, containing the heart, its great blood vessels, part of the trachea, and part of the esophagus (e-SOF-ah-gus).

Pericardium (per-e-KAR-de-um) – the membranous sac that surrounds the heart, connecting to the base of the greater vessels superior to the heart.

Pulmonary (PUL-mo-nar-e) **Artery** – the blood vessel that transports blood from the right ventricle to the lungs.

Pulmonary Circulation – the transport of blood from the right ventricle to the lungs where it is oxygenated and then returned to the left atrium.

Pulmonary Veins – the vessels that transport oxygenated blood from the lungs to the left atrium.

Sternum (STER-num) – the breastbone.

Substernal Notch – a general term for the lowest region on the sternum to which the ribs attach.

Systemic (sis-TEM-ik) **Circulation** – the portion of the circulatory system that transports blood from the left ventricle out to the body's tissues and back to the heart.

Vascular – referring to the blood vessels.

Ventricle (VEN-tri-kl) – a lower chamber of the heart. There is a right ventricle (sends blood to the lungs) and a left ventricle (sends oxygenated blood to the body).

Venae Cavae (VE-ne KA-ve) – the superior vena cava and the inferior vena cava. These two major veins return blood from the body to the right atrium.

THE HEART

This chapter introduces you to the **circulatory system.** This system is composed of the:

- Heart—acting as a pump to circulate the blood
- Arteries—the vessels that carry blood away from the heart
- Veins—the vessels that return blood to the heart
- Capillaries—the vessels where exchange between the blood and the body's tissues takes place
- Blood—the fluids and cells that are circulated to carry oxygen and nutrients to and wastes away from the body's tissues.

More will be said about this system in Chapter 7. For now, concentrate on the relationship between the circulatory system and the lungs and brain.

As you progress into this chapter, remember that an uncorrected airway obstruction can lead to respiratory arrest and that respiratory arrest will lead quickly to cardiac arrest. The process of dying may be reversed if resuscitative measures are initiated promptly and carried out effectively.

Anatomy of the Heart

The human heart is a muscular organ about the size of your fist. It is located in the center of the thoracic cavity, in an area called the **mediastinum** (me-de-as-TI-num or me-de-ah-STI-num). This portion of the thoracic cavity contains the heart, its large blood vessels, part of the trachea, and part of the **esophagus** (e-SOF-ah-gus), the tube leading from the throat to the stomach.

The heart is surrounded by a membranous sac called the **pericardium** (per-e-KAR-de-um) or **pericardial sac.** This sac protects the heart as it beats within the chest cavity.

There are two upper chambers of the heart called the right and left **atria** (A-tree-ah). The **right atrium** (A-tree-um) receives blood returning from the entire body. The **left atrium** receives oxygenated blood returning from the lungs. These two chambers are divided by a wall called the **interatrial** (In-ter-A-tre-al) **septum.*** When the right atrium is filling, so is the left atrium. When the right atrium is contracting, the left atrium is also contracting.

---

* A septum divides a large cavity or chamber to form two smaller chambers. You have a septum in your nose separating the two nostrils.

There are two lower chambers of the heart called the right and left **ventricles** (VEN-tri-kls). The **right ventricle** receives blood from the right atrium and pumps this blood to the lungs to be oxygenated. The **left ventricle** receives blood from the left atrium and pumps this blood out to the body. These two chambers are divided by the **interventricular** (IN-ter-ven-TRIK-u-lar) **septum.** Both ventricles fill and contract at the same time. Since it does more work by pumping blood out to the entire body, the left ventricle has the thickest muscle of the heart chambers.

Between each atrium and ventricle is a one-way *valve* to prevent blood in the ventricle from being forced back into the atrium. The major vessel leading from the heart to the lungs, the **pulmonary** (PUL-mo-nar-e) **artery,** also has a one-way valve so that blood does not return to the right ventricle. The major vessel leading out to the body, the **aorta** (a-OR-tah), has a one-way valve to keep blood from leaking into the left ventricle. This system of one-way valves keeps blood moving in the correct direction as it comes from the body, goes to and from the lungs, and is circulated to the body's tissues.

The beating of the heart is an automatic, involuntary process. The heart has its own "pacemaker" and a system of specialized muscle tissues that conduct electrical impulses that stimulate the heart to beat. This network is called the **conduction system.** Regulation of rate, rhythm, and force of heartbeat comes, in part, from the cardiac control centers of the brain. Nerve impulses from these centers are sent to the pacemaker of the heart. These nerve impulses and chemicals released into the blood (e.g., epinephrine) control heart action.

Heart Function

The heart may be compared to a pump—a very efficient pump. When the average adult is *at rest,* the heart will pump 10 pints (about 5 liters) of blood each minute. Since the body is not at rest all day, the heart's actions pump more than 16,000 pints of blood each day. In an average lifetime, this human pump is required to beat over 2.5 billion times in order to move over 450 million pints of blood. Unlike a mechanical pump, the heart accomplishes this remarkable feat without interruption. The only care that is needed is to maintain a healthy body. Lack of exercise, poor diet, smoking, and stress are its greatest enemies.

Blood from the body returns to the heart by way of the superior and inferior **venae cavae**

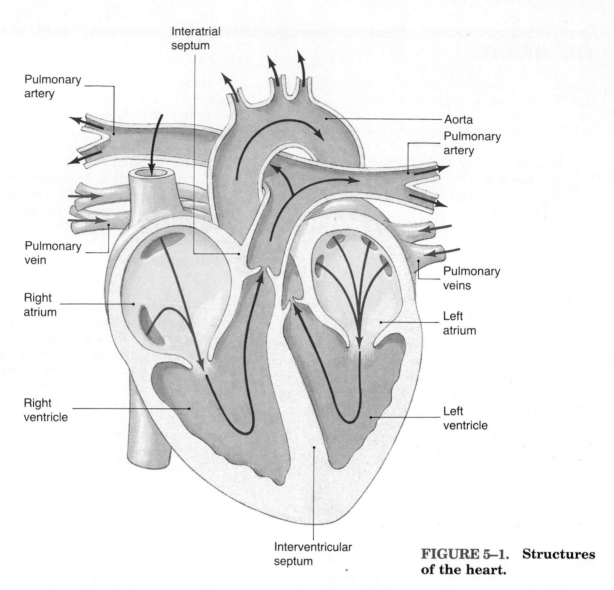

Interatrial septum

Pulmonary artery

Pulmonary vein

Right atrium

Right ventricle

Aorta
Pulmonary artery

Pulmonary veins

Left atrium

Left ventricle

Interventricular septum

FIGURE 5–1. Structures of the heart.

(VE-ne KA-ve) to enter the right atrium. It is sent from this chamber into the right ventricle through a one-way valve that prevents return to the atrium. When the right ventricle contracts, it sends blood by way of the **pulmonary artery** to the lungs, where carbon dioxide is given up from the blood and oxygen is taken from the alveoli. This oxygenated blood is sent by way of the **pulmonary veins** back to the heart to enter the left atrium, which sends this blood through a one-way valve into the left ventricle. The left ventricle contracts to send blood through the aorta out to the body.

As you can see, there are two circulatory systems functioning at the same time. One is called **pulmonary circulation,** where blood is sent from the heart to the lungs and back to the heart. The other is called **systemic** (sis-TEM-ik) **circulation.** This is the flow from the heart, out to the entire body and back to the heart. In its flow, the blood delivers oxygen to the tissues and picks up carbon dioxide.

The Heart–Lung–Brain Relationship

There is a close relationship between the functions of the heart, the lungs, and the brain. This relationship may be seen as follows:

- A patient develops respiratory arrest. Usually, the heart will continue to pump blood for several minutes; however, the blood being pumped to the brain will not contain enough oxygen for the brain. This, combined with the effects of the lack of oxygen needed by the heart muscles, will cause the heart to beat improperly and then stop beating altogether. Without oxygenated blood, the brain will die.

- The patient is breathing, but his heart stops beating. When the heart stops beating, cessation of effective breathing is almost immediate. Blood will not be sent to the lungs to

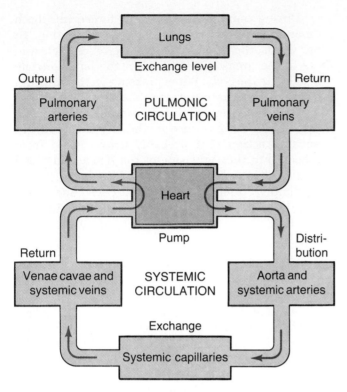

FIGURE 5–2. **The heart pumps blood through pulmonary and systemic circulation.**

pick up oxygen, nor will the blood be sent to the body's tissues. Without oxygen, the brain will die.

In Chapter 4 we defined clinical death and biological death. Remember, when the patient stops breathing, soon his heart will stop beating. When the patient's heart is not beating and he is not breathing, this is **clinical death.** This condition may be reversed. Once the patient's brain cells begin to die, this is **biological death,** which usually occurs within 10 minutes after clinical death. This is not reversible. You will study how to try to prevent a patient in clinical death from reaching biological death. Later, we will consider what factors may delay biological death, thus allowing you to resuscitate a patient who has been clinically dead for more than 10 minutes.

CPR

CPR is **cardiopulmonary** (KAR-de-o-PUL-mo-ner-e) **resuscitation.** This basic life support measure is applied when a patient's heart and lung actions have stopped. During CPR, you will have to:

- Maintain an open airway.
- Breathe for the patient.
- Force the patient's blood to circulate.

Remember, basic life support is concerned with the ABCs of emergency care, where:

- A = Airway
- B = Breathing
- C = Circulation

CPR is a procedure involving the ABCs of emergency care. Artificial ventilations are not effective unless there is an open airway. Artificial ventilation is not effective unless the blood is circulating. Circulating blood will not be effective unless the blood is oxygenated.

Remember that bleeding can prevent proper and adequate circulation. If a patient has lost too much blood, then CPR will not be effective. When bleeding is very profuse, as in the case of a severed major artery, CPR may speed up the patient's blood loss, causing biological death to occur. Even though such a case is rare, you may have to quickly ensure a reduction of this blood loss (see Chapter 7) before effective CPR can be initiated.

How CPR Works

In Chapter 4 we discussed rescue breathing (pulmonary resuscitation). Providing oxygen to the patient will do little good unless the blood is circulating. In CPR, the patient's blood is forced to circulate by the rescuer applying external chest compressions. This is known as artificial circulation.

Artificial circulation can be produced by laying the patient on a hard surface on his back and compressing the chest over the midline of the sternum. It is believed that this action causes pressure changes to take place within the thoracic cavity that help to force blood movement. The pressure created in the chest cavity is transferred to the blood vessels outside the chest. Due to thick muscular walls and other properties, the pressure transmitted is greater in the arteries than it is in the veins. The difference in pressure between the arteries and veins and the resistance offered by one-way valves in the veins probably forces the blood to flow from the arteries into the capillaries. This allows oxygenated blood to flow through the body's vital organs, including the brain.

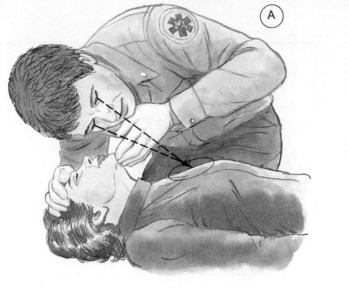

(A)

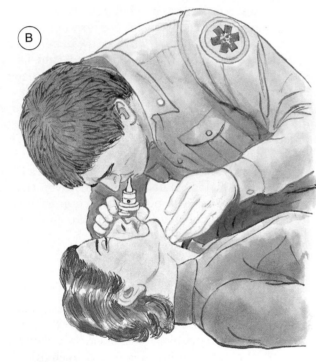

(B)

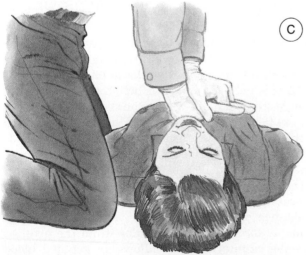

(C)

FIGURE 5–3.   The ABC technique of CPR.

During compression, blood is forced into both pulmonary circulation and systemic circulation. In other words, the blood leaves the right ventricle and flows to the lungs, while blood in the left ventricle is sent out to the body. When pressure on the sternum is released, the elastic nature of the chest wall causes the sternum to return to its normal position. The release of excess pressure in the thorax results in a sucking action that probably draws blood from the body into the right side of the heart and blood from the lungs into the left side of the heart.

Simply stated, compress the chest and blood is circulated; release compression and the heart fills with blood.

NOTE: The pumping action produced by CPR is only 25% to 33% as effective as normal heart action. To partially counter this deficiency, supplemental oxygen is provided as soon as possible for all patients with cardiac arrest. The oxygen delivery system should provide at least 90% oxygen to ensure that as high a level of oxygen as possible will reach the tissues. Even though supplemental oxygen is significant in basic life support, *do not* delay or stop CPR in order to set up an oxygen delivery system.

In one-rescuer CPR, a set number of external chest compressions are given to the patient, then

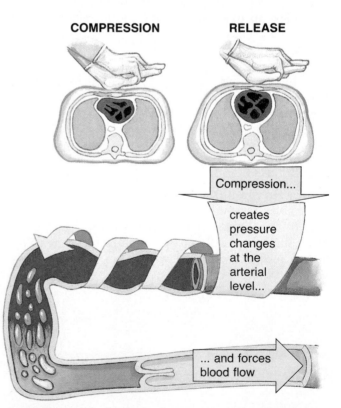

COMPRESSION   **RELEASE**

Compression...

creates pressure changes at the arterial level...

... and forces blood flow

FIGURE 5–4.   During CPR, compressions cause pressure changes that cause the blood to circulate.

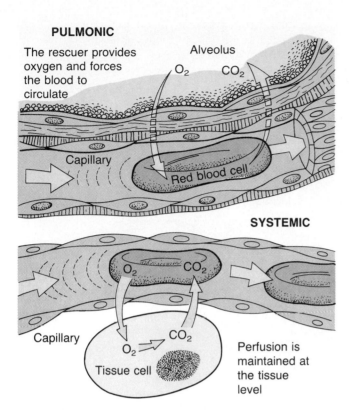

PULMONIC

The rescuer provides oxygen and forces the blood to circulate

Alveolus

O_2 CO_2

Capillary

Red blood cell

SYSTEMIC

Capillary

O_2 CO_2

O_2 → CO_2

Tissue cell

Perfusion is maintained at the tissue level

FIGURE 5–5.   CPR provides the patient with oxygen and forces the blood to circulate.

breaths are provided. These breaths, known as **interposed** (or CPR) **ventilations,** provide the patient with oxygen.

When to Use CPR

First, the patient must be in **cardiac arrest.** This means that his heart has stopped beating completely (cardiac standstill) or, because of shock, severe bleeding, heart damage, or the actions of certain drugs, the heart beats too weakly to circulate blood (cardiovascular collapse). It is possible that the patient's heartbeats are so irregular and uncoordinated that there is no effective output (ventricular fibrillation).

Should the patient be breathing at the time of cardiac arrest, within 30 to 45 seconds he will go into respiratory arrest. A patient needing CPR will be unresponsive. He will not be breathing and will have no carotid pulse or a pulse so slow, weak and irregular that it indicates a critical lack of circulation.

The Techniques of CPR

When to Begin CPR

The decision to begin CPR must come from the results of the primary survey. The events leading to the beginning of CPR should be:

1. ESTABLISH UNRESPONSIVENESS—Is the patient responsive? Gently shake the patient's shoulder and shout, "ARE YOU OKAY?" Patients requiring immediate CPR will be unresponsive.

   NOTE: If you are working by yourself, call out for help if the patient is unresponsive.

2. REPOSITION THE PATIENT (see Chapter 4), if necessary.

3. ESTABLISH AN OPEN AIRWAY—This should be done by the head-tilt, chin-lift, or jaw-thrust maneuvers. Usually at this time, you can easily check to see if the patient is a neck breather.

4. CHECK FOR BREATHING—Use the LOOK, LISTEN, and FEEL method, taking 3 to 5 seconds to determine if the patient is breathing. A patient who is breathing does not need immediate CPR. If the patient is in respiratory arrest, you should . . .

5. DELIVER TWO BREATHS—Use rescue breathing techniques. Allow for deflation between breaths. If you note an upper airway obstruction, begin the techniques used to clear the airway. If the patient's airway is clear and he is still in respiratory arrest after you have provided two breaths . . .

6. CHECK FOR A CAROTID PULSE—Maintain the head tilt with one hand on the patient's forehead and use your other hand to feel for a carotid pulse. If there is no pulse, after 5 to 10 seconds of palpation, the patient is in *cardiac arrest* and you should . . .

7. BEGIN CPR.

NOTE: If you are acting alone, have someone alert the EMS dispatcher as soon as you establish pulselessness. Make certain that this person informs dispatch that the patient has no pulse and CPR has been started. In many areas, dispatch will be able to send an advanced cardiac life support unit to the scene if it is known that the patient is in cardiac arrest.

Positioning the Patient

The cardiac arrest patient must be placed on a hard surface, such as the floor or ground or a spine board. If the patient is in bed or on an ambulance stretcher, a spine board, backboard, serving tray, or similar rigid object should be placed under his back. *Do not delay CPR to retrieve a rigid object.* Instead, move

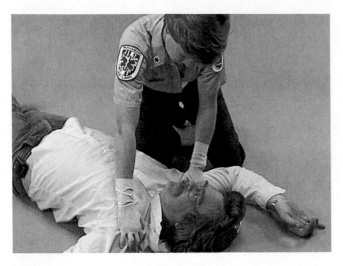

FIGURE 5–6. Establish unresponsiveness and properly position the patient for CPR.

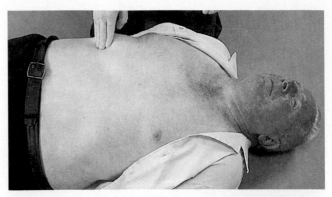

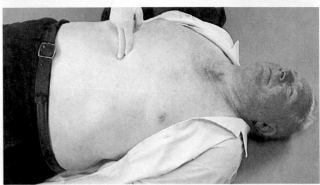

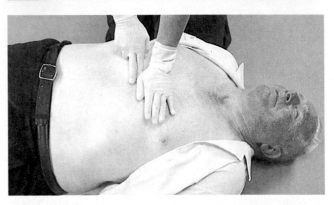

FIGURE 5–7. Finding the notch where the ribs connect to the sternum will enable you to locate the CPR compression site.

the patient to the floor. CPR cannot be delayed because of patient injury. If you are alone, *do not* try to immobilize the spine or splint fractures before initiating CPR. It is critical that CPR be started as soon as possible.

The CPR Compression Site

The heart is located in the mediastinum, between the sternum and the spinal column. The upper seven pairs of the ribs attach to the sternum. These, along with the **clavicles** (KLAV-i-kuls), or collarbones, support the sternum over the heart.

To be effective and prevent serious injury to the patient, external chest compressions *must* be delivered to the **CPR Compression site.** The technique of locating the CPR compression site requires you to begin by positioning yourself shoulder level at the patient's side, having your knees in toward the patient. Use the index and middle fingers of your hand closest to the patient's feet to locate the lower *margin* (border) of the rib cage. This is called the **costal margin.** Do this on the side of the chest closest to your knees. Move your fingers along the rib cage until you find the point where the ribs meet the sternum (lower center of the chest). This area is called the **substernal notch** (Figure 5–7). Keep your middle finger at this notch and your index finger resting over the lower end of the sternum. If you now move your other hand to the midline of the sternum and place the thumb side of this hand against the positioned index finger of your lower hand, you will be directly over the CPR compression site. The heel of your hand should be on the midline of the sternum.

Providing Chest Compressions

Remember that the patient is lying on his back on a hard surface. You are kneeling beside the patient, with your knees in toward the patient. Your knees should be spread apart, about shoulder width. Having found the CPR compression site, you should:

1. Place the hand that was closest to the patient's head directly on the CPR compression site.
2. Position the hand used to locate the substernal notch directly over the first hand. The heels of both hands should be parallel to one

another and the fingers of both hands must be pointing away from your body.

3. Your fingers may be extended, or they may be interlaced, but you must KEEP YOUR FINGERS OFF THE PATIENT'S CHEST to avoid injury to the patient.

4. Straighten your arms and lock the elbows. You must not bend the elbows when delivering or releasing compressions.

5. Make certain that your shoulders are directly over your hands (directly over the patient's sternum). This will allow you to deliver compressions straight down onto the site. Keep both of your knees on the ground or floor.

6. Deliver compressions STRAIGHT DOWN, with enough force to depress the sternum of a typical adult *1.5 to 2 inches.*

7. Fully release pressure on the patient's sternum, but *do not* bend your elbows and *do not* lift your hands from the sternum. Your movement should be at the level of your waist and hips. Make sure that you return your shoulders to their original position. The patient's chest should completely relax on the upstroke. RELEASE SHOULD TAKE AS MUCH TIME AS COMPRESSION. This is known as the 50:50 rule: *50% compression, 50% release.*

Providing Ventilations

Ventilations are **interposed** (provided between) after a set number of compressions. You are to use the same techniques that you learned for rescue breathing. The mouth-to-mask, mouth-to-mouth, mouth-to-nose, or mouth-to-stoma methods can be used as needed. (In the mouth-to-mouth procedure, remember to pinch closed the patient's nostrils, form a tight seal with your mouth, and force air into the lungs until you see the chest rise and feel resistance from the patient's lungs.) Take 1 to 1.5 seconds per ventilation.

Rates of Compressions and Ventilations

- COMPRESSIONS = a rate of 80 to 100 per minute, providing 15 compressions every 9 to 11 seconds
- VENTILATIONS = 2 breaths after every 15 compressions, delivered at 1 ventilation every 1 to 1.5 seconds.
- RATIO = 15 compressions per 2 ventilations

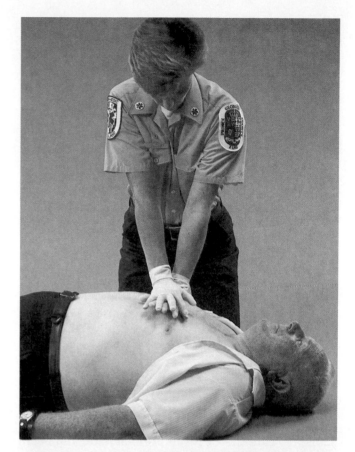

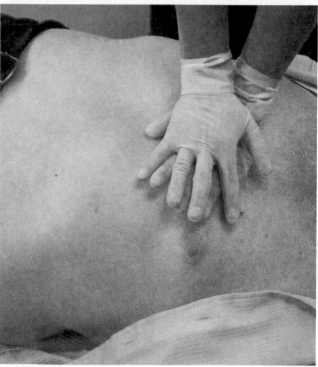

FIGURE 5–8. Positioning the hands for CPR. The arms must be straight, the elbows locked, and the shoulders over the compression site.

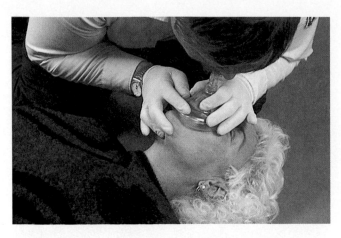

FIGURE 5–9. Providing ventilations.

During one-rescuer CPR, time is taken away from compressions in order to provide ventilations. Even though you are delivering compressions at the rate of 80 to 100 per minute, usually only 60 compressions are delivered in 1 minute. To be certain that you are delivering compressions at the correct rate, you should say:

"One-and, two-and, three-and, four-and, five-and, . . ." until you reach 15 compressions. At that point, you can deliver two quick interposed ventilations, relocate the CPR compression site, and begin the next set of 15 compressions.

Once you begin CPR, *do not interrupt* the process for more than 7 seconds. The only exceptions to this rule at the basic life support level is when you are moving a patient up or down stairs or you are acting alone when off duty and must activate the EMS System. A maximum interruption of 15 seconds is recommended. This interruption may go as high as 30 seconds for moving a patient up or down a flight of stairs.

Checking the Pulse

CPR should be carried out for approximately ONE MINUTE, or four cycles of 15 compressions and 2 interposed ventilations. Then you should check for a carotid pulse. At the same time, you should determine if the patient is breathing. *Do not* stop CPR for more than 7 seconds. If the patient has a pulse but is not breathing, begin pulmonary resuscitation, taking care to check every few minutes for a carotid pulse. If the patient is not breathing and does not have a pulse, provide two breaths and start a new cycle of compressions and ventilations, checking for a carotid pulse every few minutes.

Effective CPR

If CPR is effective, you must be able to see the patient's chest rise during interposed ventilations and someone else can feel a carotid pulse each time you deliver a compression. In addition to these events, any of the following may be noticed:

- Pupils constrict.
- Skin color improves.
- Heartbeat returns spontaneously.
- Spontaneous, gasping respirations.
- Arms and legs move.
- Attempts are made to swallow.
- Consciousness returns.

Keep in mind that you can provide effective CPR but the patient will usually not spontaneously regain heartbeat and breathing. The majority of patients will require special advanced life support and other medical procedures before they can regain heart and lung function. As an EMT, you are providing CPR to keep a clinically dead patient biologically alive. Effective CPR does not mean that the patient lives. Many patients who have received the best possible resuscitation efforts will not recover.

Ineffective CPR

Ineffective CPR refers to the application of improper resuscitative techniques. The patient's chances for survival greatly improve if CPR is done efficiently.

When CPR efforts are not effective, it is usually because of one or more of these problems:

- The patient's *head* is not placed in the proper head-tilt position for ventilations.
- The patient's *mouth* is not opened wide enough for air exchange.
- There is not an effective seal made against the patient's *mouth or nose*.
- The patient's *nose* is not pinched shut during mouth-to-mouth ventilations.
- The patient's *mouth* is not closed completely during mouth-to-nose ventilations.
- The patient is not lying on a *hard surface*.
- The rescuer's *hands* are incorrectly placed.
- There are prolonged (more than 7 seconds) *interruptions* of external chest compressions.
- The *chest* is not sufficiently compressed.
- The compression *rate* is too rapid or too slow.
- Compressions are *jerky*, not smooth with 50% of the cycle being compression and 50% being the release of compression.

Note that the first five problems relate to ventilation, as discussed in Chapter 4.

Complications of CPR

Injury to the rib cage is the most common complication of CPR. When the hands are placed too high on the sternum, fractures to the upper sternum and the clavicles may occur. If the hands are too low on the sternum, the xiphoid may be fractured or driven down into the liver, producing severe lacerations (cuts) and profuse internal bleeding. When the hands are placed too far off center, or when they are allowed to slip from their position over the CPR compression site, the ribs or their cartilage attachments may be fractured. This may happen unless

Lungs

Heart

Spleen

Liver

Stomach

Too far right:
May fracture ribs and
cause lacerations to
lung and liver.

Too far left:
May fracture ribs and
cause lacerations to
lung and heart

Too high:
May fracture collar
bone

Too low:
May depress xiphoid
process into liver

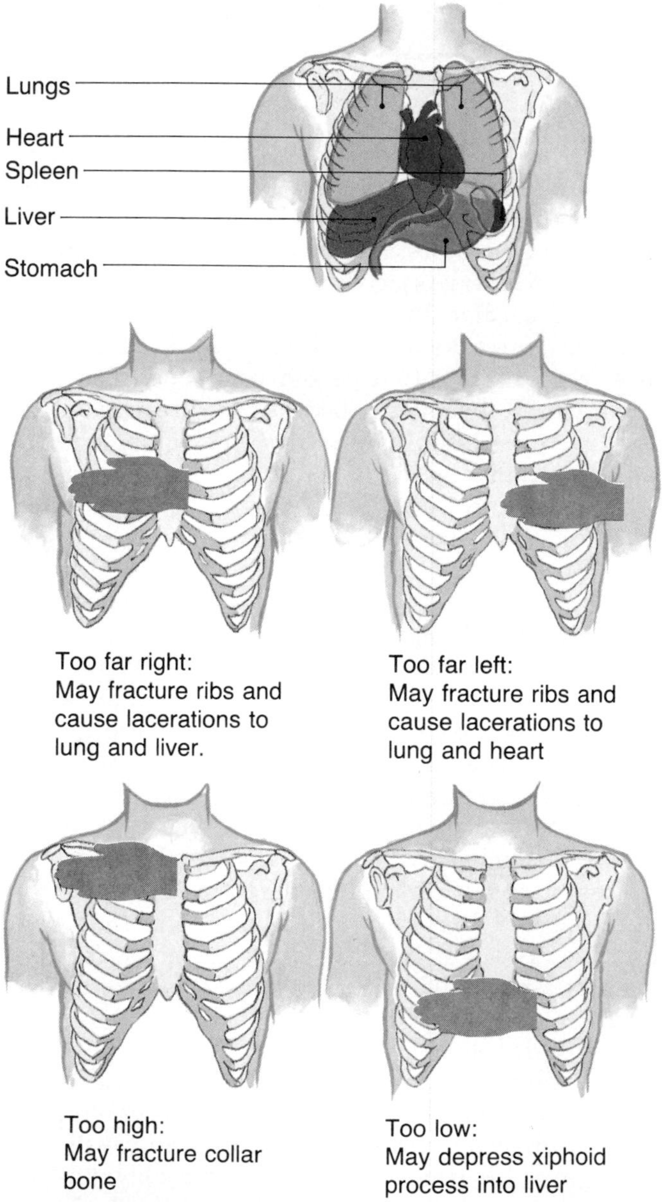

FIGURE 5–10. Improper positioning of the hands during CPR can damage the rib cage and underlying organs.

care is taken to properly locate the CPR compression site ("land-marking").

Even when CPR is correctly performed, cartilage attached to the ribs may separate or ribs may be fractured. In such cases, *do not* stop CPR. Simply reassess your hand position and compression depth and continue with CPR. It is far better that the patient suffer a few broken ribs and live than die because you did not continue to perform CPR for fear of inflicting additional injury.

Often, when CPR is performed on elderly patients the first few compressions will separate rib cartilage. When this happens, you may hear a "crunch" as you apply a compression. *Do not* stop CPR. Again, reassess your hand position and the depths of your compressions and continue with CPR.

The problem of gastric distention that is associated with pulmonary resuscitation (see pp. 124–125) also may occur when performing CPR. *Do not* attempt to relieve this distention unless suction equipment is ready for immediate use. Reposition the patient to establish an open airway and closely watch the rise and fall of his chest when providing ventilations. Be on the alert for vomiting and regurgitation. Often, a slight decrease in the volume of the ventilation will reduce gastric distention.

Other complications may result from improper CPR efforts, but most are easy to avoid by following American Heart Association guidelines.

Beginning and Terminating CPR

There are special cases when you should not resuscitate a patient. These include cases in which you detect cardiac arrest and any of the following:

- A line of lividity—This patient has been dead for over 15 minutes (no hypothermia) and blood has pooled in the dependent body parts. The process may continue for up to 10 hours. An irregular, *reddish* skin discoloration occurs where gravity has caused the blood to sink and collect. Utilizing this sign requires special training that is usually not part of an EMT–Basic program.
- Rigor mortis—This is the stiffening of the body and its limbs that occurs after death, usually within 4 to 10 hours.
- Obvious mortal wounds—These include decapitation, incineration, a severed body, and injuries that are so extensive that CPR cannot be effectively performed (e.g., severe crush injuries to the head, neck, and chest).
- Obvious decomposition.

In addition to the above, there is the special case of the stillborn infant who has died hours prior to birth (see p. 456). This patient may have blisters on the skin, a very soft head, and a strong disagreeable odor. CPR should not be started for this patient. As in all other cases, if you are in doubt, radio for a physician's advice.

When dealing with a patient in cardiac arrest, your duty as an EMT is to begin CPR *immediately*. Even though the patient may have a terminal illness or he may be very old, you cannot decide to withhold CPR. Bystanders may ask you not to begin CPR. Family members may say that the patient would not want your help, but you have no *proof* of this. Even though many states are now recognizing that resuscitation may violate certain persons' rights to die with dignity, you cannot accept hearsay evidence. It would be rare, but it is possible that the people at the scene want the patient to die for less noble reasons. You must have written documentation that is accepted by your EMS System (follow local guidelines). This documentation must be immediately available. You cannot delay starting CPR while someone searches for the document. Once CPR is started, it should be stopped only with a physician's order or if the criteria below have been met.

At the hospital, the physician's written order sheet can be used for such cases by the professional medical staff, but in the field, only a physician (with proper identification) who accepts the responsibility for the patient while at the scene, or through radio or telephone communications, may order you not to perform CPR. Some EMS Systems will keep records with dispatch that will indicate that a patient has requested resuscitation not be started. Your instructor can inform you of the laws for your state. YOU MUST FOLLOW LOCAL PROTOCOLS.

CPR is most effective if started immediately after the beginning of cardiac arrest. If a patient has been in arrest for more than ten minutes, resuscitation efforts usually are not effective. However, there are documented cases of adults who were in arrest for more than ten minutes being resuscitated with no major brain damage. Some have survived after being in arrest for well over 30 minutes. Cold temperatures appear to prolong the time someone can be in arrest before biological death occurs. Cold water is even more effective in delaying biological death. Also keep in mind that children and infants may tolerate longer periods of cardiac arrest than can adults.

Do not refuse to begin CPR because someone has been in cardiac arrest for more than 10 minutes. The moment the patient was seen to collapse and the moment of cardiac arrest are not usually the same. A patient can be unconscious with minimum effective lung and heart action for quite some time before actual cardiac arrest occurs.

Once you have started CPR, you *must* continue to provide CPR until:

- Spontaneous circulation occurs . . . then provide artificial respiration as needed.
- Spontaneous circulation and breathing occur.
- Another trained rescuer can take over for you.
- You turn care of the patient over to a physician or a medical facility.
- You are too exhausted and cannot continue.

If you turn the patient over to another rescuer, this person must be trained to your level or above. This does not mean that the person has to be an EMT. The new rescuer must have certification (American Heart Association or American Red Cross) in basic cardiac life support. Certified First Responders can take over CPR for you. If you do turn over resuscitation to a person who is certified, but not an EMT, it should be because you are exhausted, you need to set-up oxygen delivery equipment, or there are other patients who have life-threatening emergencies. You must supervise this person, since you are still responsible for the patient. In cases in which you turn over care to a physician or a medical facility, you should, when practical, obtain a written record of this change.

Many students have fears of having to stop CPR because of exhaustion. As a member of the EMS System, you have to be realistic about patient care and know when you have done all you can for a patient. If you are isolated and have provided CPR for 30 minutes to an hour and are too exhausted to go on, remember that there are physical limitations to the care you can provide. Few patients having received CPR for such a long period of time will survive. You will have done all you could for the patient and should not feel guilty at having to stop CPR.

You lessen the chances of physical exhaustion if you learn to control **rescuer hyperventilation.** When providing CPR, you establish an irregular pattern of breathing for yourself. This may cause you to begin to breathe very quickly and deeply, unable to regain control. You can help prevent this by keeping in good physical condition and learning not to try to take a breath with each compression. You have to learn to establish a normal breathing rate when delivering external chest compressions.

Interrupting CPR

Once you begin CPR, you may interrupt the process for no more than 7 seconds to check for pulse and breathing or to reposition yourself and the patient. The first recommended interruption comes after one minute when you check for pulse and breathing. You should continue to check for these vital signs every few minutes.

In addition to these built-in interruptions, you may interrupt CPR to:

- Move a patient onto a stretcher—7 seconds maximum
- Move a patient down a flight of stairs—30 seconds maximum
- Find assistance or phone for help—30 seconds maximum after performing CPR for 1 minute
- Allow for advanced cardiac life support measures to be initiated—usually no more than 15 seconds per interruption
- Suctioning to clear an obstructed airway

One-Rescuer CPR

Scan 5–1 shows all the techniques of one-rescuer CPR for the adult patient. Follow this page step by step as you practice on the adult manikins provided for your training.

There is one situation that you should practice for in addition to one-rescuer CPR as we have presented it here in this section. What if you are off duty and acting alone? The American Heart Association states that you should call out for help if you find the patient is unresponsive. The person who is helping should activate (phone) the EMS System if you do not detect a pulse. Call out for help and have someone phone while you begin CPR. Direct the person to call 911 or the local emergency number, depending on your location. Tell the person to state that it is an emergency, give the address, state CPR is being performed, and request an ambulance.

If there is no one on hand to help you, perform CPR for ONE MINUTE, quickly telephone for help, and return to providing CPR. Of course, the telephone must be very close at hand. Interruption of CPR in complicated situations should not last longer than 30 seconds. If no telephone is near, perform CPR until someone can take over for you or you are too exhausted to go on.

Two-Rescuer CPR

Advantages

CPR efforts are more effective when two rescuers work together. The patient receives more oxygen, circulation and blood pressure improve since chest compressions are not interrupted for as long, and the problem of rescuer fatigue is lessened.

Should you find yourself providing CPR while off duty, you may be able to have a bystander assist you in the two-rescuer method. However, be certain that the bystander has been trained by the American Heart Association or the American Red Cross and is currently certified in the two-rescuer procedure. Too often, people wish to help thinking they know the procedure based on what they have seen on television, without the benefit of training in CPR. If you begin two-rescuer CPR with the aid of a bystander and find that the volunteer is unable to perform properly and you cannot quickly correct the problem, stop the two-rescuer procedure and begin one-rescuer CPR.

If you wish to join another member of the EMS System who has initiated CPR, you should:

1. Ask to help.
2. Allow the first rescuer to complete a cycle of 15 compressions and 2 ventilations.
3. Assume the responsibility for compressions and allow the first rescuer to become the ventilator.

If CPR has been started by someone who is certified but not part of the EMS System and you join this person to start CPR:

1. Identify yourself and state that you are an EMT and you are ready to perform two-rescuer CPR.
2. While the first rescuer is providing compressions, spend five seconds checking for a carotid pulse produced by each compression. This is to determine if the compressions being delivered are effective. Inform the first rescuer if there is or is not a pulse being produced.*
3. You should say, "Stop compressions" and check for spontaneous pulse and breathing. This should take 5 seconds. The first compressor can count this time off out loud.

---

* If the first rescuer cannot deliver effective compressions, you will have to take over for him once CPR is resumed.

1

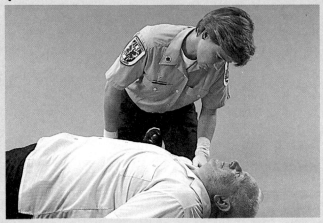

Establish unresponsiveness and reposition

2

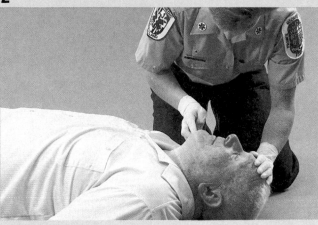

Open airway

3

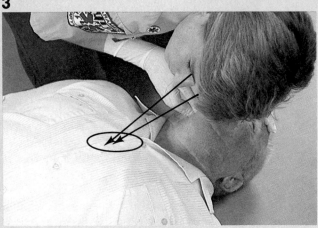

Look, listen, and feel (3–5 seconds)

4

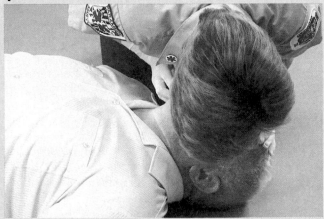

Ventilate twice (1–1.5 sec/ventilation). When practical, use a pocket face mask.

5

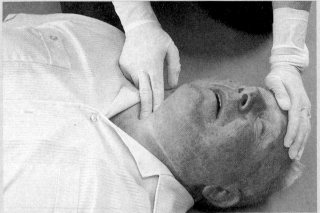

No pulse (5–10 sec.)

6

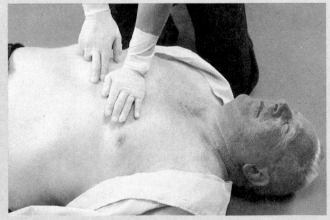

Locate compression site

7

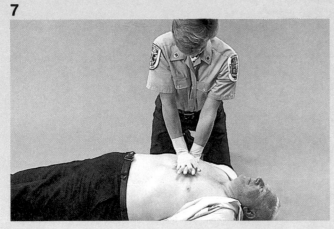

Position hands

8

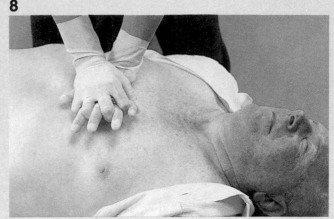

Begin compressions

Compressions delivered at a rate of
80–100/minute (15 per 9–11 sec.)

9

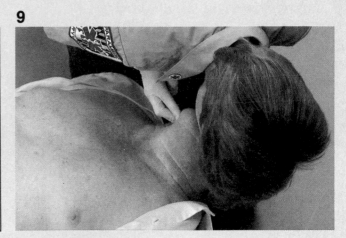

Ventilate twice

10

Provide 2 ventilations every 15
compressions (1–1.5 sec/ventilation)

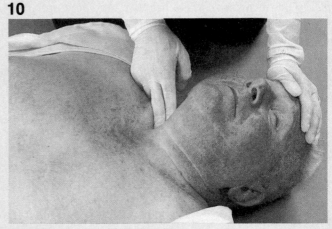

Recheck pulse after 4 cycles, and then every few
minutes

NOTE: When alone, call out for help if patient is unresponsive. If off duty, have
someone call dispatch after checking for pulselessness.

4. If there is no pulse, you should ventilate once and state, "No pulse. Continue CPR."
5. The switch from one-rescuer to two-rescuer CPR should take place after the first rescuer has completed a cycle of 15 compressions and 2 interposed ventilations.
6. The first rescuer resumes compressions, and the second rescuer provides an interposed ventilation after every fifth compression. If desired, the second rescuer can start compressions and allow the first rescuer to provide the ventilations.

NOTE: If you are off duty and arrive after CPR has been started, let the first rescuer know that you know CPR and that you are an EMT. If you find that the first rescuer does not know CPR, stop him and take over, providing one-rescuer techniques.

Compressions and Ventilations

For the two-rescuer method, the rate of compressions is 5 compressions every 3 to 4 seconds. The EMT delivering interposed ventilations (the **ventilator**) provides one full breath after every fifth compression to provide a rate of 12 breaths per minute.

- COMPRESSIONS = 80 to 100 per minute, delivering 5 compressions every 3 to 4 seconds
- VENTILATIONS = delivering 1 per 5 compressions
- RATIO = 5 compressions per 1 ventilation

The compressor counts out loud saying, "one and two and three and four and five, breathe," starting the cycle again with, "one and two. . . ." For each second counted, the compressor delivers a compression to the CPR compression site. The ventilator delivers a full breath after each fifth compression. The compressor must pause to allow the ventilator 1 to 1.5 seconds to deliver the interposed ventilation.

NOTE: If the ventilator misses a breath, he should not wait for the next fifth stroke to provide the ventilation. Instead, he should deliver this missed ventilation on the upstroke of the next compression.

Two-Rescuer CPR Procedure

The complete procedure is shown in Scan 5–2. Both rescuers are shown on the same side of the patient to allow you to see what each person is doing. The procedure goes more smoothly if the rescuers are on opposite sides of the patient, as in Figure 5–11.

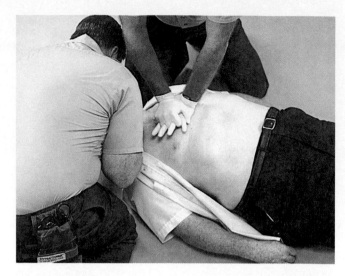

FIGURE 5–11. Opposite-side positioning in two-rescuer CPR.

This is particularly true when position changes are taking place. Once in the ambulance, the procedure will have to be done with one rescuer providing ventilations with supplemental oxygen while positioned at the patient's head.

After the first minute of CPR and every few (three to four) minutes thereafter, the ventilator should check to see if the patient has a carotid pulse and note any spontaneous breathing. Since compressions cannot be delivered while trying to detect a spontaneous carotid pulse, this check should not last longer than 5 seconds. If a pulse is detected, the ventilator should say, "Stop compressions" and rescue breathing should be provided if needed. If there is no pulse, the ventilator should say, "Continue CPR."

Changing Positions

If the compressor becomes tired and wants to change positions, or if the ventilator indicates he wishes a position change, the change is controlled by the compressor (SCAN 5–3). The ventilator is told at the beginning of the next compression cycle. The compressor will say, "CHANGE. One and two and three and four and five, BREATHE." The ventilator will provide one full breath, and the two rescuers will quickly change positions.

During the change, it is recommended that the airway be opened and a carotid pulse and breathing be checked by the compressor as he moves to the ventilator position. These checks should be done simultaneously, taking no more than 5 seconds. If the changes take place every 2 minutes or less, a check of pulse and breathing does not have to be done on every change.

SCAN 5–2 TWO RESCUER CPR

1

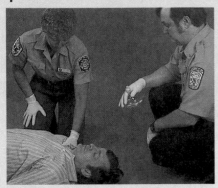

Determine unresponsiveness. Reposition patient.

2

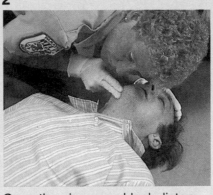

Open the airway and look, listen, and feel (3–5 sec.)

3

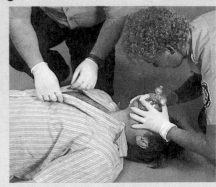

Ventilate twice (1–1.5 sec/ ventilation)

4

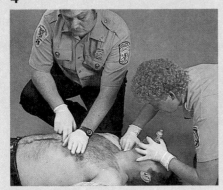

Determine pulselessness. Locate CPR compression site.

5

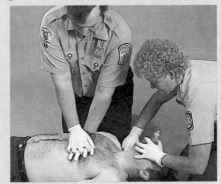

Say "no pulse." Begin compressions.

6

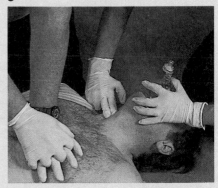

Check compression effectiveness. Deliver five compressions in 3–4 seconds. (rate = 80–100/minute)

7

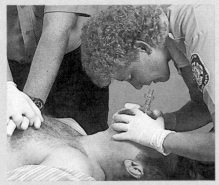

Ventilate once. (1–1.5 sec./ ventilation) Stop for ventilation

8

Continue with one ventilation every five compressions.

9

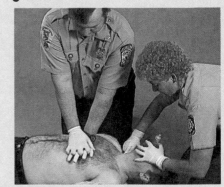

After ten cycles, reassess breathing and pulse. No pulse—ventilate and say "continue CPR." Pulse—say, "stop CPR."

NOTE: Assess for spontaneous breathing and pulse for 5 seconds at the end of the first minute, and then every few minutes thereafter.

SCAN 5–3 CHANGING POSITIONS

1

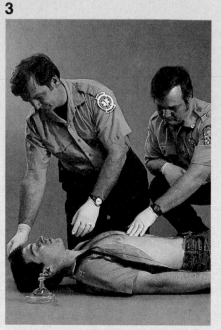

When fatigued, the compressor calls for the switch. Give a clear signal to change.

2

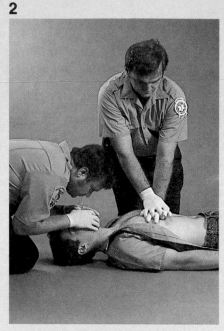

Compressor completes fifth compression. Ventilator provides one ventilation.

3

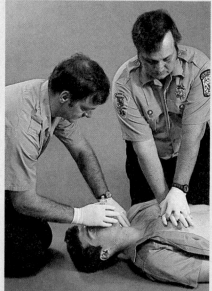

Ventilator moves to chest and begins to locate compression site. Compressor begins move to head.

4

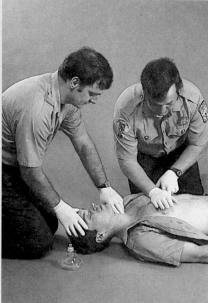

New compressor finds site. New ventilator checks carotid pulse (5 seconds).

5

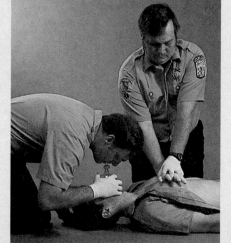

New ventilator says, "no pulse," and ventilates once (1–1.5 seconds), using his own pocket face mask.

6

New compressor delivers five compressions (3–4 seconds) at a rate of 80–100 per minute. New ventilator assesses compressions.

NOTE: Both rescuers shown on the same side of the patient for purpose of clarity.

CPR Techniques for Infants and Children

The techniques of CPR for infants and small children are essentially the same as those used for adults. You will have to:

1. Establish unresponsiveness.
2. Correctly position the patient.
3. Open the airway (head-tilt, chin-lift, or jaw-thrust).
4. Establish respiratory arrest (3 to 5 seconds).
5. Provide artificial ventilations and clear the airway, if necessary.
6. Establish the lack of pulse in 5 to 10 seconds.
7. Provide external chest compressions and interposed ventilations.
8. Do frequent assessments of pulse and breathing. This is to be done after every ten cycles of compressions and interposed ventilation.

Some procedures and rates differ when the patient is an infant or a child. If younger than one year of age, the patient is considered to be an infant. Between one and eight years of age, the patient is considered to be a child. Over the age of eight years, adult procedures apply to the patient. Keep in mind that the size of the patient can also be an important factor. A very small nine-year old may have to be treated as a child.

Positioning the Patient

When CPR must be performed, adults, children, and infants are placed on their backs on a hard surface.

Opening the Airway

- INFANT—use the head-tilt, chin-lift technique, but apply only a slight tilt. Too great a tilt may close off the airway; however, make certain that the opening is adequate (note chest rise during ventilation). Always be sure to support the infant's head.
- CHILD—the same caution applies to small children as to infants. Larger children can have their airways opened by standard head-tilt, chin-lift, or jaw-thrust techniques.

Establishing a Pulse

- INFANT—For infants, you should use the **brachial** (BRAY-key-al) **pulse.** This is the pulse that can be felt when compressing the

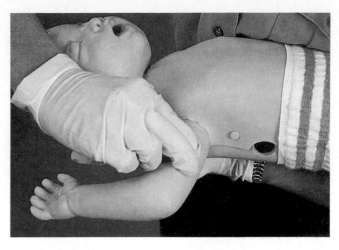

FIGURE 5–12. For infants, determine circulation by feeling for a brachial pulse.

major artery of the upper arm, the brachial artery. *Do not* use the carotid or radial pulse. You can find the brachial pulse by:

1. Locating the point halfway between the infant's elbow and shoulder
2. Placing your thumb on the lateral side of the upper arm at this midway point
3. Placing the tips of your index and middle fingers at the midway point on the medial surface of the infant's upper arm. You will feel a groove in the muscle at this location.
4. Pressing your index and middle fingers in toward the bone, taking care not to exert too much pressure. To do so may collapse the artery, stopping circulation to the lower arm and perhaps causing you to miss feeling the pulse.
5. Take 5 to 10 seconds to determine pulselessness.

- CHILD—determine circulation by finding a carotid pulse.

External Chest Compressions

- INFANT—apply compressions to the midline of the sternum, directly between the nipples. Use the tips of two or three fingers to deliver the compressions. The index finger should be on the midline and one finger width below an imaginary line directly between the nipples (intermammary line). The infant's sternum should be depressed 0.5 to 1 inch.
- CHILD—compressions are applied using the heel of one hand. The compression site is the mid sternum, located using the same pro-

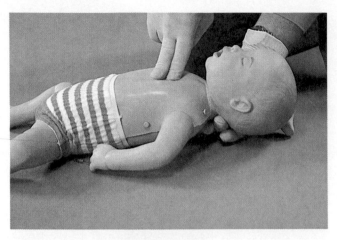

Infants: Use tips of fingers and light pressure.

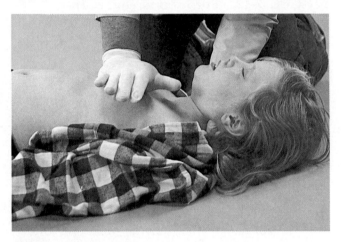

Children: Use heel of one hand only.

FIGURE 5–13. External chest compressions for infants and children.

cedure that is applied to the adult patient. The child's sternum should be depressed 1 to 1.5 inches.

Ventilations

- INFANT—the rescuer should provide a slow, gentle breath of air using the mouth-to-mouth and nose or approved mouth-to-mask or other accepted safe technique. It is essential to watch the rise and fall of the infant's chest. The rescuer should deliver just enough air to cause the infant's chest to rise, taking 1 to 1.5 seconds per ventilation.
- CHILD—a slow, gentle breath is provided to the child patient, taking 1 to 1.5 seconds per ventilation. Again, only enough air is delivered to cause the patient's chest to rise. Mouth-to-mouth or mouth-to-nose techniques are usually employed. If the patient is a small child, you may have to use the

mouth-to-mouth and nose method. The use of a pocket face mask or other accepted device is recommended.

CPR Rates

- INFANT—deliver compressions at the rate of at least 100 per minute (5 compressions in at least 3 seconds). Interpose a slow, gentle breath every five compressions to give a ratio of 5:1.
- CHILD—deliver compressions at the rate of 80 to 100 per minute. Interpose a slow, gentle breath every five compressions to give a ratio of 5:1.

NOTE: To establish the correct rate for infants, count: "One, two, three, four, five, breathe." Provide the interposed ventilation immediately after "five." For children, count: "One and two and three and four and five, breathe." Provide the interposed ventilation immediately after "five."

CPR: Moving Patients

Ideally, CPR should not be interrupted for more than seven seconds. However, when CPR is being performed and the patient must be moved for safety reasons or for transport, interruptions may be longer (SCAN 5–4). Interruptions should last no longer than 15 seconds; however, it may be necessary to interrupt the procedure for up to 30 seconds under special circumstances.

Major problems occur when moving a patient up or down a stairway or along a narrow hallway. It is necessary to provide the patient with effective CPR before the interruption. On signal, the patient is moved as quickly as possible and effective CPR is resumed beginning with a ventilation at the next level, or at the end of the narrow hallway. Note that compressions can be delivered during the move, when it is safe to do so. Ventilations provided by a bag-valve-mask unit or positive pressure can be delivered during the move (see Chapter 6).

CPR *must be continued* once the patient is loaded into the ambulance. The procedure should continue uninterrupted during transport and transfer until the emergency department staff takes over CPR or the physician on duty tells you to stop your CPR efforts.

NOTE: There are special situations which require CPR and other basic life support measures. These include near-drownings, electric shocks, accidents producing crushing chest injuries, drug overdoses, and toxic gas inhalations. The problems of resuscita-

SCAN 5—4 CPR SUMMARY

ONE RESCUER	FUNCTIONS	TWO RESCUER
	• Establish unresponsiveness • Position patient • Open airway • Look, listen, and feel (for 3–5 seconds)	
	• Deliver 2 breaths (1–1.5 sec/ventilation)	
	• Check carotid pulse . . . (5–10 seconds) If no pulse . . . • Begin chest compressions	

	DELIVER COMPRESSIONS		
	80–100/min (15/9–11 sec)	80–100/min (5/3–4 sec)	

	DELIVER VENTILATIONS		
	2/15	1/5 (Pause to allow ventilations)	
	• Do 4 cycles • Check pulse	• Ventilator checks effective- ness	
	CONTINUE PERIODIC ASSESSMENT		

Changing Positions

• Compressor—signal to change; provide 5 compressions • Ventilator—one ventilation	New ventilator checks pulse provides 1 ventilation (uses new mask)	Continue CPR sequence

NOTE: Wear gloves and use either a pocket mask with one-way valve or bag valve mask.

tion as they relate to these special problems will be covered later in this textbook.

CAUTION: CPR skills can be quickly lost when not practiced on a regular basis. As an EMT, be certain to practice CPR on infant and adult manikins. Ideally, you should be recertified in CPR once every year. One way to stay efficient in the technique is to become a CPR instructor for the American Heart Association or the American Red Cross and teach CPR to the public.

SUMMARY

When someone stops breathing and the heart stops beating, clinical death occurs. Within approximately 10 minutes, biological death can result.

There is a vital relationship between breathing, circulation, and brain activities. If one stops functioning, it will affect the other two.

When a patient's heart stops beating, he is in cardiac arrest. He will be unresponsive and there will be no breathing and no pulse.

You should determine breathing by the look, listen, and feel method. Circulation is determined by feeling for a carotid pulse. If the patient is an infant (under one year of age), then feel for a brachial pulse.

If a patient is in cardiac arrest, you should take the ABC approach: A = airway, B = breathe, and C = circulate.

To perform one-rescuer CPR (see SCAN 5–4):

1. Establish the patient's unresponsiveness.
2. Correctly position the patient and open the airway.

   CAUTION: *Do not* overextend the head-tilt for infants and small children.

3. Determine that the patient is not breathing. If he is not . . .
4. Provide two quick breaths and evaluate breathing. Clear the airway if necessary.
5. Determine that there is no breathing and no carotid pulse (or brachial pulse for the infant).
6. Find the CPR compression site:
   - ADULT: one finger-width superior to the substernal notch
   - CHILD: along the midline of the sternum, located using the same procedure applied to the adult patient.

- INFANT: along the midline of the sternum, with the index finger one finger width below an imaginary line drawn between the nipples.

7. Correctly position your hands for compressions:
   - ADULT: The heel of your hand closest to the patient's head is placed on the CPR compression site. Your other hand is placed on top of this hand so that the heels of both hands are parallel and the fingers are pointing away from your body. Your fingers can be extended or interlaced, but YOU MUST KEEP YOUR FINGERS OFF THE PATIENT'S RIBS.
   - CHILD: Deliver compressions with the heel of one hand positioned the same as with an adult patient.
   - INFANT: Deliver compressions with the tips of two or three fingers, positioned over the infant's sternum. The tip of your index finger should be one finger width below an imaginary line between the nipples.
8. Provide external chest compressions:
   - ADULT: Depth = 1.5 to 2 inches, 1 to 1.5 seconds per ventilation
     Rate = 80 to 100/minute
   - CHILD: Depth = 1 to 1.5 inches
     Rate = 80 to 100/minute
   - INFANT: Depth = 0.5 to 1 inch
     Rate = at least 100/minute
9. Provide ventilations:
   - ADULT: Two breaths after every 15 compressions, 1 to 1.5 seconds per ventilation
   - CHILD: One slow, gentle breath after every 5 compressions, 1 to 1.5 seconds per ventilation
   - INFANT: One slow, gentle breath after every 5 compressions, 1 to 1.5 seconds per ventilation. It is essential to watch for the patient's chest to rise.
10. Check for a carotid pulse after 1 minute. Use the brachial pulse if the patient is an infant. If no pulse and no breathing, continue CPR, checking for a pulse every few minutes. If there is a pulse, but no breathing, stop compressions and provide rescue breathing. Continue to monitor pulse. If patient breathes or tries to breathe, re-check pulse.

NOTE: The patient will not continue to breathe unless there is heart action.

You should not stop CPR for more than 7 seconds unless it is to move the patient. For such cases, do not stop CPR for more than 15 to 30 seconds. After providing CPR for 1 minute, the single rescuer procedure may be interrupted for 30 seconds to activate the EMS System. Continue CPR until heart or heart and lung functions start, until you are relieved by another trained person, care is transferred over to a physician or the staff of the emergency department, or you cannot continue because of exhaustion.

CPR is effective when the patient's chest rises and falls during ventilations and someone else can detect a carotid pulse produced with each external chest compression.

When a patient is in cardiac arrest, START CPR IMMEDIATELY, even if you worsen existing injuries or may cause injuries such as fractured ribs. Without CPR, the patient will go quickly from clinical to biological death.

In two-rescuer CPR (See Scan 5–4):

- Compressions = 80 to 100 per minute (5 compressions in 3 to 4 seconds)
- Provide 1 ventilation every 5 compressions. The compressor must pause to allow for adequate ventilation.
- The compressor counts the one to five cycle.
- The ventilator checks the effectiveness of compressions.
- The compressor commands the change of positions.
- Check for a spontaneous carotid pulse and spontaneous breathing every few minutes.
- Do not interrupt CPR for more than 7 seconds except to move the patient (a 30-second interruption is the maximum).
- If you miss a breath, deliver the ventilation on the upstroke of the next compression.

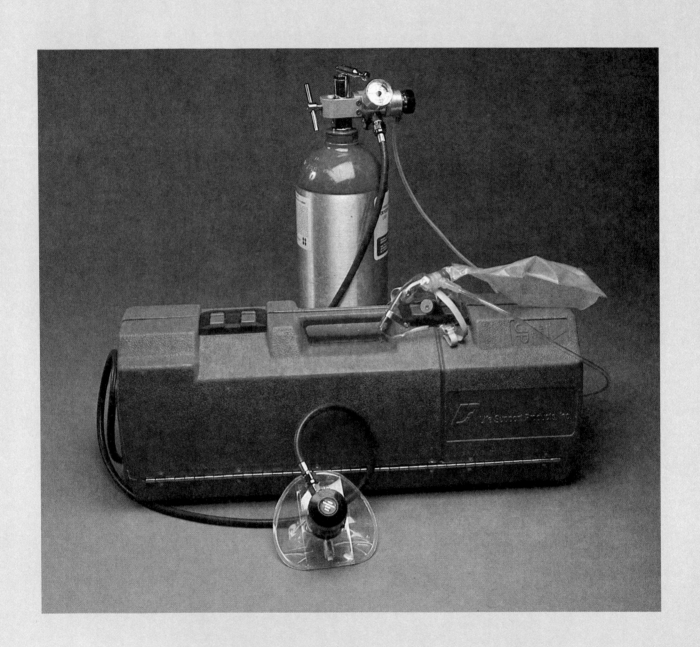

Breathing Aids and Oxygen Therapy

OBJECTIVES   As an EMT, you should be able to:

1. Define and identify oropharyngeal and nasopharyngeal airways. (p. 164, p. 166)

2. State the major advantage of using airway adjuncts. (p. 163)

3. Describe how to insert an oropharyngeal airway and a nasopharyngeal airway. (pp. 164–165, p. 166)

4. Describe how to provide artificial ventilation when using each of the above airways. (p. 165, p. 166)

5. State the importance of having suction equipment ready for immediate use when providing emergency care. (p. 167)

6. Describe, step by step, the techniques of suctioning. (p. 168)

7. Define and identify a pocket face mask and describe how this device is used to assist in ventilating a patient. (p. 170)

8. List and define the parts of a bag-valve-mask system. (p. 171)

9. Describe how to use the bag-valve-mask to provide ventilation. (p. 172)

10. State the advantages and the disadvantages of oxygen therapy. (pp. 172–175)

11. Define *hypoxia* and list several causes of this condition. (pp. 173–174)

12. Define *D, E, and M oxygen cylinders* and state how to determine the expected duration of flow for any given cylinder. (p. 176)

13. Define *pressure regulator* and describe how to connect this device to an oxygen supply cylinder. (pp. 177–178)

14. Compare and contrast the Bourdon gauge flowmeter, the pressure-compensated flowmeter, and the constant flow selector valve. Describe how to connect a flowmeter to an oxygen delivery system. (pp. 178–179)

15. Describe the correct procedures for the field use of a humidifier, stating when this device is to be used. (p. 179)

16. Identify a nasal cannula, a simple face mask, a partial rebreathing mask (reservoir mask), a nonrebreathing mask (reservoir mask), and a Venturi mask. (pp. 180–182)

17. State how the percentage of oxygen delivered by the above five devices increases in relation to every additional 1 liter per minute of oxygen flow. (p. 180)

18. For each of the above oxygen delivery devices state the range of percentage of oxygen delivered, the approximate range of liter per minute flow needed, and the typical patients for whom each device can be used. (p. 181)

19. State how the bag-valve-mask unit can be used to deliver nearly 100% oxygen to a nonbreathing patient. (p. 183)

20. Define *positive-pressure resuscitator* and *demand valve resuscitator* and describe how these devices can be used to ventilate the nonbreathing patient. (p. 183)

21. Describe, step by step, how to set up oxygen equipment, administer oxygen to a patient, and perform the procedures for discontinuing the administration of oxygen. (pp. 183–186)

SKILLS   As an EMT, you should be able to:

1. Determine if an airway adjunct is needed, insert the proper-sized device, and provide ventilation.

2. Correctly use both fixed (installed) and portable suction equipment.

3. Provide ventilation with a bag-valve-mask unit, with and without the device being connected to an oxygen supply system.

4. Use a pocket mask to provide ventilation.

5. Select the correct oxygen delivery device for a patient.

6. Properly set up oxygen equipment, deliver oxygen to a patient, and discontinue the administration of oxygen.

7. Assemble, test, disassemble (when appropriate), and clean all equipment used to ensure an airway, suction, provide ventilation, and deliver oxygen to a patient.

TERMS   you may be using for the first time:

Airway Adjunct – a device placed in a patient's mouth or nose in order to help maintain an open airway. Those inserted in the mouth help to hold the tongue in place.

• **Oropharyngeal** (or-o-fah-RIN-je-al) **Airway** – a curved airway adjunct inserted through the patient's mouth into the pharynx.

• **Nasopharyngeal** (na-zo-fah-RIN-je-al) **Airway** – a flexible breathing tube inserted through the patient's nose into the pharynx.

Atelectasis (at-i-LEK-tah-sis) – complete or partial collapse of the alveoli of the lungs.

Bag-Valve-Mask Device – a hand-held unit with a self-refilling bag, directional valve system, and face mask. The bag is squeezed to deliver atmospheric air to the patient. This unit can be set up to deliver nearly 100% oxygen when connected to a supplemental oxygen supply system.

Chronic Obstructive Pulmonary Disease (COPD) – a group of diseases and conditions including emphysema, chronic bronchitis, and black lung. Delivery of more than 28% oxygen to such patients can lead to respiratory arrest. See Chapter 14 for more specifics.

D, E, and M Cylinders – the most commonly used oxygen cylinders. D cylinders contain 350 liters of oxygen, E cylinders contain 625 liters of oxygen, and M cylinders contain 3,000 liters of oxygen.

Demand Valve Resuscitator – an oxygen-powered breathing device that will deliver oxygen when the patient attempts an inspiration.

Flowmeter – a Bourdon, pressure-compensated device or constant flow selector valve used to indicate the flow of oxygen in liters per minute.

Humidifier – a device connected to the flowmeter to add moisture to the dry oxygen coming from the cylinder.

Hypoxia (hi-POK-se-ah) – an inadequate supply of oxygen reaching the body's tissues.

Oxygen Delivery Device – typically one of four face masks or a nasal cannula.

Oxygen Toxicity – uncommon, rarely fatal effect of oxygen on a patient who has received too high a concentration of the gas for too long a period of time.

Pocket Face Mask – a device with a one-way valve to aid in mouth-to-mouth resuscitation that can be used with supplemental oxygen when fitted with an oxygen inlet.

Positive-Pressure Resuscitator – a manually triggered, oxygen-powered breathing device.

Pressure Regulator – a device connected to an oxygen cylinder to reduce cylinder pressure to a safe working level (a safe pressure for delivery of oxygen to a patient).

Suction Device – a vacuum-, air-, or oxygen-powered device that is used to remove blood, secretions, or other fluids from a patient's mouth, throat, or stoma. Electrical-, oxygen-, and manual-powered units are available.

AIDS TO BREATHING

It is vitally important that the EMT know how to provide basic life support without using any special devices. Establishing and maintaining an open airway, providing artificial ventilation, and the technique of CPR can be accomplished without equipment. Initiating basic life support is usually done this way. Should equipment not be on hand, or should it fail, the EMT can continue basic life support using the techniques presented in Chapters 4 and 5.

Even though basic life support is possible without equipment, more effective emergency care can be accomplished when devices are used to maintain an open airway, clear the airway, assist in ventilation, and provide oxygen. Their use provides more oxygen to the exchange levels of the patient's lungs (alveoli) and greatly reduces rescuer fatigue. It is critical that an EMT know how to use and maintain the aids to breathing and the oxygen delivery equipment carried on ambulances.

REMEMBER: *Never* delay resuscitation measures in order to locate, retrieve, and set up special equipment or oxygen delivery devices. Always have your equipment ready for immediate use.

Keep in mind that new responsibilities come with the use of equipment in basic life support:

- YOU must be sure that the equipment is clean and that it is operational *prior to use*. This should be done for every shift and after every run.
- YOU must select the proper equipment for the patient receiving care.
- YOU must monitor the patient more closely once you begin to use any airway device, ventilation-assist device, or oxygen delivery system.
- YOU must make certain that the equipment is properly discarded, cleaned, or tested after its use.

Airways

WARNING: Oropharyngeal (or-o-fah-RIN-je-al) airways are only to be used on *unconscious* patients who do not display a gag reflex. These devices can induce vomiting in the conscious individual. This vomitus can be aspirated into the patient's lungs, causing serious airway obstruction and damage. As little as 2 ounces of vomitus in the lungs can cause a fatal form of pneumonia. Also, oropharyngeal airways can induce some degree of vocal cord spasms

or bronchospasms in a conscious patient. *Never* use an oropharyngeal airway on a conscious patient. *Never* practice the use of airways on anyone. Manikins should be used for developing skills with airways.

Once you gain access to a patient and begin the primary survey, your first course of action is to establish an open airway. This airway must be maintained throughout all care procedures. Once the airway has been opened by the head-tilt, chin-lift, or jaw-thrust maneuvers, it can be kept open more easily by an airway adjunct. You must guard against improper head movement if there is any chance of spinal injury. If a trauma patient is unconscious, the EMT is to assume there is spinal injury and use the jaw-thrust technique.

Rules for Using Airway Adjuncts

NOTE: A variety of devices are called "airway adjuncts." In this discussion, only those devices that are part of the standard EMT–Basic course will be considered.

1. Use an airway on all unconscious patients who do not exhibit a gag reflex.
2. Open the patient's airway before use.
3. Use on nonbreathing, unconscious patients. Any gagging by the patient indicates that the adjunct airway inserted through the mouth cannot be used. Remove the device immediately if the patient exhibits a gag reflex.
4. Take great care not to push the patient's tongue back into the throat.
5. Constantly monitor the patient for spontaneous breathing or gag reflex.
6. Remove the device immediately if the patient exhibits a gag reflex or vomits.
7. Wear gloves while inserting the airway.

NOTE: Because of the danger of vomiting, many EMS Systems have restricted the use of the oropharyngeal airway to unresponsive, nonbreathing patients. Some systems *do allow* for the use of this oral airway for certain *conscious* medical patients (e.g., severe stroke) and trauma patients (e.g., facial injury preventing the use of nasal airways). You *must* follow your local protocols. If an airway is inserted into the mouth of a conscious patient, constant monitoring with suction equipment that is immediately available must be part of the protocol.

Oropharyngeal Airways

Once a patient's airway is opened, an oropharyngeal airway can be inserted to help keep it open. "Oro-" refers to the mouth. "Pharyngeo-" refers to the throat. An **oropharyngeal airway** is a curved device, usually made of plastic, which can be inserted through the patient's mouth to extend back into the throat. The oropharyngeal airway has a *flange* that fits against the patient's lips. The rest of the device holds down the tongue as it curves back to the throat.

The proper use of an oropharyngeal airway greatly reduces the chances of the patient's airway becoming obstructed. When a patient becomes unconscious, the muscles relax. The tongue will slide back into the pharynx and obstruct the airway. Even though a jaw-thrust or head-tilt, chin-lift maneuver will help open the airway of a patient, the tongue may return to its obstructive position once the maneuver is released. Sometimes, even when the jaw-thrust or head-tilt is maintained, the tongue will "fall back" into the pharynx.

There are standard sizes of oropharyngeal airways (Figure 6–1). Many manufacturers make a complete line, ranging from sizes for infants to various sizes of adult airways. An entire set should be carried in one case to allow for quick, proper selection.

The device *cannot* be used effectively unless you select the correct airway size for the patient. An airway of proper size will extend from the center of the patient's mouth to the angle of the lower jaw bone (mandible). This can be used as the way to size the airway, or you can simply measure from

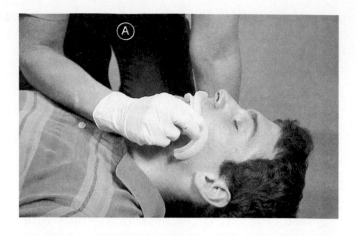

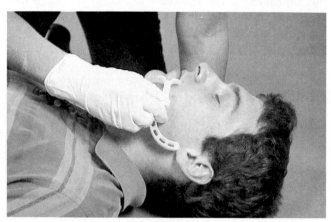

FIGURE 6–2. The airway is chosen and is checked for correct size.

the corner of the patient's mouth to the tip of the ear lobe on the same side of the face (Figure 6–2). *Do not* use an airway until it has been properly sized. If the airway is not the correct size, *do not* use it on the patient.

Inserting the Airway

1. Place the patient on his back. When caring for a medical patient with no indications of spinal injury, the neck may be hyperextended. If there are possible spinal injuries, use the jaw-thrust maneuver, moving the patient no more than necessary to ensure an open airway (the airway takes priority over the spine). Extreme care must be taken.
2. Cross the thumb and forefinger of one hand and place them on the upper and lower teeth at the corner of the patient's mouth. Spread your fingers apart to open the patient's jaws. Hold the mouth open using these same fingers.

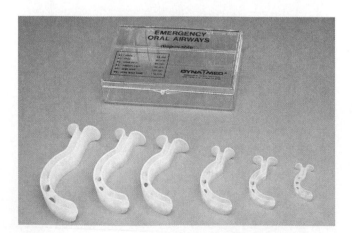

FIGURE 6–1. Various sizes of oropharyngeal airways.

3. Position the correct size airway so that its tip is pointing toward the roof of the patient's mouth (Figure 6–3).

4. Insert the airway and slide it along the roof of the patient's mouth, past the soft tissue hanging down from the back (the uvula), or until you meet resistance against the soft palate. Be certain not to push the patient's tongue back into the throat. In a few cases, you may have to use a tongue blade (tongue depressor) to hold the tongue in place. Any airway insertion is made easier by using a tongue blade. Watch what you are doing when inserting the airway. This procedure should not be performed by "feel" only.

5. GENTLY rotate the airway 180 degrees. This will position the tip so that it is pointing down into the patient's throat (Figure 6–4).

6. Place the nontrauma patient in a maximum head-tilt position. Minimize all movements of the head if there are possible spinal injuries.

7. Check to see that the flange of the airway is against the patient's lips (Figure 6–5). If the airway is too long or too short, remove the airway and replace it with the correct size.

8. Provide mouth-to-adjunct ventilation as you would provide mouth-to-mouth or mouth-to-mask ventilation (Figure 6–6).

9. Monitor the patient closely. If there is a gag reflex, remove the airway at once. Removal is accomplished by the reversal of the insertion procedures.

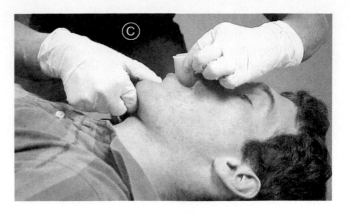

FIGURE 6–4.   The airway is rotated into position.

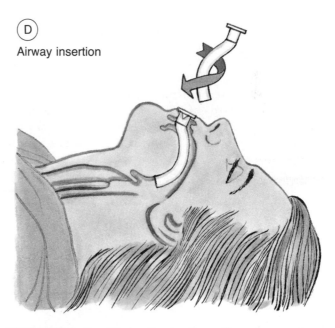

Airway insertion

FIGURE 6–5.   Note that when the airway is properly positioned, the flange rests against the patient's lips.

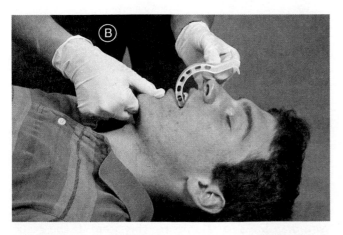

FIGURE 6–3.   The airway is inserted with the tip pointing to the roof of the patient's mouth.

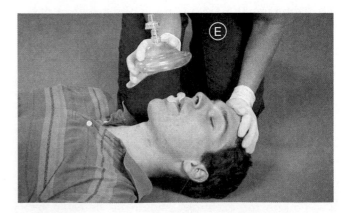

FIGURE 6–6.   The patient is ready for ventilation.

NOTE: Some EMS Systems allow an oropharyngeal airway to be inserted with the tip pointing to the side of the patient's mouth. The device is rotated 90 degrees so that its tip is pointing down into the patient's throat. Do not use this approach unless it is part of the protocol for your EMS System.

A major disadvantage of the oropharyngeal airway is that there is not a perfect size for every patient. In some cases, the closest fit may be too small and partially block the airway. If the device is too large it may fall forward and push the tongue back into the pharynx, blocking the airway again. However, for the vast majority of patients, you will be able to insert an oropharyngeal airway.

Nasopharyngeal Airways

The use of this type of airway is growing in popularity. Many EMTs are in favor of its use since the device tends not to stimulate a gag reflex, thus making it a practical airway adjunct for conscious patients. The soft, flexible tube is inserted through the nose rather than the mouth, eliminating the difficulties and hazards of trying to reposition the head and pry open the patient's mouth, and allows for an airway insertion in cases in which there is oral cavity injury.

Inserting the Airway

1. Select a nasopharyngeal airway that visually appears to be smaller in diameter than the opening of the patient's nostril. This is approximately the diameter of the little finger. Determine the size by measuring from the tip of the patient's nose to the tip of his ear lobe.
2. Lubricate the outside of the tube with a water-based lubricant before its insertion. *Do not* use a petroleum jelly or any other type of non-water-based lubricant. These can damage the tissue lining the nasal cavity and the pharynx.
3. Gently push the tip of the nose upward. Keep the patient's head in a neutral position. The airway is inserted through the right nostril (when possible) and moved along the floor of the nasal cavity. The convex curve of the airway should be upward, toward the patient's forehead. The bevel should be toward the nasal septum.
4. Once the airway is in place, the flange should rest firmly against the patient's nostril. Adequate air exchange should be detected by the look, listen, and feel method.

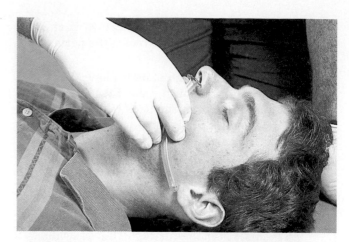

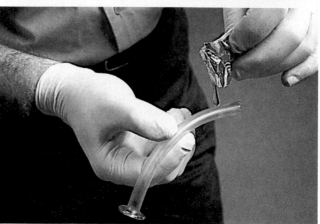

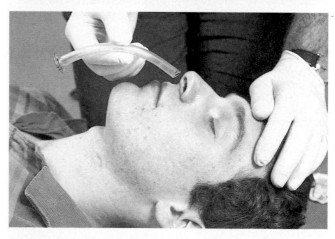

FIGURE 6–7. Inserting a lubricated nasopharyngeal airway.

Do not attempt to insert the tube if there are indications of nasal injury or cerebrospinal fluid flowing from the nose. If there is resistance when inserting the nasopharyngeal tube, *do not* force it into the nose. Pull the tube out and try the other nostril (you may have to relubricate the tube). If the resistance is such that you cannot easily insert the tube, do not continue your attempts. Successful insertion may be possible with a smaller size tube.

NOTE: The esophageal obturator airway is presented in Appendix 1.

Suction Devices

To this point, we have discussed body positioning and finger sweeps as the primary techniques to remove blood, vomitus, phlegm, and other secretions from a patient's mouth and throat. Fixed and portable mechanical suction devices are available to supplement these manual methods.

Fixed (Installed) Systems

A fixed (installed) suction system should be in every ambulance (Figure 6–8). This type of system is powered by the vacuum produced by the engine manifold or by an electrically operated vacuum pump. To be effective, a fixed system must furnish an air intake of at least 30 liters per minute at the open end of

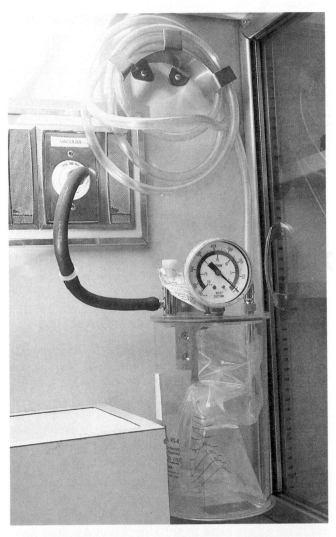

FIGURE 6–8. Fixed (installed) suction unit for ambulance patient compartments.

a collection tube. This will occur if the system can generate a vacuum of no less than 300 mmHg when the collecting tube is clamped.

A fixed system should have a nonbreakable collection bottle; a large diameter, nonkinking, noncollapsing collection tube long enough to reach the patient; several rigid suction tips; a variety of catheters for clearing the throat; and water for rinsing the system. There must be some means for controlling the suction. Most suction catheters and suction tips have a finger port (air vent) that can be sealed and unsealed by the rescuer's finger in order to control suction.

Portable Suction Units

National standards require EMTs to know how to operate and use portable suction units.

There are many different types of portable suction devices. The main difference among these units is the suction source. The unit used should provide an air flow of no less than 20 liters per minute and a vacuum of 300 mmHg that can be obtained within 4 seconds of clamping the tube.

- Oxygen- or air-powered units—Most oxygen-powered resuscitators are equipped with a special device (Venturi) that develops a vacuum for suctioning. These units deplete oxygen at a great rate. Portable air-powered units are in use. These devices may be more efficient than the oxygen-powered type and are excellent for working in confined areas, such as vehicular wreckage. Some of the older units are gas powered, using freon as a source.
- Electrically powered units—These are highly efficient devices capable of developing a vacuum of up to 600 mmHg. Some units have a converter so that they can be operated by a rechargeable battery or 110-volt sources.
- Manual-powered units—These have a simple rubber bulb aspirator or a hand- or foot-operated device to produce a vacuum for suctioning. Some of these units are not as efficient as air- or electrically powered units, but they have proved to be dependable and very durable.

All portable suction equipment must use thick-walled, nonkinking, wide-bore tubing. The collection bottle is to be nonbreakable. The vacuum pressure and the flow through the tubing has to be adequate for pharyngeal suctioning.

Portable units have to have semi-rigid or rigid suction tips. Various sizes of sterile, semi-rigid, disposable suction catheters should be available to allow

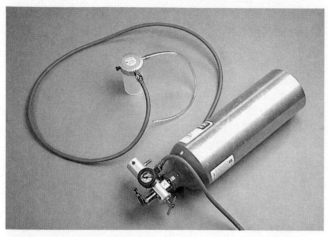

A

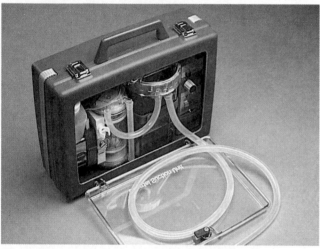

B

FIGURE 6–9. *A.* **Oxygen-powered portable suction unit.** *B.* **A portable suction unit that is powered by electricity.**

for suctioning of the mouth, throat, and stoma. The primary device now in use is the rigid suction tip. Rigid pharyngeal suction tips, sometimes referred to as tonsil suction tips (Yankauer suction tips), can be used for suctioning the throat; however, special care is required since their use may cause conscious patients to vomit.

Techniques of Suctioning

There are many variations in the technique of suctioning. A suggested procedure is presented in Scan 6–1.

Since suctioning requires you to have your fingers around and sometimes inside the patient's mouth, you should wear gloves to protect yourself from contact with blood and body fluids. In case the patient involuntarily bites down, many squads carry

commercial "bite blocks." *Do not* insert these blocks if there are loosened teeth. A bite block can be held between the patient's upper and lower teeth in cases in which care requires you to insert your gloved fingers into the patient's mouth. Some rescuers have reported success using an oropharyngeal airway that has been turned on its side as a bite block.

When inserting a catheter into a patient's mouth, *do not* apply suction. Begin to suction once the catheter has reached its proper depth, that is, once you are clear of the oral tissues and the pharynx has been reached. Use great care when suctioning a conscious patient. If you insert the catheter too deeply, it will trigger the gag reflex and the patient may vomit. Suctioning should take place *only* while you are withdrawing the catheter.

When suctioning a breathing patient, *never* suction longer than you can comfortably hold a normal breath. This would be about 15 seconds, although some systems have set a limit of 10 seconds. *Do not* suction the nonbreathing patient for more than 5 seconds at a time before attempting to ventilate him. After ventilating the patient, suctioning may continue.

During insertion of the catheter and suctioning, care must be taken to protect the soft tissues of the patient's mouth and throat. Make certain that you do not "jab" the patient's soft tissues during suctioning. Avoid any prolonged contact with the patient's tissues by rolling the catheter between your gloved fingers.

While suctioning, periodically you may have to clear debris from the catheter. Have water on hand to allow for frequent rinsing. If the materials found are too large to enter and pass through the catheter, or the catheter repeatedly clogs, change from a standard catheter to a tonsil suction tip. If the particles are still too large, remove the tip and continue suctioning using the tubing. When appropriate, use your gloved fingers to clear out foreign materials found in the patient's mouth.

NOTE: On rare occasions, severe head injuries that cause open fractures to the base and floor of the skull may expose brain tissue directly to the airway. If you are suctioning the back of the throat of a patient with a severe head injury and note what appears to be exposed brain tissues or open wounds in the throat, suction the mouth only. Do not suction the exposed tissues or probe into the wound sites. *Never try to suction away attached tissues.*

If there are no indications of possible spinal injury, the conscious patient should be suctioned after turning his head to the side. Should spinal injuries be possible, you should suction without turning the patient's head unless the obstruction is life

SCAN 6–1 TECHNIQUES OF SUCTIONING

1

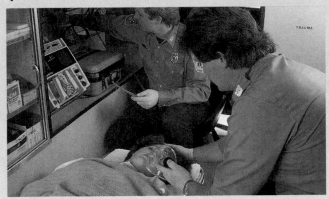

Position yourself at the patient's head and turn the patient to the side.

2

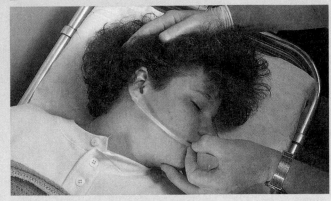

Measure suction catheter: the distance between the patient's earlobe and the corner of the mouth, or center of the mouth to the angle of the jaw.

3

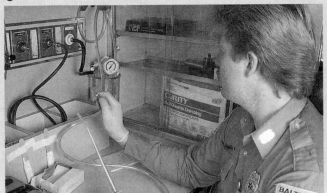

Turn unit on and test for suction.

4

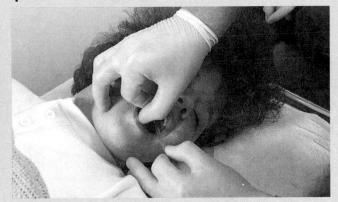

Open the patient's mouth by the crossed-finger technique and clear mouth.

Place the rigid pharyngeal tip so that the convex (bulging out) side is against the roof of the patient's mouth. Insert the tip to the beginning of the throat. **Do not** push the tip down into the throat or into the larynx.

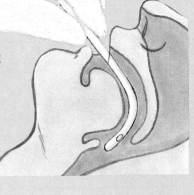

5

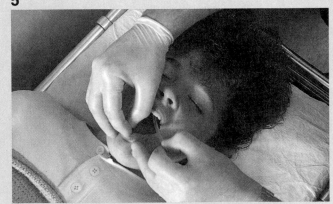

Apply suction **only** after the tip of the catheter or the rigid tip is in place.

NOTE: Suction is controlled by placing your finger over the port in the catheter or rigid suction tip.

threatening and all other methods have failed. Once the patient's head, neck, and spine are immobilized, you can turn the entire immobilized patient on his side. *Do not* delay suctioning to immobilize the patient.

There are times when it might be necessary to provide suctioning for a conscious patient. Talk to the patient to keep him calm. Let him know what you are going to do and what you are doing. *Do not* insert the catheter tip too deeply. To do so may set off the patient's gag reflex and induce vomiting. After suctioning, remember to reassure the patient.

Ventilation-Assist Devices

Two devices, the pocket face mask and the bag-valve-mask device, can be used to assist with ventilation. Even though there are times when you will use these devices apart from an oxygen supply, they are best used with supplemental oxygen.

NOTE: When using the pocket face mask or the bag-valve-mask device, the patient's chest must rise and his color should improve. If this does not happen, reposition the patient and reestablish an open airway. If ventilations continue to fail, use a different method of ventilation.

The Pocket Face Mask

The **pocket face mask** is a modification of a resuscitator facepiece. It is made of soft collapsible material and can be carried in the rescuer's pocket. The mask is available with or without an oxygen inlet. Mouth-to-mask ventilations are provided through a chimney on the mask. If oxygen is being delivered, the EMT can simultaneously ventilate the patient with air from his own lungs and the oxygen source. The oxygen delivered by this simultaneous method ranges from 40% to 45% at 10 liters per minute. Some masks will provide nearly 80% oxygen during the simultaneous method when a flow of 15 liters per minute is supplied.

One distinct advantage of the pocket face mask is that it allows the rescuer to use both hands to maintain the proper head-tilt and to hold the mask firmly in place. This device can be used without inserting an oropharyngeal airway when the airway is open and time is critical or when no such airway is available; however, when possible, an airway should be inserted.

Another advantage of the pocket face mask is that its use may greatly reduce the chances of the rescuer contracting a contagious disease from the patient. The best protection is provided by a pocket face mask that has a one-way valve. For this reason, even when a different form of ventilation-assist even-

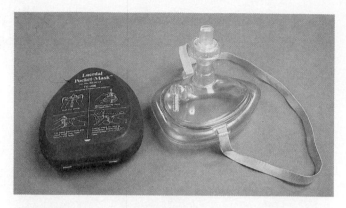

FIGURE 6–10. Pocket face masks. Note the chimney with one-way valve for mouth-to-mask ventilations.

tually will be used for the patient, it is better to start pulmonary resuscitation using the pocket face mask rather than mouth-to-mouth techniques, provided the use of the mask will not delay the start of the procedure.

To provide mouth-to-mask ventilation, you should:

1. Position yourself at the patient's head and open the airway. If necessary, clear the patient's airway. You should insert an oropharyngeal airway to keep the patient's airway open.

2. Position the mask on the patient's face so that the apex (top of the triangle) is over the bridge of the nose and the base is between the lower lip and the prominence of the chin.

3. Hold the mask *firmly* in place while maintaining the proper head-tilt:
   - Both thumbs on the sides of the mask
   - Index, third, and fourth fingers of each hand grasping the lower jaw on each side, between the angle of the jaw and the ear lobe to lift the jaw forward

4. Take a deep breath and exhale into the port of the mask chimney. Watch for the patient's chest to rise.

5. Remove your mouth from the chimney and allow for passive exhalation. Continue the cycle as you would for mouth-to-mouth ventilations.

The Bag-Valve-Mask Ventilator

The hand-held unit commonly used to ventilate a nonbreathing patient is the **bag-valve-mask unit.** The bag-valve-mask device may also be referred to

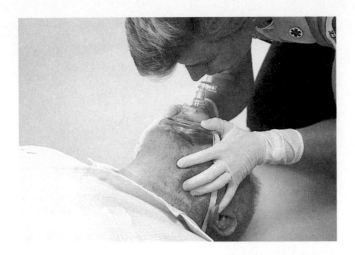

FIGURE 6–11. Providing mouth-to-mask ventilations. Note the placement of the EMT's hands.

as a bag-valve-mask unit, system, resuscitator, ventilator, or BVM. Some EMS Systems also use the bag-valve-mask unit to assist patients with shallow and failing respirations (e.g., drug overdose patients). This device comes in neonatal (newborn) size, pediatric size, and adult sizes (Figure 6–12).

WARNING: It may be very difficult to use the bag-valve-mask device properly. The primary problem is keeping an effective seal between the patient's face and the mask. To use this device properly requires considerable practice. There have been so many problems caused by the ineffective use of this device that some EMS Systems now require that it be used by two rescuers. One rescuer holds the mask in place while the other rescuer squeezes the bag. In many state protocols, the pocket face mask with supplemental oxygen is replacing the bag-valve-mask system.

WARNING: You must use the appropriate-sized unit for the patient. Use of an adult unit on infants and children may lead to severe lung damage. Pediatric units are in use that have "pop-off" valves to help prevent over-inflation of the lungs.

REMEMBER: When providing mouth-to-mouth ventilations, you are delivering 16% oxygen to the patient. The bag-valve-mask unit will deliver 21% oxygen from the atmosphere, but some of this gain is lost if there is reduced ventilatory volume when compared with the mouth-to-mouth method. When possible, use this device with supplemental oxygen. The bag-valve-mask system can deliver from 50% (oxygen delivery source) to nearly 100% oxygen (oxygen delivery source and a reservoir).

Many different types of bag-valve-mask systems are available; however, all have the same basic parts as shown in Figure 6–13. The bag must be a self-refilling shell bag (no sponge rubber). It should have a non-jam, one-way valve system that has been calibrated at 15 liters per minute inlet flow. The valve should be nonrebreathing and not subject to freezing in cold environments. There should be no pop-off valve except for pediatric models. Most units have a standard 15/22-mm respiratory fitting to accept a variety of masks or endotracheal tubes for advanced life support and paramedic use.

All bag-valve-mask units used in your EMS System must have an oxygen inlet and a reservoir must be available.

WARNING: The facepiece used on a bag-valve-mask unit must be transparent so that the EMT can see the patient's mouth. This is required so that you can see any vomitus or dislodged airway obstructions. When a clear facepiece is used, the EMT can

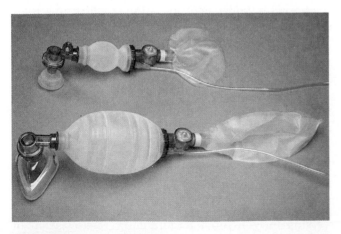

FIGURE 6–12. Pediatric and adult bag-valve-mask units.

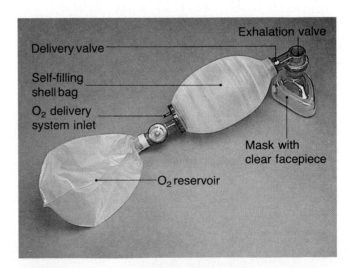

Delivery valve

Self-filling shell bag

O₂ delivery system inlet

Exhalation valve

Mask with clear facepiece

O₂ reservoir

FIGURE 6–13. The typical bag-valve-mask system.

see cyanosis (blue coloring) at the lips, which indicates the patient needs oxygenation. The best facepiece is one that has an air-inflated cuff to help maintain the mask-to-face seal.

The mechanical workings of a bag-valve-mask device are simple. When the bag is squeezed, air is delivered to the patient through a one-way valve. The air inlet to the bag is closed during delivery. When the hand-squeeze on the bag is released, a passive exhalation by the patient can occur. This air from the patient's lungs cannot reenter the bag. It passes through an exhalation valve into the atmosphere. While the patient is exhaling, air from the atmosphere or oxygen-rich air from the reservoir refills the bag. Older adult unit bags will hold 1,000 to 1,200 milliliters (ml) of air, with most newer models holding about 1,600 ml of air. Unless used properly, insufficient amounts of air will be delivered to the patient. If the two-rescuer technique is used, as much as 800 ml can be delivered to the patient. This is the minimum acceptable ventilation (AHA) for the nonbreathing patient.

When using the bag-valve-mask device, you should:

1. Position yourself at the patient's head and establish an open airway. If necessary, clear the patient's airway.
2. Insert an oropharyngeal airway.
3. Be certain to use the correct size mask for the patient. The apex or top of the triangular mask should be over the bridge of the nose. The base of the mask should rest between the patient's lower lip and the prominence of the chin.
4. Be certain to hold the mask firmly in position, with:
   • The thumb holding the upper part of the mask
   • The index finger between the valve and the lower cushion
   • The third, fourth, and fifth fingers on the lower jaw, between the chin and ear. This may vary slightly depending on the size of the rescuer's hands. With some units, you will have to hold your palm over the facepiece and hook your fingers under the patient's jaw (Figure 6–14).
5. With your other hand, squeeze the bag ONCE EVERY 5 SECONDS. The squeeze should be a full one, causing the patient's chest to rise. For children, squeeze the bag

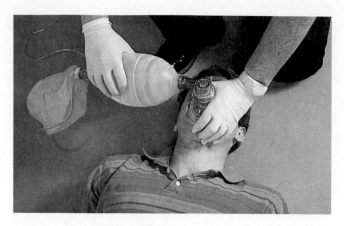

FIGURE 6–14. Hand positioning for using the bag-valve-mask.

once every 4 seconds. If ventilating an infant, squeeze the bag once every 3 seconds. (Make certain that you use the correct size mask.)
6. Release pressure on the bag and let the patient passively exhale and the bag refill from the atmosphere or oxygen source.

Two problems are often experienced when using a bag-valve-mask device. As noted earlier, a common problem is caused by an improper seal between the patient's face and the mask. Another problem is a failure of the unit to ventilate the patient because of an airway obstruction that must be cleared. It should be rare for the bag, valve, or mask to be the problem. This is because a good EMT knows how to disassemble, clean, reassemble, and test the units before they need to be used in the field.

The bag-valve-mask can be used during two-rescuer CPR (Figure 6–15). More effective care can be rendered if the unit is used with supplemental oxygen (see p. 183). The EMT should squeeze the bag quickly and smoothly, after the fifth upstroke.

OXYGEN THERAPY

The Importance of Supplemental Oxygen

It is critical that an EMT know how to maintain oxygen equipment, when to administer oxygen, and how to administer oxygen to patients. Patients receiving oxygen during pulmonary resuscitation or CPR stand a much better chance of surviving. The

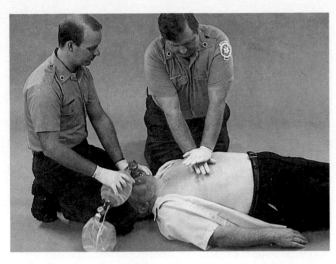

FIGURE 6–15. Two-rescuer CPR using a bag-valve-mask system.

same holds true for patients with internal bleeding, severe external blood loss, head injury, and major fractures. Heart attack and some stroke patients also do better when given high concentrations of oxygen. Administering oxygen may keep a patient from developing shock or prevent his shock from worsening. Since serious shock is a possibility with many trauma and medical emergency patients, providing oxygen therapy is a major skill required of all EMTs.

A patient may require oxygen for a variety of reasons:

- Respiratory Arrest—the patient is not breathing and there is failure to take oxygen into the lungs and rid the body of carbon dioxide.
- Cardiac Arrest—failure to pump blood to carry oxygen to the tissues. Keep in mind that respiratory arrest occurs along with cardiac arrest.
- Major Blood Loss—there is less oxygen being carried by the blood since there has been a reduction in the number of red blood cells, and the volume of blood is reduced, forcing the heart to work harder. All major trauma patients require oxygen.
- Heart Attack and Heart Failure—the ability to pump oxygenated blood efficiently is greatly reduced.
- Lung Disease or Injury—the ability to take in and exchange oxygen is seriously reduced.
- Airway Obstruction—even partial obstruction causes the amount of oxygen reaching the lungs to be greatly reduced.

- Stroke—remember that the brain requires a constant supply of oxygen. If this supply is stopped or reduced, vessels in the brain can quickly constrict to cause an irreversible form of shock and brain cells will start to die very quickly.
- Shock—since shock is the failure of the cardiovascular system to provide sufficient blood to all the vital tissues, all cases of shock can reduce the amount of oxygenated blood reaching the tissues.
- Major Head Injuries—airway obstruction and trauma to the cardiovascular system can reduce the supply of oxygenated blood to the brain.

When you are caring for a patient who is able to breathe, atmospheric air provides no more than 21% oxygen to the patient. This is usually as much as the patient needs, provided that the airway is open, the exchange surfaces of the lungs are working properly, there is enough oxygen carrying components in the blood, and the patient's cardiovascular system is properly circulating blood to all the body tissues. When any of these factors fail, a higher concentration of oxygen delivered to the patient's lungs may be required so that an adequate level of oxygen will reach the body's tissues.

Providing oxygen to the nonbreathing patient by mouth-to-mouth techniques puts 16% oxygen into his lungs. This would be enough oxygen to keep the patient alive if all other body functions were normal and there were no injuries. When the patient is not breathing and is in cardiac arrest, CPR can be applied, but the efficiency of CPR to circulate the blood is less than a third of that of a healthy, beating heart. Body tissues thus receive only the minimum oxygen required for short-term survival. Oxygen therapy, however, may provide for nearly 90% oxygen to reach the lungs. With more oxygen in the patient's blood, some of this inefficiency associated with basic life support is improved and the patient has a better chance for survival.

Always remember that oxygen is a medication. This means that you will have to decide if it is needed, how much to provide, what results are expected, and what harm may be done. The use of oxygen is a special responsibility that can be given only to someone of professional status.

Hypoxia

Hypoxia (hi-POK-se-ah) is a decrease in the supply of oxygen in the body tissues. Sometimes the term *anoxia* (an-OK-se-ah) is used to mean the same thing; however, this term means a complete lack of oxygen. There are several major causes of hypoxia, including:

- Respiratory insufficiency—too little oxygen is exchanged between the alveoli (al-VE-o-li), the microscopic air sacs of the lungs, and the blood (hypoxic hypoxia). This can be due to the air itself, as in cases of hypoxia produced by the rarefied air of high altitudes. The oxygen in the air can be reduced, as in fire, or may be contaminated with toxic gases. Breathing such air will lead to hypoxia.

  Damage to the lungs through injury (e.g., pneumothorax) or through disease (e.g., emphysema) also may prevent the proper amount of oxygen from reaching the blood. Chest injuries may produce this form of hypoxia.

  The overdose of certain drugs (e.g., morphine, phenobarbitol) can lead to respiratory insufficiency caused by a significant decline in respiratory effort.

- Circulatory insufficiency—a reduction of blood flow due to heart attack, heart failure, cardiovascular collapse, obstructed blood vessels, or blood loss can lower the amount of oxygen picked up from the lungs or circulated to the tissues (circulatory hypoxia).

- Hemoglobin insufficiency—when there is not enough hemoglobin in the red blood cells, if the hemoglobin is not free to pick up oxygen (as in carbon monoxide poisoning), or if the ability to pick up and carry oxygen is reduced (as with certain pain killer medications), hypoxia can occur (hemic hypoxia).

- Cellular exchange problems—even if a sufficient amount of oxygen is delivered to the tissues, it must be taken into the cells or hypoxia will occur (cellular hypoxia). Certain poisons, such as cyanide, can prevent oxygen exchange between the bloodstream and the cells. Drug and alcohol abuse also can cause this form of hypoxia.

As an EMT, your concern will be to prevent hypoxia from developing or becoming worse and, when possible, to reduce the level of hypoxia. There are some cases of lung disease in which you will have to modify the oxygen therapy delivered to the patient (see Chapter 14, Section One). However, in most cases in which oxygen is required, you will be delivering the maximum oxygen needed to prevent or to control hypoxia. Remember, if hypoxia is allowed to continue the patient may suffer brain damage or develop respiratory arrest.

The Disadvantages and Hazards of Oxygen Therapy

There are certain hazards associated with the administration of oxygen. These hazards can be grouped as nonmedical and medical.

The *nonmedical* hazards of oxygen therapy include:

1. The oxygen used in emergency care is stored under pressure, usually 2,000 to 2,200 pounds per square inch (psi) or greater in a full cylinder. If the tank is punctured, or if a valve breaks off, the supply tank can become a missile (damaged tanks have been able to penetrate concrete walls). Imagine what would happen in the passenger compartment of an ambulance if such an oxygen cylinder-related accident occurred.

2. Oxygen supports combustion, causing fire to burn more rapidly. It can saturate towels, sheets, and clothing, greatly increasing the risk of fire.

3. Under pressure, oxygen and oil do not mix. When they come into contact, a severe reaction occurs, which, for our purposes, can be termed an explosion. This is seldom a problem, but it can easily occur if you try to lubricate a delivery system or gauge with petroleum products, or allow for contact with a petroleum-based adhesive (e.g., adhesive tape).

The *medical* hazards of oxygen therapy include:

1. Oxygen toxicity—destruction of lung tissue due to high concentrations of oxygen provided for a long period of time. This is *not* a consideration in EMT-level emergency care.

2. Air sac collapse—the alveoli of the lungs react to oxygen in a fashion similar to the way the pupils of the eyes react to light. If the concentration of oxygen is low, the alveoli expand. If the concentration of oxygen is high, the alveoli constrict. If too high a concentration of oxygen is given for too long a period of time, the alveoli may collapse and never be able to regain their normal size. This collapse is one form of a condition

known as **atelectasis** (at-i-LEK-tah-sis). In severe cases whole sections of a lung may collapse. The condition can be fatal, but it is *not* a problem in prehospital emergency care.

3. Infant eye damage—occurs when infants are given too much oxygen, particularly the premature infant. Scar tissue will form behind the lens of the eye (retrolental fibroplasia), leading to impaired vision or permanent blindness. This is caused by too much oxygen in the bloodstream, not as a result of direct exposure of the eyes to high concentrations of oxygen. This should never be a problem in field situations.

4. Respiratory arrest—this problem occurs with patients having chronic obstructive pulmonary disease (COPD), including emphysema, chronic bronchitis, and black lung. When given oxygen in too high a dosage (above 28%), these patients can develop respiratory depression or arrest.

As an EMT, you probably will not see oxygen toxicity or alveolar collapse. The time required for such conditions is too long to cause any problems during standard field emergency care. Damage to the eyes of a premature infant can be prevented by delivering oxygen to a tent of aluminum foil that has been placed over the patient's head. The amount of time the infant will be breathing the high level of oxygen is shorter than the time required to cause damage to his eyes. In addition to the exposure time, most cases of eye damage have been associated with concentrations of oxygen above 40%. The tent delivery of oxygen usually does not maintain this high a level of oxygen. For more on the delivery of oxygen to the infant patient, see Chapter 16.

You can cause serious problems for some COPD patients if you deliver too high a concentration of oxygen. In healthy individuals, the primary control center for respiration is in the brain. This center reacts to the amount of carbon dioxide in the blood. The higher the concentration of carbon dioxide, the more rapid the ventilations. Most patients with COPD have, *over a period of time*, maintained an increase in blood carbon dioxide level. This can lead to a condition known as **hypoxic drive.** At a certain point, the primary center for respiration will no longer respond to the high carbon dioxide level in the blood. Secondary centers, located in the carotid arteries (*carotid bodies*) take over the major control of respiration. These centers react to the level of oxygen in the blood. High concentrations of oxygen will cause the patient to slow down his respirations. If you provide too much oxygen quickly to the patient, the carotid centers will shut down. Since the primary center in the brain is not functioning normally, the patient will stop breathing. For more on COPD, see Chapter 14, Section One.

REMEMBER: Never deliver more than 28% oxygen to a COPD patient whose problem is respiratory failure that is related directly to his COPD. Most EMS Systems recommend no more than 24% oxygen, with constant monitoring of the patient. When the patient is in respiratory arrest, cardiac arrest, respiratory distress not caused by the COPD, shock, or the possibility of developing shock (due to illness or injury) or is having a possible heart attack or stroke, he should receive the amount of oxygen required to care for the problem (usually started at 4 to 6 liters per minute). Once this type of patient is placed on oxygen, *do not* leave the patient unattended. If the conscious COPD patient slows down or stops his respirations, you can remind him to breathe. If the unconscious patient stops breathing, then resuscitation with supplemental oxygen should be started immediately. Resuscitation is best done with the highest concentration of oxygen available.

RULE: *Never* withhold oxygen if it is needed by any patient. If uncertain, radio the medical facility for directions.

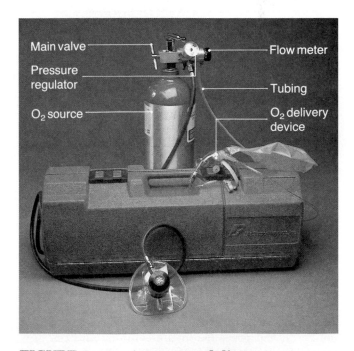

FIGURE 6–16. An oxygen delivery system.

Equipment and Supplies for Oxygen Therapy

A field oxygen delivery system for the breathing patient includes an oxygen source, pressure regulator, flowmeter, and a delivery device (face mask or cannula). The delivery system is the same for a non-breathing patient, but a device must be added to allow the EMT to force oxygen into the patient's lungs. This is known as positive-pressure ventilation.

Oxygen Cylinders

Outside a medical facility, the standard source of oxygen is a seamless steel or lightweight alloy cylinder filled with oxygen under pressure, equal to 2,000 to 2,200 psi when the cylinders are full. Cylinders come in various sizes, identified by letters. Those in common use in emergency care include:

> • D cylinder—contains about 350 liters of oxygen
> • E cylinder—contains about 625 liters of oxygen
> • M cylinder—contains about 3,000 liters of oxygen

Fixed systems on ambulances include the M cylinder and larger cylinders:

> • G cylinder—contains about 5,300 liters of oxygen
> • H cylinder—contains about 6,900 liters of oxygen.

The United States Pharmacopeia has assigned a *color code* to distinguish compressed gases. Light green and white cylinders have been assigned to all grades of oxygen. Stainless steel and aluminum cylinders are not painted. Regardless of the color, always check the label to be certain you are using medical grade oxygen.

You cannot tell if an oxygen cylinder is full, partially full, or empty by lifting or moving the cylinder. Part of your duty as an EMT is to make certain that the oxygen cylinders you will use are full and ready before they are needed to provide care. The length of time you can use an oxygen cylinder depends on the pressure in the cylinder and the flow rate. The method of calculating cylinder duration

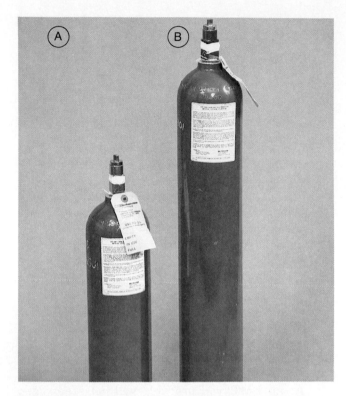

FIGURE 6–17. *A.* D cylinder. *B.* E cylinder. These cylinders still have the suppliers' plastic wrappers over the outlets. Do not use adhesive tape.

is shown in Table 6–1. Oxygen cylinders should *never* be allowed to empty below the *safe residual*. The safe residual for an oxygen cylinder is determined when the pressure gauge reads 200 psi. At this point there is not enough oxygen in the cylinder to allow for proper delivery to the patient. Prior to the 200 psi reading, you must switch to a fresh cylinder.

SAFETY is of prime importance when working with oxygen cylinders. You should:

- NEVER drop a cylinder or let it fall against any object. Make certain that the cylinder is well secured, preferably in an upright position.
- NEVER allow smoking around oxygen equipment in use. Clearly mark the area of use with signs that read "OXYGEN—NO SMOKING."
- NEVER use oxygen equipment around an open flame.
- NEVER use grease, oil, or fat-based soaps on devices that will be attached to an oxygen supply cylinder. Take care not to handle these devices when your hands are greasy.

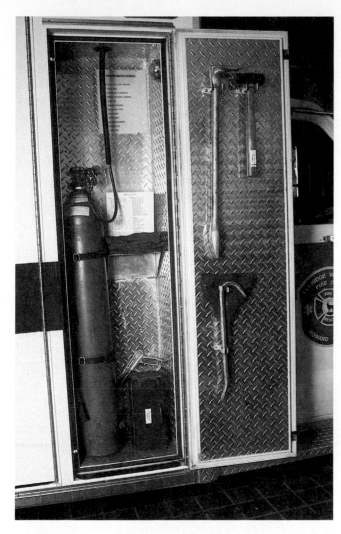

FIGURE 6–18. Larger cylinders are used for fixed systems on ambulances.

Table 6–1. OXYGEN CYLINDERS: DURATION OF FLOW

SIMPLE FORMULA

$$\frac{\text{Gauge pressure in psi} - \text{the safe residual pressure} \times \text{constant}}{\text{Flow rate in liters/minute}} = \frac{\text{duration of flow in minutes}}{}$$

RESIDUAL PRESSURE = 200 psi

CYLINDER CONSTANT (based on size)

D = 0.16	G = 2.41
E = 0.28	H = 3.14
M = 1.56	K = 3.14

Determine the life of an M cylinder that has a pressure of 2000 psi and a flow rate of 10 liters/minute.

$$\frac{(2000 - 200) \times 1.56}{10} = \frac{2808}{10} = \begin{array}{l}281 \text{ minutes} \\ \text{or 4 hours and} \\ 41 \text{ minutes}\end{array}$$

Use greaseless tools when making connections.

- NEVER use adhesive tape to protect an oxygen tank outlet or to mark or label any oxygen cylinders or oxygen delivery apparatus. The oxygen can react with the adhesive and debris and cause a fire.
- NEVER try to move an oxygen cylinder by dragging it or rolling it on its side or bottom.
- ALWAYS use the pressure gauges, regulators, and tubing that are intended for use with oxygen.
- ALWAYS use nonferrous metal oxygen wrenches for changing gauges and regulators or for adjusting flow rates. Other types of metal tools may produce a spark should they strike against metal objects.
- ALWAYS ensure that valve seat inserts and gaskets are in good condition. This prevents dangerous leaks. Gaskets on D and E oxygen cylinders should be replaced each time a cylinder change is made.
- ALWAYS use medical grade oxygen. Industrial oxygen contains impurities. The cylinder should be labeled "OXYGEN U.S.P." The oxygen must not be more than 5 years old.
- ALWAYS open the valve of an oxygen cylinder fully, then close it half a turn to prevent someone else from thinking the valve is closed and trying to force the valve open. The valve does not have to be turned fully to be open for delivery.
- ALWAYS store reserve oxygen cylinders in a cool, ventilated room, properly secured in place.
- ALWAYS have oxygen cylinders hydrostatically tested every 5 YEARS. The date a cylinder was last tested is stamped on the cylinder. Some cylinders can be tested every 10 years. These will have a star after the date (e.g., 4M86☆).

Pressure Regulators

The pressure in an oxygen cylinder is too high to be delivered to a patient. A pressure regulator must be connected to the cylinder to provide a safe working pressure of *30 to 70 psi.*

On cylinders of the E size or smaller, the pressure regulator is secured to the cylinder valve assembly by a yoke assembly. The yoke is provided with pins that must mate with corresponding holes in the valve assembly. This is called a *pin-index safety system*. Since the pin position varies for different gases, this system prevents an oxygen delivery system from being connected to a cylinder designed to contain another gas.

Cylinders larger than the E size have a valve assembly with a threaded outlet. The inside and outside diameters of the threaded outlets vary according to the gas in the cylinder. This prevents an oxygen regulator from being connected to a cylinder containing another gas. In other words, a nitrogen regulator cannot be connected to an oxygen cylinder, and vice versa.

Cylinder pressure can be reduced in one or two steps (Figure 6–19). For a one-step reduction, a single-stage pressure regulator is used. A two-step reduction requires a two-stage regulator. Most regulators used in emergency care are the single-stage variety. This type will allow for the use of a demand valve (see p. 183).

Before connecting the pressure regulator to an oxygen supply cylinder, stand to the side of the main valve opening and open (crack) the cylinder valve slightly for just a second to clear dirt and dust out of the delivery port or threaded outlet.

NOTE: You must maintain the regulator inlet filter. It has to be free of damage and clean to prevent contamination of and damage to the regulator.

Flowmeters

A flowmeter allows control of the flow of oxygen in liters per minute. It is connected to the pressure regulator. Most jurisdictions keep the flowmeter permanently attached to the pressure regulator.

Three major types of flowmeters are available (Figure 6–20). For emergency care use in the field, the pressure-compensated flowmeter is considered to be superior to the Bourdon gauge flowmeter; however, it is more delicate than the Bourdon gauge and must be operated in an upright position. For these reasons, many EMS Systems use the pressure-compensated flowmeter for fixed oxygen systems only.

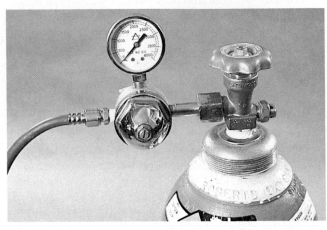

A

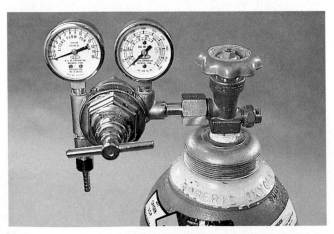

B

FIGURE 6–19. *A.* **Single-stage regulator.** *B.* **Two-stage regulator for D and E size cylinders.**

- Pressure-Compensated Flowmeter (Thorpe tube–type flowmeter)—This meter is gravity dependent and must be in an upright position to deliver an accurate reading. The unit has an upright, calibrated glass tube in which there is a ball float. The float rises and falls according to the amount of gas passing through the tube. This type of flowmeter indicates the actual flow at all times, even though there may be a partial obstruction to gas flow (as from a kinked delivery tube). If the tubing collapses, the ball will drop to show the lower delivery rate. This unit is not practical for many portable delivery systems.
- Bourdon Gauge Flowmeter—This unit is a pressure gauge calibrated to indicate flow in liters per minute. The meter is fairly inaccurate at low flow rates and has often been criticized as being unstable. It is rugged and will operate at any angle. It is a useful gauge for most portable units.

  The major fault with this type of flowmeter is its inability to compensate for back pressure. A partial obstruction (as from kinked tubing) will be reflected in a reading that

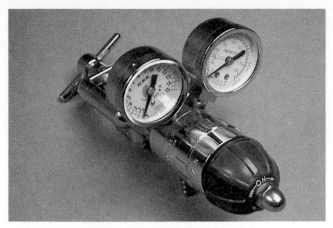

A

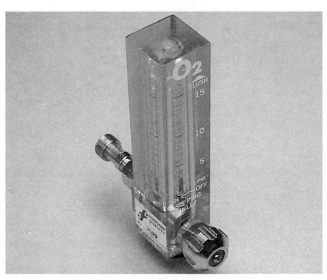

B

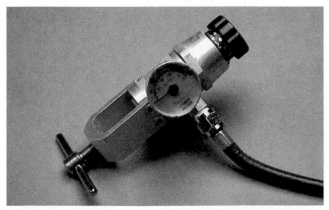

C

FIGURE 6–20. *A*. **Bourdon gauge flowmeter (pressure gauge).** *B*. **Pressure-compensated flowmeter.** *C*. **Constant flow selector valve.**

is higher than the actual flow. The gauge may read 6 liters per minute and only be delivering 1 liter per minute. This type of gauge contains a filter that can become clogged, causing the gauge to read higher than the actual flow. Inspect and change the filter as recommended by the manufacturer.

• Constant Flow Selector Valve—This new type of flowmeter is gaining in popularity. This device has no gauge. It allows for the adjustment of flow in liters per minute in stepped increments (2, 4, 6, 8, . . . 15 liters per minute). When using this type of flowmeter, *make certain* that it is properly adjusted for the desired flow and monitor the meter to make certain that it stays properly adjusted. This type of meter should be tested for accuracy as recommended by the manufacturer.

Humidifiers

NOTE: Many EMS Systems no longer use humidifiers. They have been found to have a problem with contamination. Those that do use humidifiers typically use disposable devices and have strict guidelines for the source of water used to fill the reservoir. Single-use, prefilled units may be available in your EMS System. Usually the use of a humidifier is not critical if transport to a medical facility is relatively short. However, a humidifier is recommended for long transports (25 minutes or longer) and for patients having severe repeated asthma attacks (status asthmaticus; see p. 399).

A humidifier can be connected to the flowmeter to provide moisture to the dry oxygen coming from the supply cylinder (Figure 6–21). Dry oxygen can dehydrate the mucous membranes of the patient's airway and lungs. In most short-term use the dry nature of the oxygen being delivered is not a problem; however, the patient is usually more comfortable when given humidified oxygen. This is particularly true if the patient has COPD.

A humidifier is usually no more than a nonbreakable jar of water attached to the flowmeter. Oxygen passes (bubbles) through the water to become humidified. As with all oxygen delivery equipment, the humidifier must be kept clean. The water reservoir can become a breeding ground for algae, harmful bacteria, and dangerous fungal organisms. Always use fresh water in a clean reservoir for each patient.

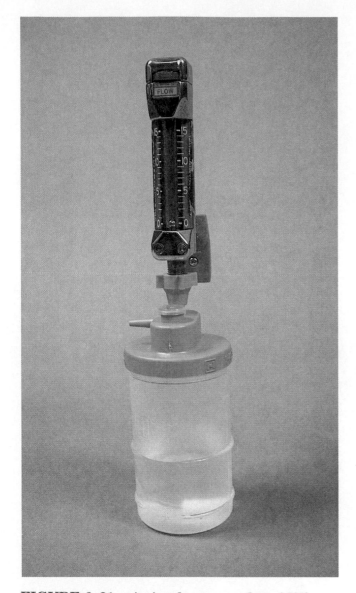

FIGURE 6–21. A simple oxygen humidifier.

Oxygen Delivery Devices

There are five oxygen delivery devices in common use for the emergency care of breathing patients (Table 6–2). The nasal cannula and four types of face masks provide a wide selection of devices for oxygen delivery. Many EMS Systems are using the nasal cannula to start oxygen therapy on breathing medical emergency patients who are not in distress. If shock appears to be a problem, or if the patient is very cyanotic or has very labored breathing, a face mask is used. These same systems use one of the four types of face masks to begin oxygen therapy for breathing trauma patients.

There is a simple rule to determine the percentage of oxygen being delivered to a patient:

> For every 1 liter per minute increase in oxygen flow, you deliver approximately a 4% increase in the concentration of oxygen.

If you know a particular device will give 24% oxygen at 4 liters per minute, an increase to 5 liters per minute will deliver a concentration of approximately 28% oxygen.

The five major oxygen delivery devices for breathing patients include:

1. Nasal Cannula—There are two types, one with an elastic band for holding the device in place and the newer design having a slip-loop to secure around the patient's ears and chin (Figure 6–22). Both types deliver oxygen into the patient's nose by way of two small plastic prongs that curve back into the nostrils. The efficiency of the device is greatly reduced by nasal injuries and by colds and other types of nasal airway obstruction. In common usage, a flow rate of 4 to 6 liters per minute will provide the patient with 36% to 44% oxygen. The relationship of oxygen concentration to liter per minute flow is as follows:

Liters/minute	% Oxygen
1	24
2	28
3	32
4	36
5	40
6	44

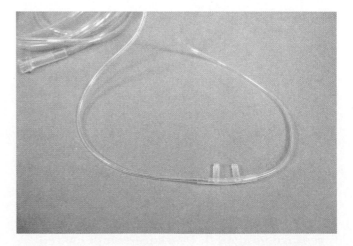

FIGURE 6–22. A loop type nasal cannula.

At 4 liters per minute and above, the patient's breathing patterns prevent the delivery of the stated percentages. At 5 liters per minute, there is a rapid drying of the nasal membranes. After 6 liters per minute, the device does not deliver any useful higher concentration of oxygen and proves to be very uncomfortable for most patients.

This delivery device is very helpful when the patient is afraid of using a face mask and refuses its application.

NOTE: The nasal cannula can be used for COPD patients who are in respiratory distress if a flow rate no greater than 2 to 3 liters per minute is maintained. Since there are many variables to be considered when using a nasal cannula, the Venturi mask is the delivery device of choice for COPD patients. When in doubt, follow your local guidelines.

2. Simple Face Mask—This is a soft, clear plastic mask that will conform to the contours of the patient's face (Figure 6–23). There are small perforations in the mask to allow atmospheric air to enter and the patient's exhaled air to escape. The mask is used to deliver moderate concentrations of oxygen (35% to 60%) with a flow rate of 6 to 8 liters per minute. The infant-sized face mask can be used on a stoma.

CAUTION: Always start with 6 liters per minute of flow when using this mask. If you start with less, carbon dioxide can build up in the mask. At a flow of 1 liter per minute,

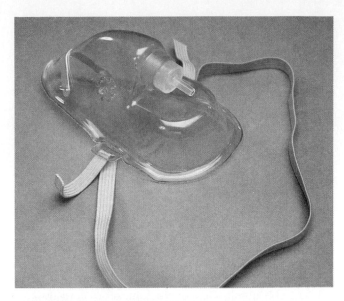

FIGURE 6–23. A simple face mask.

the patient is getting less oxygen than he would from atmospheric air.

3. Partial Rebreathing Mask—This device combines a face mask and a reservoir bag (Figure 6–24). The mask will only function properly if it is well fitted to the patient's face. Oxygen should be in the reservoir before you place the mask on the patient's face. The reservoir bag must be filled with enough oxygen so that it does not collapse by more than one third when the patient inhales. Part of the patient's oxygen enriched exhaled air will enter the reservoir bag to be mixed with oxygen, the rest will escape through perforations

Table 6–2. **OXYGEN DELIVERY DEVICES**

Oxygen Delivery Device	*Flow Rate**	*% Oxygen Delivered*	*Special Use*
Nasal cannula	1 to 6 LPM	24 to 44	Most medical patients
Simple face mask	Start at 6 LPM . . . can go as high as 15 LPM, but 8 LPM more practical	35 to 60	Preferred on trauma patients with no indications of developing shock
Partial rebreathing mask	6 to 10 LPM	35 to 60	Trauma patients
Nonrebreathing mask	Start with 8 LPM, practical high is 12 LPM	80 to 95	Good for severe non-COPD hypoxia and shock patients. Provides high oxygen concentrations
Venturi mask	4 to 8 LPM	24 to 40 (delivers as indicated on adaptor)	COPD patients and long-term use

* LPM, liters per minute.

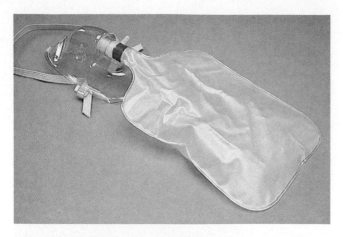

FIGURE 6–24. A partial rebreathing mask.

stead, it escapes through a flutter valve in the facepiece.

This mask will provide concentrations of oxygen ranging from 80% to 95%. The minimum flow rate is 8 liters/minute. Depending on the manufacturer and the fit of the mask, the maximum flow can range from 12 to 15 liters/minute. New design features allow for one emergency port in the mask so that the patient can still receive atmospheric air should the oxygen supply fail. This feature keeps the mask from being able to deliver 100% oxygen but is a necessary safety feature. The mask is excellent for use in shock and for severely hypoxic patients who do not suffer from COPD.

NOTE: Some devices are made so that they can be rebreathing or nonrebreathing masks, depending on a valve adjustment.

in the mask. Concentrations of 35% to 60% can be delivered when flow rates are between 6 and 10 liters per minute.

4. Nonrebreathing Mask—Excluding the bag-valve-mask system used with oxygen and the demand valve resuscitator, the nonrebreathing mask is the EMT's best way to deliver high concentrations of oxygen (Figure 6–25). This device *must* be placed properly on the patient's face to provide the necessary seal to ensure high concentration delivery. The reservoir bag must be inflated before the mask is placed on the patient's face. To inflate the reservoir bag, use your finger to cover the exhaust portal or the connection between the mask and the reservoir. The reservoir must always contain enough oxygen so that it does not deflate by more than one third when the patient takes his deepest inspiration. This can be maintained by the proper flow of oxygen. Air exhaled by the patient does not return to the reservoir. In-

5. Venturi Mask—This mask is specifically designed for use when low concentrations of oxygen (24% to 40%) are required (Figure 6–26). The oxygen is delivered into the mask by way of a jet that pulls in atmospheric air to mix it with the oxygen. The flow is rapid enough to flush out the carbon dioxide that tends to accumulate in a face mask.

Various-sized color-coded adaptors can be attached to the device to control the oxygen flow to the patient. Standard sizes include 3, 4, and 6 liter per minute adaptors. If a 4-liter adaptor is in place and you attempt to deliver 8 liters of oxygen per minute, the jet will draw in more atmospheric air to mix with the oxygen. This "Venturi effect"

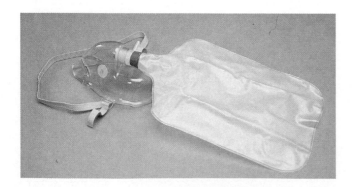

FIGURE 6–25. A nonrebreathing mask.

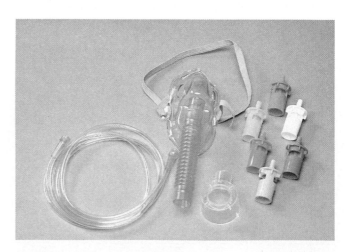

FIGURE 6–26. A Venturi mask.

draws in enough air so that only 4 liters of oxygen per minute reaches the patient.

NOTE: The Venturi is the only face mask recommended for COPD patients. Delivery concentrations should begin at 24%.

Administering Oxygen

Scans 6–2 and 6–3 will take you step by step through the process of administering oxygen and discontinuing the administration of oxygen.

WARNING: *Do not* attempt to learn on your own how to use oxygen delivery systems. You should work with your instructor and follow his directions for the specific equipment you will be using.

Administering Oxygen to a Nonbreathing Patient

Remember that a pocket face mask with an oxygen inlet can be connected to a high flow oxygen source and used in combination with your own ventilations to deliver 40% to 45% oxygen to the patient. Some masks can provide 50% oxygen at a flow rate of 10 liters per minute.

Most EMS Systems currently use the bag-valve-mask device with 100% oxygen under pressure and the manually controlled demand valve resuscitator with 100% oxygen under pressure in ventilating the nonbreathing patient.

NOTE: Before using either of these two devices, an airway should be inserted.

WARNING: These devices can be used for two-rescuer CPR, but may be a problem for one-rescuer CPR. Even with face straps, the face mask will not remain in place and keep a tight seal. The delay between compressions and proper ventilation may be too great for efficient one-rescuer CPR. The use of this mask for CPR requires much practice.

The Bag-Valve-Mask and Oxygen This device can be connected to an oxygen supply system by tubing that joins the oxygen inlet of the bag-valve-mask unit to the outlet of the flowmeter. Most newer devices have an oxygen reservoir attached to the bag to improve efficiency. The bag-valve-mask device used with oxygen will deliver from 35% to 40% oxygen. With a reservoir added, it can deliver 90% to 95% oxygen for pulmonary resuscitation and for interposed ventilations during two-rescuer CPR. The reservoir is recommended.

NOTE: The adult bag-valve-mask unit should not have a pressure-release valve.

Maintain a tight mask-to-face seal, squeeze the bag to deliver oxygen, and release the bag to allow for passive expiration. There is no need to remove the mask to allow for expirations. Keeping a proper seal requires special skills that can only be developed through practice.

Use the highest possible flow rate of oxygen (15 liters per minute). Squeeze the bag every 5 seconds for adults, 4 seconds for children, and 3 seconds for infants.

This device can also be used to assist the breathing efforts of a severely hypoxic patient or one who has failing, shallow respirations (as in drug overdose).

The Demand Valve Resuscitator

Commonly called a *demand valve*, the entire device is a *demand valve resuscitator*. It will deliver nearly 100% oxygen to the patient's lungs if the face mask is properly sealed to the patient's face. When an inspiration occurs, the device will deliver oxygen and then shut off flow as soon as an expiration begins. Most new demand valve resuscitators are part of a multiple function resuscitator (see p. 187).

WARNING: *Do not* use this device on infants and children. Exercise extreme caution if the device must be used on a COPD patient: It may cause severe lung damage. Follow your local guidelines.

The Positive-Pressure Resuscitator Most positive-pressure resuscitators have a control button on top of the valve unit to which the facepiece is attached. When the EMT depresses the control button, oxygen flows into the face mask at a high rate (up to 150 liters per minute in some models). The patient's lungs will inflate until a preset pressure is reached (about 40 mmHg) or until the control button is released. You *must* keep one hand free to seal the mask properly to the patient's face. Stay alert for gastric distention. Observe the rise of the patient's chest to determine if too little or too much volume is being delivered. *Do not* depend on the device to always deliver in accordance with its preset pressure. It should not be used on breathing patients.

NOTE: There have been many problems experienced by EMTs using this device in field emergency care. Difficulties may occur with the mask seal, even when two hands are used. Many rescuers have reported problems with overventilation and underventilation. The positive-pressure resuscitator is no

SCAN 6–2 PREPARING THE O₂ DELIVERY SYSTEM

1

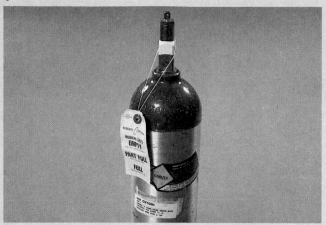

Select desired cylinder. Check label, "Oxygen U.S.P."

2

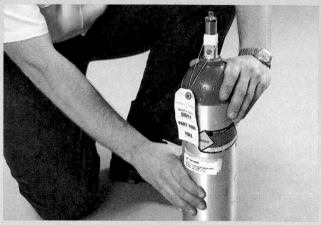

Place the cylinder in an upright position and stand to one side.

3

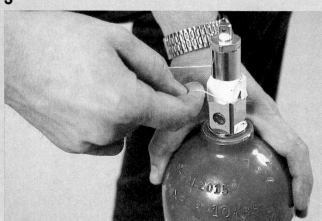

Remove the plastic wrapper or cap protecting the cylinder outlet.

4

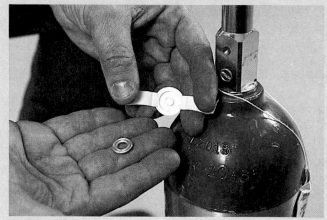

Keep the plastic washer (some set-ups).

5

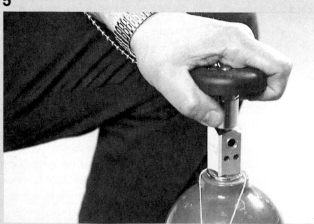

"Crack" the main valve for one second.

6   PIN   DISS

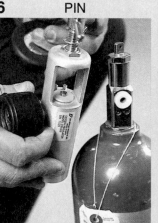 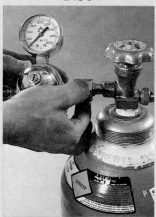

Select the correct pressure regulator and flowmeter.

7

Place cylinder valve gasket on regulator oxygen port.

8

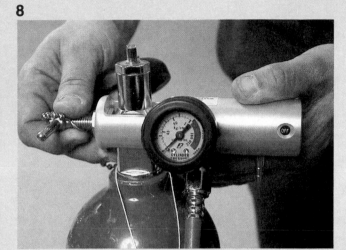

Make certain that the pressure regulator is closed.

9   PIN   DISS

Align pins, for DISS, thread by hand.

10

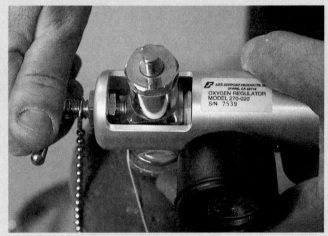

Tighten T-screw for pin-index.

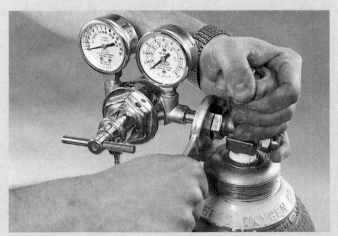

Tighten with a wrench for DISS.

11

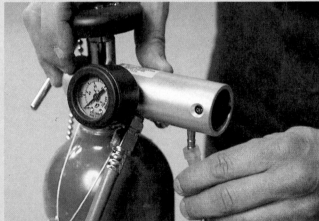

Attach tubing and delivery device.

SCAN 6–3 ADMINISTERING OXYGEN

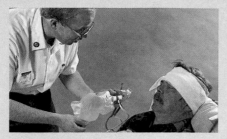

1 Explain to patient the need for oxygen

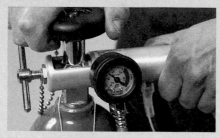

2 Open main valve—adjust flowmeter

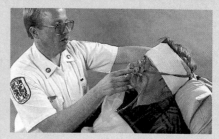

3 Place oxygen delivery device

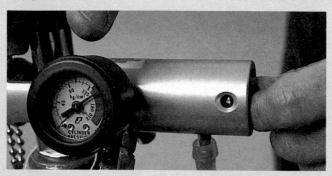

4 Adjust flowmeter

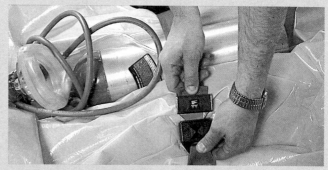

5 Secure during transfer

Discontinuing Oxygen

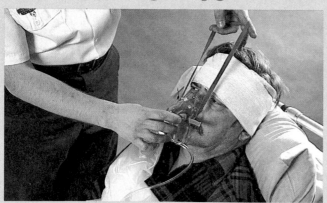

1 Remove delivery device

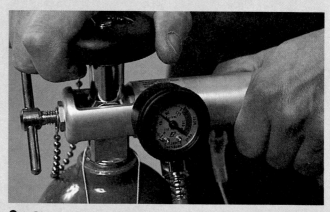

2 Close main valve

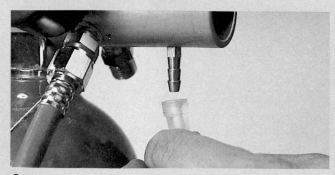

3 Remove delivery tubing

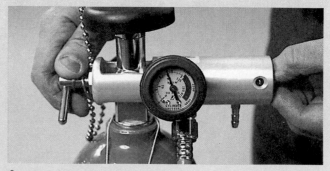

4 Bleed flowmeter

longer used by many EMS Systems. It has been replaced with multiple-function resuscitators.

Multiple-Function Resuscitator At present, federal regulations and national guidelines require resuscitators to have manual controls. Many resuscitators are made to function in the manually triggered positive-pressure mode as previously described, or in the patient demand mode (see p. 183). These devices, known as positive-pressure demand valve resuscitators, are highly recommended. They must be able to deliver 100 liters per minute of 100% oxygen at 50 psi. A constant flow rate of 40 liters per minute is recommended to reduce the chances of gastric distention (in the manually triggered mode).

When used for the breathing patient, the resuscitator functions in the demand mode. A valve assembly opens as the patient inhales, allowing him to receive oxygen flow until the end of the inhalation. As the patient exhales, this valve assembly closes and the exhaled air is released into the atmosphere.

The nonbreathing patient is resuscitated in the positive-pressure mode. When the button on top of the valve is depressed, oxygen is forced into the patient's lungs. Even though a relief valve to prevent overventilating the lungs is part of the system, the rescuer should carefully watch the patient's chest expand as oxygen is delivered. The button should be released when the rescuer sees the patient's chest expand.

WARNING: *Do not* use the positive-pressure, demand-valve, or multiple-function resuscitator on infants or children. Use these devices with caution on the COPD patient. They can cause severe lung damage for this type of patient.

NOTE: For CPR, you should employ a manually controlled resuscitator. During two-rescuer CPR, a ventilation should be provided after the fifth upstroke. To be effective in CPR, a resuscitator *must* deliver a flow rate of not less than 40 liters per minute.

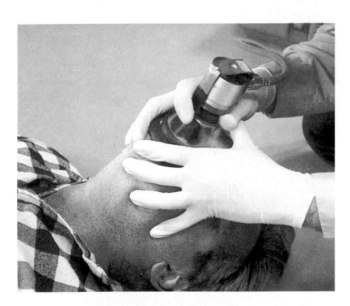

- **BREATHING PATIENT**
  Demand valve model delivers
  as patient starts
  an inspiration

- **NONBREATHING PATIENT**
  Manually triggered positive
  pressure mode delivers when
  rescuer depresses control
  button

FIGURE 6–27. **Multiple-function (demand valve, positive pressure) resuscitator.**

SUMMARY

The EMT should never delay resuscitation measures to locate, retrieve, and set up special equipment or oxygen delivery systems. When practical to do so, airway adjuncts, ventilation assist devices, and supplemental oxygen should be used when they are needed.

Airway adjuncts can be used to maintain an open airway. There are two major types, oropharyngeal and nasopharyngeal.

Oropharyngeal airways will help keep the tongue from slipping back into the throat. These airways should be used for *unconscious* patients who have no gag reflex. Before insertion, the airway adjunct must be measured to ensure that it is the correct size. The airway is inserted with the tip toward the roof of the mouth and then rotated into position. Once inserted, the flange must be against the patient's lips.

Nasopharyngeal airways must be lubricated with a water-based lubricant. These devices can be used for a conscious patient. Before inserting the device, be sure to explain to the patient what you are going to do.

Fluids can be removed from a patient's mouth and throat using a fixed or portable suction system. Suction is not to begin until the rigid tip or catheter is in place, at the back of the throat. Do not suction the nonbreathing patient for more than 5 SECONDS before providing ventilations.

Common ventilation assist devices include the bag-valve-mask and the pocket face mask. When using the bag-valve-mask device, one hand must hold the facepiece firmly in place. Air is delivered by squeezing the bag. For the nonbreathing adult patient, the rate is ONCE EVERY 5 SECONDS. Better results may occur when one rescuer can hold the mask with both hands and another rescuer squeezes the bag. The pocket face mask has a chimney on the mask to allow for mouth-to-mask ventilations.

Oxygen administration is essential for patients in respiratory arrest or cardiac arrest. Realize that other types of patients also will do better if placed on oxygen therapy; these include patients suffering from blood loss, major fractures, head injury, shock, lung disease or injury, heart attack, stroke, and heart failure. Atmospheric air contains 21% oxygen. The air provided by mouth-to-mouth techniques only delivers 16% oxygen to the patient. REMEMBER, OXYGEN IS A MEDICATION.

Hypoxia is a low concentration of oxygen at the tissue level. This can be caused by respiratory insufficiency (hypoxic hypoxia) due to the air itself, lung disease, lung injury, or chest injury. Circulatory insufficiency (circulatory hypoxia) can be due to blood loss or problems with the heart and blood vessels. There may not be enough hemoglobin in the red blood cells (hemic hypoxia) to carry the required amount of oxygen. Problems with cellular exchange (cellular hypoxia) may prevent oxygen from entering the cells.

Oxygen can be dangerous because it is stored under pressure, it supports combustion, and it can detonate if mixed with oil. Medical problems can be caused by prolonged use of high concentrations of oxygen, including lung damage (oxygen toxicity), collapsed alveoli (atelectasis), and damage to a premature infant's eyes (retrolental fibroplasia).

Of major concern to the EMT is the effect of too much oxygen on some chronic obstructive pulmonary disease (COPD) patients (emphysema, chronic bronchitis, black lung). When given oxygen above 28% in concentration, such patients may develop respiratory arrest. Most systems recommend delivery of oxygen at 24% using a Venturi face mask or nasal cannula. If the COPD patient's problem is not respiratory distress related to his COPD, provide the concentration of oxygen appropriate for the situation, but stay alert for the reduction of respiratory rate.

Three sizes of oxygen cylinders are commonly used: D, E, and M. When full, oxygen is stored under pressure equal to 2,000 to 2,200 psi. You can calculate the length of time you can use a cylinder. The formula, residual pressure, and constants are given in Table 6–1 on page 177.

A pressure regulator is used to reduce the pressure in an oxygen cylinder to a safe working pressure (30 to 70 psi). E size and smaller cylinders use the pin-index safety system. Larger cylinders use threaded outlets to prevent the wrong regulator or gas being used. Remember to "crack" the cylinder valve before use to clear the delivery port or threaded outlet.

A flowmeter allows the control of oxygen flow in liters per minute. The gravity-dependent, ball float meter is a pressure-compensated flowmeter that measures actual flow. The Bourdon gauge flowmeter is a calibrated gauge that measures flow in liters per minute. This gauge cannot compensate for back-pressure. The constant flow selector valve has no gauge. It can be adjusted for flow in liters per minute.

Oxygen used for medical purposes is a dry gas. Moisture can be added by using a humidifier.

There are five commonly used oxygen delivery devices for the breathing patient:

- Nasal cannula—24% to 44% oxygen delivered to the nose; 28% may be the maximum delivered to the lungs.
- Simple face mask—35% to 60% oxygen delivered
- Partial rebreathing mask—35% to 60% oxygen delivered
- Nonrebreathing mask—80% to 95% oxygen delivered
- Venturi mask—24% to 40% oxygen delivered

If you begin with the minimum flow rate and concentration of oxygen delivered by Venturi mask, the oxygen delivered will INCREASE 4% FOR EVERY ADDITIONAL LITER PER MINUTE FLOW.

The nasal cannula and Venturi mask can be used for COPD patients if the concentration of oxygen delivered is approximately 24%. NEVER WITHHOLD NEEDED OXYGEN.

The simple face mask requires a flow rate of no less than 6 liters per minute. The minimum flow rate for the non-rebreathing mask is 8 liters per minute.

A demand valve resuscitator with oxygen under pressure can be used to assist breathing patients who have failing respirations. Oxygen can be administered to the nonbreathing patient by using a pocket face mask with the oxygen inlet connected to a high flow oxygen source, a bag-valve-mask ventilator with supplemental oxygen (a reservoir is recommended), or a positive-pressure resuscitator with manual control.

The multifunction, positive-pressure demand valve resuscitator can be operated in the positive-pressure mode for nonbreathing patients or the demand mode for breathing patients.

A positive-pressure device can be used during two-rescuer CPR. It should be manually controlled.

Before using any of these devices, insert an adjunct airway. Wear latex or rubber gloves to avoid contact with the patient's blood or body fluids.

Do not use the demand-valve, positive-pressure, or multifunction resuscitator on infants and children.

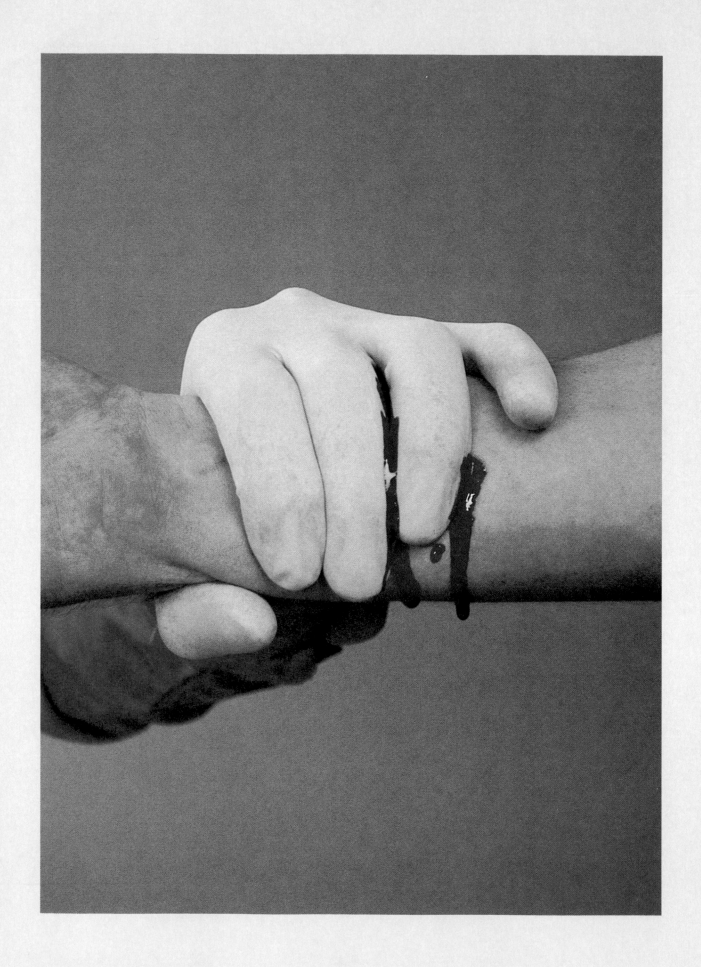

Basic Life Support III:
Bleeding and shock

SECTION ONE:
Basic Procedures

WARNING: Avoid direct contact with patient blood and body fluids. Wear latex or rubber gloves, and any additional protective gear as required by your EMS System.

OBJECTIVES   As an EMT, you should be able to:

1. List the FIVE major functions of blood. (p. 193)

2. List the THREE major types of blood vessels and describe the functions of each. (p. 194)

3. Classify bleeding as external or internal and relate the types of blood vessels to the THREE kinds of external bleeding. (p. 194)

4. Relate profuse bleeding to the primary survey and basic life support. (p. 195)

5. List EIGHT methods of controlling external bleeding. (p. 195)

6. Describe the direct pressure control of profuse bleeding and mild bleeding. (pp. 195–197)

7. Describe the application of a pressure dressing. (pp. 196–197)

8. Describe the use of elevation in the control of external bleeding and note when this procedure should *not* be used. (p. 197)

9. Define *arterial pressure point* and list and locate the major pressure point sites used in EMT-level emergency care. (pp. 197–198)

10. Describe, step by step, the use of pressure points to control bleeding from the upper and lower limbs. (p. 198)

11. Describe how a blood pressure cuff can be used to control bleeding. (p. 198)

12. Explain why tourniquets are used only after other methods of controlling profuse bleeding have failed. (pp. 198–199)

13. Describe, step by step, the procedures for applying a tourniquet, including all precautions for the procedure. (pp. 199–200)

14. List the symptoms and signs of internal bleeding and state FOUR factors that may cause difficulties when trying to detect this type of bleeding. (pp. 200–201)

15. List at least TEN conditions associated with internal bleeding. (p. 201)

16. Describe, step by step, the EMT-level procedures for controlling internal bleeding. (p. 202)

17. Define shock and match the causes of shock to the types of shock. (pp. 202–204)

18. List the symptoms and signs of shock. (pp. 204–205)

19. Describe, step by step, the procedures used in the prevention and the care for shock. (pp. 205–207)

20. Describe anaphylactic shock in terms of what it is, how serious it is, and what causes it. (pp. 207–208)

21. List the symptoms and signs of anaphylactic shock. (p. 208)

22. Compare the care provided in anaphylactic shock with the care provided for other types of shock. (pp. 208–209)

23. Describe how to reduce a patient's chances of fainting. (p. 209)

SKILLS   As an EMT, you should be able to:

1. Evaluate the seriousness of bleeding and the approximate blood loss.

2. Control external bleeding by:
   A. Direct pressure
   B. Direct pressure and elevation
   C. Arterial pressure point
   D. Rigid splinting
   E. Air splints (when carried)
   F. Blood pressure cuff
   G. Tourniquet

3. Survey for internal bleeding and apply the measures required to control this type of bleeding.

4. Survey for shock and anaphylactic shock.

5. Apply the measures needed to prevent shock and to care for shock.

6. Apply the measures needed to care for anaphylactic shock.

7. Carry out the procedure used to help prevent fainting.

NOTE: Pneumatic anti-shock garments (PASG) will be covered in Section Two of this chapter.

TERMS   you may be using for the first time:

Anaphylactic (an-ah-fi-LAK-tik) **Shock** – the most severe type of allergic reaction in which a person develops shock when he encounters a substance to which he is allergic. This is a true, life-threatening emergency.

Artery – any major blood vessel carrying blood away from the heart.

Capillary – the thin-walled, microscopic blood vessels where oxygen/carbon dioxide and nutrient/waste exchange with the tissues takes place.

Coma – a state of complete unconsciousness, the depth of which may vary.

Cyanosis (sigh-ah-NO-sis) – when the skin, lips, tongue, earlobes, nailbeds, and/or the mucous membranes turn blue or gray owing to insufficient oxygen in the blood.

Embolism (EM-bo-liz-m) – a moving blood clot or foreign body, such as fat or an air bubble inside a blood vessel.

Femoral (FEM-o-ral) **Artery** – the major artery supplying the thigh. Some types of external bleeding from the lower extremity can be controlled by applying pressure to the femoral artery pressure point.

Formed Elements – red blood cells, white blood cells, and platelets.

Hemorrhage (HEM-o-rej) – internal or external bleeding.

Liter (LE-ter) – metric measurement of liquid volume that is equal to 1.057 quarts. One pint is almost equal to one-half liter.

Perfusion – the constant flow of blood through capillaries.

Plasma (PLAZ-mah) – the fluid portion of the blood. It is the blood minus the formed elements.

Platelet (PLATE-let) – the formed elements of the blood that release chemical factors needed to form blood clots.

Shock – the reaction of the body to the failure of the cardiovascular system to provide an adequate supply of blood to all vital parts of the body.

Temporal Artery – the major artery in the region of the temple. Some types of external scalp bleeding can be controlled by applying pressure to the temporal pressure point.

Vein – any major blood vessel returning blood to the heart.

BLEEDING

The Blood

Blood is a living tissue made up of plasma (PLAZ-mah) and formed elements. The **plasma** is a watery, salty fluid that makes up over half the volume of the blood. The **formed elements** are:

- Red blood cells—also called RBCs, erythrocytes, and red corpuscles. Their primary function is to carry oxygen to the tissues and carbon dioxide away from the tissues.
- White blood cells—also called WBCs, leukocytes, and white corpuscles. They are involved in destroying microorganisms (germs) and producing substances called antibodies that help the body resist infection.
- Platelets (PLATE-lets) — membrane-enclosed fragments of specialized cells. When these fragments rupture, they release chemical factors needed to form blood clots.

The functions of blood are:

- TRANSPORTATION OF GASES—to carry oxygen from the lungs to the tissues and to carry carbon dioxide from the tissues to the lungs.
- NUTRITION—to carry food substances from the intestine or storage tissues (fatty tissue, the liver, and muscle cells) to the rest of the body tissues.
- EXCRETION—to carry wastes away from the tissues to the organs of excretion (kidneys, large intestine, skin, and lungs).
- PROTECTION—to defend against disease-causing organisms by engulfing and digesting (eating) them, or by producing antibodies against them (immunity).
- REGULATION—to carry hormones, water, salt, and other chemicals that control the functions of organs and glands. The regulation of body temperature is aided by the blood, which carries excessive body heat to the lungs and skin surface.

The volume of blood differs from person to person, based on body size (Table 7–1). The typical adult

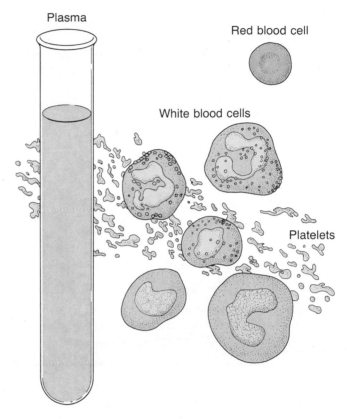

FIGURE 7–1. **The major components of blood.**

Table 7–1. **BLOOD VOLUMES**

Patient	Total Blood Volume	Lethal Blood Loss if Not Replaced (rapid)
Adult male (154 pounds)	5.0 to 6.6 liters	2.0 liters
Adolescent (105 pounds)	3.3 to 4.5 liters	1.3 liters
Child (early to late childhood . . . depends on size)	1.5 to 2.0 liters	0.5 to 0.7 liter
Infant (newborn, normal weight range)	300+ milliliters	30 to 50 milliliters

NOTE: One liter equals about two pints. One milliliter is about the same as 20 drops from a medicine dropper.

male has from 5.0 to 6.6 liters of blood, or between 10 to 12 pints (about 7% of the body weight). The loss of blood volume is very significant, not only in terms of the loss of formed elements but also in loss of plasma. Keep in mind that each person has a minimum volume of blood that is needed in circulation to keep the cardiovascular system working efficiently enough to maintain life.

A general classification of blood volume can be based on the age of the patient. An infant may have only 300 milliliters (ml) of blood (1 ml equals about 20 drops from a medicine dropper, 15 ml equals 1 tablespoon). Depending on size, children have from 1.5 to 2 liters of blood. Adolescents usually have from 3.3 to 5.0 liters of blood depending on their size.

Blood Vessels

The major types of blood vessels are:

- Arteries—carry blood away from the heart
- Capillaries—where oxygen/carbon dioxide and nutrient/waste exchange takes place
- Veins—carry blood back to the heart

As the heart beats, it circulates blood. Except for a few special cases in the body, blood moves through arteries, to capillaries, to veins, and back to the heart. These pulsations are most noticeable in the arteries. Blood travels at its greatest speed and under the greatest pressure in these vessels. Arterial blood is sent ultimately through the thin-walled, microscopic capillaries. When moving through capillaries, the flow is constant and the blood does not pulsate. This constant flow is called **perfusion** and is essential for the life of all tissues.

NOTE: A reduction of blood volume greatly affects perfusion. The failure of this constant flow of blood

can lead to tissue death. The brain and nerve cells are very sensitive to decreased perfusion.

Classifying Bleeding

The term **hemorrhage** (HEM-o-rej) means bleeding. Bleeding can be classified as external or internal. In addition, bleeding can be classified as to the type of vessel losing the blood. At the EMT-level of care, this is done only for external bleeding.

External bleeding (Figure 7–3) is classified as:

- Arterial Bleeding—the loss of blood from an artery. The blood loss is often rapid and profuse, as blood spurts from the wound. Usually, the spurting blood pulsates as the heart beats. The color of the blood is bright red.
- Venous Bleeding—the loss of blood from a vein. The blood loss is a steady flow and can be quite heavy. The color of the blood is dark red, often appearing to be dark maroon.
- Capillary Bleeding—the loss of blood from a capillary bed. The flow is slow, often described as "oozing." The color of the blood is red, usually less bright than arterial blood.

In most cases, arterial bleeding is less likely to clot spontaneously than other types of bleeding. When completely severed, arteries often constrict and seal themselves off. However, if an artery is not completely severed but is torn, or has a hole in its wall, it will probably continue to bleed.

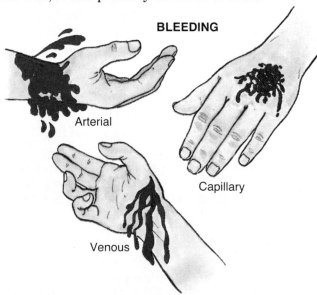

FIGURE 7–3. The three types of external bleeding.

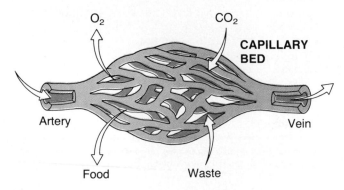

FIGURE 7–2. The blood vessels.

Veins are usually located closer to the body surface than are the arteries. Bleeding from surface veins is easier to control than arterial bleeding, even when the flow is profuse (a steady noticeable flow). Most veins will collapse when they are cut; however, bleeding from deep veins can be as profuse and as hard to control as arterial bleeding.

Open veins can suck in debris and air bubbles. This is sometimes the case with the major neck veins. When air is sucked in and forms an air bubble, known as an **air embolism** (EM-bo-liz-m), the bubble can be carried to the heart and may interfere with or stop the heart's pumping action completely. Other areas of the body that may be seriously affected by air emboli (EM-bo-li) include the lungs and the brain.

Bleeding from capillaries is slow, and clotting typically takes place within 6 to 8 minutes. This type of bleeding often involves a large area of injured skin; thus, wound contamination and the chance of infection are problems.

External Bleeding

Evaluating External Bleeding

Detecting and stopping life threatening bleeding are part of the primary survey. Priority is given to the arterial and large vein bleeding.

Estimating external blood loss requires some experience before the EMT can do so with confidence. Such estimates are important in terms of predicting possible shock, sorting patients for triage, and considering the seriousness of prolonged slow bleeding. Slow bleeding that normally could wait until the secondary survey may be a primary survey concern if it has been steady for a long period of time and blood loss has become significant. Anxious or com-

bative behavior, a decline in the patient's level of consciousness and/or a rapid pulse rate, shallow and rapid respirations, and low blood pressure detected during the taking of vital signs are valuable indicators of possible significant blood loss.

To help form a concept of blood loss, pour a pint of water on the floor next to a fellow student or a manikin. Try soaking an article of clothing with a pint of water and note how much of the article is wet and how wet it feels to your touch.

The amount of blood that can be lost before death occurs will vary from individual to individual (see Table 7–1). Usually a loss of 25% to 40% of the person's total blood volume will create a life-threatening condition. However, certain guidelines can be used that do not require calculating total blood volume. A rapid loss of 1 liter of blood by an adult must be considered to be life threatening. Depending on size, a loss of one-fourth to one-half liter of blood by a child will be life threatening. For an infant, 24 ml of blood loss *must* be viewed as life threatening. Regardless of the apparent volume of blood loss, if the patient has any of the indications of shock (pp. 204–205), then the bleeding must be classified as serious.

Controlling External Bleeding

NOTE: All patients with serious bleeding should be given oxygen as soon as possible. (*Do not* delay your efforts to control serious bleeding to retrieve oxygen equipment.) These patients should be transported as soon as possible.

The eight major methods used to control external bleeding are:

1. Direct pressure
2. Elevation
3. Pressure points
4. Splinting
5. Inflatable splints (air splints)
6. Pneumatic anti-shock garments or pneumatic counterpressure devices. (see Section Two)
7. Applying a tourniquet.
8. Blood pressure cuff (used as a tourniquet)

Direct Pressure   The most acceptable method of controlling external bleeding is by pressure applied directly to the wound (Figure 7–5). Direct pressure can be applied by your hand, by a dressing and your hand, by your fingers placed in a wound, or by a pressure dressing. Always wear protective gloves.

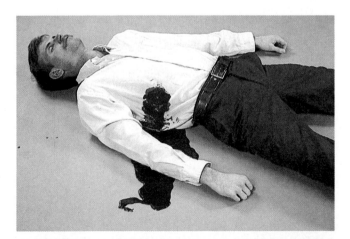

FIGURE 7–4. Estimating external blood loss: one-half liter (approx. 1 pint).

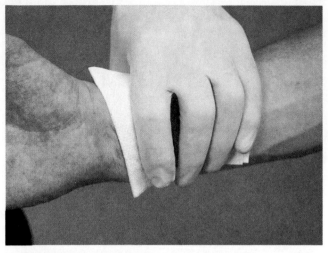

Apply pressure with dressing.

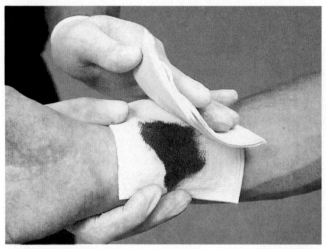

Apply additional dressing if necessary.

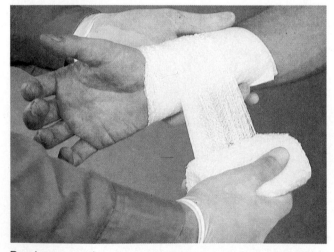

Bandage wound.

FIGURE 7–5. Direct pressure is applied until bleeding is controlled.

When bleeding is MILD, you should:

1. Apply pressure to the wound, preferably with a sterile dressing held against its surface. (A clean handkerchief or cloth can be used if a sterile dressing is not immediately available.)
2. Pressure held firmly on the wound for 10 to 30 minutes will usually stop the bleeding. Your role is to control the bleeding and limit additional significant blood loss.
3. Once bleeding is controlled, secure the dressing in place with bandaging.
4. NEVER remove a dressing once it is in place. To do so may restart bleeding or cause additional injury to the site. Apply another dressing on top of the blood-soaked one and hold them both in place. Continue this procedure until bleeding is controlled, or until you deliver the patient to the staff of a medical facility.

If bleeding is PROFUSE, you should:

1. NOT waste time trying to find a dressing.
2. Place your gloved hand directly on the wound and exert firm pressure.
3. Keep applying steady, firm pressure until the bleeding is controlled.
4. Once bleeding is controlled, a dressing can be bandaged in place to form a pressure dressing.

A **pressure dressing** can be applied to establish enough direct pressure to control most bleeding. Several sterile gauze pad dressings are placed on the wound. A bulky dressing is placed over the gauze pads. An efficient bulky dressing for a severely bleeding wound is the combined, or multitrauma, dressing. Sanitary napkins also can be used. The dressings should be held in place with a self-adherent roller bandage wrapped tightly over the dressing and above and below the wound site. Enough pressure must be created to control the bleeding.

NOTE: After controlling the bleeding from an extremity using a pressure dressing, check for a distal pulse to be certain that the dressing has not restricted blood flow in the treated limb. If you do not feel a pulse, you may have to adjust the pressure to reestablish circulation. Frequent checks of the distal pulse should continue throughout your care

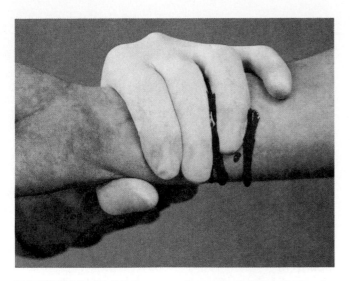

FIGURE 7–6. In cases of profuse bleeding, *do not* waste time hunting for a dressing.

for the patient. In some cases, the severing of a major artery will stop the circulation needed to produce a pulse.

The dressings *should not* be removed once they are applied. In cases where bleeding continues, more pressure can be added using the palm of your hand, or a tighter bandage can be applied. In some cases, you may have to create more bulk by adding additional dressings. In rare cases, you may have to remove a blood-soaked bulky bandage leaving the initial dressing in place so that bleeding can be controlled by direct pressure (see page 196).

A variety of dressings can be used in emergency situations. Some of these are shown in Figure 7–7.

Be aware that, in certain areas of the body, you may be unable to apply an effective pressure dressing, as when bleeding is from the armpit. You may have to maintain pressure by holding your hand directly over the wound. Even though you may be

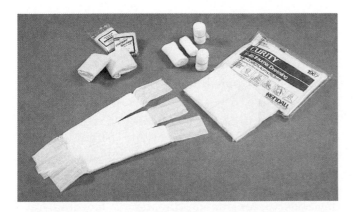

FIGURE 7–7. Dressings for use in emergencies.

contaminating the wound, the risk of uncontrolled bleeding far outweighs that of possible infection.

REMEMBER: Direct pressure is usually the quickest and most efficient means of controlling external bleeding.

Elevation This method is used along with direct pressure. When an injured extremity is elevated so that the wound is above the level of the heart, gravity helps to reduce blood pressure, thus bleeding is slowed (Figure 7–8). This method should *not* be used if there are possible fractures or dislocations to the extremity, objects impaled in the extremity, or possible spinal injury. To use elevation, you should:

1. Apply direct pressure to the site of bleeding.
2. Elevate the injured extremity. If the forearm is bleeding, simply elevate the forearm. You do not have to elevate the entire limb.

Pressure Points If direct pressure or direct pressure and elevation fail, your next approach may be the use of pressure points. A **pressure point** is a

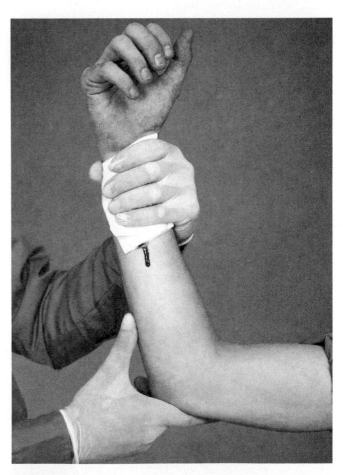

FIGURE 7–8. Combine direct pressure and elevation.

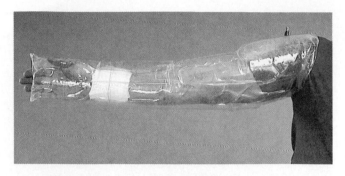

FIGURE 7–9. Air splints can be used to control bleeding from an extremity.

site where a main artery lies near the surface of the body and directly over a bone (these correspond well to pulse sites). These 6 sites (3 on each side) are used to control profuse bleeding in field emergency care. These sites are the:

> • Brachial (BRAY-ke-al) Artery—for bleeding from the upper limb.
> • Femoral (FEM-o-ral) Artery—for bleeding from the lower limb.
> • Temporal Artery—for bleeding from the scalp.

The use of pressure points requires skill on the part of the rescuer. Unless you know the exact location of the point and how much pressure to apply, the pressure point technique is of no use.

REMEMBER: Pressure point techniques are to be used only after direct pressure or direct pressure and elevation have failed to control the bleeding.

Bleeding from the Upper Extremity Apply pressure to a point over the brachial artery. To find the artery, hold the patient's arm out at a right angle to his body, with the palm facing up. (This angle will provide the best results but may be reduced if a 90-degree extension is not possible.) Find the groove between the biceps muscle and the arm bone (humerus), about midway between the elbow and the armpit. Cradle the upper arm in the palm of your hand and position your fingers into this medial groove. You can now compress the brachial artery against the underlying bone by pressing your finger into this groove. If pressure is properly applied, you will not be able to feel a radial pulse. If the wound is to the distal end of the limb, bleeding may not be effectively controlled by this method. This is because blood is being sent to this region from many smaller arteries that have branched off of the major arteries in the limb.

Bleeding from the Lower Extremity Apply pressure to a point over the femoral artery. Locate this artery on the medial side of the thigh where it joins the lower trunk. You should be able to feel pulsations at a point just below the groin. Place the heel of your hand over the site and exert pressure downward toward the bone until it is obvious that the bleeding has been controlled. You will need more pressure than that applied for the brachial artery pressure point. Considerable force must be exerted if the patient is very muscular or obese. If pressure is properly applied, a distal pulse cannot be felt. This method may not control bleeding for distal wounds (see the above discussion on bleeding from the upper extremity).

Splinting The splinting of fractures will be covered in Chapters 9 and 10. Often, when a fractured extremity is splinted, bleeding associated with the fracture may be controlled. This occurs when the sharp ends of broken bones are stabilized, preventing additional damage to blood vessels at the injury site.

Inflatable Splints (Air Splints) These devices may serve to control internal and external bleeding from an extremity, even when there is no fracture. They are useful when a severe laceration (cut) extends over the length of the extremity. The pressure produced by the splint is actually a form of direct pressure. The application of these splints will be covered in Chapter 9.

Blood Pressure Cuff This device can be applied as a tourniquet to control apparently life-threatening arterial bleeding from an extremity. The cuff is placed above the wound (between the wound and the heart) and inflated to the pressure required to control the bleeding. This is usually in the 150-mmHg range for persons with normal blood pressure. A dressing and bandage is secured after the bleeding is controlled. The cuff can safely be left inflated for 30 minutes or more; however, it must be closely monitored to make certain that cuff pressure is not lost. The use of the blood pressure cuff may prove to be the only way to control bleeding for patients who are trapped in wreckage.

A blood pressure cuff can be used after a dressing has been applied to make a pressure dressing (see p. 196).

Pneumatic Anti-Shock Garments (PASG) These are covered in Section Two of this chapter.

Tourniquet A tourniquet applied to a bleeding extremity is an extreme measure. THIS PROCEDURE IS A LAST RESORT, used only when other methods to control life-threatening bleeding have failed. The application of a tourniquet could lead to eventual loss of the limb. An amputated extremity may leave you with no other choice than to apply a tourniquet; however, direct pressure, elevation, and pressure points work to control most bleeding, including many amputations.

NOTE: Tourniquets are used only for wounds of the extremities. DO NOT apply a tourniquet on or below the elbow, or on or below the knee.

Clean-edged amputations often do not require the application of a tourniquet. This is because many of the injured blood vessels seal shut as a result of spasms produced in their muscular walls (vasospasms). Bulky pressure dressings are very effective in controlling the bleeding associated with this type of injury. Rough-edged amputations, usually produced by crushing or tearing injuries, often bleed freely since the nature of the injury does not allow for effective vasospasms. These types of amputations may require the application of a tourniquet to control profuse bleeding; however, direct pressure is usually very effective.

ONCE A TOURNIQUET IS IN PLACE, IT SHOULD NOT BE LOOSENED. Loosening of the tourniquet may dislodge clots and precipitate enough additional bleeding to cause severe shock, which can then lead to death. A slowly developing form of **tourniquet shock** can occur due to harmful substances released by severely injured tissues. These substances are held back by the tourniquet, only to be released in high concentration each time the tourniquet is loosened. The sudden release of blood can cause such a pronounced variation in circulation that a rapidly developing form of tourniquet shock may occur. If you keep a tourniquet in place, the patient has a better chance for survival, even if it means the loss of a limb.

REMEMBER: A tourniquet is a last-resort measure to be used for profuse bleeding in an extremity. Once a tourniquet has been applied, it should not be loosened.

NOTE: Many physicians recommend that the blood pressure cuff be used as a tourniquet when direct pressure with bulky dressings does not control bleeding resulting from amputation.

If a commercially made tourniquet is not available, a makeshift one may be prepared from a cravat bandage, a stocking, a wide belt, or some other soft, flat material. The ideal width of the tourniquet is 2 to 3 inches.

WARNING: Among the items that should *not* be used are ropes, pieces of wire, or other small-diameter materials that could cut into the patient's skin and soft tissues.

When possible, have another rescuer apply pressure point and direct pressure techniques while you apply the tourniquet. To apply a tourniquet, you should:

1. Select a place between the heart and the wound, as close as possible to, but not flush with, the edge of the wound. This should be within 2 inches of the wound. If the wound is on a joint, apply the tourniquet above the joint (toward the heart).
2. Place a pad made from a dressing (a roll of gauze bandage) or a folded handkerchief over the main supplying artery before applying the constricting band. This will help protect the site and will apply additional pressure over the artery.
3. If a commercial tourniquet is used, carefully place it around the limb at the site and pull the free end of the band through the buckle or friction catch and draw this end tightly over the pad. You should tighten the tourniquet to the point where bleeding is controlled. *Do not* tighten the tourniquet beyond this point.

   If you are using a cravat or other piece of material, carefully slip the material around the injured limb and tie a knot with the ends of the tourniquet. The knot should be over the pad. A stick, rod, or similar device

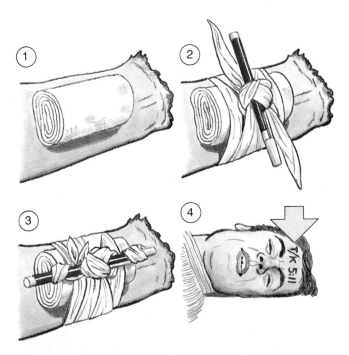

FIGURE 7–10. Application of a tourniquet.

should be inserted into the knot and used to tighten the tourniquet. Turn the device until bleeding is controlled. *Do not* tighten beyond this point. Tape or tie the tightening device in place.

4. KEEP THE TOURNIQUET IN PLACE. DO NOT LOOSEN.

5. Attach a notation to the patient to indicate that a tourniquet has been applied and the time of application. If a tag is not available, mark the patient's forehead in ink. Write "TK" and the time of application. This notation *must* be written so that the tourniquet does not go unnoticed by the emergency department staff. Make certain that you do not cover the extremity to which the tourniquet has been applied. This is done for the visual monitoring of the effectiveness of the tourniquet and to ensure that the tourniquet does not go unnoticed by others who render care.

NOTE: It is the EMT's responsibility to advise the emergency department staff of the application of a tourniquet.

There may be instances in which you arrive at a scene and find that bystanders have applied a tourniquet. Most EMS Systems have standard operating procedures that *must* be followed in such cases. Sometimes, a responsive patient will be able to tell you if he thought the bleeding was serious. Since the bystanders applied the tourniquet, they may or may not be a good source of information. Obviously, they thought the bleeding was serious, but they may have applied the tourniquet thinking this is a proper procedure for all bleeding. If the EMT can judge from interviews and observations that a tourniquet was not necessary, the tourniquet can be released slowly while applying direct pressure to the wound site. Remember, this can only be done if it is allowed in your EMS System. Check with your instructor. It is usually best to leave all tourniquets in place.

Cryotherapy   This is the treatment of an injury with cold, a basic technique used for centuries. Cold therapy is used for bruises, dislocations, sprains, burns, and minor bleeding. The application of cold will reduce pain, minimize swelling, and reduce bleeding by constricting blood vessels. Cryotherapy is not useful by itself, but it can be used in combination with other bleeding control techniques. Chemical cold packs and splints inflated with cryogenic liquids make cold therapy available in field situations.

When using cryotherapy, the cold pack should not be allowed to come into direct contact with the skin. Wrap the pack in a cloth cover or towel so that there is a barrier between it and the skin. It is recommended that the cold pack be left in place no more than 20 minutes at a time. This is done to avoid the development of frostbite.

Internal Bleeding

Significance

A small *contusion* (bruise) is an example of internal bleeding. By itself, a small bruise is of minor importance. Other cases of internal bleeding can produce enough blood loss to bring about shock, heart and lung failure, and eventual death. Internal injury, rupturing of blood vessels in the chest and abdomen can produce internal bleeding that causes death in a matter of minutes or seconds. Crushing injuries, ruptured or lacerated organs and blood vessels, bleeding ulcers, severely bruised tissues, and fractured bones can all produce serious internal blood loss.

Internal bleeding can occur with wounds that are deep enough to sever major arteries and veins. A deep chest or abdominal wound can cut through many blood vessels, causing blood to flow freely into the body cavity. Any cut into muscle or the fracturing of bone also will cause blood loss. Often, such serious internal bleeding is accompanied by only minor external bleeding. If the patient is not properly assessed, the internal bleeding may be considered only minor or missed entirely.

Be alert to the fact that many cases of internal bleeding occur when there are no cuts in the skin or cavity walls. **Blunt trauma,** an injury produced by an object that was not sharp enough to penetrate the skin, may cause major internal bleeding. The force is carried into the body, rupturing vessels and organs. Patients who are thrown against dashboards, steering wheels, armrests, and other objects in motor vehicle accidents can suffer from internal injuries that produce serious internal bleeding. Knowing the mechanism of injury is important in detecting internal bleeding.

Life-threatening internal bleeding may occur when there are no signs of obvious external injury. In blunt trauma situations, a minor externally visible bruise may be the only indication that an abdominal organ has been ruptured. Also, a blow delivered to one side of the body may cause internal bleeding on the opposite side. For example, a blow to the right side of the abdomen may rupture the spleen (on the left side of the body) and release a liter or more of blood.

REMEMBER: The secondary survey is of major importance in detecting internal bleeding.

Detecting Internal Bleeding

Assume internal bleeding whenever you detect:

- Wounds that have penetrated the skull
- Blood or bloody fluids in the ears or nose
- Vomiting or coughing up blood (coffee-ground or frothy red in appearance)
- Bruises on the neck
- Bruises on the chest or the signs of possible rib fracture
- Wounds that have penetrated the chest or abdomen
- Areas of bruised or swollen abdomen
- Abdominal tenderness, rigidity, or spasms (the patient may guard the abdomen)
- Blood in the urine
- Rectal or vaginal bleeding
- Bone fractures, especially the pelvis and the long bones of the arm and thigh.

NOTE: The items listed above follow the physical examination of the secondary survey.

As an EMT, you should learn to associate internal bleeding with the symptoms and signs of shock, which will be considered later in this chapter. For now, consider the patient assessment procedures.

Related to internal bleeding, you will find some of the symptoms of shock, including:

- Anxiety or restlessness
- Weakness
- Thirst
- Complaints of feeling cold

The signs of shock are closely associated with internal bleeding, including:

- Restlessness (a reliable early sign) or combativeness
- Altered level of consciousness
- Breathing—rapid, possibly becoming shallow
- Pulse—rapid and weak
- Blood pressure—a marked drop, usually to 90/60 mmHg or lower (usually a late sign)
- Skin—pale, cool, and clammy, often with profuse sweating (usually found first at the extremities)

- Eyes—pupils may be dilated
- Body—shaking and trembling (rare)

REMEMBER: You may detect internal bleeding by looking for mechanisms of injury, wounds and injuries that often produce internal bleeding, and certain symptoms and signs of shock.

Evaluating Internal Blood Loss

Special tests and procedures are done at the hospital to determine the approximate amount of internal blood loss. At the scene, it is difficult for the EMT to know how serious internal bleeding may be. Consider internal bleeding to be severe if the patient is vomiting or coughing up blood. This blood may look like coffee grounds. Pink, frothy blood in the mouth or nose often indicates bleeding in the lungs. Rigidity or spasms of the abdominal wall muscles also may indicate possible severe internal bleeding. If there is penetration of the chest cavity or the abdomen consider internal bleeding to be an immediate threat to life. Blood loss of 1 liter or more must be considered anytime there is a fracture to the femur or pelvis.

Since it is very difficult to estimate internal blood loss, assume a 10% blood loss for every deep bruise the size of a man's fist that is found on the chest or abdomen. Even though this may not be true for a particular patient, it is better to overestimate the significance of possible internal bleeding.

Carefully evaluating the patient's symptoms and signs and quickly estimating internal blood loss will help you determine the possibilities of your patient developing severe shock or cardiac arrest. Remember, when there is more than one patient, the order of care and transport may be affected by internal blood loss.

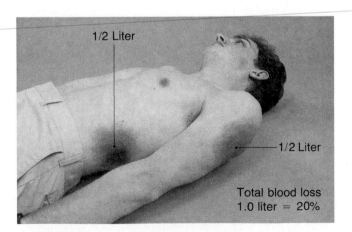

FIGURE 7–11. Estimating internal blood loss.

Controlling Internal Bleeding

Control of internal bleeding depends on the location of the injury and the cause of the bleeding. Minor internal bleeding related to a blunt injury to an extremity *may* be controlled by a pressure dressing and bandage. The pressure applied will tend to close off the ends of bleeding vessels. Extreme care must be taken, however, since a fracture may have been produced by the accident. The careless application of a pressure bandage to a closed fracture site may injure soft tissues or aggravate the fracture. Special care must be taken to avoid additional injury to the spine, chest, and pelvis.

The application of a splint to an injured extremity often will help control internal bleeding related to fractures. Inflatable splints are useful for such cases.

Injury-related or illness-induced bleeding into the thoracic or the abdominopelvic cavity may not be controllable at the accident scene, even when using pneumatic counterpressure devices.

You must continue to ensure an open airway and monitor vital signs. Patients with possible neck or spinal injuries must be given special care to avoid aggravation of these injuries. Profuse external bleeding must be cared for immediately.

When providing care for a patient with possible internal bleeding, you should:

1. Maintain an open airway.
2. Reassure the patient and provide emotional support throughout all aspects of care. A calm patient has a better chance for survival. The stress and anxiety produced by the emergency will increase the patient's pulse rate, thus increasing the bleeding rate.
3. Keep the patient lying down and at rest.
4. Control all serious bleeding. If the bleeding is in an extremity, use a snug bandage over a bulky pad applied directly over the injury site, taking care not to aggravate fractures. Remember that applying a splint serves both to immobilize an injured limb and to control bleeding.
5. PASG if indicated.
6. Position and treat for shock, as described on page 206. You may have to first immobilize fractures before positioning to complete the care for shock.
7. Administer high concentrations of oxygen as soon as possible.
8. Loosen restrictive clothing at the neck and waist.
9. Provide appropriate care for fractures.
10. Give nothing to the patient by mouth. ANTICIPATE VOMITING, having suction available for immediate use.
11. Monitor vital signs every 5 minutes.
12. Transport as soon as possible to a medical facility. Avoid rough and excessive handling. Remember, patients with bleeding into the chest and abdominal cavities are HIGH-PRIORITY PATIENTS.

SHOCK

Defining Shock

The first hour after injury is known as the *golden hour*. If advanced life support is started and the required surgery can begin during this hour, many trauma patients have an improved chance of survival. The major problem to be cared for during this hour is shock. Once shock reaches a certain level of severity, the patient *cannot* be saved.

The term shock has many meanings. In medicine, there are specific types of shock. In most cases, perfusion fails and shock results when the cardiovascular system fails to provide sufficient blood circulation to all the vital tissues of the body.

Shock *develops* from the effects of damage brought about by severe injury or illness. Shock is the body's reaction to low perfusion. The development of shock can be related to the:

- Heart—Should the heart fail to pump blood efficiently, shock will develop.
- Blood—There must be enough blood to fill the vascular system. Shock will develop if there is a loss of blood or plasma.
- Blood Vessels Dilitation—The volume of the vascular system cannot be too large for the amount of blood that is available for circulation.

Understanding the role of the blood vessels in the development of shock is important. Blood vessels can change their diameter. If an area of the body requires more blood because it is doing more work, the vessels in that area dilate, as needed, to allow greater flow. At the same time, another area of the body that does not require the extra blood flow may constrict its vessels to reduce the blood flow to help keep the system filled with blood. If you are running, blood flow to the muscles increases through dilated arteries. At the same time, blood flow to the stomach and intestines lessens because vessels supplying these organs have constricted. If all the vessels in the body dilated at once, there would not be nearly enough blood to fill the entire system, causing circulation to fail. Whenever too many vessels dilate to allow for adequate perfusion, shock develops.

The chambers of the heart and the blood vessels make up what is known as the **vascular container.** The function of this container is greatly influenced by blood loss or the failure to maintain proper vessel diameter or heart action. To function properly, this container must be filled with blood. Normally, there is enough blood to fill the vessels. The heart keeps pumping, circulating the blood to keep the vessels full. For the system to work, the heart must keep pumping adequately, there must be an adequate supply of blood, and the blood vessels must keep changing diameter to adjust to different circulation patterns. If any of these three factors fail, perfusion in the brain, lungs, and other body organs will not be adequate.

As you can see from the above, as the body reacts and develops shock, more problems are caused. For example, if blood is being lost through bleeding, the heart rate will increase in an effort to circulate blood to all the vital tissues. This action causes more blood to be lost. Immediately, the body will react to this additional blood loss by again increasing the heart rate. This process will continue, leading to the death of the patient.

At the onset of shock, the body tries to adjust to the loss of blood, improper heart activity, or the dilation of too many blood vessels. At a certain point in some types of shock, enough blood has been lost so that the system is no longer filled, no matter how hard the heart pumps or how much the blood vessels constrict. In other cases of shock, the heart becomes too inefficient in circulating blood and perfusion fails. There are also cases in which there is no loss of blood volume and the heart is performing properly, but too many vessels are dilated. For these cases, there is too much volume (capacity) in the system to be filled by the available blood. *Regardless of the mechanism, shock is the failure of the cardiovascular system to provide sufficient blood to all the vital tissues of the body.*

REMEMBER: Shock may develop if the heart fails as a pump, blood volume is lost, or blood vessels dilate to create a vascular container capacity too great to be filled by the available blood.

Types of Shock

Shock may accompany many emergency situations; thus treatment for it is included in emergency care procedures for virtually every serious injury and medical problem.

There is more than one type of shock. A patient may develop:

- *Hypovolemic* (HI-po-vo-LE-mik) *Shock*—caused by the loss of body fluids. When shock develops due to blood loss or loss of plasma (as seen in burns and crushing injuries), this form of hypovolemic shock is called hemorrhagic (HEM-or-RAJ-ik) shock. Dehydration due to diarrhea, vomiting, or heavy perspiration can lead to the development of hypovolemic shock.
- *Cardiogenic* (KAR-di-o-jen-ic) *Shock*—caused by the heart failing to pump blood adequately to all vital parts of the body.
- *Neurogenic* (NU-ro-jen-ic) *Shock*—caused by the failure of the nervous system to control the diameter of blood vessels (seen with spinal injury). Once the blood vessels are dilated, there is not enough blood in circulation to fill this new volume, causing inadequate circulation of the blood.
- *Anaphylactic* (AN-ah-fi-LAK-tik) *Shock*—a life-threatening reaction of the body to an allergen, something to which the patient is extremely allergic.
- *Psychogenic* (SI-ko-jen-ic) *Shock* (fainting)—is a nervous system reaction and is often brought about by fear, bad news, the sight of blood, or a minor injury. A sudden dilation of the blood vessels takes place and the proper blood flow to the brain is momentarily interrupted, causing the patient to faint. This is a temporary condition and is considered a self-correcting form of shock.
- *Metabolic Shock*—often associated with diarrhea, vomiting, and polyuria (excessive urination). Such conditions cause loss of body fluids and changes in body chemistry, including salt balance and acid-base balance. Failure of the adrenal, thyroid, or pituitary glands may lead to metabolic shock.
- *Septic Shock*—caused by severe infection. Toxins (poisons) are released into the bloodstream and cause blood vessels to dilate, increasing the volume of the circulatory system beyond functional limits. In addition, plasma is lost through vessel walls, causing a loss in blood volume. This type of shock is seldom

seen by the EMT in the field since the patient is usually hospitalized before it occurs.

The most common form of serious shock associated with injury is *hemorrhagic shock,* due to the loss of blood. Bleeding can be external or internal. In addition to the loss of whole blood, enough plasma may also be lost to result in a severe drop in blood volume. This is the case with burns and crushing injuries. A preexisting condition of dehydration will hasten the reaction. Be alert to this in areas of high temperatures, such as warehouses and factories. This also can be a problem if the patient was sweating profusely prior to injury, as in sports and hunting accidents. Certain strenuous work situations, such as those of dockworkers and steelworkers, may cause enough body fluid loss prior to the accident to quicken the effects of blood loss.

Cardiogenic shock is usually brought about by injuries to the heart, heart attacks, or electrical shock. Many diseases, if allowed to go untreated, may eventually do enough heart damage to cause cardiogenic shock. Be on the alert for low blood pressure, edema (swelling) of the ankles, and the signs of left heart failure (pp. 392–393).

In neurogenic shock due to nerve paralysis caused by spinal cord or brain injuries, there is no actual loss of blood but a dilation of blood vessels that increases the volume of the circulatory system beyond the point where it can be filled. Blood can no longer adequately fill the entire system, pooling in the blood vessels in certain areas of the body. Severe blows to the abdomen also can disrupt nerves, possibly bringing about neurogenic shock. This type of shock also is seen when neurologic reactions cause circulation patterns to change, as seen in some cases of hypoglycemia (low blood sugar), overexertion, or improper diet or when a diabetic takes an overdose of insulin (insulin shock).

NOTE: Some classifications of shock include the category known as respiratory shock. This is not due to a collapse of the cardiovascular system but to a failure of the lungs to provide enough oxygen for circulation to the tissues. This may be due to injured or diseased lungs or to airway obstruction. The typical patient is an adult who has a long-term respiratory disease.

Symptoms and Signs of Shock

Shock can occur very rapidly, placing the patient in a critical condition long before you arrive at the scene. In other cases, the patient may slowly develop shock as you provide care. There is a saying used by EMS personnel: "Patients can go into shock a little at a time." For such patients, you will have warning signs, but never assume that an apparently stable patient will not go into shock. Monitor your patients.

The symptoms and signs of shock usually develop in a specific order. Before considering this development, imagine that you have just arrived at an accident scene. Look over the following list of symptoms and signs and consider how they might be obtained during the patient assessment.

The symptoms of shock can include:

- A feeling of impending doom. The patient may show fear and restlessness. Your observations of such can be included as signs of shock.
- Weakness
- Nausea
- Thirst
- Dizziness
- Coolness

The signs of shock can include:

- ENTIRE BODY—look for evidence of:
  1. Restlessness
  2. Profuse external bleeding
  3. Vomiting
  4. Shaking and trembling (rare)
- LEVEL OF CONSCIOUSNESS—sudden unresponsiveness, faintness, or loss of consciousness
- PULSE—rapid and weak (usually the first sign)
- BREATHING—shallow and rapid
- BLOOD PRESSURE—marked drop (to 90/60 mmHg or lower)*
- SKIN—pale, moist, and cool. There is often profuse sweating and a clammy feel to the touch.
- EYES—lackluster, dilated pupils
- EYELIDS—pale inner surfaces (rare)
- FACE—pale, often with cyanosis at the lips and ear lobes

* Children and young adults can compensate for a loss of blood volume better than mature adults (35 years old and older). They can have a 10% blood loss and still have a normal blood pressure. At 15% to 20% blood loss, they are no longer able to compensate and may rapidly develop life-threatening shock.

- Decreased capillary refilling (more than 2 seconds). When you apply pressure to the tip of a nail bed, it will turn white. When pressure is released, it should regain its normal color in no more than 2 seconds. A simple rule to follow is that the refill should take place in less time than it takes to say "capillary refill."

All the symptoms and signs of shock are usually not present at once, nor do they occur in the order in which they may be detected during the patient assessment. In most cases, as shock develops you will see the following events:

1. **Restlessness or combativeness** is the patient's reaction to his body's attempt to compensate to the developing shock. This may be the first detectable sign in some cases. He often "feels" that something is wrong. In many cases, the patient looks afraid.

2. **Increased pulse rate** indicates that the body is adjusting to the loss of blood, plasma, or other body fluids, or that it is trying to adjust for some other cause of inefficient circulation. Unlike the rapid pulse rate associated with the stress and fear of the emergency, this increased rate will not slow down. The rate may rise significantly when the patient assumes an erect or sitting position.

3. **Increased breathing rate** occurs next, but not in all cases. The patient developing shock has inefficient circulation. This means that his tissues may not be receiving enough oxygen and that carbon dioxide is increasing at the tissue level. His body attempts to compensate by increasing the rate of breathing. This rate will not slow down as it does in cases of stress.

4. **Capillary refill time will increase and skin changes will be detected.** Skin changes start early in the development of shock, but they may not be noticed until the latter stages. The patient's skin will turn pale and his lips, nailbeds, and the membranes in his mouth will show cyanosis. Profuse sweating (diaphoresis) is usually present.

5. **Thirst, weakness, and nausea** may be noticed.

6. **Rapid, weak pulse and labored, weakened respirations** indicate that the body is failing in its attempts to compensate for the circulatory system failure.

7. **Changes in level of consciousness** may occur.

EARLY DEVELOPMENT	LOSS OF COMPENSATION	LATE DEVELOPMENT
Increased pulse rate	Skin color changes	Changes in levels of consciousness
Increased respirations	Rapid, weak pulse	Marked drop in blood pressure
Restlessness	Labored breathing	Weak pulse
Fearfulness	Weakness	Weakened respirations
Increased capillary refill time	Thirstiness	
	Nausea	

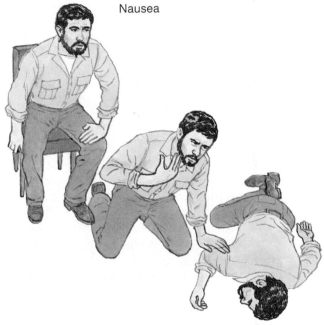

FIGURE 7–12.   The development of shock.

This may precede detection of weakened respiratory efforts. The effects of inadequate circulation to the brain will cause the patient to become confused, disoriented, sleepy, or unconscious.

8. **Drop in blood pressure**—this is a marked drop in pressure, indicating the failure of the patient's body to compensate for the developing shock. This may be delayed in children and young adults.

Preventing and Managing Shock

The same basic care should be used to keep a patient from *developing* shock and to manage a patient who is in shock. The best management for shock is prevention. When in doubt, care for shock, providing a high concentration of oxygen.

Keep in mind that a patient's body may be able to compensate for the early effects of shock (compensated shock), especially if the patient is young and in good physical condition. He may, at first, show little more than a slight increase in pulse rate. An increase in capillary refill time may be observed. Next, his systolic blood pressure may drop slightly and his diastolic pressure may increase. This type of patient will appear to be stable, but he is actually at his limit in being able to compensate. Unless he receives immediate effective care for shock, he will rapidly decline, quickly showing the symptoms and signs of life-threatening shock (decompensated shock).

When the nature of the illness or injury or the mechanism of injury indicates that shock is a possibility, care for shock, regardless of the patient's symptoms and signs.

Some specific measures must be added to our list of care procedures for the shock patient. These measures are:

1. *Ensure an adequate airway and breathing.* As in all cases, if the patient is breathing, maintain an adequate airway. If the person is not breathing, establish an airway and provide pulmonary resuscitation. STAY ALERT FOR VOMITING. If both respiration and circulation have stopped, initiate CPR measures.

2. *Control bleeding.* Use direct pressure, elevation, pressure points, splints, a blood pressure cuff, or a tourniquet as required. The loss of blood volume is life threatening for the shock patient. Apply a pneumatic counterpressure device when appropriate.

3. *Administer oxygen.* An oxygen deficiency will result from the reduced circulation taking place in shock. Provide a high concentration of oxygen. STAY ALERT FOR VOMITING.

4. *Splint fractures.* Splinting slows bleeding and reduces pain, both of which aggravate shock. AVOID ROUGH HANDLING since body motion has a tendency to aggravate shock.

5. *Position the patient.* You have three choices of patient position, depending on the patient's problem and local policies.
   • LOWER EXTREMITY ELEVATION: This is the most recommended position. Raise the patient's legs slightly, about 12 inches. If there are fractures of the lower extremities, they cannot be major and they *must* be splinted. *Do not* use this procedure if there are indications of neck or spinal injuries, head injuries, chest injuries, abdominal injuries, hip dislocations or fractures,

or pelvic fractures. *Do not* tilt the patient's entire body into a head-down position. To do so will press the abdominal organs against the diaphragm.
   • SUPINE: The patient is placed flat on his back, with adequate padding to provide comfort. This position is often used if there are serious injuries to the extremities.
   • SEMISEATED (semi-Fowler's): This position is used for conscious medical patients

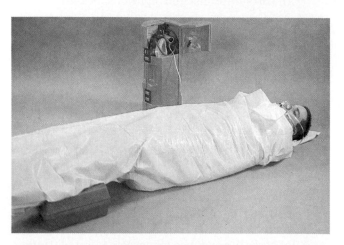

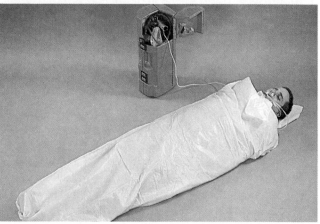

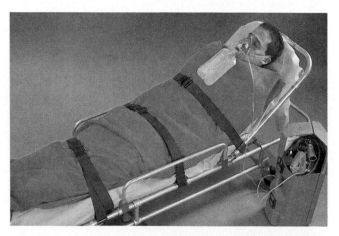

FIGURE 7–13. **Positioning the shock patient.**

with indications of respiratory or heart problems. It is not recommended for patients with the symptoms and signs of internal or external bleeding. The idea is to keep the patient as comfortable as possible and to allow him to find the position that provides for the easiest breathing.

WARNING: Regardless of the position used, monitor the patient's vital signs and be alert for vomiting.

6. REASSURE THE PATIENT.

7. Keep the patient lying still. The more at rest a shock patient remains, the better are his chances for survival. Avoid excessive and rough handling.

8. Prevent loss of body heat. You wish to keep the patient's body temperature as near to normal as possible. Place a blanket under and over the patient (ground placement of the blanket is best done when positioning the patient so as not to increase body movement). Prevent heat loss, but DO NOT ALLOW THE PATIENT TO OVERHEAT. When possible, remove any wet clothing. Do not move patients with head, neck, or spinal injury for the purpose of placing a blanket under them.

9. Give nothing by mouth. The patient in shock or developing shock may develop a dry mouth and thirst. Also, the oxygen being administered may dry the patient's oral and nasal pathways. If oxygen is to be used for long periods, the humidification of the oxygen should be considered. Do not give the patient anything to drink, including ice. Do not give any food or medications orally. To do so will probably induce vomiting.

10. Monitor the patient. You *must* take vital signs and record the results when you do the patient assessment. Check and record these signs every 5 MINUTES until you deliver both patient and information to a medical facility staff.

The use of pneumatic anti-shock garments may be part of your EMS System's protocol for certain shock patients. See Section Two of this chapter for details.

Anaphylactic Shock

Anaphylactic shock must be considered **life threatening** whenever it is encountered. There is no way for you to predict what may happen to a patient in anaphylactic shock. Severe reactions may take place immediately, or they may be delayed 30 minutes or more. A very mild allergic reaction may turn into serious anaphylactic shock in a matter of minutes. Exposure to the allergen will cause blood vessels

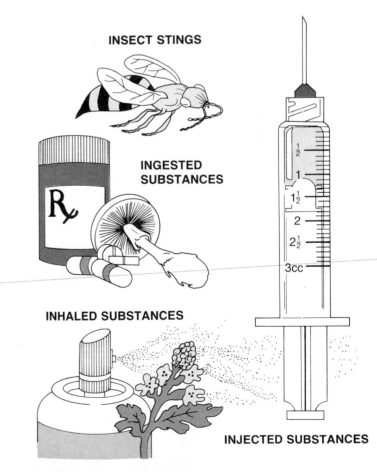

INSECT STINGS

INGESTED SUBSTANCES

INHALED SUBSTANCES

INJECTED SUBSTANCES

FIGURE 7–15. Substances that can cause anaphylactic shock.

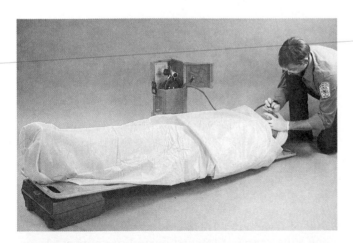

FIGURE 7–14. Managing the shock patient.

to dilate rapidly and cause a drop in blood pressure (hypotension) and the tissues that line the respiratory system may swell and obstruct the airway leading to respiratory failure.

Anaphylactic shock occurs when a person comes into contact with something to which he is extremely allergic. Causes of anaphylactic reactions include:

- INSECT STINGS—Bees, yellow jackets, wasps, and hornets can cause rapid and severe reactions.
- INGESTED SUBSTANCES—Foods such as nuts, spices, berries, fish, and shellfish and also certain drugs can cause reactions. In most cases, the effect is slower than that seen with insect stings.
- INHALED SUBSTANCES—Dust, pollens, and chemical powders can often cause very rapid and severe reactions.
- INJECTED SUBSTANCES—Antitoxins and drugs such as penicillin may cause severe reactions.
- ABSORBED SUBSTANCES—Certain chemicals, when in contact with the skin, produce severe reactions.

The symptoms of anaphylactic shock can include:

- Itching and burning skin, especially about the face, chest, and back
- Painful constriction of the chest with difficult breathing
- Dizziness
- Feelings of restlessness and anxiety
- Nausea, abdominal pain, or diarrhea
- Headache
- Temporary loss of consciousness (rare)

REMEMBER: When interviewing a patient, ask if he is allergic to anything. Check to see if that substance is at the scene or is likely to be at the scene. If you are in the patient's residence, see if there is a "Vial of Life" (Figure 7–16) or similar type of sticker on the main outside door, the closest window to the main door, or the refrigerator door. Patient information and medications can be found in such refrigerators. Look for medical identification devices to see if the patient has a known allergy.

The signs of anaphylactic shock can include:

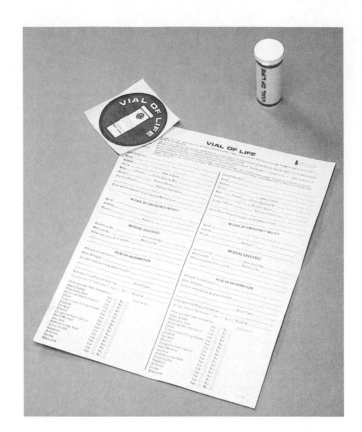

FIGURE 7–16. A "Vial of Life" sticker.

- LEVEL OF CONSCIOUSNESS—restlessness, often followed by fainting or unconsciousness
- BREATHING—difficult, sometimes with wheezing or rales
- PULSE—rapid and very weak or imperceptible
- BLOOD PRESSURE—above normal at first and then it may drop to shock level
- SKIN—obvious irritation or blotches (such as hives)
- FACE—marked swelling of the face and tongue, often with cyanosis of lips and paleness around the mouth and tongue
- VOMITING
- EXTREMITIES—often there is swelling of the ankles and/or wrists

---

Again, relate the above to the patient assessment.

Anaphylactic shock is a serious emergency requiring the injection of medications to combat the allergic reaction. Initial emergency care efforts should be directed toward basic life support. As an EMT, you should:

1. PROVIDE BASIC LIFE SUPPORT MEASURES. Maintain an open airway and perform pulmonary resuscitation or CPR as required.
2. PROVIDE A HIGH CONCENTRATION OF OXYGEN AND CARE FOR SHOCK.
3. TRANSPORT TO A MEDICAL FACILITY IMMEDIATELY. Notify the facility by radio on the way. Place the alert patient in a supine or semi-Fowler position. If the information is available, tell the staff the substance causing the reaction and the means of patient contact (e.g., sting, inhalation). Continue basic life support measures during transport. In some jurisdictions, you should provide basic life support and wait for an advanced life support response.

NOTE: Some EMS Systems are now considering the problems faced by the EMT when asked by a patient to help in administering medications at the scene. These medications, usually epinephrine or antihistamines for cases of bee sting sensitivity, are provided by physicians to persons with severe allergies. A more serious problem occurs when the patient is unconscious and the EMT finds a medical identification device and the medication is available at the scene. We give no recommendations in this text. Your instructor will inform you of the local policies for such cases.

Fainting

As noted in our classification of shock, fainting (syncope, sin-co-PE) is a self-correcting, temporary form of shock. Usually, the serious problems related to fainting are injuries that occur during falls due to the temporary loss of consciousness. Fainting may be caused by stressful situations. However, it may be an indication that the patient has blood pressure problems (sudden drop or elevation) or some other serious medical problem. Brain tumors, heart disease, undetected diabetes, and inner ear disorders are just a few medical problems that may first present themselves through fainting. Fainting in an older person is a serious sign more often than with younger patients. Often, it may indicate a serious cardiovascular problem that may prove to be *lethal*. Take the pulse and blood pressure of *anyone* who faints. If you are called to the scene of a fainting and the patient refuses additional care, recommend that he see a physician as soon as possible. In a polite but firm manner, tell the patient not to drive or operate any machinery until he has been examined by a physician. Make certain that you have the patient's witnessed refusal in writing, relay informa-

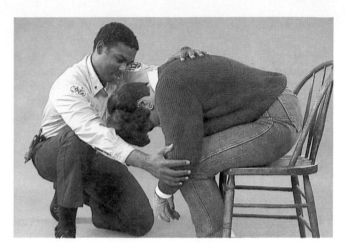

FIGURE 7–17. Protect the patient and try to prevent fainting.

tion to the medical facility and write an extensive documentation about refusal.

In all cases of fainting, protect the patient from injury and provide emotional support. You can often prevent a patient from fainting by placing him in a seated position and lowering his head to a level between the knees. *Do not* do this for patients with fractures, possible neck or spinal injuries, or severe head injuries. This procedure is *not recommended* for anyone having difficulty breathing or who has a known heart problem. Have these patients lie down with the feet slightly elevated and give emotional support. This will provide protection and may prevent fainting. If the patient is suffering from congestive heart failure or some form of COPD, a semi-seated position will provide him with comfort and allow you to protect him in case he faints.

SUMMARY

Bleeding can be classified as EXTERNAL or INTERNAL and can range from minor to life threatening.

External bleeding can be:

- ARTERIAL—profuse loss of bright red blood spurting from an artery.
- VENOUS—mild to profuse loss of dark red blood flowing steadily from a vein.
- CAPILLARY—slow loss of red blood flowing (oozing) from a bed of capillaries, as seen in minor scrapes of the skin.

The eight procedures for controlling external bleeding are:

1. DIRECT PRESSURE—where your gloved hand, a sterile dressing, or a clean cloth can be used to apply pressure directly to a wound to stop bleeding. NEVER remove a dressing that is in direct contact with a wound. A pressure dressing can be applied to stop most cases of external bleeding from a limb.

2. ELEVATION—usually used in combination with direct pressure to control bleeding from an intact extremity, when there is no spinal injury.

3. PRESSURE POINTS—using external hand pressure to compress an artery. This method is most often performed on the upper limb (brachial) and the thigh (femoral).

4. SPLINTING—stabilizing the ends of broken bones to prevent additional injury to blood vessels.

5. INFLATABLE SPLINTS—used even when there is no fracture. This method is useful for long cuts on an extremity.

6. BLOOD PRESSURE CUFF—used to control bleeding from an extremity.

7. PNEUMATIC ANTI-SHOCK GARMENTS (PASG)—useful for certain types of internal bleeding.

8. TOURNIQUET—a LAST RESORT procedure used to control bleeding from an extremity. The flat belt of a tourniquet is placed over a pad that has been set close to the wound, over the main supplying artery between the site of the wound and the patient's heart. The tourniquet belt is tightened to where the bleeding stops and is fixed in place at this point. A plainly visible note indicating a tourniquet has been placed and the time of placement must accompany the patient. ONCE THE TOURNIQUET IS IN PLACE, DO NOT LOOSEN IT.

REMEMBER: Direct pressure is the first choice in controlling bleeding.

Internal bleeding can be very serious. Look for mechanisms of injury that may cause internal bleeding, and look for wounds associated with internal bleeding. Note that fractures have internal bleeding, and examine the patient for the symptoms and signs of shock. Management of internal bleeding is basically the same as for shock. In addition, pressure dressings and splints can be applied for internal bleeding found in an extremity.

REMEMBER: Patients with serious blood loss will benefit from the administration of a high concentration of oxygen.

The symptoms of shock can include nausea, thirst, weakness, dizziness, coolness, and the feeling of impending doom.

The signs of shock can include the patient becoming unresponsive, restlessness, shaking and trembling, rapid and weak pulse, shallow and rapid breathing, marked drop in blood pressure, moist and cool skin, pale face and inner eyelids, dilated, lackluster pupils, and cyanosis at the lips or ear lobes. Increased capillary refill time may be observed.

Prevention and management of shock are basically the same. Maintain an adequate airway, control major bleeding, and splint fractures. ADMINISTER OXYGEN AS SOON AS POSSIBLE. Keep the patient at rest, lying down, and covered to stay warm but not overheated. In most cases, the patient will benefit if the lower extremities are elevated. A supine or semiseated position may be more useful, depending on the nature of the patient's illness or injury. Give nothing by mouth, monitor the patient's vital signs, and provide emotional support.

NOTE: When providing care for shock patients, monitor vital signs and BE ON THE ALERT FOR VOMITING.

Anaphylactic shock is a SERIOUS EMERGENCY. This type of shock is brought about when the patient comes into contact with a substance to which he is allergic (bee stings, insect bites, chemicals, dusts, pollens, drugs, foods).

The symptoms of anaphylactic shock include complaints of itching and burning skin, chest pains with difficult breathing, dizziness, restlessness, and nausea. The signs of anaphylactic shock can include restlessness, becoming unresponsive, difficult breathing, wheezing or rales, a rapid and very weak pulse, hives or blotchy skin, swelling of the face and tongue, cyanosis, and vomiting.

The care for anaphylactic shock includes basic life support measures and the same care as for all shock patients. Transport the patient to a medical facility immediately.

REMEMBER: Ask the patient about allergies during the interview. Be certain to look for medical identification devices. If you are in the patient's residence, check the main door, the closest window to the door, or the refrigerator door for a "Vial of Life" or similar type sticker.

Fainting is a mild form of self-correcting shock; however, it may be a sign of very serious problems. Always look for injuries caused by falls due to fainting. Take the patient's pulse and blood pressure and provide emotional support. Discourage the patient from driving or operating machinery until he is examined by a physician. Encourage the patient to see a physician.

Fainting can often be prevented by placing the patient in a seated position, protecting him from falls, and lowering his head to a level between the knees. *Do not* follow this procedure for patients having fractures, spinal injuries, heart problems, or difficult breathing; have them lay supine or with legs elevated.

Detection of bleeding and shock depends on the proper patient assessment procedures carried out by the EMT.

SECTION TWO:
Pneumatic Anti-shock Garment

OBJECTIVES As an EMT, you should be able to:

1. Define *pneumatic anti-shock garment*. (p. 211)
2. Explain how anti-shock garments work. (pp. 211–212)
3. List the indications for the use of anti-shock garments. (p. 212)
4. State the absolute contraindication for the use of the anti-shock garment. (pp. 212–213)
5. Describe how to apply an anti-shock garment. (p. 213)
6. Describe how to remove an anti-shock garment. (p. 213)

SKILLS As an EMT, you should be able to:

1. Detect rales, rhonchi, wheezes, and other major breathing sounds as required by local protocols.
2. Correctly apply an anti-shock garment.
3. Correctly remove an anti-shock garment.

ANTI-SHOCK GARMENTS

Pneumatic counterpressure means that air is used to create a pressure against something. In the case of the garments, the pressure is being applied against the flow of blood. These devices are also referred to as anti-shock garments, pneumatic anti-shock garments (PASG), military anti-shock trousers, medical anti-shock trousers, and pneumatic counter pressure device. The term *anti-shock garment* is the most popular and will be used in this chapter.

The anti-shock garment is used primarily for the patient who has developed or is certain to develop severe *hypovolemic shock*.

How Anti-Shock Garments Work

The anti-shock garment is designed to counteract hypovolemia (low circulating blood volume) and occasionally is effective against certain internal bleeding. The garment does this by developing an encircling pressure around both lower extremities, pelvis, and abdomen. This pressure slows or stops bleeding in the areas of the body that are enclosed by the pressurized garment. Bleeding is controlled by direct pressure being placed on the damaged vessel. The patient's blood pressure will elevate (circumferential compression), fluids being pushed from the extremities (translocation of fluids), and a reduction in the vascular compartment size caused by the pressure on the vessels without.

There are a number of advantages associated with the use of an anti-shock garment other than the control of further blood loss. Among the advantages are:

- The garment can be applied quickly and not inflated until it is needed.
- An anti-shock garment could serve as an air splint for a fractured pelvis and lower extremity fractures.
- Electrocardiograms and x-rays can be taken, and a Foley catheter (used to drain the urinary bladder) can be inserted while the patient is in an inflated garment.
- Intravenous lines can be started more easily in some cases due to the increase in the volume of blood in the vascular beds in the upper extremities.

Some of the disadvantages of using anti-shock garments include:

- There may be an increase of fluids in the lungs (pulmonary edema) of some elderly patients.
- There may be increased difficulty in breathing or discomfort during breathing for some patients.
- Bleeding may increase in areas not enclosed by the device.
- There may be a worsening of injury at the diaphragm (traumatic diaphragmatic herniation).
- Nausea and vomiting will increase for some patients.
- Problems can occur with defecation and urination.

Indications

Use of an anti-shock garment should be considered for patients with:

- A systolic blood pressure less than 80 mmHg
- A systolic blood pressure less than 100 mmHg and evidence of the classic signs of shock
- Profuse bleeding from injuries to the lower extremities
- Fractures of the lower extremities
- Fractures of the pelvis or femur with shock
- Closed abdominal injury, with shock
- Multiple trauma, with shock
- Pregnant patient with shock. Only the leg compartments of the garments are inflated unless there is abdominal hemorrhage. This approach may have to be taken for some obese patients.

In the past, anti-shock garments have been recommended for patients who developed cardiac arrest. This is a controversial procedure and is under study. The anti-shock garment probably increases the resistance to blood flow in the lower extremities. Some researchers believe that this may provide improved circulation to the vital organs. In addition to this, there is an increase in the pressure in the thoracic cavity. If your local EMS System protocol indicates the application of anti-shock garments for cardiac arrest patients, remember that you cannot delay or stop CPR in order to apply the garment.

Contraindications

The decision to apply the garment is the choice of the emergency department physician, the attending physician, or specific local standing orders.

Pulmonary edema is a condition in which the pulmonary blood vessels are engorged with blood and the alveoli contain excess fluids. In most cases, it is the only absolute contraindication for the application of anti-shock garments.

NOTE: In some EMS Systems, anti-shock garments can be used if the pulmonary edema is due to cardiogenic shock or occurs as a complication of anaphylactic shock.

Many EMS Systems allow EMTs to use a stethoscope to listen for fluids in the lungs and rales (an abnormal lung sound produced when air moves through fluids in the bronchial tree). They also are directed to look for distended neck veins. Other important signs and symptoms of pulmonary edema also are considered. (See page 393.)

A physician may choose not to order an anti-shock garment based on the following conditions:

- Congestive heart failure (usually not recommended)
- Heart attack (usually not recommended)
- Cerebrovascular accident (stroke), unless the patient has a low blood pressure and the symptoms and signs of shock
- Pregnancy, unless the abdominal compartment can be left uninflated. In some cases, when the inflation of the leg compartments fails to ensure vital organ perfusion, the physician may order the inflation of the abdominal compartment.

There are additional local EMS System conditional contraindications for the use of the anti-shock garment. These cases usually involve injury to the chest or abdomen and the lower extremities. The anti-shock garment can be applied in such cases only on the orders of a physician who has been informed of the patient's problems. In such cases, the garment is applied for the lower extremity injury. The abdominal compartment is not inflated. The conditional contraindications include any of the following:

- Massive bleeding into the thoracic cavity. The garment can be applied and the patient's systolic blood pressure is raised to 100 to 110 mmHg.
- Abdominal injury with evisceration. In some cases, the abdominal compartment will be

inflated after the proper dressing of the wound.

- Abdominal penetration when the object is still in the abdomen
- Impaled objects in the lower extremity
- Injury above the level of the garment that has external bleeding that cannot be controlled with a simple pressure dressing

The anti-shock garment may be ordered for all of the above situations, even when there is no lower extremity injury. Typically, the physician ordering the application of the garment will be concerned with severe hypovolemia, since this is a greater concern than the other problems suffered by the patient.

Some EMS Systems have a protocol that does not allow for the application of anti-shock garments in cases involving injury to the head. The reason is to help prevent an increase in intracranial pressure. However, some protocols now allow for the application of an anti-shock garment when there is head injury, severe hypovolemia, and the symptoms and signs of shock. Since the patient's hypovolemic shock is not due to the head injury, but to internal or external bleeding, the application of the anti-shock garment is justified. The hypovolemic shock can be treated and there is little chance of increased intracranial pressure when severe hypovolemic shock exists. Follow your local guidelines.

Applying an Anti-Shock Garment

An anti-shock garment is to be applied in accordance with local protocol. In many localities, application requires the order from a physician. The procedure for application of the garment is shown in Scan 7.1. When internal abdominal bleeding is suspected, inflate all the compartments at the same time. There are three major types of anti-shock garments in use. The plain garment does not have any pressure gauges. The one-gauge garment measures individual pressures, one compartment at a time. The three-gauge garment has a pressure gauge for each compartment.

NOTE: Vital signs are to be taken before applying an anti-shock garment. The patient's clothing should not be left on under the garment. The removal of the patient's lower outer garments improves the application of the garment and allows for the easier insertion of a Foley catheter at a later time. If this is not possible, then remove the patient's belt and any sharp objects found in the patient's trouser pockets before applying the garment. Since transport will

be required, the anti-shock garment should be placed on the patient-carrying device before the patient.

Removing an Anti-Shock Garment

The garment should be removed only when a physician is present and:

1. The physician orders the removal of the garment.
2. Intravenous correction of volume loss has begun.
3. Vital signs have just been monitored and recorded, noting that the patient is stable.
4. An operating room is available.

In some cases the garment may have to remain inflated until the patient is taken into surgery. The garment should only be deflated and removed by someone trained in its use and familiar with the type of garment being used. To remove an anti-shock garment, have someone continually monitor vital signs and:

1. Slowly deflate the abdominal compartment, checking the patient's blood pressure after each small increment of deflation. If the patient's blood pressure drops 6 mmHg or more, stop the deflation and wait for fluids or blood to be infused to stabilize the patient. If at any time the patient shows a sudden drop in blood pressure (a drop of 10 mmHg or more), the garment will have to be reinflated.
2. * Slowly deflate one leg compartment following the same procedure as above.
3. Slowly deflate the other leg compartment, following the same procedure as above.

REMEMBER: Discontinue deflation if the systolic blood pressure drops more than 6 mmHg from its previous level or if the systolic blood pressure is 100 mmHg or less. Additional intravenous infusion is needed before deflation can continue.

WARNING: Currently, many EMS Systems have no indications for the prehospital removal of anti-shock garments once they are inflated. Where removal is allowed, it is done for patients who develop shortness of breath, pulmonary edema, or hypertension.

* This time varies with different protocols. Some methods have the rescuer continue immediately with the deflation if the patient's blood pressure is stable. Other methods require 20 minutes between deflating each compartment. Follow your local protocol.

SCAN 7–1 APPLICATION OF ANTI-SHOCK GARMENT

Adult garment and inflation pedal.

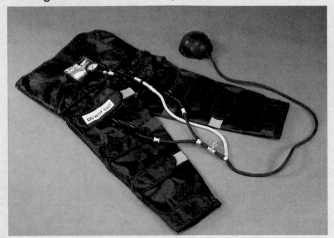

Pediatric garment.

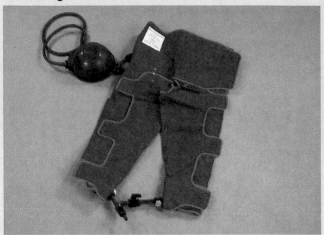

1

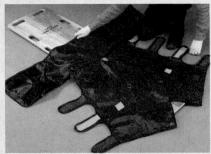

Unfold the garment and lay it flat. It should be smoothed of wrinkles.

2

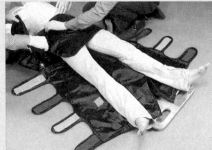

Log roll the patient onto the garment, or slip it under him. The upper edge of the garment must be just below the rib cage.

3

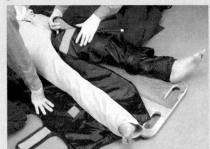

Check for a distal pulse and enclose the left leg, securing the velcro straps.

4

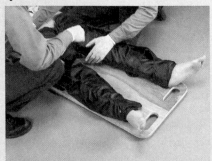

Check for a distal pulse and enclose the right leg securing the velcro straps.

5

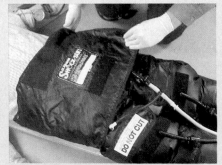

Enclose the abdomen and pelvis, securing the velcro straps.

6

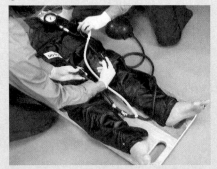

Check the tubes leading to the compartments and the pump.

NOTE: Patient's clothing remains on for demonstration purposes. In actual use, clothing should be removed. Anti-shock garment can be placed over traction splint.

7

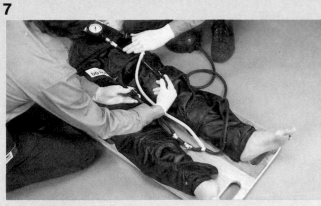

Open the stopcocks to the legs and close the abdominal compartment stopcock.

8

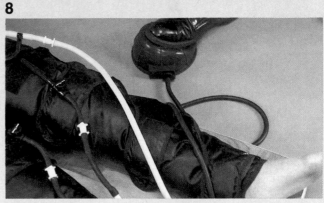

Use the foot pedal to inflate the lower compartments simultaneously, or the required lower extremity compartment. Inflate until air exhausts through the relief valves, the velcro makes a crackling noise, or the patient's systolic blood pressure is stable at 100 to 110 mmHg or higher.

9

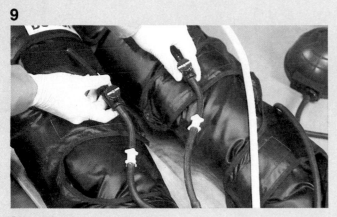

Close the stopcocks.

10

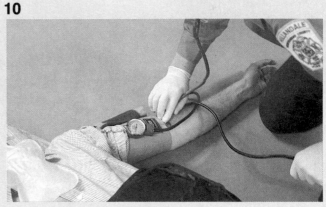

Check the patient's blood pressure.

11

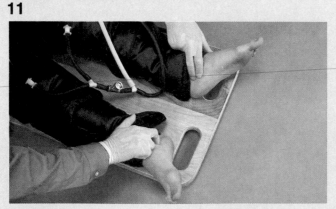

Check both lower extremities for a distal pulse.

12

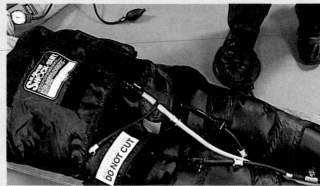

If BP is below 100 mmHg, open the abdominal stopcock and inflate abdominal compartment. Close stopcock.

NOTE: Monitor and record vital signs every 5 minutes. Add pressure to the garment as required.

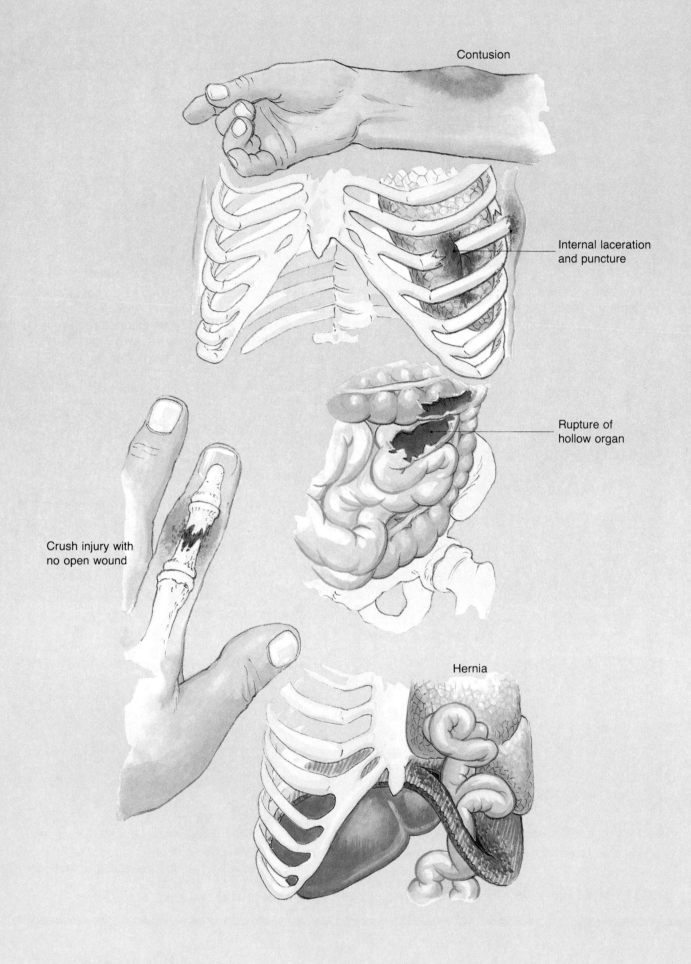

Contusion

Internal laceration
and puncture

Rupture of
hollow organ

Crush injury with
no open wound

Hernia

CHAPTER 8

Injuries I:
Soft tissues and internal organs

WARNING: Avoid direct contact with patient blood and body fluids.

OBJECTIVES As an EMT, you should be able to:

1. Define *soft tissues*. (p. 218)
2. Label and define the THREE major layers of the skin. (p. 219)
3. Define *closed* and *open wound*. (p. 220, p. 221)
4. Classify closed wounds as contusions, internal lacerations, internal punctures, crushing injuries, or ruptures. (pp. 220–221)
5. Classify open wounds as abrasions, incisions, lacerations, punctures, avulsions, amputations, or crush injuries. (pp. 221–223)
6. Cite the basic procedures used in caring for a closed wound. (p. 224)
7. Cite the basic procedures used in caring for open wounds. (pp. 224–228)
8. List the steps used in caring for wounds involving impaled objects. (p. 228–229)
9. Cite the basic procedures used in caring for avulsions, amputations, and crushing injuries. (pp. 230–232)
10. Define *dressing, multitrauma dressing, occlusive dressing,* and *bandage.* (p. 224–225)
11. State the FOUR basic rules that apply to the dressing of wounds. (p. 226)
12. State the FIVE basic rules that apply to bandaging. (p. 226–227)

SKILLS As an EMT, you should be able to:

1. Determine types of soft tissue injuries.
2. Control bleeding and provide the proper emergency care for open wounds.
3. Provide basic emergency care for closed wounds.

NOTE: Chapter 8 is an introduction to soft tissue and internal organ injuries. In many EMT courses, you will practice basic dressing and bandaging skills that apply to most soft tissue injuries before learning specific injury care. This is because modern dressing materials and self-adhering roller bandages eliminate the need for complicated bandaging techniques. Specific injuries requiring special care will be covered later in this text. Some general wound care procedures are included in this chapter to aid you during your practice sessions.

Abrasion (ab-RAY-shun) – a scratch or scrape.

Amputation – the surgical removal or traumatic severing of a body part. The most common usage in emergency care refers to the traumatic amputation of an extremity or part of an extremity.

Avulsion (ah-VUL-shun) – the tearing away or tearing off of pieces or flaps of skin and other soft tissues. This term also may be used for an eye pulled from its socket or a tooth dislodged from its socket.

Bandage – any material used to hold a dressing in place.

Contusion (kun-TU-zhun) – a bruise.

Dermis (DER-mis) – the inner (second) layer of skin found beneath the epidermis. It is rich in blood vessels and nerves.

Dressing – any material (preferably sterile) used to cover a wound that will help control bleeding and help prevent additional contamination.

Ecchymosis (EK-i-MO-sis) – the discoloration of the skin due to internal bleeding.

Epidermis (ep-i-DER-mis) – the outer layer of skin.

Evisceration (e-vis-er-A-shun) – when an organ or part of an organ protrudes through a wound opening.

Hematoma (hem-ah-TO-mah) – a swelling caused by the collection of blood under the skin or in damaged tissues as a result of an injured or broken blood vessel.

Incision – a smooth cut.

Laceration – a jagged cut.

Occlusive Dressing – any dressing that forms an airtight seal.

Puncture Wound – an open wound that tears *through* the skin and destroys underlying tissues. The path of the wound is usually a straight line. Bullet wounds are a noted exception to this fact.

Subcutaneous (SUB-ku-TA-ne-us) **Layers** – the layers of fat and soft tissues found below the dermis.

THE SOFT TISSUES

The soft tissues of the body include the skin, muscles, blood vessels, nerves, fatty tissues, and tissues that line or cover organs (Figure 8–1). The teeth, bones, and cartilage are considered hard tissues.

The most obvious soft tissue injuries involve the skin (Figure 8–2). Most people do not think of the skin as a body organ, but it is. In fact, it is the largest organ of the human body. The major functions of the skin include:

- Protection—the skin serves as a barrier to keep out microorganisms (germs), debris, and unwanted chemicals. Underlying tissues and organs are protected from environmental contact. This helps preserve the chemical balance of body fluids and tissues.

- Water balance—the skin helps prevent water loss and stops environmental water from entering the body.

- Temperature regulation—blood vessels in the skin can dilate (increase in diameter) to carry more blood to the skin, allowing heat to radiate from the body. When the body needs to conserve heat, these vessels con-

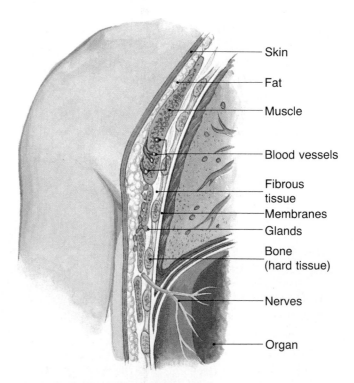

Skin

Fat

Muscle

Blood vessels

Fibrous tissue

Membranes

Glands

Bone (hard tissue)

Nerves

Organ

FIGURE 8–1. Soft tissues.

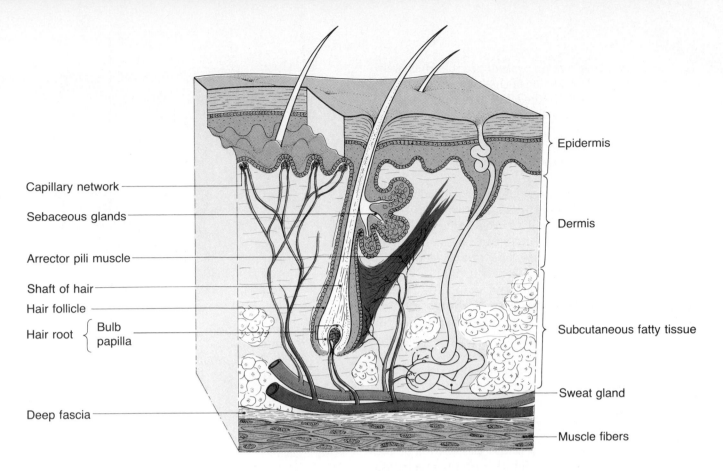

FIGURE 8–2. The skin.

strict (decrease in diameter) to prevent the heat loss. The sweat glands found in the skin produce perspiration, which will evaporate and help cool the body. The fat that is part of the skin serves as a thermal insulator.

- Excretion—salts, carbon dioxide, and excess water can be released through the skin.
- Shock (impact) absorption—the skin and its layers of fat help protect the underlying organs from minor impacts and pressures.

The outer layer of the skin is called the **epidermis** (ep-i-DER-mis). It is composed of four layers (strata) except for the skin of the palms of the hands and soles of the feet. These two regions have five layers. The outermost layers are composed of dead cells, which are rubbed off or sloughed off and are replaced. The pigment granules of the skin and living cells are found in the deeper layers. The cells of the innermost layer are actively dividing, replacing the dead cells of the outer layers.

The epidermis contains no blood vessels or nerves. Except for certain types of burns and injuries due to cold, injuries of the epidermis present few problems in EMT-level care.

The layer of skin below the epidermis is the **dermis** (DER-mis). This layer is rich with blood vessels, nerves, and specialized structures such as sweat glands, sebaceous (oil) glands, and hair follicles. Specialized nerve endings are found in the dermis. They are involved with the senses of touch, cold, heat, and pain.

Once the dermis is opened to the outside world, contamination becomes a major problem. The wound can be serious, accompanied by profuse bleeding and intense pain.

The layers of fat and soft tissue below the dermis are called the **subcutaneous** (SUB-ku-TA-ne-us) layers. Shock absorption and insulation are major functions of this layer. Again, there are the problems of tissue and bloodstream contamination, bleeding, and pain when these layers are injured.

TYPES OF SOFT TISSUE INJURY

The EMT cannot repair blood vessel and nerve damage, although additional injury can be prevented through prompt and efficient care. Controlling bleeding, protecting from additional wound contamination, and initiating certain procedures to reduce pain and prevent shock are some of the important prehospital measures taken by the EMT. There is no direct EMT-level care for muscle injury other than treating wounds and perhaps immobilizing the injured limb. However, the control of bleeding and proper wound care is critical and may be the determining factor in patient survival.

The body's organs and glands are composed of *soft tissues*. Injuries to these structures can range from minor to immediate life-threatening problems. At the EMT-level of care, little can be done directly to organ and gland injuries, but what can be done may be a major factor in patient survival.

The detection of organ and gland injury and how this knowledge affects care, priority of care, and order of transport are of great importance in emergency medicine. As an EMT, you must know the organs and major glands and where they are located. You must know which are solid organs and which are hollow so you can consider the possible types of injuries based on the mechanism of injury, extent of internal bleeding, and complications due to a ruptured organ. As you learn more about the body organs, remember to relate the organs of the abdominopelvic cavity to the abdominal quadrants (see Chapter 2).

A general classification of soft tissue injuries includes closed wounds and open wounds.

Closed Wounds

A **closed wound** is an internal injury, that is, there is no open pathway from the outside to the injured site. These wounds usually result from the impact of a blunt object. Although the skin itself may not be broken, there may be extensive crushed tissues beneath it. Closed wounds can be simple bruises, internal lacerations (cuts), and internal punctures caused by fractured bones, crushing forces, or the rupture (bursting open) of internal organs. Bleeding can range from minor to life threatening. As an EMT, you should always consider the possibility of soft tissue injuries when there are fractures and blunt trauma.

Contusions

A **contusion** (kun-TU-zhun) is a bruise. A variable amount of bleeding always occurs at the time of injury and may continue for a few hours after the trauma. Swelling at the wound site may occur immediately, or it may be delayed as much as 24 to 48 hours. This swelling is caused by a collection of blood under the skin or in the damaged tissues. A blood clot almost always forms at the injury site and is

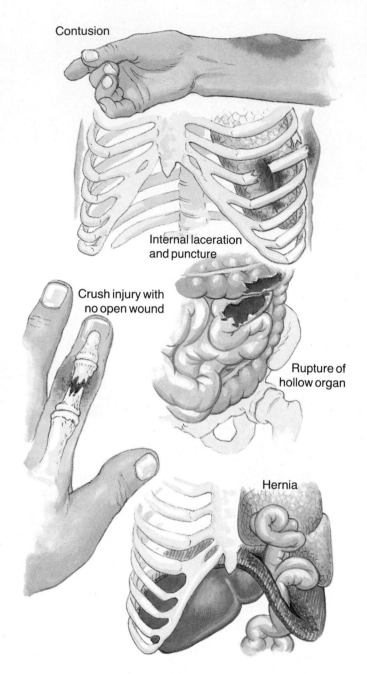

FIGURE 8–3. Classification of closed wounds.

called a **hematoma** (hem-ah-TO-mah) as blood seeps into the surrounding tissues to form the characteristic "black and blue" mark (**ecchymosis** [EK-i-MO-sis]). When you perform the patient assessment, the color of the bruise will probably be blue to reddish purple. With time, the blood at the site undergoes changes, causing the color of the bruise to turn to a brownish yellow.

Keep in mind that large bruises can mean serious blood loss and may be an indication of fractures or extensive tissue damage below the site of the bruise.

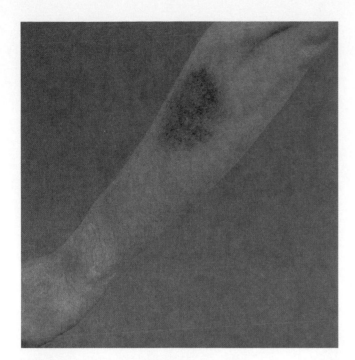

FIGURE 8–4. **Contusions are the most common form of closed wounds.**

Internal Lacerations and Punctures

When bones are fractured, sharp ends or fragments can cut or puncture internal body structures. The lungs, heart, liver, kidneys, and spleen can be lacerated by fractured ribs. Ends of fractured ribs may also puncture a lung, allowing inspired air to flow into the pleural cavity. On rare occasions, the urinary bladder can be lacerated or punctured as a result of pelvic fractures. A fractured bone can damage muscles, blood vessels, nerves, organs and glands, and other structures composed of soft tissues.

Crush Injuries and Ruptures

Force can be transmitted from the body's exterior to the internal structures, even when the skin remains intact and even in cases in which the only indication of injury is a simple bruise. This force can cause the internal organs to be crushed or to rupture and bleed internally. Contents of hollow organs can leak into the body cavities, causing severe inflammation and tissue damage.

When these types of injuries occur in the abdominal and pelvic cavities, the application of an anti-shock garment may help correct the effects of internal bleeding.

Organ coverings and cavity linings also can rupture during injury. Parts of organs or muscles may be forced through these openings; yet all the damage is internal, not directly visible on the outside of the body. This type of injury is often called a *rupture* but is actually classified as a **hernia** (her-NE-ah).

Open Wounds

Open wounds are injuries in which the skin is interrupted, exposing the tissues underneath. The cause of the interruption can come from the outside, as a laceration, or from the inside when a fractured bone end tears outward, through the skin.

Abrasion

The classification of **abrasion** (ab-RAY-shun) includes simple scrapes and scratches in which the outer layer of the skin is damaged but all the layers are not penetrated (Figure 8–5). Skinned elbows and knees, "mat burns," "rug burns," and "brush burns" are examples of abrasions. There may be no detectable bleeding or only the minor ooze of blood from capillary beds. Care should be provided to reduce wound contamination. The patient may be experiencing great pain, even though the injury is minor.

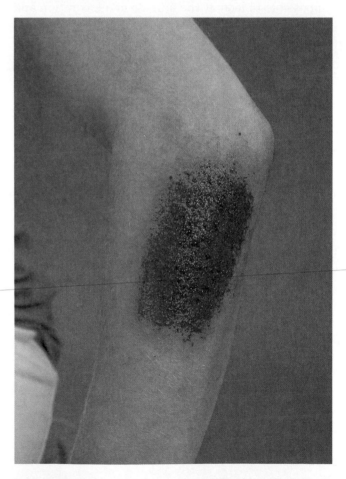

FIGURE 8–5. **Abrasions are the least serious form of open wound.**

Incisions

An **incision** is a smooth cut, usually made by a sharp object, such as a knife or razor blade. The edges of the cut skin and the underlying tissues are smooth due to the sharpness of the object inflicting the injury (Figure 8–6). If the wound is deep, large blood vessels and nerves may be severed. Bleeding from a long, deep incision may be difficult to control, but direct pressure over a dressing usually works well. The air-inflated splint can be useful in the management of this type of wound when it is applied over top of a dressing.

Lacerations

A **laceration** is a jagged cut. The tissues are snagged and torn, forming a rough edge around the wound (Figure 8–7). Often, this type of wound is caused by objects having sharp, irregular edges, such as broken glass or a jagged piece of metal. However, a laceration can also result from a severe blow or impact with a blunt object. The rough edges of a laceration tend to fall together and obstruct the view as you try to determine the wound depth. It is usually impossible to look at the outside of a laceration and determine the extent of the damage to underlying tissues. *Do not* pull apart the wound edges in an effort to see into the wound. If significant blood vessels have been torn, bleeding will be considerable, but usually less than that seen with incisions. Sometimes, the bleeding is partially controlled when blood vessels are stretched and torn. This is due to the natural curling and folding of the cut ends that aid in rapid clot formation.

Punctures

When a sharp, pointed object passes through the skin or other tissue, a **puncture wound** has occurred. Typically, puncture wounds are caused by sharp, pointed objects: nails, ice picks, splinters, or knives. Often, there is no severe external bleeding

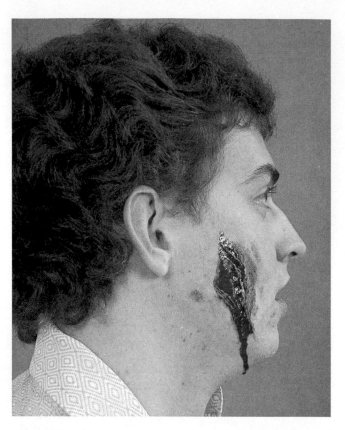

FIGURE 8–7. **The edges of a laceration are jagged and rough.**

problem, but internal bleeding may be profuse. Contamination must always be viewed as serious. There are two types of puncture wounds. A **penetrating puncture** wound can be shallow or deep. In either case, tissues and blood vessels are injured. A **perforating puncture wound** has both an *entrance wound* and an *exit wound* (Figure 8–9). The object

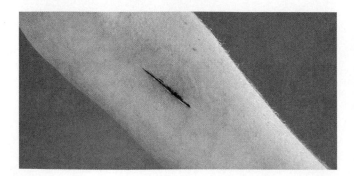

FIGURE 8–6. **The edges of an incision wound are smooth.**

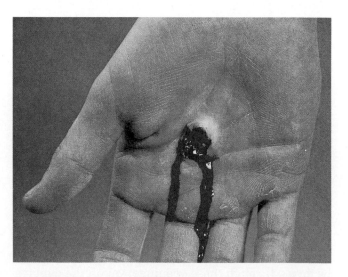

FIGURE 8–8. **A penetrating puncture wound.**

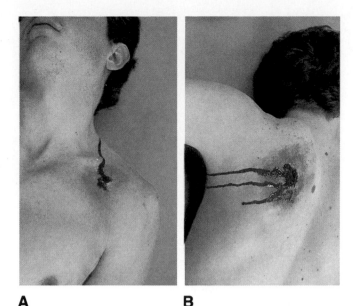

A   **B**

FIGURE 8–9. A perforating puncture wound has an entrance and exit.

causing the injury passes through the body and out to create an exit wound. In many cases, the exit wound is more serious than the entrance wound. A "through-and-through" gunshot wound may be an example of a penetrating puncture wound.

Avulsion

In an **avulsion** (a-VUL-shun), flaps of skin and tissues are torn loose or pulled off completely (Figure 8–10). When the tip of the nose is cut or torn off, this is an avulsion. The same applies to the external ear. A glove avulsion occurs when the hand is caught in a roller. In this type of accident, the skin is stripped off like a glove. An eye pulled from its socket (extruded) is a form of avulsion. The term **avulsed** is used in reporting the wound, as in "an avulsed eye," or "an avulsed ear."

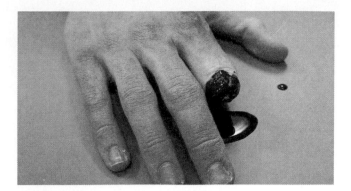

FIGURE 8–11. Amputation.

Amputation

Amputations involve the extremities. The fingers (Figure 8–11), toes, hands, feet, or limbs are completely cut through or torn off. Jagged skin and bone edges can be observed. There may be massive bleeding; however, the force that amputates a limb may close off torn blood vessels, limiting the amount of bleeding. Often, blood vessels collapse or retract and curl closed to limit the bleeding from the wound site.

Crush Injury

A **crush injury** can result when an extremity is caught between heavy items, such as pieces of machinery. Blood vessels, nerves and muscles are involved and swelling may be a major problem with resulting loss of blood supply distally. Bones are fractured and may protrude through the wound site. Soft tissues and internal organs can be crushed to produce both profuse external and internal bleeding (Figure 8–12). Sometimes, external bleeding may be mild or totally absent.

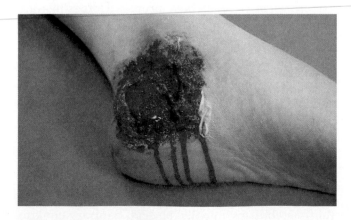

FIGURE 8–10. Avulsed skin.

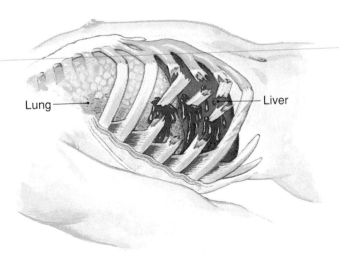

Lung — Liver

FIGURE 8–12. Both soft tissues and internal organs are damaged in crush injuries.

SOFT TISSUE WOUND CARE

Closed Wounds

Contusions are the most frequently encountered closed wounds. Most simple bruises will not require emergency care in the field; however, a bruise is an indication of possible internal injuries and related internal bleeding. Make certain that you look for large areas of bruises and any large bruises directly over body organs, such as the spleen, liver, and kidneys. Swelling and deformity at the site of a bruise should warn you of possible underlying fractures.

If you find a contusion on the head or neck, remember that there may be injury to the cervical spine. Always search for blood in the mouth, nose, and ears. Should you find a bruise on the trunk of the body, consider the possibility of chest injury. Determine if the patient is coughing up frothy red blood, which may indicate a punctured lung, and assess him for difficult breathing. Be certain to use your stethoscope to listen for equal air entry and any unusual breathing sounds. Any symptoms or signs that indicate damage to the ribs or sternum also indicate possible soft tissue injury.

If the bruise is on the abdomen, look to see if the patient has vomited. If so, is there any substances in the vomitus that looks like coffee grounds (partially digested blood)? Use the methods described in Chapter 3 to detect if the patient's abdomen is rigid or tender.

Each of these signs associated with a bruise of the trunk indicate serious internal injuries requiring special care. Later, we will cover the care you need to render in specific cases of internal injuries to the soft tissues and body organs.

When the patient's injuries allow you to do so, position the patient so that a minimum of weight is placed on a bruised area. If you believe that there is a possibility of internal injuries, MANAGE AS IF THERE IS INTERNAL BLEEDING AND CARE FOR SHOCK. Stay alert for the patient to vomit. Continue to monitor the patient for the development of shock and transport as soon as possible. Remember that most patients with internal injuries will benefit from the administration of oxygen at the highest possible concentration. When appropriate, apply anti-shock garments.

Open Wounds

There are few cases of open wound care that do not require the application of dressings and bandages. You should know the following definitions:

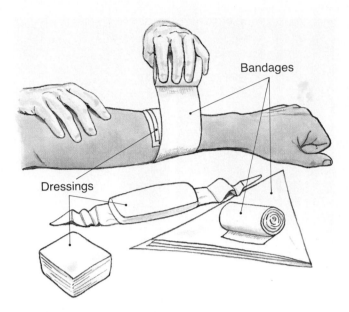

FIGURE 8–13. **Dressings cover wounds, while bandages hold dressings in place.**

- DRESSING—Any material applied to a wound in an effort to control bleeding and prevent further contamination. Dressings should be sterile.
- BANDAGE—Any material used to hold a dressing in place. Bandages need not be sterile.

WARNING: Be certain to wear latex gloves to avoid contact with the patient's blood and body fluids.

Dressings

Various dressings are carried in emergency care supplies. These dressings should be sterile, meaning that all microorganisms and spores that can grow into active organisms have been killed. Dressings also should be aseptic, meaning that all dirt and foreign debris have been removed. In emergency situations, when commercially prepared dressings are not available, clean cloth, towels, sheets, handkerchiefs, and other similar materials may have to be used.

The most popular dressings are individually wrapped sterile gauze pads, typically 4 inches square. A variety of sizes are available, referred to according to size such as 2 by 2's, 4 by 4's, 3 by 7's, and 5 by 9's.

Large bulky dressings, such as the multitrauma or universal dressings, are available when bulk is required for profuse bleeding or when a large wound must be covered. These dressings are especially useful for stabilizing impaled objects. Sanitary napkins can sometimes be used in place of the standard bulky dressings. Although not sterile, they are separately wrapped and have very clean surfaces (do not apply any adhesive surface of the napkin directly to the wound). Of course, bulky dressings can be made by building up layers of gauze pads.

NOTE: Large bulky dressings are not meant to be used to cover multiple wound sites. With the exception of closely spaced shotgun pellet wounds and other similar puncture wounds, each wound should be dressed independently to ensure proper bleeding control and dressing techniques.

The **occlusive dressing** is used when it is necessary to form an airtight seal. This is done when caring for open wounds to the abdomen,* for external bleeding from large neck veins, and for certain types of open wounds to the thorax. Sterile, commercially prepared occlusive dressings are available in two different forms. There are plastic wrap and petroleum gel-impregnated gauze occlusive dressings. Local protocols vary as to which form to use. Nonsterile wrap and foil also can be used in emergency situations. There are cases when EMTs have made their own emergency occlusive dressings from plastic credit cards, plastic bags, and aluminum foil wrappers.

WARNING: Some EMS Systems report that aluminum foil has caused lacerations of exposed abdominal organs.

Large dressings are sometimes needed in emergency care. Sterile, disposable burn sheets are commercially available. Bed sheets can be sterilized and kept in plastic wrappers to be later used as dressings. These sheets can make effective burn dressings or may be used in some cases to cover exposed abdominal organs.

Bandaging Materials

Bandages are provided in a wide variety of types. The preferred bandage is the self-adhering, form-fitting roller bandage (Figure 8–14). It eliminates the need to know many specialized bandaging techniques developed for use with ordinary gauze roller bandages.

Dressings can be secured using adhering or nonadhering gauze roller bandage, triangular bandages, or strips of adhesive tape. When necessary, you can use strips of cloth, handkerchiefs, and other such materials (Figure 8–15). Elastic bandages that are used in the general care of strains and sprains should *not* be used to hold dressings in place. They

can become constriction bands, interferring with circulation. This is very likely to occur as the tissues around the wound site begin to swell after the elastic bandage is in place.

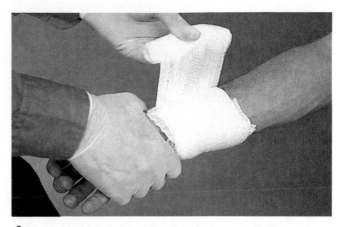

A

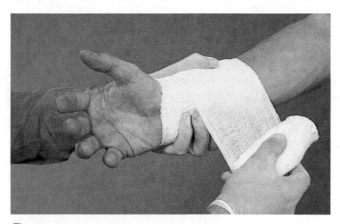

B

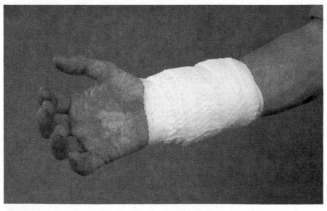

C

FIGURE 8–14. Applying a self-adhering roller bandage: (A) Secure with several overlying wraps. (B) Overlap the bandage, keeping it snug. (C) Cut and tape or tie into place.

---

* Occlusive dressings are used for open abdominal wounds to help prevent the loss of moisture.

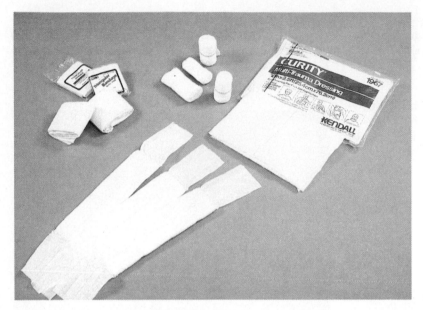

FIGURE 8–15. Materials used for dressings and bandages.

Dressing and Bandaging

The following rules apply to the general dressing of wounds:

1. USE STERILE OR VERY CLEAN MATERI-ALS—Avoid touching the dressing in the area that will come into contact with the wound. Grasp the dressing by the corner, taking it directly from its protective pack and place it on the wound.

2. COVER THE ENTIRE WOUND—The entire surface of the wound and the immediate surrounding areas should be covered.

3. CONTROL BLEEDING—With the exception of the pressure dressing, a dressing should not be bandaged into place if it has not controlled the bleeding. You should continue to apply dressings and pressure as needed for the proper control of bleeding.

4. DO NOT REMOVE DRESSINGS—Once a dressing has been applied to a wound, it *must* remain in place. Bleeding may restart and tissues at the wound site may be injured if the dressing is removed. If the bleeding continues, put new dressings over the blood-soaked ones.

There is an exception to the rule prohibiting the removal of dressings. If a bulky bandage has become blood-soaked, it may be necessary to remove the bandage so that direct pressure can be reestablished or a new bulky bandage can be added and a pressure dressing created. Protection for the wound site is better maintained if one or more simple gauze dressing pads are placed over the top of the injured tissues prior to the placement of the bulky bandage. This will allow for the removal of a bulky bandage without disturbing the wound.

The following rules apply to general bandaging.

1. DO NOT BANDAGE TOO TIGHTLY—All dressings should be held snugly in place, but they must not restrict the blood supply to the affected part.

2. DO NOT BANDAGE TOO LOOSELY—Hold the dressing by bandaging snugly, so the dressing does not move around or slip from the wound. Loose bandaging is a common error in emergency care.

3. DO NOT LEAVE LOOSE ENDS—Any loose ends of gauze, tape, or cloth may get caught on objects when the patient is moved.

4. DO NOT COVER THE TIPS OF FINGERS AND TOES—When bandaging the extremities, leave the fingers and toes exposed whenever possible to observe skin color changes that indicate a change in circulation and to allow for easier neurologic reassessment. Pain, pale or blue-colored skin, cold skin, numbness, and tingling are all indications that a bandage may be too tight. If the fingers or toes are burned, they will have to be covered.

5. COVER ALL EDGES OF THE DRESSING—This will help to reduce additional contami-

nation. The exception is found in the procedures for open chest wounds (see p. 353).

There are two special problems that occur when bandaging an extremity. First, point pressure can occur if you apply the bandage around a very small area. It is best to wrap a large area of the extremity, ensuring a steady, uniform pressure. Apply the bandage from the smaller diameter of the limb to the larger diameter (distal to proximal) to help ensure proper pressure and contact. Second, the joints of the extremity have to be considered. You can bandage across a joint, but do not bend the limb once the bandage is in place. To do so may restrict circulation, loosen the dressing and bandage, or cause both to happen. In some cases, it may be necessary to apply an inflatable or rigid splint, or to use a sling and swathe to prevent movement of the joint after bandaging.

Emergency Care for Open Wounds

Listed below are the general principles of emergency care that apply to the majority of open wounds. Make certain that you avoid direct contact with the patient's blood and other body fluids.

1. EXPOSE THE WOUND—Clothing that covers a soft tissue injury must be lifted, cut, or split away. For some articles of clothing, this is best done with scissors or a seam cutter. *Do not* attempt to remove clothing in the usual manner. To do so may aggravate existing injuries and cause additional damage and pain.

2. CLEAR THE WOUND SURFACE—Do not waste time trying to pick out embedded particles and debris from the wound. Do not clean the wound; simply remove foreign matter from its surface. Proper wound cleaning must be done by a physician. When possible, use a piece of sterile dressing to clear the wound. This will allow you to brush away large debris from the surface, protect your fingers from glass and other sharp objects, and reduce contamination from your fingers.

3. CONTROL BLEEDING—Start with direct pressure or direct pressure and elevation. When necessary, employ pressure point procedures, apply an air-inflated splint, or use a blood pressure cuff. *Remember, a tourniquet is used only as a last resort.*

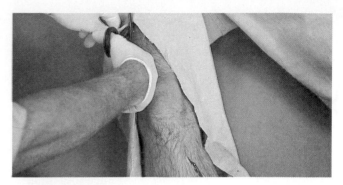

1. Expose wound.

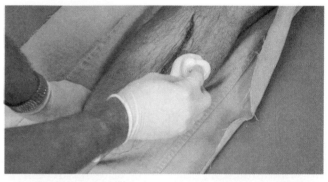

2. Clear wound surface.

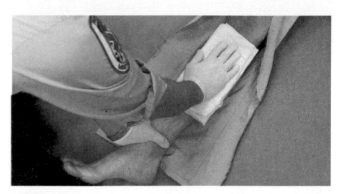

3. Direct pressure.

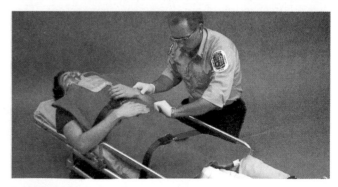

4. Keep patient at rest.

FIGURE 8–16. Care for open wounds.

4. PREVENT FURTHER CONTAMINA-TION—Use a sterile dressing, if possible. When none is available, use the cleanest cloth material at the scene.

5. BANDAGE THE DRESSING IN PLACE AFTER BLEEDING HAS BEEN CON-TROLLED—If an extremity is involved, check for a distal pulse to make certain that circulation has not been interrupted by the application of a tight bandage. With the exception of a pressure dressing, bleeding must be controlled before bandaging is started. Periodically recheck the bandage to make certain that bleeding has not restarted.

6. KEEP THE PATIENT LYING STILL—Any patient movement will increase circulation and could restart bleeding.

7. REASSURE THE PATIENT—This will help ease the patient's emotional response and perhaps lower his pulse rate and blood pressure. In some cases this may help to reduce the bleeding rate. Also, a patient who feels reassured will usually be more willing to lie still, reducing the chances of restarting controlled bleeding.

8. CARE FOR SHOCK—For all serious wounds, care for shock, including the administration of a high concentration of oxygen.

NOTE: If serious bleeding originates from an extremity, or if the wound is a long laceration on an extremity and there are no indications of a possible fracture, immobilize and elevate the injured part. An air-inflated splint can serve to help control bleeding from the forearm or lower leg. A gauze pad dressing should be placed over the top of the wound before applying the splint. Usually, the air splint will be effective only for bleeding from vessels that have been cut through their diameter (transected). This type of splint has *not* been shown to be very effective if the vessels are cut along their length (incised).

Incisions and Lacerations

Most incisions and lacerations can be cared for by bandaging a dressing in place. Some EMS Systems recommend using a butterfly bandage for minor incisions and lacerations. A gauze dressing should be bandaged over the butterfly strip.

Puncture Wounds

Use caution when caring for puncture wounds. An object that appears to be embedded *only* in the skin may actually go all the way to the bone. In such cases, it is possible that the patient may not have any serious pain. Even an apparently moderate puncture wound may cause extensive internal injury with serious internal bleeding. What appears at first to be a simple, shallow puncture wound may be only part of the problem. There also could be a severe exit wound that requires immediate care. Moderate and serious puncture wounds require you to make special efforts to reassure the alert patient. Such injuries are often frightening to the patient.

Gunshot wounds are puncture wounds that can fracture bones and cause extensive soft tissue and organ injury. The seriousness of the wound cannot be determined by the caliber of the bullet or the point of entry and exit. The bullet may have tumbled through tissues, reflected off of a bone, fragmented, or exploded inside the body. All bullet wounds are to be considered to be serious. If the bullet has penetrated the body, you *must* assume that there is considerable internal injury. As with all care, basic life support measures may be necessary for the victim of a bullet wound. To ensure control of bleeding and adequate wound care, you must search for an exit wound.

For all serious puncture wounds, care for shock, administering oxygen at a high concentration. When appropriate, immobilize the patient's spine.

Impaled Objects

As an EMT, you may have to care for patients with puncture wounds containing impaled objects. The object may be a knife, a steel rod, a shard of glass, or even a wooden stick, piercing any part of the body. Even though it is rare, you may be confronted with a long impaled object that must be shortened before care can begin or transport is possible. In such cases, contact the emergency department physician for specific directions. Usually, someone must hold the object, keeping it very stable, while you gently saw it through at the desired length. A fine-toothed saw with rigid blade support (e.g., hack saw) will have to be used.

In general, when caring for a patient with a puncture wound involving an impaled object:

1. *DO NOT REMOVE THE IMPALED OB-JECT.* To do so may cause severe bleeding when the pressure is released from any severed blood vessels. Removal of the object may cause further injury to nerves, muscles, and other soft tissues.

2. *Expose the wound area.* Cut away clothing to make the wound site accessible. Take

great care not to disturb the object. Do not attempt to lift clothing over the object; you may accidentally move it. Long impaled objects may have to be stabilized by hand during the exposure, bleeding control, and dressing steps.

3. *Control profuse bleeding by direct hand pressure if possible. CAUTION:* Position your hand so the fingers are on either side of the object and exert pressure downward. *Do not* put pressure on the object. This pressure must be applied with great care if the object has a cutting edge, such as a knife or a shard of glass; otherwise, you may cause additional injury to the patient. Be careful so that you do not injure your hands.

4. *Stabilize the impaled object with a bulky dressing.* Have another trained rescuer manually stabilize the object while you place several layers of bulky dressing around the injury site so that the dressings surround the object on all sides. Manual stabilization *must* continue until the stabilizing dressings are secured in place. Begin by placing folded multitrauma pads, sanitary napkins, or some other bulky dressing material on opposite sides of the object, along the vertical line of the body or affected limb. For long or large objects, folded towels, blankets, or pillows may have to be used in place of dressing pads. The next layer of pads should be placed on opposite sides of the object, perpendicular to the first layer. Continue this process of stacking dressing pads until as much of the object as possible has been stabilized. Once bandaged into place, the dressings will stabilize the object and exert downward pressure on bleeding vessels. Keep in mind that there is a limited amount of time that can be given to impaled object stabilization. Stay in contact with the emergency department for directions and recommendations.

5. *Adhesive strips* may hold the dressings in place; however, blood around the wound site, sweat, and body movements may not allow you to use tape. *Cloth strips* known as *cravats* can be applied, tying one above and one below the impaled object. The cravats should be wide (no less than four inches in width once folded). A thin, short, rigid splint can be used to push the cravats under the patient's back when they are needed to care for objects impaled in the trunk of the body.

6. *Care for shock and provide oxygen at the highest possible concentration.* When appropriate, the administration of oxygen and the covering of the patient to conserve body heat should be done as soon as possible. When working by yourself, these may have to be delayed while you attempt to control bleeding.

7. *Keep the patient at rest and provide emotional support.* Position the patient for minimum stress. If possible, immobilize the affected area the same as you would for a possible fracture.

8. *Carefully transport the patient as soon as possible.* Avoid any movement that may jar, loosen, or dislodge the object.

9. *Reassure the patient throughout all aspects of care.* An alert patient with an impaled object is usually very frightened.

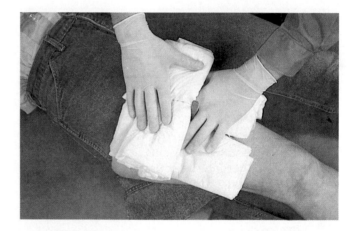

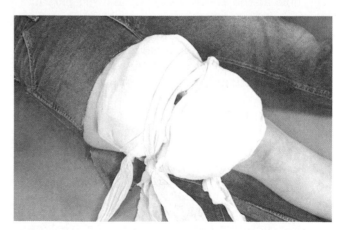

FIGURE 8–17. Impaled objects. Expose the wound, control bleeding, and stabilize the impaled object.

NOTE: Special procedures are used when caring for objects impaled in the eye and in the cheek. These procedures will be covered in Chapter 12.

Avulsions

The emergency care for avulsions requires the application of large, bulky pressure dressings. In addition, you should make every effort to preserve any avulsed parts and transport them to the medical facility along with the patient. It may be possible to surgically restore the part or use it for skin grafts.

In cases in which flaps of skin have been torn loose but not off:

1. Clear the wound surface.
2. As gently as possible, fold the skin back to its normal position.
3. Control bleeding and dress the wound using bulky pressure dressings.

Should skin or another body part be torn from the body:

1. Control bleeding and dress the wound using a bulky pressure dressing.
2. Save the avulsed part by wrapping it in a dry *sterile* gauze dressing secured in place by self-adherent roller bandage and placing the wrapped part in a plastic bag, plastic wrap, or aluminum foil, in accordance with local protocol. If none of these items is available at the scene, wrap the avulsed part in a lint-free, sterile dressing. Make certain that you label the wrapped part as to what it is and the patient's name, date, and time the part was wrapped and bagged. Your records should show the approximate time of the avulsion.
3. The avulsed part should be kept as cool as possible, without freezing. Place the wrapped and bagged part in a cooler or any other available container so that it is on top of a cold pack or a SEALED bag of ice (do not use dry ice). *Do not* immerse the avulsed part in ice, cooled water, or saline. Label the container the same as the label used for the saved part.

REMEMBER: Serious avulsions can be frightening. You must reassure the patient.

NOTE: The care of avulsed tissues is directed by local protocols, often written to match the reimplantation procedures of the hospitals in your EMS region. Some EMS Systems prefer that the dressing used to wrap the avulsed part be moistened with normal sterile saline (sterile distilled water is not recommended). This saline must be from a fresh sterile source. Keep in mind that once a sterile source of saline has been opened it is no longer considered sterile. Take great care if you use this method since the saline may carry microorganisms from your gloved hand through the dressing to the avulsed part.

Amputations

As in other external bleeding situations, the most effective method to control bleeding is a snug pressure dressing. This should be placed over the stump. Pressure point techniques or a blood pressure cuff also may be required to control bleeding. A tourniquet should not be applied unless the other methods used to control profuse bleeding have failed. When possible, wrap the amputated part in sterile dressing and secure this dressing material in place with self-adherent gauze bandage. Wrap or bag the amputated part in plastic, label it, and transport the part with the patient. The amputated part should be kept cool, in the same manner as an avulsed part.

Do not immerse the amputated part in water or saline.

Protruding Organs

Open wounds of the abdomen may be so large and deep that organs protrude through the wound opening. This is known as an **evisceration** (e-vis-er-A-shun). In such cases:

1. Administer oxygen in a high concentration as soon as possible.
2. Care for shock, positioning the patient to provide for a clear airway and minimum stress to the wound site.
3. *Do not* touch or try to replace the organ.
4. Expose the wound site, cutting away clothing. *Do not* attempt to pull away any article or piece of clothing that does not lift off easily.
5. When possible, flex the patient's uninjured legs at the hips and knees to reduce tension on the abdominal muscles.

SCAN 8-1 EXAMPLES OF GENERAL DRESSING AND BANDAGING

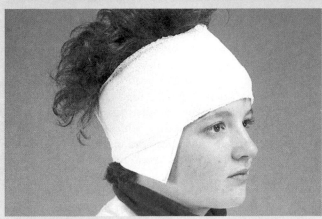

FOREHEAD (NO SKULL INJURY) OR EAR Place dressing and secure with self-adherent roller bandage.

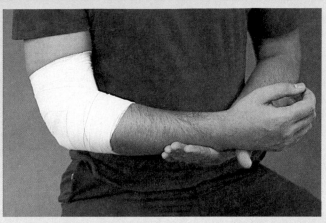

ELBOW OR KNEE Place dressing and secure with cravat or roller bandage. Apply roller bandage in Figure 8 pattern.

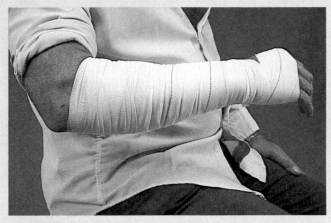

FOREARM OR LEG Place dressing and secure with roller bandage, distal to proximal. Better protection is offered if palm or sole is wrapped.

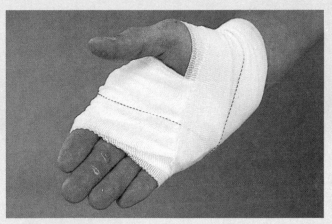

HAND Place dressing, wrap with cravat, and secure at wrist. Use same pattern for roller bandage.

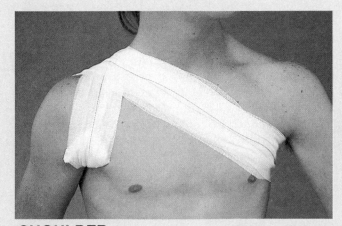

SHOULDER Place dressing and secure with Figure 8 of cravat or roller dressing. Pad under knot if cravat is used.

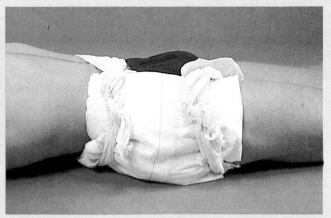

HIP Place bandage and large dressing to cover hip. Secure with first cravat around waist and second cravat around thigh on injured side.

6. Cover the exposed organ and wound opening with sterile plastic wrap (or aluminum foil—see warning on p. 225—in accordance to local protocol. Some EMS Systems apply a sterile, lint-free dressing that is soaked with sterile saline before the occlusive dressing). The dressing should extend at least two inches beyond the wound edges or the edges of the exposed organ.

7. Tape the dressing in place, sealing the edges to create an occlusive dressing. This will help prevent the loss of moisture from the internal organs, membranes, and tissues.

8. Apply a thick dressing pad or clean towel over the top of the first dressing. This will help to prevent heat loss. Hold this in place with cravats.

9. If appropriate, apply an anti-shock garment (do not place the garment on the eviscerated organs).

10. Reassure the patient through all steps of care.

If a sterile occlusive dressing is not available, make your own from the plastic wrappers of trauma pads, oxygen masks, or intravenous bags. Place the inner surface against the wound.

More specifics for this type of wound care will be presented in Chapter 13.

SUMMARY

WARNING: Avoid direct contact with patient blood and body fluids.

Soft tissue damage may be classified under closed wounds and open wounds. Remember that body organs are composed of soft tissues. Contusions are the most common form of closed wound. Abrasions and lacerations are the most common forms of open wounds.

Puncture wounds are open wounds and classified as penetrating or perforating. Perforating wounds have both an entrance wound and an exit wound.

Avulsions occur when skin or certain body parts are torn loose or from the body. Amputation is the cutting or tearing off of a finger, hand, arm, toe, foot, or leg. Crush injuries can create external and internal injury with severe tissue damage. Both in-

ternal and external bleeding are seen with such injuries.

Always care for closed wounds as if there is internal bleeding.

Use all necessary safety personal protective measures when caring for open wounds. Control bleeding as soon as possible after exposing and clearing the surface of the wound.

Remember, when caring for a patient your first priorities are airway, breathing, circulation, and the control of profuse bleeding. Once this is done, continued control of bleeding and prevention of further wound contamination are achieved by dressing the wound.

If the patient has a puncture wound, assume there are serious internal injuries with bleeding. Look for an exit wound.

Keep in mind that patients suffering from blood loss do better when you administer oxygen and treat for shock.

When dealing with an open or closed wound, keep the patient lying still and provide emotional support. Always be alert for vomiting in cases of internal injury.

Do not remove impaled objects. Control bleeding and stabilize the impaled object. Partially avulsed skin can be folded gently back to its normal position after the wound surface is cleared. If skin is torn off, preserve the part in a secured wrap of sterile gauze dressing and place it in a plastic bag. Be certain to properly label the saved part. Transport the avulsed part with the patient, keeping it cool but out of direct contact with ice or cooled water. Your EMS system may require that the sterile gauze wrap be soaked with sterile saline.

When confronted with an amputation, attempt to control bleeding by direct pressure applied to a bulky dressing held directly over the stump, or use a pressure dressing. Care for the amputated part is the same as for an avulsed part. If necessary, use pressure point techniques to help control bleeding from the stump. When an extremity is injured, the application of a blood pressure cuff may be the best way to control severe external bleeding. The last resort is a tourniquet.

Do not try to replace protruding organs. Control bleeding and cover with an occlusive dressing. Care for shock.

Dressings cover wounds and bandages hold dressings in place. Dressings can be single layered or built up into bulky dressings. Occlusive dressings are used to form airtight seals.

The procedures for dressing a wound require you to control bleeding, to use sterile or clean materials, and to cover the entire wound. *Do not* remove a dressing once it is in place.

The procedures for bandaging require you to apply the bandage so that the dressing is not too loose or too tight and to be sure that there are no loose ends. Check for a distal pulse to ensure that the bandage is not too tight. Remember, *do not* cover the patient's fingertips and toes so that you can monitor circulation in the injured limb. Make certain that you completely cover all edges of the dressing unless specific care protocols specify a different procedure.

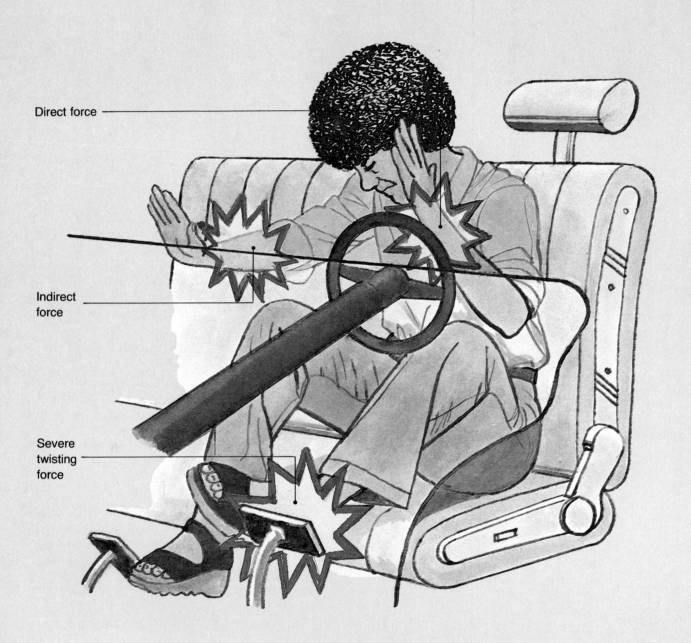

Direct force

Indirect force

Severe twisting force

Injuries II:
Musculoskeletal injuries—the upper extremities

OBJECTIVES   **As an EMT, you should be able to:**

1. List the FOUR major functions of the skeletal system. (pp. 238–239)
2. Define *bone*, *joint*, *ligament*, and *tendon*. (p. 239, pp. 246–247)
3. Label the major anatomical structures of a long bone. (p. 239)
4. Describe the special healing properties of bone. (p. 239)
5. Define *axial* and *appendicular skeleton*. (p. 240)
6. Distinguish between cranium and face. (p. 240)
7. Name and label the FIVE major divisions of the spinal column. (p. 242)
8. Define *thorax* in terms of its skeletal components. (p. 240 and p. 242)
9. Locate and name the major bones of the extremities. (pp. 243–244)
10. Define *open fracture* and *closed fracture*, listing symptoms and signs associated with both. (p. 245, pp. 247–248)
11. Define *angulated fracture*, noting when special care should be provided for this type of fracture. (p. 245, p. 253)
12. Define *dislocation*, *sprain*, and *strain*. (pp. 246–247)
13. State the basic care provided for given injuries of the upper extremities, include soft and rigid splinting procedures. (pp. 256–264)
14. Describe the procedures used to determine nerve and vascular function for the upper extremities. (p. 254, p. 257)

SKILLS   **As an EMT, you should be able to:**

1. Assess injuries to the upper extremities based on symptoms and signs.
2. Provide soft tissue care for injuries to the upper extremities.
3. Provide care for injuries to the bones and joints of the upper extremities, including:
   • Fractures and dislocations of the pectoral girdle

235

- Fractures of the humerus
- Fractures and dislocations of the elbow
- Fractures of the forearm and wrist
- Fractures of the hand, including the fingers
4. Use the basic splints that are a part of EMT-level care at the accident scene, including:
  - Soft splints (sling and swathe, pillow splints)
  - Upper extremity splint set
  - Lower extremity splint set
  - Traction splints
- Inflatable splints
5. Straighten closed angulated fractures, when appropriate.
6. Evaluate nerve and vascular function of the upper extremities.
7. Make and use noncommercial splints for emergency situations.
8. Provide total patient care for patients with fractures.

TERMS you may be using for the first time:

Angulated Fracture – a break to a bone causing the limb or joint to take on an unnatural shape or bend.

Appendicular (AP-en-DIK-u-ler) **Skeleton** – that part of the skeleton in the upper and lower extremities.

Articulation (ar-TIK-u-LAY-shun) – formation of a joint where two or more bones come together.

Axial (AK-si-al) **Skeleton** – the skull, spine, ribs, and sternum.

Cervical (SER-ve-kal) **Vertebrae** – relating to the seven vertebrae in the neck.

Closed Fracture – a broken bone with no associated opening in the skin.

Coccyx (KOK-siks) – the four fused vertebrae that form the terminal bone of the spine; the "tailbone."

Cranium (KRAY-ni-um) – the bones forming the brain case of the skull.

Crepitus (KREP-i-tus) – a grating sensation or sound made when fractured bone ends rub together.

Dislocation – injury causing the end of a bone to be pulled or pushed from its joint.

Ligament – tissue that connects bone to bone.

Lumbar (LUM-bar) **Vertebrae** – relating to the five vertebrae of the midback.

Open Fracture – either a broken bone with the ends or fragments tearing outward through the skin or a penetrating wound with an associated fracture.

Periosteum (per-e-OS-te-um) – the white fibrous membrane covering a bone.

Sacral (SA-kral) **Vertebrae** – the five fused vertebrae of the lower back.

Splinting – the process used to immobilize fractures and dislocations so that there is a minimum of movement to the bone and to the joints above and below the bone.

Sprain – a partially torn ligament.

Strain – the overstretching or mild tearing of a muscle.

Tendon – tissue that connects muscle to bone.

Thoracic (tho-RAS-ik) **Vertebrae** – relating to the 12 vertebrae to which the ribs attach.

Traction – to pull gently along the length of an extremity prior to splinting.

Traction Splinting – to use a special splint to apply a constant pull along the length of a lower extremity. This helps to stabilize the fractured bone and may reduce muscle spasms.

NOTE: The study of medicine that deals with musculoskeletal injury and disease is orthopedics. The term comes from *ortho-* (to straighten or correct) and *pedio-* (pertaining to the child). The term literally means to straighten the child. The first orthopedists provided care for the deformities of children.

THE MUSCULOSKELETAL SYSTEM

Many students have an interest in extremity injuries and eagerly await the part of their training in which they will study injuries to the bones and joints. A few hours of disciplined study enable them to learn the names and locations of the bones, how to classify and detect probable fractures, and how to apply

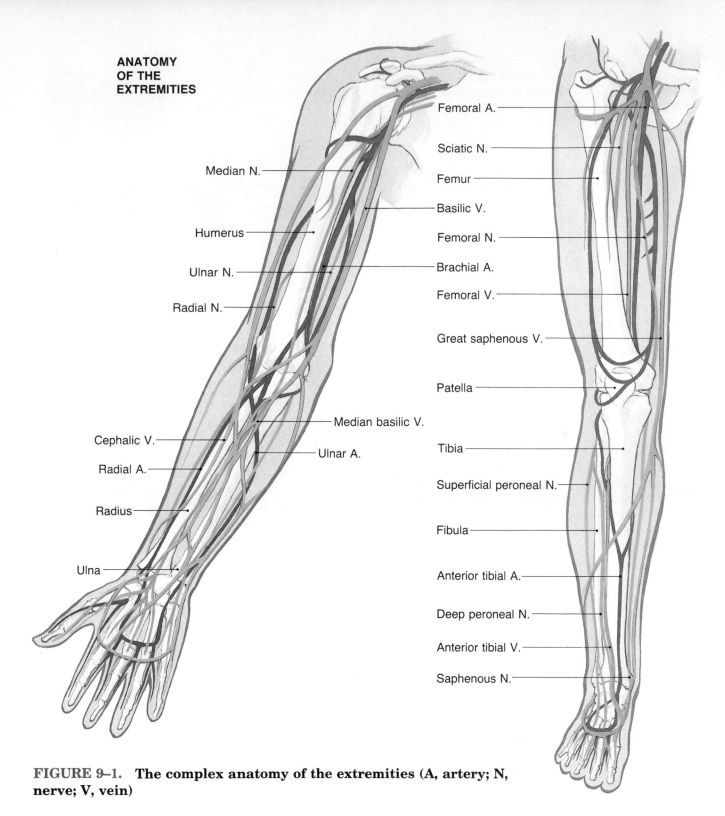

ANATOMY
OF THE
EXTREMITIES

Median N.

Humerus

Ulnar N.

Radial N.

Cephalic V.

Radial A.

Radius

Ulna

Median basilic V.

Ulnar A.

Femoral A.

Sciatic N.

Femur

Basilic V.

Femoral N.

Brachial A.

Femoral V.

Great saphenous V.

Patella

Tibia

Superficial peroneal N.

Fibula

Anterior tibial A.

Deep peroneal N.

Anterior tibial V.

Saphenous N.

FIGURE 9–1. **The complex anatomy of the extremities (A, artery; N, nerve; V, vein)**

splints to these injuries. However, while they are learning this new information, some students may neglect what they have been taught about soft tissues. The muscles, nerves, connective tissues, and blood vessels are no longer considered as they should be in care procedures. This can carry over into the field: some EMTs become so concerned about detecting and caring for fractures that they fail to notice other injuries or give fractures too high a priority.

REMEMBER: When a bone is fractured, the damage to blood vessels, nerves, and other soft tissues may be of greater significance than the fracture. Proper care of bone and joint injuries *must* include efficient soft tissue care.

Figure 9–1 shows the major blood vessels and muscles, along with a few of the major nerves found in the upper and lower limbs. As an EMT, you do not need to know *every* structure found in an extremity. However, you will need to remember how complex these structures are and consider the damage that may be done to soft tissues in cases of possible fracture or dislocation.

Bones are a part of a more complex system called the musculoskeletal system. This system is composed of all the bones, joints, muscles, tendons, ligaments, and cartilages in the body.

Muscles

Muscles are involved with *body movement*, with *moving food*, *fluids*, or *blood* through structures in the body, with *body posture*, and with helping to make up certain body *structures* (e.g., the wall of the intestine). Most references to the musculoskeletal system are referring to the muscles involved with body movement.

There are three types of muscles in the body (Figure 9–2):

- SKELETAL MUSCLE—this is *voluntary muscle*, meaning that its actions are controlled by conscious thought. It is fast to contract and fast to relax and be ready for its next contraction. Skeletal muscle connects to bones directly or by way of tendons.
- SMOOTH MUSCLE—this is *involuntary muscle*, meaning that its actions cannot be controlled by conscious thought. It is slow to contract and slow to relax and be ready for its next contraction. With the exception of the heart, smooth muscle helps to make up the walls of internal organs.
- CARDIAC MUSCLE—a highly specialized form of *involuntary muscle* that makes up the walls of the heart. When the body is at rest, cardiac muscle can contract and relax and be ready for its next contraction in approximately 0.8 second.•

The *diaphragm* is a special type of voluntary muscle. Even though you can have conscious control of its contractions, you cannot hold your breath for too long a period of time before involuntary nervous system control takes over.

Most of the emergency care of muscle injury is associated with care of soft tissue injury and possible fractures. Dressing open wounds, immobilizing the injured part, and treating for shock are the basic care procedures for serious muscle injuries.

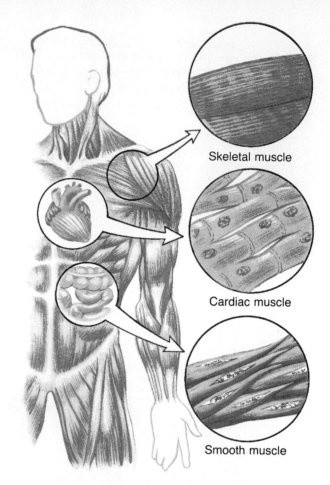

FIGURE 9–2. The three types of muscles.

The Skeletal System

The skeletal system is made up of all the bones and joints in the body.

Bones are not simply mineral deposits that require less care than other living tissues of the body. If you do not realize that bones are hard yet somewhat flexible living structures, you may find yourself providing improper care.

Functions of the Skeletal System

The skeletal system provides the body with four major functions. The bones *support*, creating a framework to give the body form and to provide a rigid structure for the attachment of muscles and other body parts. Bones **articulate** (ar-TIK-u-late) or connect to other bones to form joints, most of which are movable. Acting with muscles, bones and their joints allow for *body movement*. Bones also provide *protection* for the vital organs. The skull protects the brain; the spinal column encloses and protects the spinal cord; the ribs protect the heart, lungs, liver, stomach, and spleen; and the bones of the pelvis protect the urinary bladder and the internal reproductive organs. Bones also protect a soft tissue called marrow that is found within them. Some bones have red bone marrow that contains cells involved in *blood cell production.*

The Anatomy of Bone

Bones are classified according to their appearance (Figure 9–3). There are long, short, flat, and irregular bones. The bones found in the arm and thigh are examples of **long bones.** The major **short bones** of the body are in the hands and feet. Among the **flat bones** are the sternum, shoulder blades, and ribs. The vertebrae of the spinal column are examples of **irregular bones.**

The outward appearance of a typical long bone creates the impression that it is a simple, rigid structure, made of the same material throughout. Most people are aware that bone contains calcium, making it very hard. Bone also contains protein fibers that give it a degree of flexibility. The strength of our bones is a combination of this hardness and flexibility. As we age, there is less protein being formed in the bones and less calcium being stored. As a result, bones become brittle and fracture more easily than when we are young.

Bones are covered by a strong, white, fibrous material called the **periosteum** (per-e-OS-te-um). Blood vessels and nerves pass through this membrane as they enter and leave the bone. When bone is exposed as a result of injury, the periosteum becomes visible. You may see fragments of bones and foreign objects on this covering, but do not remove them. If they have pierced this tissue, the objects may be held firmly in place and offer a great deal of resistance to any pulling or sweeping efforts. In addition, you will not be able to tell if the object has entered the bone or is impaled in an underlying blood vessel or nerve.

The typical long bone has a **shaft** that is cylindrical in shape. The shafts of bones appear to be straight, but each bone has its own unique curvature. When the end of a bone is involved in forming a ball-and-socket joint, it will be rounded to allow for rotational movement. This rounded end is called the **head** of the bone. It is connected to the shaft by the **neck.** The ends of bones forming joints are covered with cartilage called **articular cartilage.** Bone marrow is contained in the center of bones. In long bones, this is found in a marrow cavity known as the **medullary** (MED-u-lar-e) **canal.**

The Self-Healing Nature of Bone

Before discussing fractures and emergency care procedures, let us examine how a broken bone repairs itself. Understanding this process will give you an appreciation of why a broken bone must be immobilized *quickly* and must *remain* immobilized to heal properly.

The first effect of an injury to a bone is the swelling of soft tissues and the formation of a blood clot in the area of the fracture. Both are due to the destruction of blood vessels in the periosteum and the bone and to the loss of blood from adjacent damaged vessels. Interruption of the blood supply causes death to the cells at the injury site. Cells a little farther from the fracture site remain intact, and within a few hours of the trauma, they begin to divide rapidly to form a mass of new tissue that eventually grows together to form a collar of tissue that completely surrounds the fracture site. New bone is generated from this mass to eventually heal the damaged bone. The whole process can take weeks or months, depending on the bone that has been fractured, the type of fracture, and the health and age of the patient. Should the fractured bone be mishandled early in care, more soft tissues may be damaged, requiring a longer period for the formation of a tissue mass and replacement of the bone. If the bone ends are disturbed during regeneration, proper healing will not take place and a permanent disability may result.

The Human Skeleton

There are 206 bones in the human body. Each bone is a part of one of the two major divisions of the skeletal system (Figure 9–4):

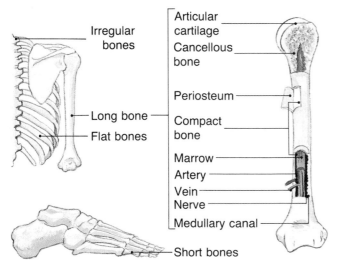

Irregular bones
Long bone
Flat bones
Short bones

Articular cartilage
Cancellous bone
Periosteum
Compact bone
Marrow
Artery
Vein
Nerve
Medullary canal

FIGURE 9–3. The anatomy of bone and classification by shape.

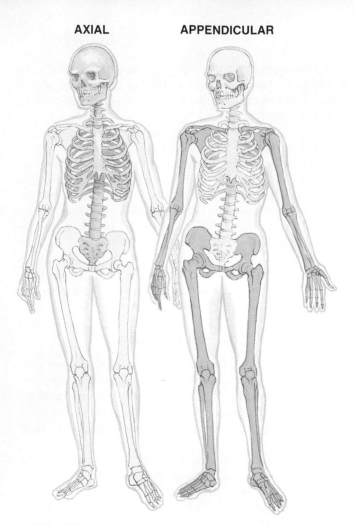

FIGURE 9–4.   The major divisions of the skeletal system.

- AXIAL (AK-si-al) SKELETON—all the bones forming the upright axis of the body, including the skull, spinal column, sternum, and ribs.
- APPENDICULAR (AP-en-DIK-u-ler) SKELETON—all the bones forming the upper and lower extremities, including clavicles, scapulae, arms, forearms, wrists, hands, pelvis, thighs, legs, ankles, and feet.

The Axial Skeleton

The axial skeleton is composed of the *skull*, the *vertebral* (VER-te-bral) *column* or spinal column, the *ribs*, and the *sternum* (Figure 9–5). It makes up the longitudinal axis of the human body.

The Skull   The skull is made up of 22 bones that form the **cranium** (KRAY-ni-um) and the **face** (Figure 9–6). The 8 bones of the cranium are classified

as flat bones and are irregular in shape. These bones begin to fuse together strongly at approximately 2 years of age to produce immovable joints, forming the rigid brain case surrounding the cranial cavity (see Chapter 2). The point at which two bones of the cranium articulate (join together) is known as a **suture.** The fusion is not complete in infants, causing "soft spots" (fontanelles) in a baby's cranium (Figure 9–7). This is why one must be careful in applying any pressure to the skull of an infant. Whenever care procedures call for you to support the head of an infant, spread your fingers to reduce pressure, avoiding these "soft spots."

The cranium forms the forehead and upper orbits, the top and back of the skull, and the sides of the upper skull. In addition, its bones fuse to form an internal structure called the **cranial floor.** This is the inferior wall of the brain case, containing numerous small openings to provide passageways for nerves and blood vessels that lead to and from the brain.

NOTE: Many people use the term *skull* to mean cranium. In most cases, when you hear that a patient has a skull fracture, you can be certain that the cranium is the injury site.

The remaining 14 bones of the skull form the face. These bones are highly irregular in shape, but when fused together, they give the face its characteristic shape. As in the case of the cranium, the facial bones are fused into immovable joints, except for the lower jaw or **mandible** (MAN-di-bl). The anatomy of the face will be discussed in Chapter 11.

The Spinal Column   The spinal column is made up of 33 irregularly shaped bones known as **vertebrae** (VER-te-bre). This column of bones gives support to the head and upper body, provides a point of attachment for the pelvis, and protectively houses the spinal cord within the spinal cavity (see Chapter 2). Each bone has a posterior spinous process, many of which can be felt along the midline of a person's back.

The vertebrae are connected by *ligaments*. Located between each two vertebrae is a *disk* of cartilage, hard enough in composition to prevent collapse, yet soft enough to serve as a cushion. Since the spinal cord must be protected and an upright posture is to be maintained, spinal column movement is limited. The spinal column has five divisions (Figure 9–8).

The Thoracic Cage   The thoracic cage is composed of 12 pairs of ribs, 12 thoracic vertebrae, and the sternum.

There are 12 pairs of ribs in the human body, the same for both male and female. All of the ribs

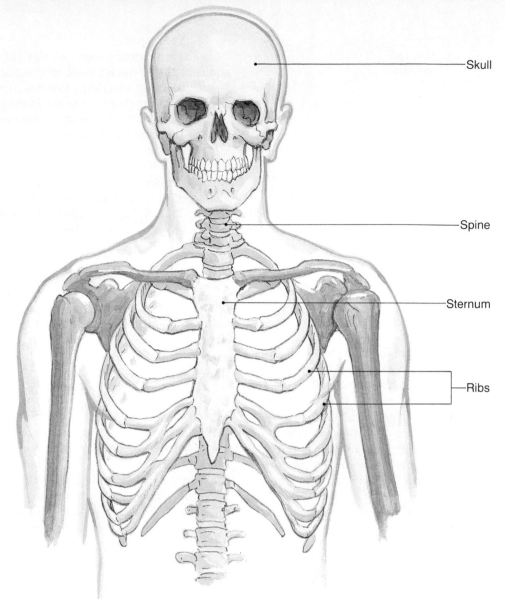

FIGURE 9–5. **The axial skeleton.**

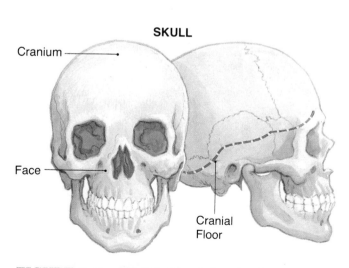

SKULL

FIGURE 9–6. **Divisions of the skull.**

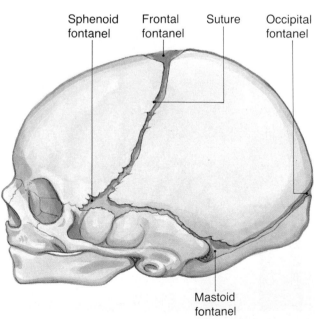

FIGURE 9–7. **The infant skull.**

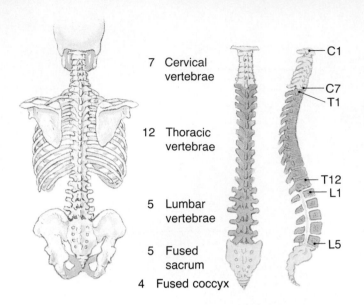

7 Cervical
  vertebrae

12 Thoracic
   vertebrae

5 Lumbar
  vertebrae

5 Fused
  sacrum

4 Fused coccyx

C1

C7
T1

T12
L1

L5

FIGURE 9–8. Anatomy of the spine.

connect posteriorly to the thoracic vertebrae. The upper 7 pairs of ribs attach directly to the sternum by way of cartilage. The next 3 pairs of ribs connect to the cartilage of the seventh pair of ribs. The term *floating ribs* is given to the last two pairs of ribs. These ribs are connected to the spine, but they do not attach to the sternum or the cartilages of the ribs located above them. Anteriorly, all the ribs are palpable, except for the first pair, which lie behind the clavicles.

The points of attachment for rib pairs 6 through 10 can be easily felt on each side of the sternum. The cartilage attachment points on each side are referred to as the **costal** (KOS-tal) **margin.** The costal margins combine to form the **costal arch.**

The sternum is part of the axial skeleton. In addition to the attachment of the ribs, the sternum also articulates with the clavicles. A visible depression occurs at this point known as the **jugular notch** (*suprasternal notch*). The lower extension of the sternum is the **xiphoid process.**

The chest surrounds and protects the lungs and the pleura, the heart and the pericardial sac, part of the trachea, part of the esophagus, and the great blood vessels (aorta and superior and inferior venae cavae). The rib cage extends downward to offer protection to portions of the liver, gallbladder, stomach, and spleen.

The Appendicular Skeleton

The appendicular skeleton is composed of the upper and lower extremities. In this chapter, we will consider, in detail, the structures making up the upper extremities. The lower extremities are covered in Chapter 10.

The Upper Extremities As an EMT, you will be expected to know the medical names for the major bones in the body. This will allow you to communicate better with the other members of the patient care team and to use materials available for your continuing education. Should you ever forget the medical name of a bone when presenting information to the emergency department staff, use the common name of the bone. This is better than losing your credibility by using the incorrect term.

The bones of the upper extremities are shown in Figure 9–10.

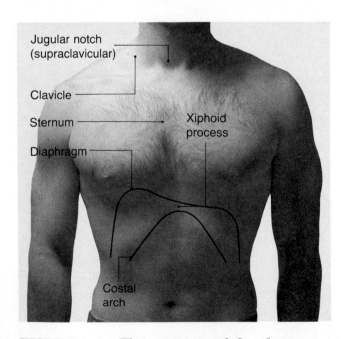

Jugular notch
(supraclavicular)

Clavicle

Sternum

Diaphragm

Xiphoid
process

Costal
arch

FIGURE 9–9. The anatomy of the chest.

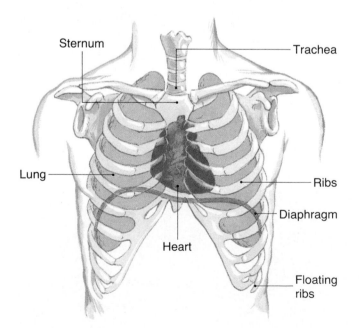

Sternum

Trachea

Lung

Ribs

Diaphragm

Heart

Floating
ribs

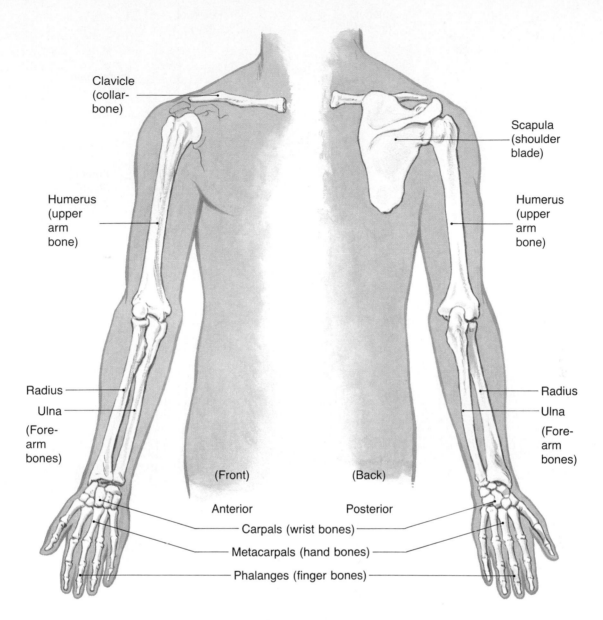

Clavicle
(collar-
bone)

Scapula
(shoulder
blade)

Humerus
(upper
arm
bone)

Humerus
(upper
arm
bone)

Radius

Ulna

(Fore-
arm
bones)

Radius

Ulna

(Fore-
arm
bones)

(Front)

(Back)

Anterior

Posterior

Carpals (wrist bones)

Metacarpals (hand bones)

Phalanges (finger bones)

THE UPPER EXTREMITIES

COMMON NAME	ANATOMICAL NAME
Shoulder girdle	Pectoral girdle (pek-TOR-al): clavicle, scapula, and head of humerus
Collarbone (1/side)	Clavicle (KLAV-i-kul)
Shoulder blade (1/side)	Scapula (SKAP-u-lah)
Arm bone (1/limb, from shoulder to elbow)	Humerus (HU-mer-us)
Forearm bones (2/limb, from elbow to wrist: 1/medial, 1 lateral	Ulna (UL-nah) — medial Radius (RAY-de-us) — lateral
Wrist bones (8/wrist)	Carpals (KAR-pals)
Hand bones (palm bones, 5/palm)	Metacarpals (meta-KAR-pals)
Finger bones (14/hand)	Phalanges (fah-LAN-jez)

FIGURE 9–10. Bones of the upper extremity.

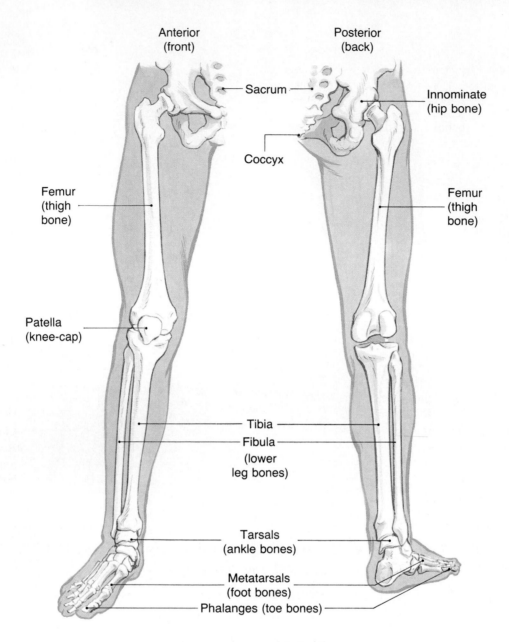

Anterior
(front)

Posterior
(back)

Sacrum

Innominate
(hip bone)

Coccyx

Femur
(thigh
bone)

Femur
(thigh
bone)

Patella
(knee-cap)

Tibia

Fibula
(lower
leg bones)

Tarsals
(ankle bones)

Metatarsals
(foot bones)

Phalanges (toe bones)

THE LOWER EXTREMITIES

COMMON NAMES	*ANATOMICAL NAMES*
Pelvic girdle (pelvis or hips)	Innominate on each side made up of the fused ilium, ischium, and pubis bones, as well as sacrum and coccyx posteriorly
Thigh bone (1/limb)	Femur (FE-mer)
Kneecap (1/limb)	Patella (pah-TEL-lah)
Leg bones (shin bones, 2/leg, 1 medial, 1 lateral)	Tibia (TIB-e-ah) — medial Fibula (FIB-yo-lah) — lateral
Ankle bones (7/foot)	Tarsals (TAR-sals)
Foot bones (5/foot)	Metatarsals (meta-TAR-sals)
Toe bones (14/foot. some peole have two bones in their little toe, others may have three)	Phalanges (Fah-LAN-jez)

FIGURE 9–11. Bones of the lower extremity.

NOTE: When a physician uses the term *arm*, it is to make reference to the upper arm or humerus. The lower arm is the forearm. The entire structure, from shoulder to fingertips, is the upper extremity.

The Lower Extremities The bones of the lower extremities are shown in Figure 9–11.

NOTE: To a physician, the hip is the joint formed by the pelvis and the head of the femur. Many patients commonly refer to the lateral pelvis as their hip. The medical staff will call the upper leg the *thigh* and the lower leg the "leg." From pelvis to the tips of the toes is the lower extremity.

INJURIES TO BONES AND JOINTS

Structures of the musculoskeletal system are subject to injury in the form of fractures, dislocations, sprains, and strains.

Fractures

By definition, a **fracture** is any break in a bone, including chips, cracks, splintering, and complete breaks. There are two basic types of fractures (Figure 9–12).

A **closed fracture** occurs when a bone is broken but there is no penetration extending from the

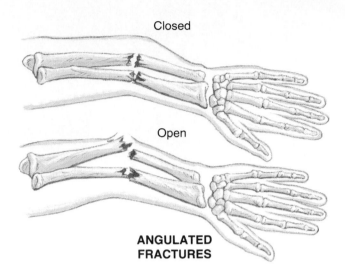

FIGURE 9–13. Angulated fractures.

fracture through the skin. In other words, pieces of bone have not been forced outward to rip through the skin. In many cases of closed fracture, soft tissue damage is minor. In some cases, because of bone end displacement or bone splintering, soft tissue damage may be great, with the damage being difficult to detect. Internal bleeding may be profuse.

An **open fracture** can occur in one of two ways. First, a bone can be fractured with soft tissues damaged from the fracture outward through the skin. Pieces of bone may actually pierce through the skin. Second, a penetrating wound can produce fractures. The wound is open from the skin to the injured bone.

An **angulated fracture** involves a broken bone, with the limb or joint taking on an abnormal shape (the humerus may be bent or twisted between the shoulder and the elbow). Angulated fractures can be mild or very severe, occurring with both open and closed fractures.

There is another classification of fractures that is based on x-ray appearance (Figure 9–14). Obviously, this is not part of the knowledge, skills, and equipment of the EMT. However, you will hear these terms at the medical facility when discussing fractures. The x-ray–based classification is:

- Greenstick—an incomplete fracture, so called because it looks like a green stick that is bent but not broken. Some fibers are separated, while others remain intact. This type of fracture is common in infants and children whose bones are still soft and pliable.
- Transverse—a break straight across the shaft of a bone.
- Oblique—a break that forms an angle to the shaft.

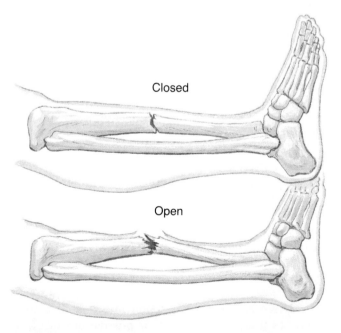

FIGURE 9–12. Basic types of fractures.

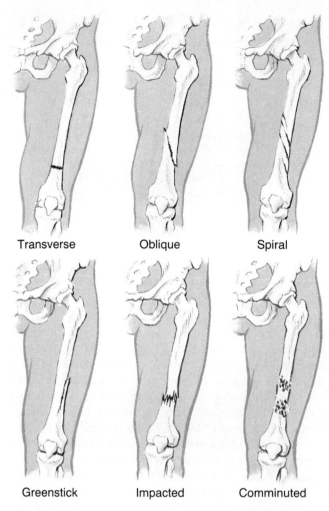

Transverse   Oblique   Spiral

Greenstick   Impacted   Comminuted

FIGURE 9–14.   Classifications of fractures.

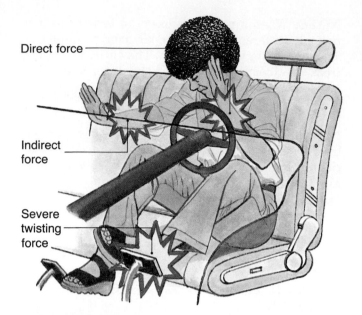

Direct force

Indirect force

Severe twisting force

FIGURE 9–15.   Bones may be fractured in a variety of ways.

foot is caught and twisted with enough force to fracture a leg bone. *Aging* and *bone disease* can increase the risk of fractures (pathologic fractures), with bones being broken even during minor accidents.

Fractures may be hard to detect. When assessing a patient, you should always consider if the mechanism of injury is the type that might cause broken bones, the age of the patient, and the general health of the patient.

Other Injuries

The most severe injuries to bones are fractures. Severe injuries to joints can be the result of fractures, dislocations, or a combination of both. Joints occur wherever two or more bones articulate. The resulting joint can be immovable, as seen when two bones join together to form part of the cranium. Most joints are movable joints, such as the hinge joint of the elbow and the ball-and-socket joint of the hip.

A movable joint consists of the ends of the two joining bones, with these ends usually covered by articular cartilage. The highly movable joints in the body are **synovial** (si-NO-ve-al) **joints** (Figure 9–16). They are surrounded by a fibrous **joint capsule** and contain membranes that produce a slippery fluid (synovial fluid) to lubricate joint movements. Injury to synovial joints can include damage to the capsule, the bone ends, and the ligaments that hold the bone ends in place.

Dislocations occur when one end of a bone making up a joint is pulled or pushed out of place. Usually, the dislocated bone is pulled from its socket.

- Spiral—a fracture having the appearance of a spring. The break twists around the shaft of the bone.
- Comminuted—a fracture in which the bone is fragmented. A severe crush injury may cause a bone to break into many pieces.
- Impacted—a fracture in which the ends of broken bones are jammed into each other.

Causes of Fractures

The force necessary to fracture a bone can be applied in a variety of ways. *Direct force* can fracture a bone at the point of contact. A person may be struck by the bumper of an automobile and suffer a fracture at the point where the leg was hit. *Indirect force* also can fracture bones. This happens when forces are carried from the point of impact to the bone, as when a person falls on his hand and receives a broken arm or clavicle. *Twisting forces*, as in sports injuries, can cause bones to break. Such injuries often occur in football and skiing accidents when a person's

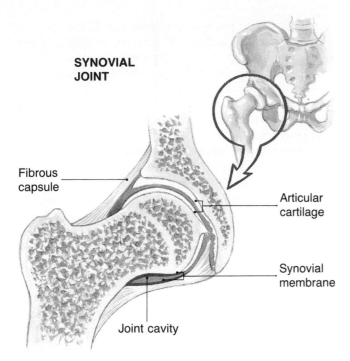

SYNOVIAL
JOINT

Fibrous
capsule

Articular
cartilage

Synovial
membrane

Joint cavity

FIGURE 9–16. **The anatomy of a synovial joint.**

Soft tissue injury can be very serious, including damage to blood vessels, nerves, and the joint capsule. Major blood vessels and nerves tend to be well protected in most parts of the body. However, in a movable joint these structures lie close to the bones forming the joint.

Ligaments connect bone to bone, holding the ends in place to help form and strengthen joints (Figure 9–17). When ligaments are torn, **sprains** occur. These are different from strains, where muscles or the tendons that connect muscle to bone are stretched or where mild tearing of the muscle takes place.

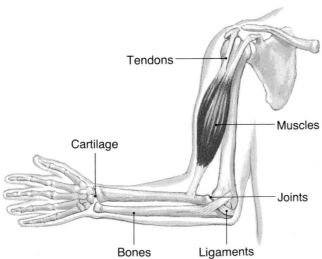

Tendons

Muscles

Cartilage

Joints

Bones

Ligaments

FIGURE 9–17. **Ligaments, tendons, and joints.**

NOTE: You will often have to treat all musculoskeletal injuries to the extremities as possible fractures. Dislocations, sprains, and some strains are difficult to distinguish from fractures. In certain cases, you will be able to tell that a dislocation has taken place. Most of the time, you will have to *assume* that any severe injury to an extremity is a possible fracture and treat it accordingly.

Symptoms and Signs of Injury to Bones and Joints

The symptoms and signs of a fracture can include:

- The patient says that he felt a bone break or heard the bone snap.
- Tenderness and pain—Pain is often severe and constant. The patient may hold the injured part, attempting to prevent additional pain from being produced by movement (guarding). The tissues directly over the fracture will be very tender. You should gently touch the area along the line of a bone in order to determine whether or not there is a possible fracture and the exact location of the injury site. *Do not* probe into or near the edges of open fractures. *Point tenderness* at the injury site is a strong indicator of a possible fracture.
- Deformity—If a part of a limb appears different in size, shape, or length than the same part on the opposite side of the patient's body, you must assume that there is a fracture. If a bone or a joint appears to have an unusual angle, consider this deformity to be a reliable sign of fracture. Gently feel along the patient's limbs noting any lumps, fragments, or ends of fractured bones.
- Swelling and discoloration—These begin shortly after injury. Discoloration may start as a reddening of the skin. Black and blue bruises will usually not occur for several hours.
- Crepitus (KREP-i-tus)—The patient tells you that he heard noises or felt a grating sensation when he moved a limb. This sound or sensation is known as crepitus. It is caused when the broken bone ends rub together. *Do not* ask the patient to move the limb so that you may hear the noise. Crepitus also can be a sign. When the patient moves, you may hear a grating sound or feel unusual vibrations through the patient's skin. If you detect crepitus, *do not* ask the patient to move again so that you can confirm the sign.

- Loss of function—The patient may not be able to move a limb or part of a limb. Sometimes he will be able to move a limb, but the movement will produce intense pain. If the patient reports that he can move the arm but not the fingers, or if he can move the leg but not the toes, there may be a fracture that has caused damage to adjoining nerves and blood vessels.
- Loss of distal pulse—This is very serious, indicating the interruption of circulation.
- Loss of sensation—Displaced bones or bone fragments may have injured nerves.
- Numbness or tingling sensations—Displaced bones or bone fragments may have injured blood vessels or nerves.
- Exposed bone—Fragments or the ends of fractured bone may be visible where they break through the skin in some cases of open fractures.
- False motion—When the patient moves, the injured bone will display abnormal motion along the shaft, indicating that the bone has been fractured into separate segments. *Do not* ask the patient to move in order to check for this sign.
- Muscle spasms in the injured extremity.

NOTE: Any of the above symptoms or signs gives you enough evidence to assume that there is a fracture.

Dislocations typically produce an obvious deformity of the joint. Swelling at the joint is a common sign. Usually there is pain, which increases with

Signs of fractures
- Deformity
- Swelling
- Discoloration
- Loss of use
- Tenderness and pain
- Crepitus (grating)

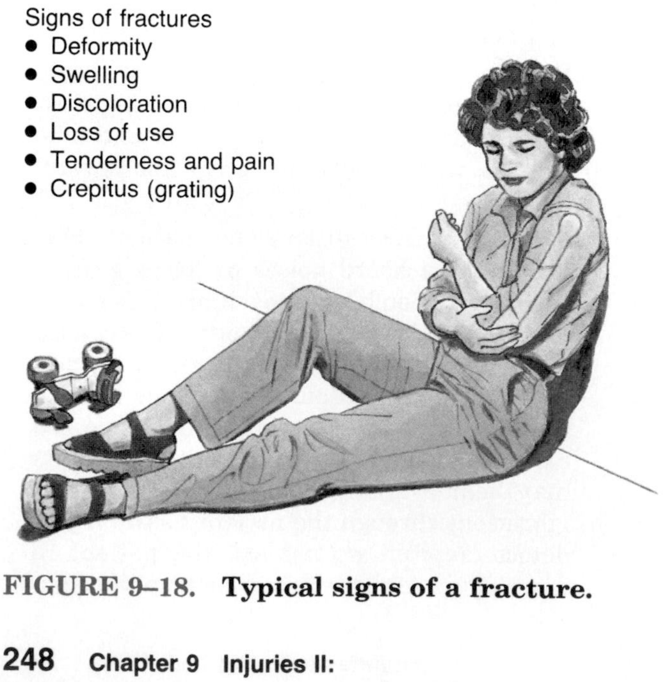

FIGURE 9–18. **Typical signs of a fracture.**

movement. The patient may lose use of the joint or may complain of a "locked" or "frozen" joint. If the patient's only sign is deformity at a joint, a dislocation is more likely than a fracture. However, you *must* still consider a fracture to be a possibility. Even when you believe that a dislocation has occurred, you cannot rule out a *combined injury* of dislocation and fracture.

Sprains can sometimes be difficult to tell from fractures and dislocations. In most cases there is swelling and discoloration and the patient complains of pain on movement. There may be considerable swelling and deformity associated with dislocations and fractures. A typical sprain should not have the deformity but may have the swelling due to soft tissue injury. As an EMT, you should manage suspected sprains as if they were fractures.

The only sign of a strain may be pain. Even when you think that you are dealing with an obvious strain, you should keep the patient at rest and ask him not to move any part of the injured extremity. Remember, with the conditions at the accident scene, the diagnostic equipment you carry, and your level of training, you cannot rule out the possibility of a fracture.

Complications

Muscle is often damaged when there are injuries to the joints and bones. In addition to this damage, injuries such as lacerations, punctures, damage from impaled objects, and serious contusions can occur to muscle. The principles of soft tissue injury care must be applied to open wounds involving muscles. Splinting is often desirable even when there are no indications of fractures. Immobilizing the limb will help prevent additional injury to muscle tissue and help control internal bleeding.

Fractures and dislocations can cause blood vessels to be lacerated or pinched shut (Figure 9–20). The major arteries of the extremities lie close to the bones, especially at the joints. As part of the care provided, you must take a distal pulse when evaluating the extent of injury and after you splint an extremity. No pulse indicates a lack of circulation below the injury site and may mean extensive tissue death will take place unless blood flow is reestablished within a reasonable length of time.

Other signs can indicate impaired circulation. Capillary refill should be evaluated as a standard procedure before and after splinting. Carefully examine the skin at the distal end of the injured limb and compare what you find with the same area on the opposite side of the body. If the skin color has turned blue (cyanosis) or pale (pallor), or the skin

TYPE	DISLOCATION Joint deformity	SPRAIN Ligament Torn	STRAIN Muscle over- stretched

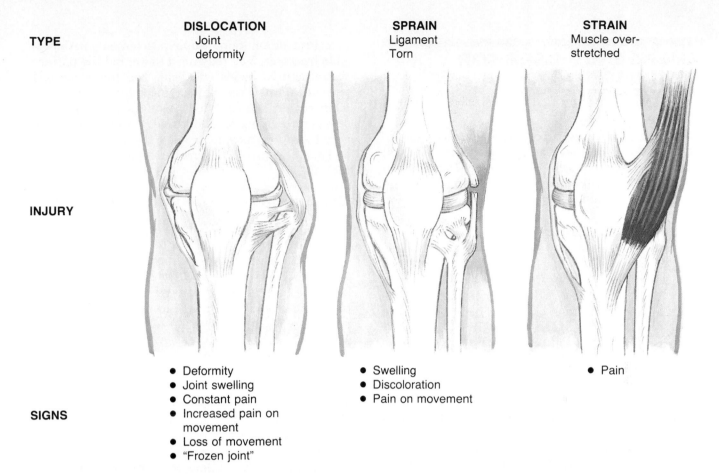

INJURY			

SIGNS	• Deformity • Joint swelling • Constant pain • Increased pain on movement • Loss of movement • "Frozen joint"	• Swelling • Discoloration • Pain on movement	• Pain

FIGURE 9–19. Injuries other than fractures.

is cold by comparison to the uninjured limb, circulation is probably inadequate. Next, exert pressure over a nailbed on the injured limb, then release the pressure. The nailbed should appear white (blanched) for a brief moment, then regain color as the capillaries refill. If **capillary refilling** does not take place within 2 seconds, there may be impaired

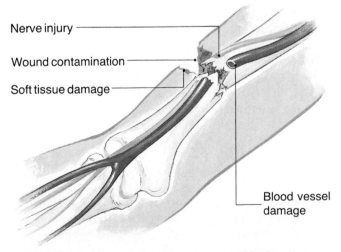

Nerve injury

Wound contamination

Soft tissue damage

Blood vessel damage

FIGURE 9–20. Complications with fractures.

circulation. This is not a very reliable sign if the patient has been exposed to a cold environment.

Just as blood vessels can become cut or have too much pressure placed on them, so too can the nerves running through the extremities. Even when there is no spinal damage, the patient with nerve damage due to a fracture may be unable to move his fingers or toes, depending on the site of the injury. A fracture of the humeral shaft can interrupt the radial nerve, limiting the patient's ability to extend the hand at the wrist. Elbow injuries can damage the ulnar nerve, limiting muscular action or sensation in the hand, particularly in the fourth (ring) and fifth (little) fingers. Lack of movement at the ankles with no response to stimulus along the superior surface of the foot is seen in some cases of fibula fractures in which nerves are damaged.

In the case of open fractures, a common complication is *contamination*. *Do not* reach into the wound or try to clean the surface of the exposed bone. In the case of long bone open fractures, contamination is a major problem in the long-term care of the patient. Improper initial care can lead to serious infection. Detached bone fragments outside the body should be cared for and transported the same as an avulsed tissue.

EMERGENCY CARE FOR INJURIES TO THE EXTREMITIES

While some fractures, especially open fractures, appear gruesome and very serious, few present a real threat to life. Your unhurried but efficient action may mean the difference between a rapid and complete recovery and a long, painful hospitalization and rehabilitation. When dealing with fractures, one of your main duties is to immobilize the injured limb. No matter how near the medical facility, fractures and dislocations should be immobilized to prevent aggravation of the injury. Of course, basic cardiac life support situations and certain critical multiple injuries may necessitate transport before such care can be rendered.

Total Patient Care

Many untrained people arrive at the scene of an accident and try to start caring for fractures. When caring for a person with an injury to the bone or joint of an extremity, it is first necessary to resolve other more serious problems. Remember to conduct a primary survey and a secondary survey with an interview. You must detect life-threatening problems and correct these problems as quickly as possible. An open airway, respiration, pulse, and control of bleeding must be ensured before starting care of fractures. Detecting neck and spinal injuries is more important than detecting extremity fractures. As with all patients, you must take the necessary steps to reduce the chance of the patient developing shock. Both open chest wounds and open abdominal wounds should be cared for before you worry about fractures. Serious burns, especially those that may compromise respirations, should be cared for before fractures to the extremities, even if the fractures are major.

There also is an order of care in terms of fractures:

1. First priority—fractures of the spine.
2. Second priority—fractures to the head, rib cage, and pelvis.
3. Lowest priority—fractures of the extremities. Fractures of the lower limbs are cared for before those to the upper limbs. The order of priority after the pelvis is the femurs, joints, and other long bones.

Provide emotional support to patients with possible fractures. You may need to remind the patient that fractured bones will heal. Tell the concerned patient that new techniques in the care of fractures often reduce the time a patient spends wearing a cast and receiving rehabilitative therapy. Your emotional support may help keep the patient at rest and help to control blood pressure, pulse, and breathing rate.

General Care for Skeletal Injuries

The proper time to care for a specific bone or joint injury is when the patient is reasonably stable. Be certain that serious bleeding is controlled and that all open wounds have been dressed with sterile dressings. The general care procedures for suspected fractures and dislocations are shown in Scan 9–1. The exceptions to this approach will be covered under specific care procedures.

Repositioning Limbs

A realistic approach must be taken when splinting a patient's possible fractures. In some cases, especially those involving motor vehicle accidents, it will be necessary to slightly reposition a limb or perhaps the entire patient to allow for splinting to take place, or to allow for the patient to be removed from the debris or wreckage after splinting is completed. Variations in splinting procedures occur when the questions of straightening a limb or straightening an angulated fracture are considered.

Each EMS System has its own protocols for the repositioning of limbs and straightening of angulated fractures. These protocols are formulated after considering typical response and transport times, the specialized training of the EMTs, methods of splinting and the types of splints used, the type of medical facility that will receive the patient, and the care procedures that will be used at the medical facility. All EMS Systems recognize that some movement of a limb may be necessary to allow for a splint to be applied. Usually, a combination of two or more of the following protocols will be used. Your instructor will explain which of these protocols are followed in your EMS System. Check off these protocols as you are provided with the information concerning your EMS System. YOU MUST FOLLOW LOCAL PROTOCOLS.

- Place angulated long bone fractures (no joint involvement) in anatomical position before splinting or traction is applied unless there is an associated dislocation or resistance is met. (Seek recommendation of emergency department physician.)

Unless shock or other injuries require immediate transport, **DO NOT** move the patient until all fractures have been immobilized. Reassure the patient throughout the care process, explaining procedures when necessary.

1

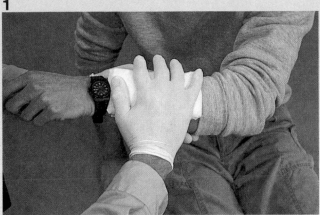

Control serious bleeding and dress open wounds.

2

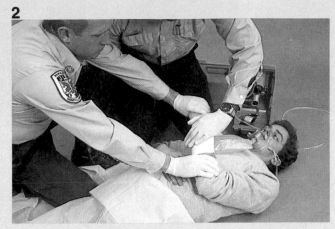

Begin to treat for shock as soon as possible. Provide a high concentration of oxygen when appropriate.

3

ASSESS THE INJURY:

- Gather symptoms
- Tenderness and pain
- Deformity
- Swelling and discoloration
- Crepitus
- Loss of function, distal pulse, or sensation
- Numbness or tingling
- Exposed bone
- False motion
- Muscle spasms.

4

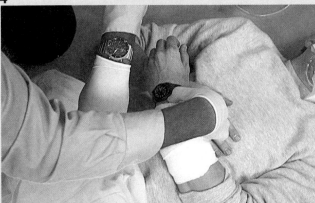

Check for the impairment of circulation. Palpate the distal pulse and evaluate capillary refill.

5

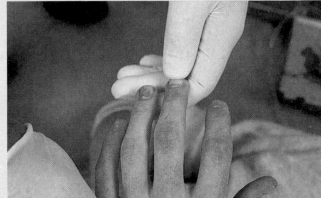

Check nerve function. Check for sensitivity to touch and for finger or toe movement and slight hand or foot movement.

(Scan continues on next page)

6

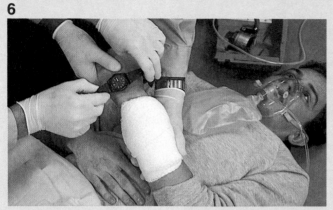

Remove or cut away clothing around site. Remove jewelry on injured limb.

7

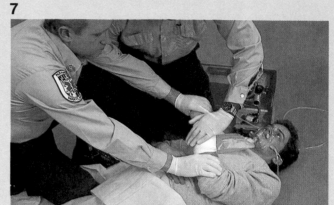

When appropriate, **gently** move fractured limbs to the splinting position . . . only if there is no resistance or severe pain.

8

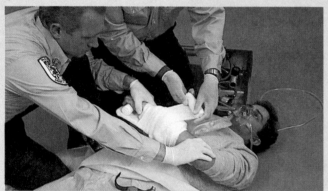

When necessary, straighten any severely angulated closed fractures that can be straightened **safely.**

9

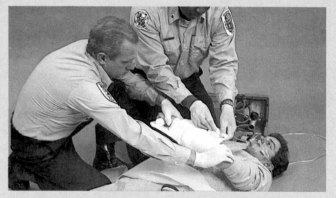

Apply manual traction (tension) and maintain throughout the splinting process. Immobilize dislocated joints, but **do not** attempt to reduce (straighten) any dislocation.

10

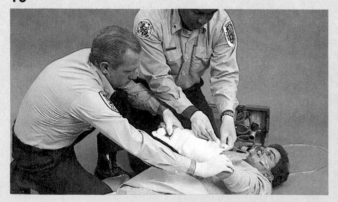

Splint firmly but do not impair circulation. Wrap distal to proximal. Immobilize joints immediately above and below the fracture site.

11

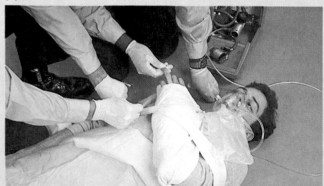

Leave fingers and toes exposed. Monitor circulation and nerve function. Continue to treat for shock, and assess vital signs.

- If pulse is absent distal to long bone injury, splint as above and expedite transport.
- Splint all dislocations in the position in which they are found.

When in doubt as to the correct protocol, contact the Emergency Department physician. Such contact is recommended for any case that involves a patient who does not have a distal pulse or has evidence of nerve damage.

Straightening Angulated Fractures

Straightening angulations of closed long bone fractures is within the scope of EMT-level care. If appropriate, slightly angulated closed fractures of the extremities can usually be straightened and immobilized with few problems. However, severely angulated fractures can pose serious problems. Angulations make splinting and transport more difficult. They can pinch or cut through nerves and blood vessels and usually are painful for the patient.

WARNING: DO NOT ATTEMPT TO STRAIGHTEN ANGULATED FRACTURES OF THE SHOULDER OR WRIST. Major nerves and blood vessels pass through these joints, close to the major bones. Attempts to straighten dislocations may cause serious, even permanent, damage. DO NOT ATTEMPT TO STRAIGHTEN ANY DISLOCATED JOINT.

Gently attempt to straighten the limb, stopping if there is any resistance, crepitus, or significant increase in pain.

If your effort fails, do not make a second attempt to straighten the limb. If the joint shows evidence of a crush injury, do not attempt to straighten it. Whenever there is no distal pulse, transport the patient as soon as possible.

Open angulated leg fracture—Once the wound has been covered with a sterile dressing, it is appropriate to attempt to return the extremity to the anatomical position and splint as for closed fractures.

The patient's pain may increase during the process of straightening an angulation. This will be temporary, with the pain lessening and muscle spasms being reduced as splinting is completed. The procedure for straightening closed angulated fractures *other* than those to the shoulders, elbows, wrists, or knees is as follows:

1. CAREFULLY cut away clothing that lies over the fracture site.
2. Upper Limb: Grasp the limb above and below the fracture site and apply smooth, steady

tension along the long axis of the limb. Hold the limb so that you maintain alignment and tension until your partner can apply a splint.

Lower Limb: Have your partner hold the limb firmly in place while you apply tension below the break. Maintain tension and alignment until a splint has been applied. If the limb must be lifted, the fracture site must be supported.

NOTE: If a firm resistance is felt while you are applying tension, crepitus occurs, or the patient experiences a significant increase in pain, *do not* try to correct the angulation. Attempt to correct the angulation only once. Be certain that your actions do not displace a joint. Any additional attempts require a physician's approval.

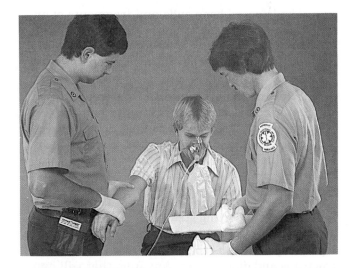

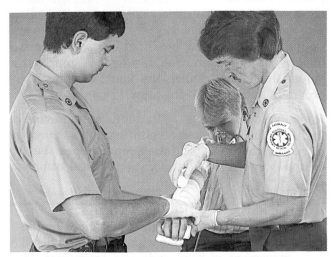

FIGURE 9–21. Procedure for straightening an angulated closed fracture.

patient when the splint is removed have led some EMS systems to drop air-inflated splints from their approved equipment lists.

The second type of soft splint consists of items such as pillows, blankets, towels, and dressings. Soft splinting usually is *not* the most effective form of splinting, but the process does help to immobilize fractures and dislocations. One of the most useful soft splinting techniques is the application of a sling and swathe (see Scan 9–2). In cases such as fractures to the foot, the soft splint is preferred over the rigid splint.

Traction splints are used to immobilize broken bone ends of a fractured femur so that further damage is avoided. Traction is the application of just enough force to stabilize the broken bone. It is not the stretching or moving of the fractured bone until the ends are aligned. When a bone breaks completely, the normal tendency of the muscles to contract often causes bone ends to slip past one another, or "override." When muscles are large and powerful, as in the thigh, the tendency is more pronounced. Patient movement and the movement necessary during transport can increase the override and cause serious soft tissue damage, including a closed fracture becoming an open fracture (a Scan on traction splinting appears in Chapter 10).

There will be times when you do not have enough splints at the scene of an accident or you are responding while you are off duty and do not have any commercial splints. You will have to make your own splints from materials at the scene (Figure 9–25). Your emergency splints may be soft splints such as pillows or rolled blankets, or they may be rigid splints made from a variety of materials. You can use pieces of lumber, plywood, compressed wood products, cardboard, rolled newspapers or magazines, umbrellas, canes, broom handles, shovel handles, sporting equipment (a catcher's or hockey goalie's shin guards have been used), or tongue depressors (for fractured fingers). Some of these items can be found at the scene of a typical accident. Ask bystanders to help you find something that can be used as a splint. Give them suggestions and ask if they have any ideas. Having bystanders check the trunks of their cars usually produces results. Tell them you are looking for something rigid and long enough to hold the fractured bone and the joints immediately above and below this bone.

In some cases, it will be necessary to splint the injured limb to an unaffected limb, thus using the patient's own body as a splint. For example, an injured finger may be taped to an adjoining uninjured finger, or it may be necessary to tie a patient's lower limbs together.

Splinting the Upper Extremities

There are eight basic rules to keep in mind as you apply splints for injuries to the extremities:

- WHEN IN DOUBT, SPLINT.
- Patients with possible fractures or dislocations should be treated for shock and, when appropriate, administered a high concentration of oxygen.
- Always be sure that a rigid splint is padded before it is applied to a patient.
- When securing a splint to an extremity, wrap it from distal to proximal.
- Be certain that you have not disrupted vascular or nerve function during the splinting process. Check the distal pulse, capillary refill, and nerve function *before* and *after* splinting. Remember to record your findings. Monitor these factors and distal skin color and temperature during transport.
- Splint the forearm and hand with the hand in its position of function.
- When possible, elevate an injured extremity after it is immobilized to reduce swelling.
- Continue to check air-inflated splints to be certain that they have not lost or gained pressure. Altitude or temperature changes will affect splint pressure. Leaks may occur from punctures or the deterioration of valves or zippers.

Musculoskeletal (orthopedic) injuries can be frightening to the patient. Always reassure the conscious patient, explaining what you must do. Many

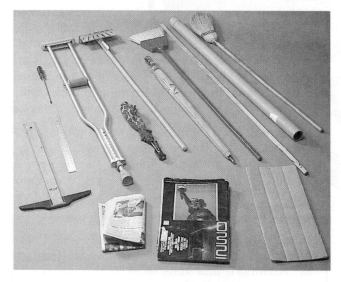

FIGURE 9–25. You must know how to make emergency splints.

patients assume that a splint means that they definitely have a fracture. Unless the fracture is obvious, let patients know that you are suspicious of a fracture and the splinting process is a precaution.

Most of the following section is done as a series of scansheets. You are responsible for knowing how to care for injuries to the entire upper extremity.

The Shoulder Girdle

Symptoms and Signs

1. Pain in the shoulder may indicate several types of injury. Look for specific signs.
2. A dropped shoulder, with the patient holding the arm of his injured side against the chest often indicates a fracture of the clavicle or scapula (Figure 9–26).
3. All the bones of the shoulder girdle can be felt except the scapula. Only the superior ridge of the scapula, called the spine, can be easily palpated. Injury to the scapula is rare, but must be considered if there are indications of a severe blow striking the back over top of this bone.
4. Check the entire shoulder girdle:
   - Check for deformity where the clavicle attaches to the sternum—possible fracture or dislocation.
   - Feel for deformity where the clavicle joins the scapula (acromioclavicular joint, ak-KRO-me-o-KLAV-ik-u-lar)—possible dislocation.
   - Feel and look along the entire clavicle for deformity—possible fracture.
   - Note if the head of the humerus can be felt or moves in front of the shoulder—possible anterior dislocation. This displacement also may be due to a fracture.

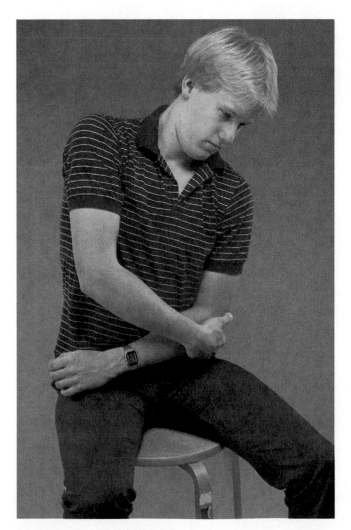

FIGURE 9–26. Fractured clavicle, noted by "dropped" shoulder.

Emergency Care

1. Check for a radial pulse on the injured side. If there is no pulse, immobilize and transport as soon as possible.
2. Determine for nerve function by checking for feeling and movement of the fingers on the injured side. If there is possible nerve damage, immobilize and transport as soon as possible.
3. It is not practical to use a rigid splint for injuries to the clavicle, scapula, or the head of the humerus. Use a sling and swathe (see Scan 9–2).
4. If there is evidence of a possible anterior dislocation of the head of the humerus, place a thin pillow between the patient's arm and chest before applying the sling and swathe.
5. *Do not* attempt to straighten or reset any dislocations.

NOTE: Sometimes a dislocated shoulder will reduce itself ("pop back into place"). When this happens, you should check for a distal pulse and nerve function. Apply a sling and swathe and transport the patient. The patient must be seen by a physician. Be certain to note the self-reduction on the patient form and to report the event to the emergency department staff.

Scans 9–2 through 9–6 complete your study of the upper extremities.

SCAN 9–2 SLING AND SWATHE

A sling is a triangular bandage used to support the shoulder and arm. Once the patient's arm is placed in a sling, a swathe can be used to hold the arm against the side of the chest. Commercial slings are available. Roller bandage can be used to form a sling and swathe. Velcro straps can be used to form a swathe. Use whatever materials you have on hand, provided they will not cut into the patient.

1

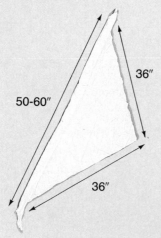

The sling should be in the shape of a triangle.

2

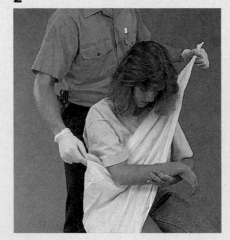

Position the sling over the top of the patient's chest as shown. Fold the patient's injured arm across the chest.

3

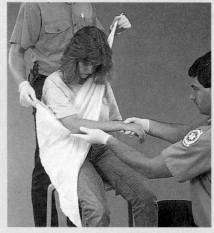

If the patient cannot hold his arm, have someone assist until you tie the sling.

4

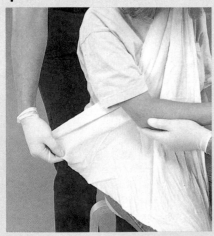

One point of the triangle should extend behind the elbow on the injured side.

5

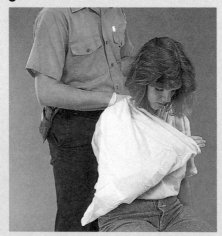

Take the bottom point of the triangle and bring this end up over the patient's arm. When you are finished, this point should be taken over top of the patient's injured shoulder.

6

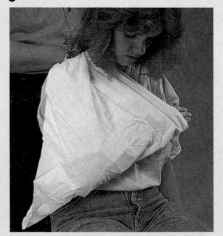

Draw up on the ends of the sling so that the patient's hand is about four inches above the elbow (exceptions are discussed later).

7

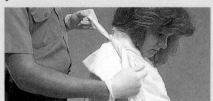

Tie the two ends of the sling together, making sure that the knot does not press against the back of the patient's neck. The area can be padded with bulky dressings or sanitary napkins.

8

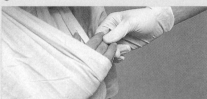

Leave the patient's fingertips exposed to detect any color or skin temperature changes that indicate the lack of circulation.

9

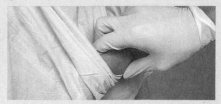

Check for a radial pulse. If the pulse has been lost, take off the sling and repeat the procedure. Check neurologic function. Repeat sling procedure if necessary.

10A

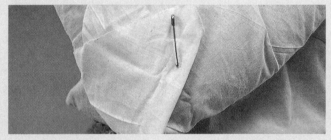

Take hold of the point of material at the patient's elbow and fold it forward, pinning it to the front of the sling. This forms a pocket for the patient's elbow.

10B

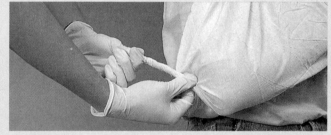

If you do not have a pin, twist the excess material and tie a knot in the point.

11

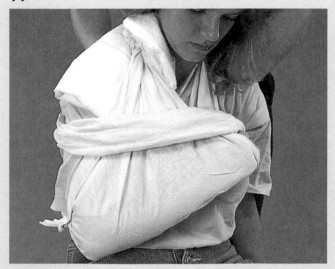

A swathe can be formed from a second piece of triangular material. This swathe is tied around the chest and the injured arm, over the sling. Do not place this swathe over the patient's arm on the uninjured side.

12

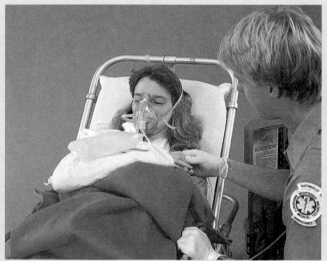

- Assess distal pulse and neurologic function.
- Treat for shock.
- Provide a high concentration of oxygen.
- Continue to reassure patient.
- Take vital signs.

SCAN 9–3 INJURIES TO THE HUMERUS— SOFT SPLINTING

SIGNS: Injury to the humerus can take place at the proximal end (shoulder), along the shaft of the bone, or at the distal end (elbow). Deformity is the key sign used to detect fractures to this bone in any of these locations; however, assess for all signs of skeletal injury. Follow the rules and procedures for care of an injured extremity.

1

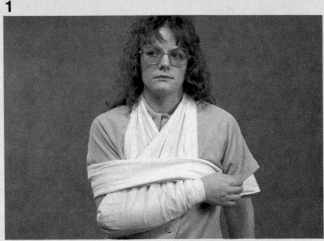

NOTE: RIGID SPLINTING IS PREFERRED.
Fracture at proximal end. Gently apply a sling and swathe. If you have only enough material for a swathe, bind the patient's upper arm to his body, taking great care not to cut off circulation to the forearm.

2

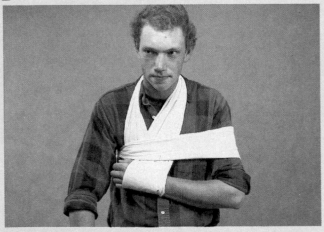

Fracture of the shaft. Use rigid splints whenever possible; otherwise, gently apply a sling and swathe. The sling should be modified so that it supports the wrist only.

3

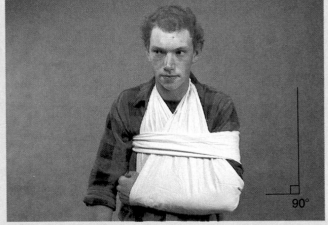

Fracture at distal end. Gently apply a full sling and swathe. Do not draw the hand upward to a position four inches above the elbow. Instead, keep elbow flexion as close to a 90° angle as possible.

WARNING:

Before applying a sling and swathe to care for injuries to the humerus, check for nerve function and circulation. If you do not feel a pulse, attempt to straighten any slight angulation if the patient has a closed fracture (follow local protocol). Otherwise, prepare for immediate immobilization and transport. Should straightening of the angulation fail to restore the pulse or function, splint with a medium board splint (36 inches), keeping the forearm extended. If there is no sign of circulation or nerve function, you will have to attempt a second splinting. If this fails to restore circulation and nerve function, transport immediately. Do not try to straighten angulation of the humerus if there are any signs of fracture or dislocation of the shoulder or elbow.

SCAN 9—4   ARM AND ELBOW FRACTURES AND DISLOCATIONS

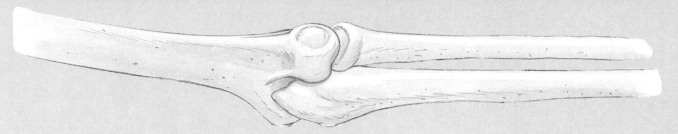

The elbow is a joint and not a bone. It is composed of the distal humerus, and the proximal ulna and radius forming a hinge joint. You will have to decide if the injury is truly to the elbow. Deformity and sensitivity will direct you to the injury site.

Care If there is a distal pulse, the elbow should be immobilized in the position in which it is found. The

joint has too many nerves and blood vessels to risk movement. Be certain to check for circulation and nerve impairment before and after splinting. When a distal pulse is absent, make one attempt to gently straighten the limb after contacting the emergency department physician. Do not force the limb into its normal anatomical position.

Elbow in or Returned to Bent Position

1

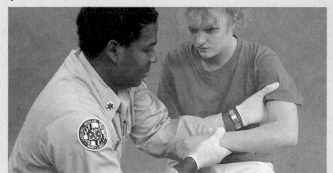

Slight repositioning of the limb may be necessary to allow for proper splinting. **Do not** continue if you meet resistance or significantly increase the pain.

2

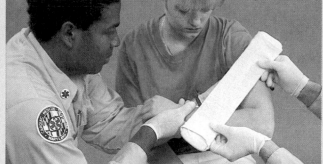

Use a padded board splint that will extend 2 to 6 inches beyond the arm and wrist when placed diagonally.

3

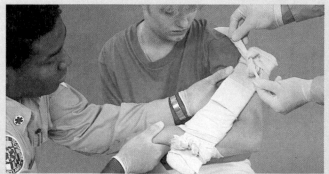

Place the splint so it is just proximal to the shoulder and to the wrist. Use cravats to secure to the forearm, then the arm.

4

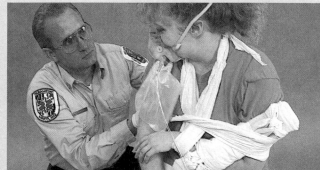

A wrist sling can be applied to support the limb; keep the elbow exposed. Apply a swathe if possible.

(Scan continues on next page)

Elbow Injury-Elbow in Straight Position

1

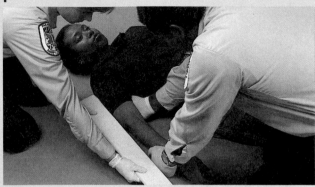

Use a padded board splint that extends from under the armpit to a point past the fingertips.

2

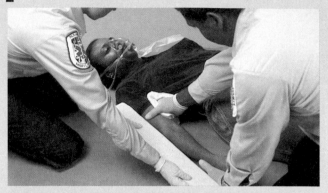

Pad the armpit, and place a roll of bandages in the patient's hand to help maintain position of function.

3

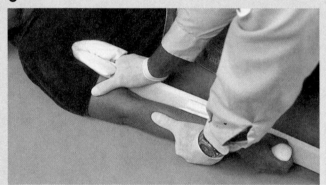

Place padded side of board against medial side of limb. Pad all voids.

4

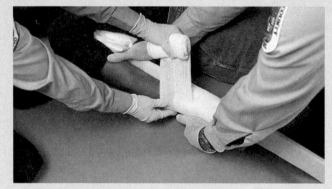

Secure splint, bandaging from distal to proximal. Leave finger tips exposed. Reassess distal pulse and neurologic signs.

5

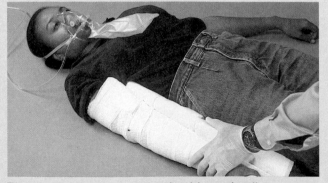

Place pads between patient's side and splint.

6

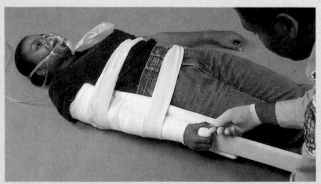

Secure splinted limb to body with two cravats . . . avoid placing over suspected injury site.

SCAN 9–5 INJURIES—FOREARM, WRIST, AND HAND

SIGNS:

- Forearm—deformity and tenderness. If only one bone is broken, deformity may be minor or absent.
- Wrist—deformity and tenderness, with the possibility of a Colles (KOL-ez) fracture that gives a "silverfork" appearance to the wrist.
- Hand—deformity and pain. Dislocated fingers are obvious.

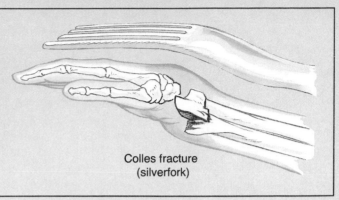

Colles fracture
(silverfork)

CARE: Check for circulation and nerve impairment before and after splinting. Fractures occurring to the forearm, wrist, or hand can be splinted using a padded rigid splint that extends from the elbow, past the fingertips. The patient's elbow, forearm, wrist, and hand all need the support of the splint. Tension must be provided throughout splinting. Roller bandage should be placed in the hand to ensure the position of function. After rigid splinting, apply a sling and swathe.

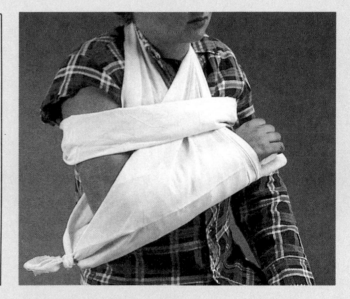

ALTERNATIVE CARE: Fractures of the hand and dislocations of the wrist can be cared for with soft splinting by placing the hand in the position of function and tying the forearm, wrist, and hand between the fold of one pillow or between two pillows.

An injured finger can be taped to an adjacent uninjured finger, or splinted with a tongue depressor. Some Emergency Department physicians prefer that care be limited to a wrap of soft bandages. Do NOT try to "pop" dislocated fingers back into place.

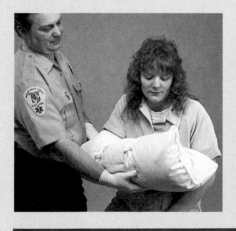
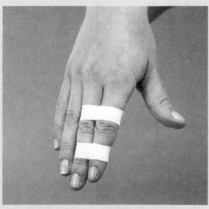
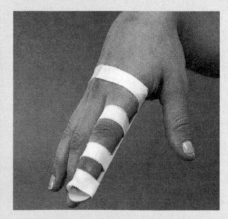

SCAN 9—6 AIR-INFLATED SPLINTS

WARNING! Air-inflated splints may leak. Make certain that the desired pressure is maintained. When applied in cold weather, an inflatable splint will expand when the patient is moved to a warmer place. Variations in pressure also occur if the patient is moved to a different altitude. Occasionally monitor the pressure in the splint with your fingertip. Air-inflated splints may stick to the patient's skin in hot weather.

1

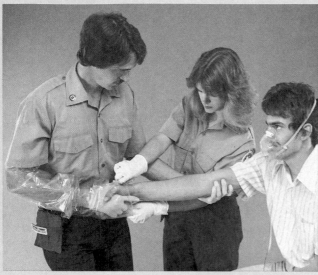

Slide the uninflated splint up your forearm, well above the wrist. Use this same hand to grasp the hand of the patient's injured limb as though you were going to shake hands.

2

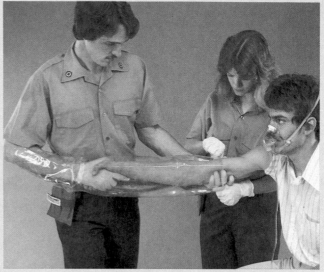

While holding his hand in this fashion, gently slide the splint over your hand and onto his limb. The lower edge of the splint should be just above his knuckles. Make sure the splint is properly placed and free of wrinkles.

3

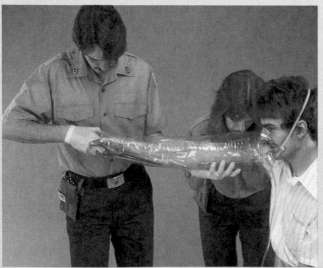

Continue to hold the patient's hand while you have your partner inflate the splint by mouth to a point where you can make a slight dent in the plastic when you press your thumb against the splint surface.

4

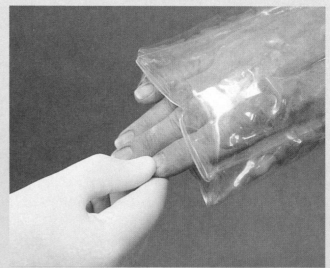

Monitor the patient's fingernail beds and fingertips for indications of circulation impairment. Continue to assess neurologic function.

SUMMARY

As an EMT, you should never become so preoccupied with fractures that you forget to conduct a primary survey and a secondary survey with an interview. Remember that an open airway, breathing, circulation, and bleeding are your first priorities. Shock, neck, spinal, chest, abdominal, and head injuries, and serious burns are all to be treated before fractures.

Remember, soft tissues are damaged when bones are injured.

The bones, joints, and muscles make up the musculoskeletal system. There are three types of muscle: skeletal, smooth, and cardiac. Skeletal muscle is considered when studying musculoskeletal injuries.

The skeletal system is involved with body support, body movement, organ protection, and certain aspects of blood cell production. There are two major divisions to the skeletal system: the axial skeleton and the appendicular skeleton. The upper and lower extremities are part of the appendicular skeleton.

Each upper extremity consists of the scapula, clavicle, humerus, ulna, radius, carpals, metacarpals, and phalanges.

Each lower extremity consists of the femur, patella, fibula, tibia, tarsals, metatarsals, and phalanges, with each femur joining with the pelvis.

If a part of a fractured bone tears through the patient's skin, the injury is an open fracture. This also is the case when a penetrating wound accompanies a fracture. If the fractured bones do not tear through the patient's skin to open the fracture to the outside, the injury is a closed fracture. You should apply sterile dressings, when possible, to all open fractures of the extremities.

When a bone is broken, it will often bend or twist to form an angulated fracture. Angulations can be straightened by grasping the limb above and below the site of the fracture and gently pulling with the hand you have placed below the site. Basically, fractures should be realigned unless they involve a joint. *Do not* attempt to straighten dislocations. Splint dislocations in the position they are found.

Any break of a bone is a fracture. A dislocation occurs when a bone is pulled out from a joint. Partially torn ligaments produce sprains. Stretching or minor tearing of muscles produces strains.

The symptoms and signs of fracture may include deformity, swelling, discoloration, tenderness, pain, loss of function, loss of distal pulse, crepitus, the sound of breaking bone, and exposed bone. Dislocation usually has pain, deformity, swelling, and loss of function. Sprains normally have swelling, discoloration, and pain on movement. Pain is usually the only sign of strain.

There are some SPECIAL SIGNS that you need to know, including:

- Dropped shoulder = clavicular fracture.
- Head of humerus bone out of socket = anterior dislocation of the shoulder.

Splinting is used to immobilize fractures. The process can be carried out using rigid splints, soft splints, or traction splints. In some cases, it may be necessary to splint one body part to another.

The application of a splint can help to prevent or reduce the severity of complications such as pain, soft tissue damage, bleeding, restricted blood flow, and closed fractures becoming open fractures. WHEN IN DOUBT, SPLINT.

Remember to cut away, remove, or lift away the patient's clothing over the injury site before splinting. Control bleeding and dress open wounds. Remove all jewelry from the affected limb. Check for a distal pulse and assess nerve function before and after splinting. When possible, straighten closed angulated fractures. All rigid splints should be padded before they are secured to the patient.

Patients with possible fractures and dislocations need to be reassured throughout the care process. Remember to care for shock and administer a high concentration of oxygen. When possible, an injured limb should be elevated once it is splinted to reduce swelling.

A rigid splint should immobilize the bone and the joints directly above and below the injured bone.

Whenever possible, immobilize all fractures and dislocations before moving the patient.

As an EMT, you must be able to use noncommercial splints. Consider lumber, plywood, rolled newspapers and magazines, compressed wood products, sporting equipment, canes, umbrellas, cardboard, and tool handles when you need to make an emergency splint.

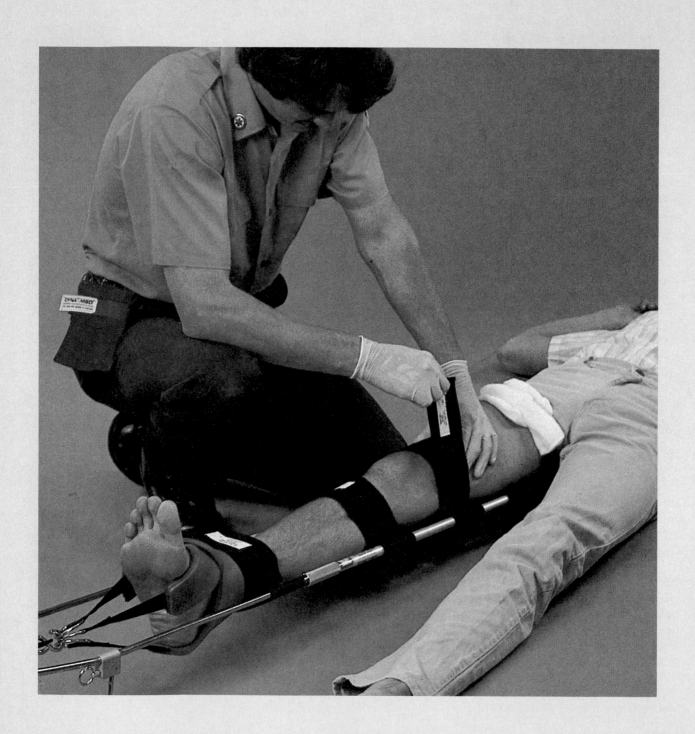

CHAPTER 10

Injuries II:
The lower extremities

OBJECTIVES As an EMT, you should be able to:

1. Locate and name the major bones of the lower extremities. (p. 269)
2. Explain, in terms of its anatomy, why special consideration is given to injury to the bones of the pelvis. (pp. 268–269)
3. Relate the significance of the muscle mass of the thigh to the care procedures for a fractured femur. (p. 269)
4. State the basic care provided for given injuries of the lower extremities, including soft and rigid splinting procedures. (pp. 271–293)
5. Describe the procedures used to determine nerve and vascular function for the lower extremities. (p. 271)
6. Describe how an EMT can determine if a patient has a possible fracture of the pelvis, an anterior dislocation of the hip, or a posterior dislocation of the hip. (pp. 273–276)
7. Describe, step by step, traction splinting procedures. (pp. 276–283)

SKILLS As an EMT, you should be able to:

1. Identify injuries to the lower extremities based on symptoms and signs.
2. Provide soft tissue care for injuries to the lower extremities.
3. Provide care for injuries to the bones and joints of the lower extremities, including:
   - Pelvic fractures
   - Hip fractures
   - Anterior and posterior hip dislocations
   - Fractures of the femur
   - Fractures and dislocations of the knee
   - Fractures of the leg
   - Fractures and dislocations of the ankle
   - Fractures of the foot
4. Use the basic splints that are a part of EMT-level care at the accident scene, including:
   - Soft splints (pillow splints)
   - Lower extremity splint set

- Inflatable splints
- Traction splints

5. Properly straighten closed angulated fractures, when appropriate.
6. Evaluate nerve and vascular function for the lower extremities.

7. Make and use noncommercial splints for emergency situations.
8. Provide total patient care for patients with injury to the lower extremities.

TERMS you may be using for the first time:

Achilles (ah-KEL-ez) **Tendon** – the common term for the tendon that connects the posterior lower leg muscles to the heel. The anatomical term is *calcaneal* (kal-KA-ne-al) *tendon.*

Condyles (KON-dials) – the large, rounded projections at the distal end of the femur and the proximal end of the tibia. Some persons refer to these as the sides of their knees.

Iliac (IL-e-ak) **Crest** – the upper, curved boundary of the ilium.

Ilium (IL-e-um) – the upper portions of the pelvis, forming the wings of the pelvis.

Ischium (IS-ke-em) – the lower, posterior portions of the pelvis.

Pubic (PYOO-bik), **Pubis** (PYOO-bis) – the middle (medial), anterior portion of the pelvis.

Traction Splinting – to use a special splint to apply a constant pull along the length of a lower extremity. This helps to stabilize the fractured bone and reduce muscle spasms in the limb.

THE LOWER EXTREMITIES

The basic anatomy of the lower extremities was presented in Chapter 9. You need to know that the lower extremities are composed of the pelvis and the two lower limbs (Figure 10–1). Each limb consists of the femur, patella, tibia, fibula, tarsals, metatarsals, and phalanges. The joint between the pelvis and the head of the femur is the hip. The knee joint is the distal femur, the proximal tibia, and the patella. The distal tibia and fibula join with the tarsals to form the ankle.

The Pelvis

The pelvis is sometimes called the pelvic girdle. It is composed of two large hip bones, one on each side. Each large hip bone is made up of three bones fused together tightly (Figure 10–2):

1. Ilium (IL-e-em)—Each ilium forms an upper "wing" of the pelvis. If you ask someone to place his hands on his hips, he will usually place them over the ilia (plural of ileum) of the pelvis.
2. Ischium (IS-ke-em)—Each ischium forms the lower, posterior portion of the pelvis. Part

of the ischium can be felt as a ridge of bone underneath the muscles of the buttock.
3. Pubis (PYOO-bis) or Pubic (PYOO-bik) Bone—The right and left pubic bones join to form the medial, anterior section of the pelvis.

The pelvic bones join with the sacrum and coccyx of the spine to encircle the pelvic cavity.

All injuries involving the bones of the pelvis must be considered to be serious. Patients with possible pelvic bone injury must be seen by a physician as soon as possible. Four anatomical factors makes this special caution necessary:

1. The pelvis surrounds and protects the urinary bladder, part of the large intestine, and the internal reproductive organs. Injury to the pelvic bones also may mean injury to the internal organs and frequently severe internal bleeding.
2. Many major nerves are associated with the pelvis. The spinal cord does not pass through the entire spinal column. It stops at the level of the lower border of the first lumbar vertebra. A large number of nerves originate from

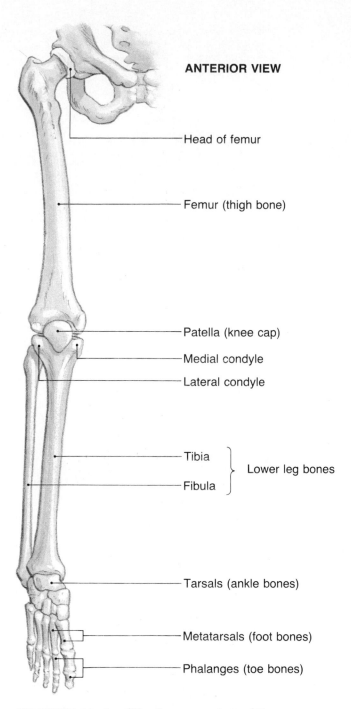

ANTERIOR VIEW

— Head of femur

— Femur (thigh bone)

— Patella (knee cap)

— Medial condyle

— Lateral condyle

— Tibia
— Fibula } Lower leg bones

— Tarsals (ankle bones)

— Metatarsals (foot bones)

— Phalanges (toe bones)

FIGURE 10–1. The lower extremities.

this level, sweeping downward like a horse's tail (see Figure 10–3). Injury to the ilia also may mean injury to many of these nerves.

3. The pelvis joins with the sacrum. If there is injury to the pelvis, there may be injury to the spine. There is a *rule* to follow in EMT-level care: if the mechanism of injury produced enough force to damage the strong bones of the pelvis, then *assume* that there is also spinal injury.

4. The lower limbs join with the pelvis. This means that major arteries, veins, and nerves must be associated with the pelvis and the hip joints. Damage to the pelvic bones or the joints with the femurs may mean significant blood vessel damage and blood loss or serious nerve injury.

As noted, the pelvic bones are very strong bones; however, the force applied to these bones during motor vehicle accidents and falls may produce serious injury. About 3% of all fractures involve the pelvis, with the percentage increasing for elderly patients. Fractures to the pelvis are second to skull fractures in terms of complications and death. Depending on the location of the fracture site and its severity, the mortality rate for pelvic fractures is from 5% to 20%. The most serious complication is usually severe internal bleeding that rapidly leads to hypovolemic shock.

The Femur

The femur is a large, strong bone. Since a great force is required to damage this bone, there may be associated injury to the hip joint, pelvis, or spine in accidents involving the femur. Large blood vessels and nerves pass close to the hip joint and are associated with the femur and the large muscles of the thigh and leg. If the mechanism of injury produced enough force to fracture the femur, there is a strong possibility that circulation and nerve function in the lower extremity could be impaired. Internal and/or external bleeding may be *severe*, with a blood loss of 1 pint or more occurring rapidly.

The large muscle mass of the thigh must be considered when assessing and providing care for lower extremity injury. External bleeding from deep arteries in the thigh may be difficult to control because of the barrier created by this muscle mass. Direct pressure, applied to avoid a possible fracture site, must be forceful enough to overcome this barrier and compress the femoral artery. The femoral artery pressure point site may be utilized.

The large muscles of the thigh can complicate fractures to the femur. Contractions of the thigh muscles may cause the ends of a completely fractured femur to ride over one another, complicating splinting procedures. You must check for the signs of open fracture and never assume that a wound on the thigh is of external origin. A traction splint will be necessary to overcome the actions of the thigh muscles and to provide adequate immobilization.

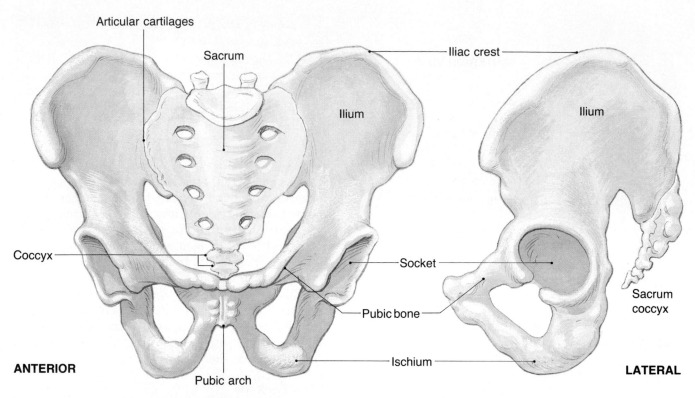

FIGURE 10–2. **The bones of the pelvis.**

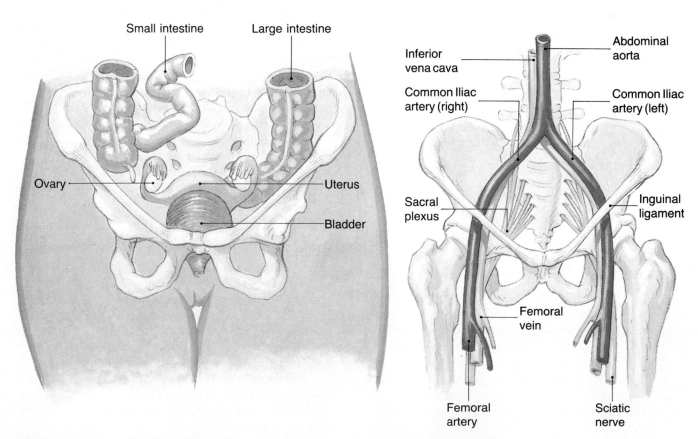

FIGURE 10–3. **Injury to the pelvis may damage internal organs and major blood vessels and nerves.**

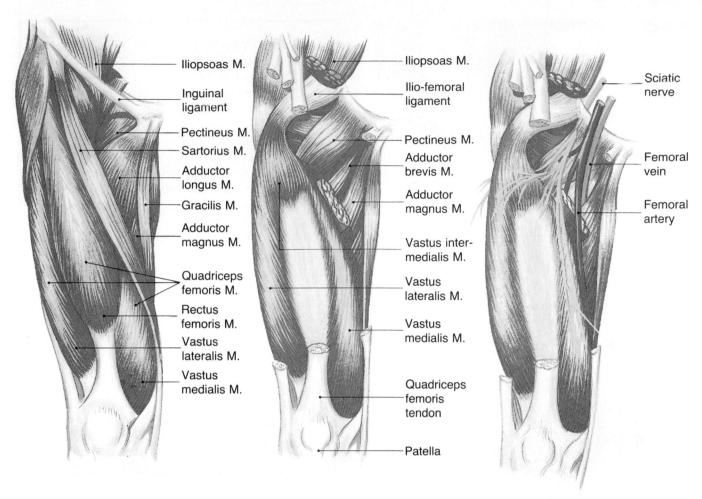

Iliopsoas M.
Inguinal ligament
Pectineus M.
Sartorius M.
Adductor longus M.
Gracilis M.
Adductor magnus M.
Quadriceps femoris M.
Rectus femoris M.
Vastus lateralis M.
Vastus medialis M.

Iliopsoas M.
Ilio-femoral ligament
Pectineus M.
Adductor brevis M.
Adductor magnus M.
Vastus inter-medialis M.
Vastus lateralis M.
Vastus medialis M.
Quadriceps femoris tendon
Patella

Sciatic nerve
Femoral vein
Femoral artery

FIGURE 10–4. **Injury to the femur is complicated by the muscle mass of the thigh and its major vessels and nerves.**

SPLINTING THE LOWER EXTREMITIES

The basic rules for patient care and the splinting of the upper extremities also apply to the lower extremities (see Chapter 9). Special consideration must be given to assessment of a distal pulse and nerve function, providing manual traction, use and application of a traction splint, and procedures to protect possible spinal injuries.

Pulse Assessment

Circulation must be assessed beyond (distal to) the injury site. One of two pulse sites can be used:

- Posterior Tibial Pulse—This site is recommended if the patient's shoe cannot be removed and there is no serious injury to the posterior ankle. The pulse site can be found on the medial side of the limb, posterior to the "ankle bone." To feel the pulse, apply pressure using the tips of two fingers placed in the groove found between the ankle bone and the **Achilles** (ah-KEL-ez) **tendon** (see Figure 10–5).

- Dorsalis Pedis Pulse—This site is on the anterior surface of the foot, lateral to the tendon of the great toe. The pulse may be felt by applying pressure with the tips of two fingers. The patient's shoe must be removed for proper pulse assessment. As noted in Chapter 3, this pulse site is more reliable than the posterior tibial but may be difficult to feel.

Manual Traction

Depending on injury site, manual traction is applied in one of two ways and is maintained until the completion of splinting.

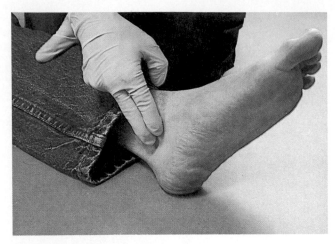

A

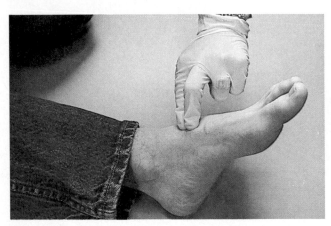

B

FIGURE 10–5. Establishing distal pulse. A. Posterior tibial. B. Dorsalis pedis.

1. Kneel alongside the injured limb, with your knee that is closest to the patient's head kept at the level of his knee.
2. Using the hand closest to the patient's head, grasp the back of the patient's thigh above the knee. This would be just above the rounded distal ends of the femur known as the femoral *condyles* (KON-dials). These rounded ends form what most persons call the "sides" of their knees.
3. Grasp the injured leg at the calf with your other hand, below the fracture site and as close to the ankle as possible while still providing support for the injury site.
4. Warn the conscious patient that there may be a temporary increase in pain. While supporting the knee and thigh, use the hand at the distal end of the limb to apply manual traction. Sometimes the patient will tell you that the limb feels better after you have applied manual traction.
5. At the same time that you are applying manual traction, gently lift the limb so that the heel is about ten inches off the ground. This lift will allow the splint to be secured to the leg without having to reposition the limb.

Thigh Injuries

The weight of the thigh and its strong muscle mass requires that manual traction be applied with the

Leg Injuries

Manual traction is applied in the same fashion that was used for the upper extremities (see Chapter 9). The EMT uses one arm to stabilize the patient's limb at the fracture site and the other arm to provide the manual traction. The manual traction should not be applied until you and your partner are ready to apply the splint. This is because the procedure of manual traction *must* be a continuous one until the splint takes over for the rescuer. Since providing manual traction to a lower limb is a tiring procedure, splinting must be done immediately to avoid the loss of traction. Whenever possible, three rescuers should be involved so that one person can lift and support the limb, the second person can apply manual traction, and a third person can apply the splint.

If the fracture is to the tibia or fibula:

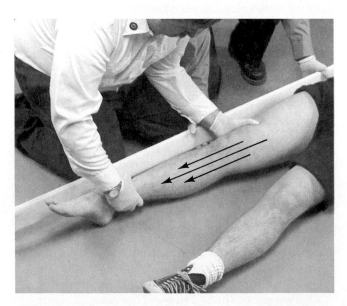

FIGURE 10–6. Applying manual traction for leg fractures.

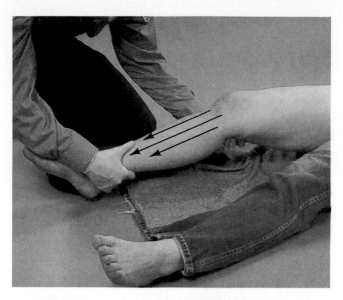

FIGURE 10–7. **Applying manual traction to the thigh.**

pulling action of two hands (Figure 10–7). When possible, another person should support the thigh while manual traction is applied.

1. Kneel alongside of the injured limb, with your knee closest to the patient's head at the level of his knee. This should be a comfortable position since care procedures and splinting of the injured limb may take some time.
2. Using the hand closest to the patient's head, grasp the back of the thigh above the femoral condyles. The fracture site will have to be supported.
3. Using your free hand, grasp the injured limb above the ankle, leaving room for the ankle strap that is used for traction splinting.
4. Use both hands to apply traction.
5. At the same time, gently lift the patient's limb so that the heel is about 10 inches off the ground.
6. Brace yourself to hold manual traction through the traction splinting process. Some rescuers have found that they can place the knee that is closest to the patient's ankle against the elbow of the arm used to grasp the ankle.

NOTE: The traction splint should not be applied if there are lower leg fractures on the same limb.

Spinal Protection

After splinting, the patient should be placed on a rigid surface to help protect and support the spine. The long spine board or orthopedic (scoop-style) stretcher can be used, in accordance with local protocols (see Chapters 11 and 23). This procedure should be done for all injuries to the pelvis, hip, and femur. The orthopedic stretcher is useful for injuries to the pelvis and hip. The long spine board is recommended for patients with injuries to the femur, after splinting has been completed.

INJURIES OF THE LOWER EXTREMITIES

Injuries to the Pelvis

Fractures of the pelvis may occur with falls, in motor vehicle accidents or when a person is crushed by being squeezed between two objects. Pelvic fractures may be the result of direct or indirect force.

WARNING: Indications of pelvic fractures mean that there may be serious damage to internal organs, blood vessels, and nerves. Internal bleeding may be profuse leading to shock. Provide the highest possible concentration of oxygen as soon as possible, care for shock, and monitor vital signs. Any force strong enough to fracture the pelvis also can cause injury to the spine.

Symptoms and Signs

- Complaint of pain in pelvis, hips, groin, or back. This may be the only indication, but it is significant if the mechanism of injury indicates possible fracture. Usually, obvious deformity will be associated with the pain.
- Painful reaction when pressure is applied to wings of pelvis (iliac crest) or to the pubic bones (see p. 100).
- Patient complains that he cannot lift his legs when lying on his back (*Do not* test for this, but do check for sensation.)
- The foot on the injured side may turn outward (lateral rotation). This also may indicate a hip fracture.
- The patient has an unexplained pressure on the urinary bladder and the feeling of having to void the bladder.

NOTE: It may be very difficult to tell a fractured pelvis from a fractured hip. When there is doubt, care for the patient as if there is a pelvis fracture in order to protect blood vessels and nerves associated with the joint. Remember, there may be spinal injuries.

Emergency Care

1. MOVE THE PATIENT AS LITTLE AS POSSIBLE. Any moves should be done so that the patient moves as a unit. Never lift the patient with the pelvis unsupported.
2. Determine the status of circulation and nerve function distal to the injury site.
3. Straighten the patient's lower limbs into the anatomical position if there are no serious injuries to the hip joints and lower limbs and if it is possible to do without meeting resistance or causing excessive pain. WARNING: DO NOT USE A LOG ROLL TO MOVE A PATIENT WITH A SUSPECTED PELVIC FRACTURE.
4. Prevent additional injury to the pelvis by stabilizing the lower limbs. Place a folded blanket between the patient's legs, from the groin to the feet and bind them together with wide cravats. Thin rigid splints can be used to push the cravats under the patient. The cravats can then be adjusted for proper placement:
   - Upper thigh
   - Above knee
   - Below knee
   - Above ankle
5. Assume that there are spinal injuries and immobilize the patient on a long spine board or use an orthopedic stretcher (see Chapters 11 and 23). When securing the patient, avoid placing the straps or ties over top of the pelvic area.
6. Reassess distal circulation and nerve function.
7. Care for shock, providing a high concentration of oxygen.
8. Transport the patient as soon as possible.*
9. Monitor vital signs.

* Some EMS Systems allow for adjustments to be made prior to transport. Once the patient is in the ambulance and prepared for transport, the EMT is allowed to make adjustments to improve patient comfort and reduce muscle spasms of the abdomen and lower limb. This can be done by gently flexing the patient's legs and placing a pillow under the knees. If you are allowed to follow this protocol, a warning must be issued since the patient may have associated spinal injuries.

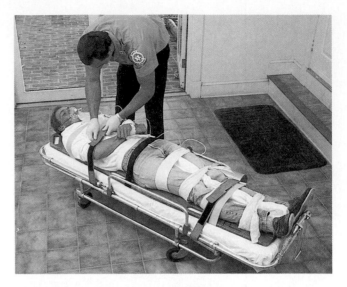

FIGURE 10–8. Immobilizing a patient with pelvic injuries on a long spine board.

NOTE: Be alert for shock and possible injury to the internal organs. Anti-shock garments may be ordered for such cases (see Chapter 7, Section Two). The garment should be placed prior to moving the patient onto the spine board.

Hip Dislocation

It is difficult to tell a hip dislocation from a fracture to the proximal femur. Conscious patients will complain of intense pain with both types of injury.

Signs

- Anterior hip dislocation—the patient's entire lower limb is rotated *outward* and the hip is usually *flexed*.
- Posterior hip dislocation (most common)— the patient's leg is rotated *inward*, the hip is flexed, and the knee is bent. The foot may hang loose (footdrop), and the patient is unable to flex the foot or lift the toes. Often, there is a lack of sensation in the limb. These signs indicate possible damage to the **sciatic** (si-AT-ik) **nerve** caused by the dislocated femoral head. This injury often occurs when a person's knees strike the dashboard during a motor vehicle accident.

Emergency Care

1. Check for circulation and nerve impairment.
2. Move patient onto a long spine board. Some systems use a scoop-style stretcher. When

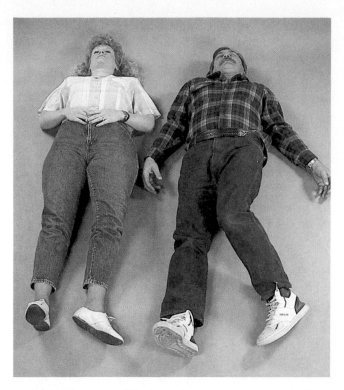

FIGURE 10–9. Signs of anterior and posterior hip dislocation.

this device is used, the limb should be immobilized (see Step 3) prior to placing the patient on the stretcher.

3. Immobilize the limb with pillows or rolled blankets.
4. Secure the patient to the board with straps or cravats.
5. Reassess circulation and nerve function. IF PULSE OR SENSORY PROBLEM, NOTIFY MEDICAL FACILITY and transport immediately.
6. Care for shock, providing a high concentration of oxygen.
7. Transport carefully, monitor vital signs, and continue to check for nerve and circulation impairment.

NOTE: If the head of the femur slides or pops back into place, note this on the patient form and report the event to the emergency department staff so that the previous dislocation does not go unnoticed.

Hip Fractures

A hip fracture is a fracture to the uppermost portion of the femur, not to the pelvis. The fracture can occur to the femoral head, femoral neck, or at the proximal end of the femur, just below the neck of the bone. Direct force (motor vehicle accidents) and twisting forces (falls) can cause a hip fracture. Elderly people are more susceptible to this type of injury due to brittle bones or bones weakened by disease. Consider the pathophysiology that may have caused the fall in an elderly patient.

Symptoms and Signs

- Pain is localized, but some patients complain of pain in the knee.
- Sometimes the patient is sensitive to pressure exerted on the lateral prominence of the hip (greater trochanter).
- Surrounding tissues are discolored. This may be delayed.
- Swelling is evident.
- Patient is unable to move limb while on his back.
- Patient complains about being unable to stand.
- Foot on injured side *usually* turns outward; however, it may rotate inward (rarely).
- Injured limb may appear shorter.

Emergency Care

Be certain to check for nerve and circulatory impairment. This must be continued during transport. The patient should be managed for shock and be administered oxygen at a high concentration. It is recommended that the patient be placed on a spine board or orthopedic stretcher after splinting.

One of the following methods can be used to stabilize a hip fracture:

- Bind the legs together: Place a folded blanket between the patient's legs and bind the legs together with wide straps, Velcro-equipped straps, or wide cravats. Carefully place the patient on a long spine board and use pillows to support the lower limbs. Secure the patient to the board. An orthopedic stretcher can be used in place of the long spine board.
- Padded boards: Push cravats or straps under the patient at the natural voids (small of the back and back of the knees) and readjust them so that they will pass across the chest, the abdomen, just below the belt, below the crotch, above and below the knee, and at the ankle. Use thin splints to push the cravats or straps under the patient to avoid the unnecessary moving of the patient.

  Splint with two long padded boards. Ideally, one padded board should be long enough

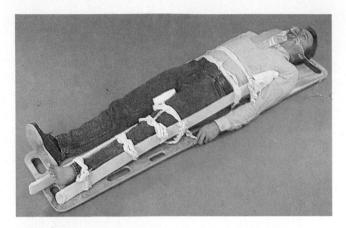

FIGURE 10–10. Long board splinting for a fractured hip.

to extend from the patient's armpit to beyond the foot. Splint with another padded board that is long enough to extend from the crotch to beyond the foot. Cushion with padding in the armpit and crotch and pad all voids created at the ankle and knee. Secure the boards with the cravats or straps.

- Traction splinting (see SCANS 10–1 A and B and 10–2)*: This procedure is acceptable for most patients. Many systems recommend this method for the elderly patient only if transport is to take more than 30 minutes or will be very rough.

    Traction splinting usually reduces patient pain and will help reduce muscle spasms in the lower limb.

- Apply an anti-shock garment if indicated as per local protocols (see Chapter 7, Section Two). Usually, this requires a fall in blood pressure.

Femoral Shaft Injuries

Symptoms and Signs

- Pain, often intense
- Often there will be an open fracture with deformity and sometimes with the end of the bone protruding through the wound. When the injury is a closed fracture, there will be deformity with possible severe angulation.
- The injured limb may appear to be shortened.

* Most EMS Systems restrict the use of the traction splint to the care for patients who have possible fractures to the *shaft* of the femur.

WARNING: Studies of mechanisms of injury indicate that pediatric patients with fractured femurs often have injury to internal organs.

Emergency Care

As soon as possible, the patient should be managed for shock and provided a high concentration of oxygen. Check circulatory and nerve impairment, then apply a **traction splint.** See SCANS 10–1 A and B and 10–2 for the procedures and variations in procedures for applying a traction splint. Whenever possible, three rescuers should be used to apply the splint. This allows one rescuer to support the injury site when the limb is lifted to place the splint.

If traction splint is not available, bind the legs together after placing them in anatomical position and checking for pulse and sensation.

NOTE: Most of the splints in use today require that the patient's shoe be removed for proper traction splinting. With some older splints, the patient's shoe may remain in place if neurologic and pulse assessment is possible, the shoe will not prevent the ankle hitch from being properly placed, and it will not slip off after mechanical traction is applied.

Knee Injuries

The knee is a *joint* and not a single bone. Fractures can occur to the distal femur, to the proximal tibia and fibula, and to the patella (kneecap). What may appear to be a dislocation may prove to be a fracture or a combined fracture and dislocation. Even if you believe that the patient has suffered a dislocated patella and the kneecap has repositioned itself, realize that other damage may be hidden. Always manage as if there is a fracture and transport.

Symptoms and Signs

- Pain and tenderness
- Deformity with obvious swelling

Emergency Care

DO NOT ATTEMPT TO STRAIGHTEN ANGULATIONS if there is evidence of dislocation of the knee. Remember to check for circulatory and nerve impairment. If there is no indication of dislocation, an attempt may be made to place the leg in anatomical position if this is required to move or otherwise manage the patient. DO NOT FORCE THE LEG. Stop if there is any resistance or increase in pain for the patient. Make only one attempt to straighten the leg. If this attempt fails, call the emergency department physician.

SCAN 10–1A   THE HARE TRACTION SPLINT—PREPARING THE SPLINT

1

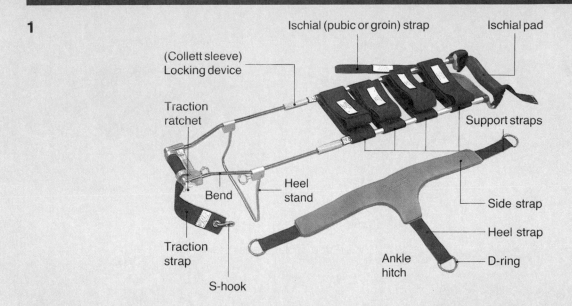

Ischial (pubic or groin) strap

Ischial pad

(Collett sleeve) Locking device

Traction ratchet

Support straps

Bend

Heel stand

Side strap

Traction strap

Heel strap

Ankle hitch

D-ring

S-hook

2

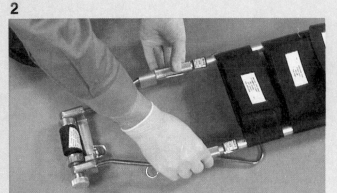

Loosen sleeve locking device.

3

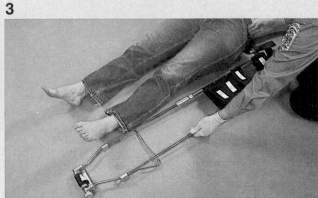

Place next to uninjured leg—ischial pad next to iliac crest.

4

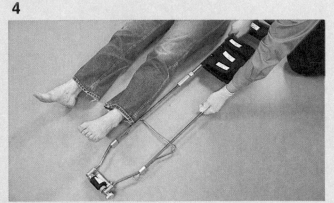

Hold top and move bottom until bend is at heel.

5

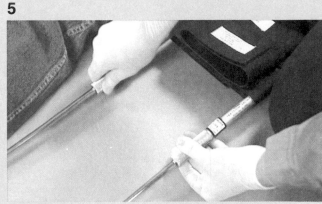

Lock sleeve.

NOTE: Some splints in use are measured by placing the ring at the level of the bony prominence that can be felt in the middle of each buttock (ischial [IS-ki-al] tuberosity) and the distal end of the splint placed 8 to 10 inches beyond the foot.

(Scan continues on next page.)

6

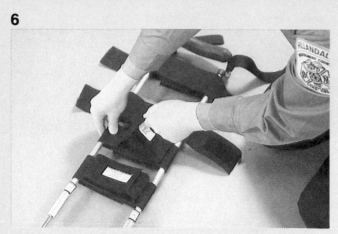

Open support straps.

7

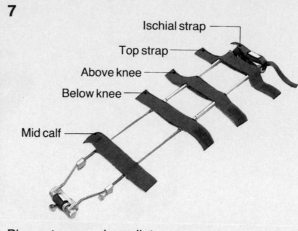

Ischial strap
Top strap
Above knee
Below knee
Mid calf

Place straps under splint.

8

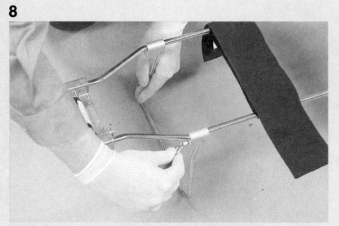

Extend and position heel stand.

9

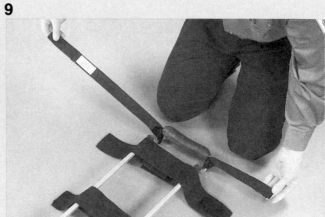

Release ischial strap. Attached ends should be next to ischial pad.

10

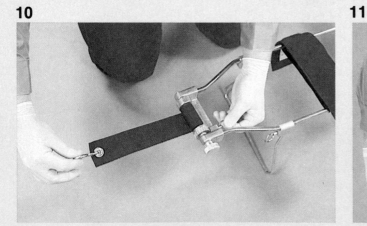

Pull release ring on ratchet and . . .

11

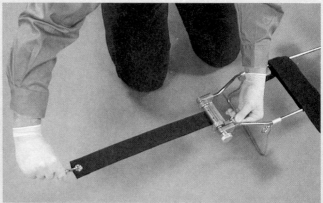

. . . Release the traction strap.

NOTE: Traction splints vary depending on the manufacturer. Learn to use the equipment supplied in your area and keep up to date with new equipment as it is approved for use.

SCAN 10–1B TRACTION SPLINTING

WARNING: Do not attempt to manually correct angulated fractures of the femur.

1

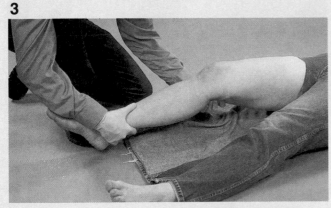

EMT 1 stabilizes limb, assesses nerve function, and palpates distal pulse while EMT 2 cuts trouser leg to expose injury site. Open wounds are dressed.

2

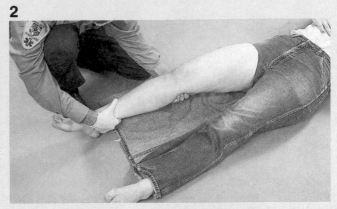

EMT 1 applies manual traction, pulling with both hands and lifting limb about 10 inches off ground.

3

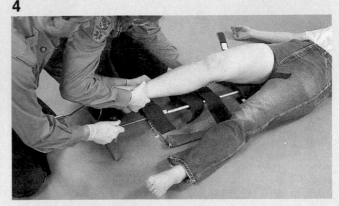

EMT 1 braces self and holds traction throughout splinting.

4

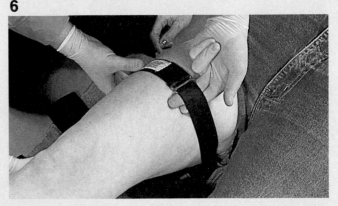

EMT 2 places splint with ischial pad against bony prominence of buttocks (ischial tuberosity).

5

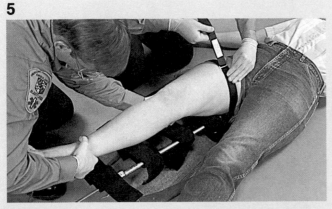

EMT 2 attaches ischial strap—over groin and thigh. (Be careful of genitalia.) Some systems require padding under the strap.

6

Buckle strap and test tightness—two fingers should fit under buckle.

(Scan continues on next page)

7

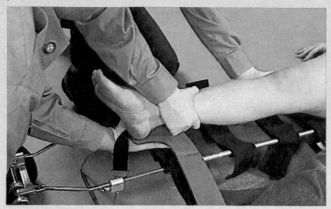

EMT 2 wraps sized ankle hitch—base of "T" at heel . . . top of "T" at ankle.

8

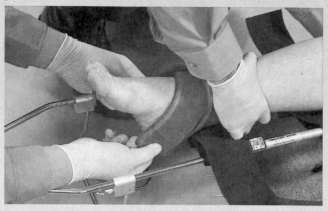

Side straps are crossed over ankle.

9

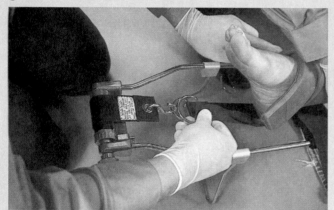

EMT 2 inserts S-hooks into D-rings, starting with heel ring.

10

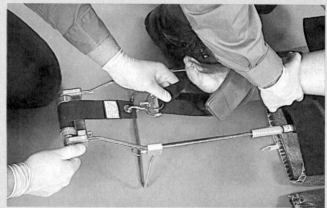

EMT 2 begins to apply mechanical traction while EMT 1 gently lowers limb onto splint.

11A

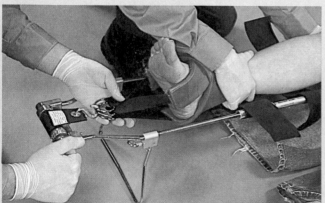

Apply full traction: conscious patient—until manual traction is equalled and pain and muscle spasms are reduced.

11B

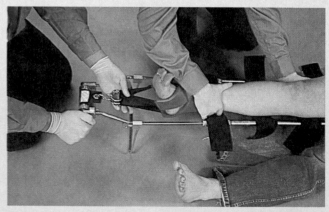

Apply full traction: unconscious patient—until splint equals manual traction . . . The injured limb will be about the same length as the uninjured one.

12

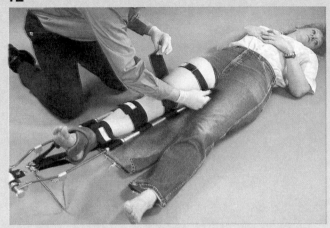

Remaining straps are snugly applied.

13

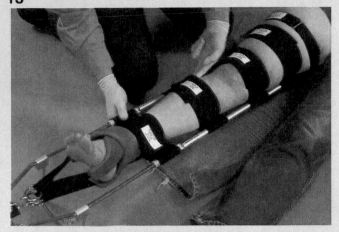

Check all straps. Patient's foot should be upright.

14

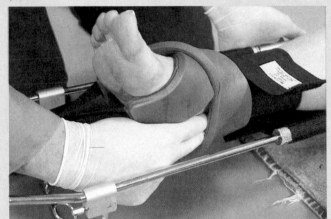

Reassess neurologic function and distal pulse.

15

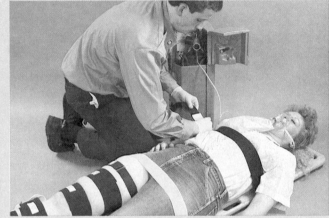

Place patient on long spine board.

16

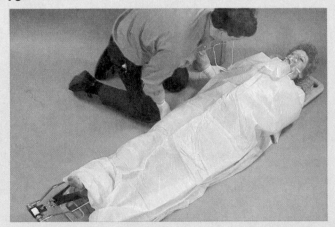

Care for shock and continue to provide a high concentration of oxygen.

17

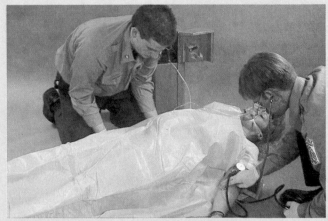

Continue to monitor splint and vital signs.

SCAN 10–2 TRACTION SPLINTING

Variations

1

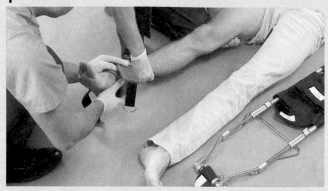

Some systems attach the ankle hitch prior to applying manual traction. EMT 1 should apply the hitch while EMT 2 stabilizes the limb.

2A

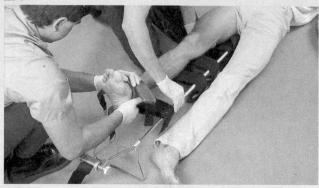

While EMT 1 applies manual traction, EMT 2 can support the injured thigh and position the splint.

2B

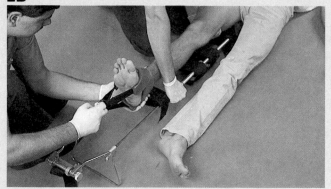

Some systems allow manual traction to be applied by grasping the D-ring and ankle.

3

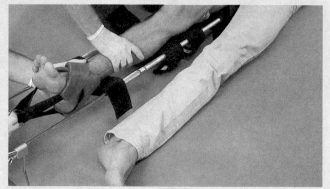

EMT 1 maintains manual traction and lowers the limb onto the cradles of the splint.

4

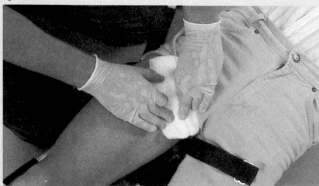

While EMT 1 maintains manual traction, EMT 2 applies padding to the groin area before securing the ischial strap. Note: Some EMS systems do not apply padding in order to reduce slippage.

5

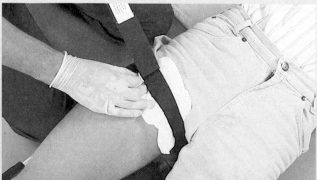

EMT 2 secures the ischial strap, connects the ankle hitch to the windlass, tightens the ratchet to equal manual traction, and secures the cradle straps.

The Sagar Splint

1

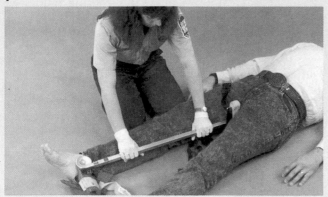

Splint will be placed medially.

2

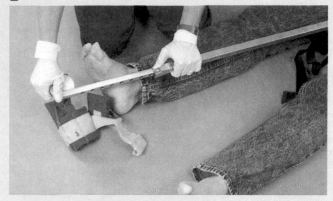

Length should be from groin to 4 inches past heel. Unlock to slide.

3

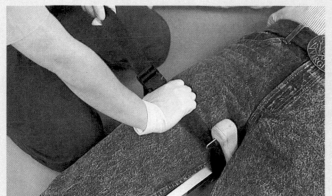

Secure thigh strap.

4

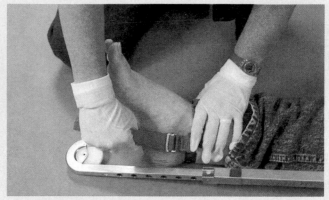

Wrap ankle harness above ankle (malleoi) and secure under heel.

5

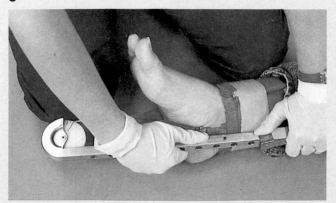

Release lock and extend splint to achieve desired traction (in pounds on pulley wheel).

6

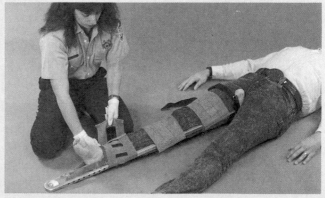

Secure straps at thigh, lower thigh and knee, and lower leg. Strap ankles and feet together. Secure to spine board.

Once splinting is done, monitor the patient. If there is a loss of distal pulse, a loss of sensation, or if the foot becomes discolored (white, mottled or blue, or a loss of tone) and turns cold, transport the patient without delay. Notify the emergency department while en route.

- Knee Bent—Immobilize in the position in which the leg is found if resistance and pain prevent straightening. Tie two padded board splints to the thigh and above the ankle so that the knee is held in position (Scan 10–3). A pillow can be used to support the leg.
- Knee Straight or Returned to Anatomical Position—Immobilize with two padded board splints or a single padded splint and an ankle hitch (Scans 10–4 through 10–6). When using two padded boards, one medial and one lateral offer the best support. Remember to pad the voids created at the knee and ankle.

Injuries to the Leg

Symptoms and Signs

- Pain and tenderness
- Swelling (other deformity is often absent)

Emergency Care

1. Check for circulatory and nerve impairment.
2. Splint by using an air-inflated splint, a gutter splint, the two-splint method, or a single splint with an ankle hitch.
   - Apply an air-inflated splint (Figure 10–11). Slide the uninflated splint over your hand and gather it in place until the lower edge clears your wrist. Grasp the patient's foot with one hand and his leg just above the injury site using your free hand. While maintaining manual traction, have your partner slide the splint over your hand and onto the injured leg. Your partner must make sure that the splint is relatively wrinkle free and that it covers the injury site. Continue to maintain traction while your partner inflates the splint. Test to see if you can cause a slight dent in the plastic with fingertip pressure. Remember to check periodically to see that the pressure in the splint has remained adequate and

has not decreased or increased. Note that there are problems associated with the use and removal of this type of splint. See the warnings in Chapter 9 (p. 264) concerning the use of air-inflated splints.
   - You can immobilize the fracture using two rigid board splints (Scan 10–7).
   - A single splint with an ankle hitch can be applied (Scan 10–8).

Regardless of the technique used, you *must* check for circulation and nerve function after immobilization is completed, care for shock, administer a high concentration of oxygen, and monitor distal pulse, neurologic function, and vital signs.

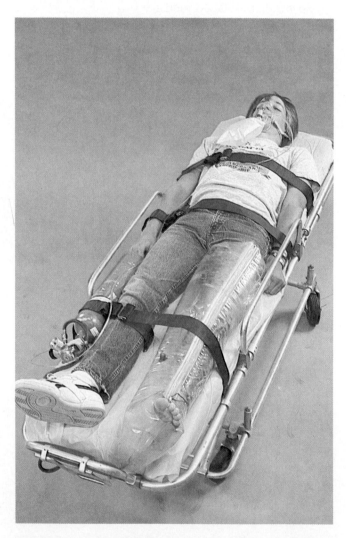

FIGURE 10–11. Using an air-inflated splint for lower leg fractures.

SCAN 10–3 KNEE INJURIES—BENT KNEE

Two Splint Method

If there is a distal pulse and neurologic function, or the limb cannot be straightened without meeting resistance or causing severe pain, knee injuries should be splinted with the knee in the position in which it is found.

1

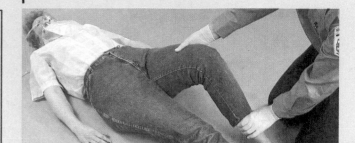

Without applying traction, attempt to place the knee in anatomical position if allowed to do so in your EMS system. If this fails . . .

2

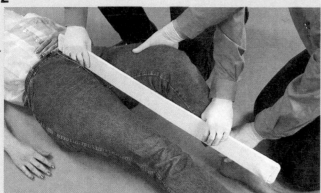

The splints should be equal and extend 6–12″ beyond the mid thigh and mid calf.

3

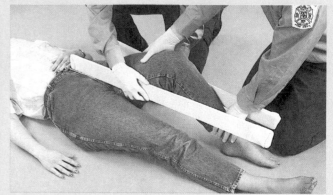

Place padded side of splints medially and laterally.

4

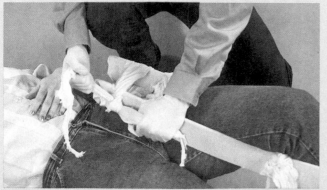

Use folded cravats . . . Tie two to each end of the splints. Tie knots over board.

5

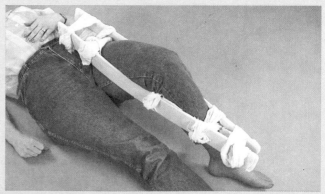

Slip another cravat through the knee void and tie the boards together.

SCAN 10–4 KNEE INJURIES—KNEE STRAIGHT

Single Splint Method

1

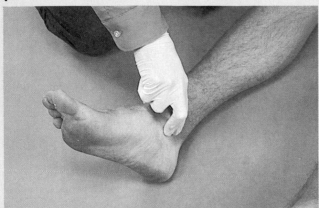

Assess distal pulse and nerve function.

2

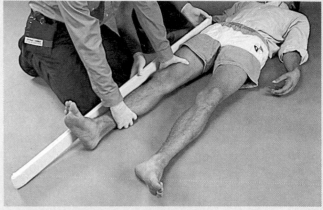

Use a padded board splint that extends from buttocks to 4″ beyond heel.

3

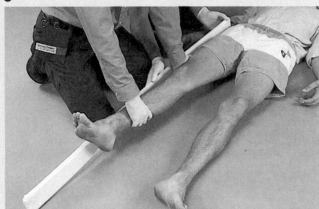

Stabilize and lift the limb.

4

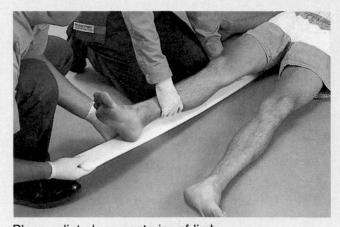

Place splint along posterior of limb.

5

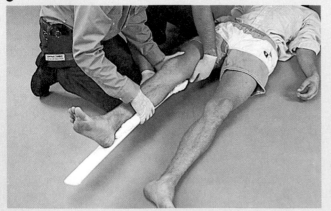

Pad voids.

6

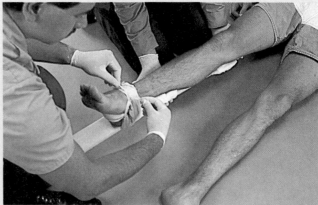

Apply an ankle hitch (see Scan 10.5).

7

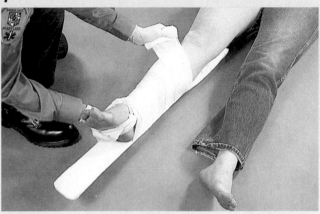

Use 6″ self-adherent roller bandage . . . Apply distal to proximal, or use cravats.

8

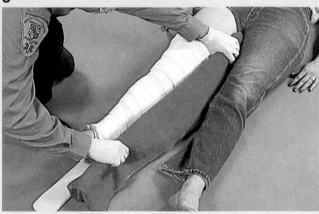

Place folded blanket between legs . . . groin to feet.

9

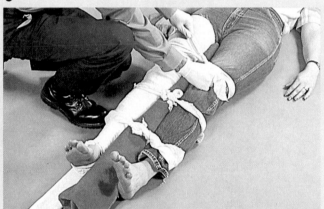

Tie thighs, calves, and ankles together . . . knot over uninjured limb.

10

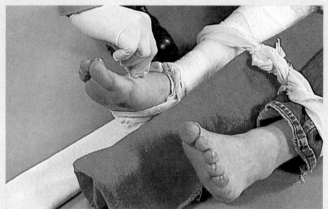

Reassess distal pulse and nerve function.

11

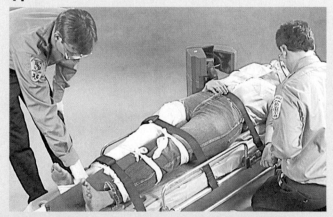

Care for shock and continue to provide a high concentration of oxygen.

12

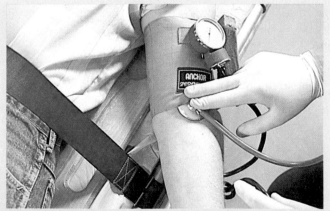

Monitor distal pulse and vital signs.

SCAN 10—5 THE ANKLE HITCH

The ankle hitch can be used with a single padded board splint to immobilize injured knees and legs. It is made with a 3-inch-wide cravat.

1

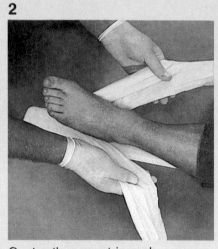

Kneel at distal end of injured limb.

2

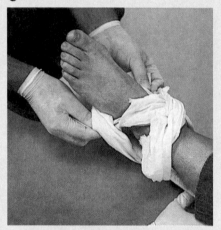

Center the cravat in arch.

3

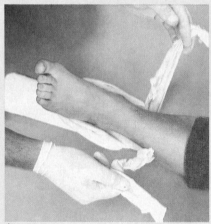

Place cravat along sides of foot and cross cravat behind ankle.

4

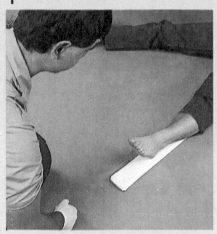

Cross the cravat ends over top of ankle.

5

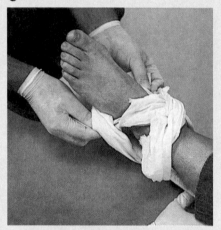

A stirrup has been formed.

6

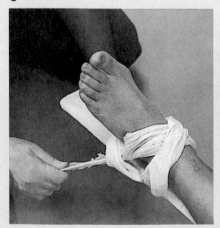

Thread ends through stirrup.

7

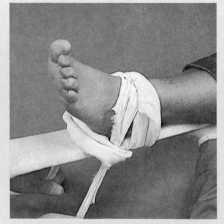

Pull ends downward to tighten.

8

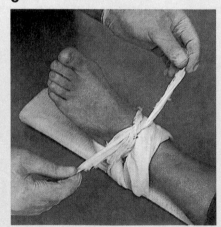

Pull upward and tie over ankle wrap.

SCAN 10–6 KNEE INJURIES—KNEE
STRAIGHT OR RETURNED—Two Splint Method

1

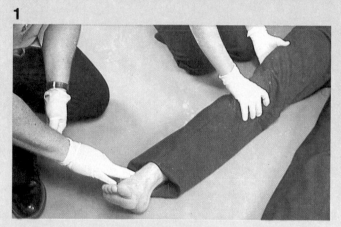

Assess distal pulse and nerve function.

2

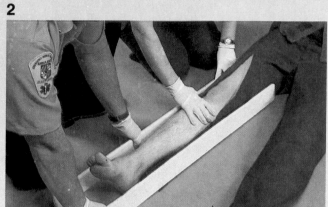

Select two padded board splints. Medial = groin to 4″ beyond foot. Lateral = iliac crest to 4″ beyond foot.

3

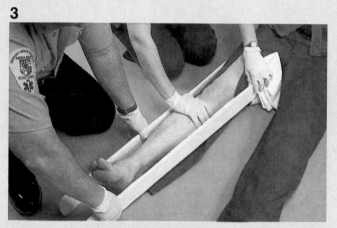

Stabilize the limb and pad groin.

4

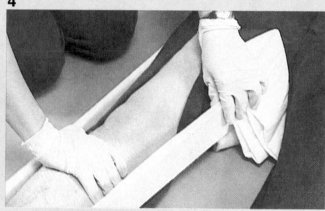

Position splints.

5

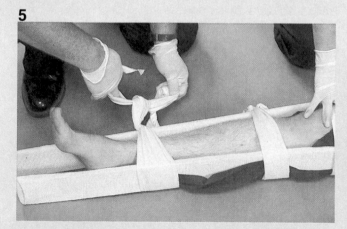

Secure splints at thigh, above and below knee, and at mid calf. Pad voids.

6

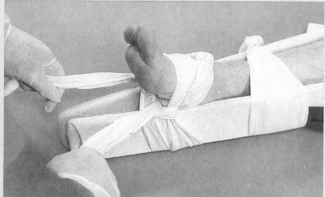

Cross and tie two cravats at the ankle or hitch the ankle.

Remember to reassess distal pulse and nerve function. Care for shock and continue to provide a high concentration of oxygen.

1

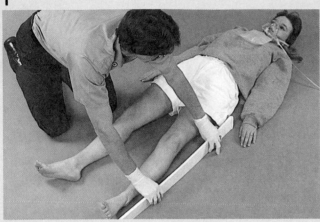

Measure splint—it should extend above the knee and below the ankle.

2

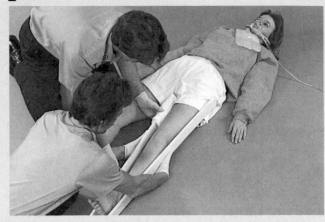

Apply manual traction and place one splint medially and one laterally . . . padding is toward the leg.

3

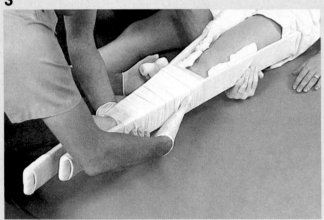

Secure splints distal to proximal, padding voids.

4

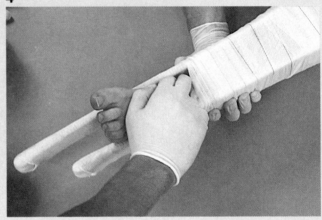

Reassess distal pulse and nerve function.

5

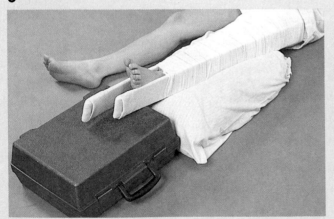

Elevate once immobilized

6

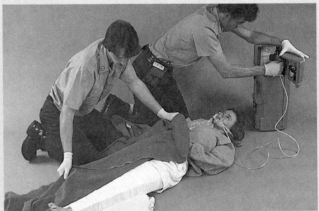

Care for shock and continue to administer a high concentration of oxygen.

SCAN 10–8 LEG INJURIES—SINGLE SPLINT METHOD

1

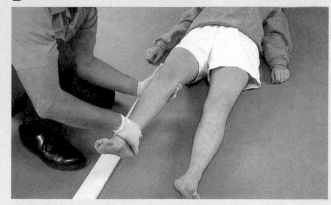

Measure splint—it should extend from mid thigh to 4 inches below ankle.

2

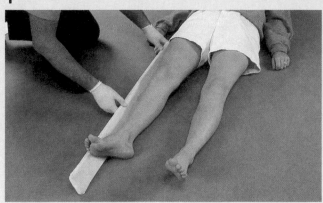

Apply manual traction and lift limb 10 inches off ground.

3

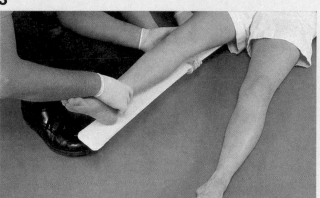

Place splint along the posterior of the limb, at mid thigh.

4

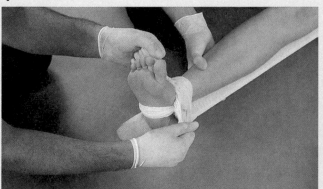

Apply ankle hitch (see scan 10.5).

5

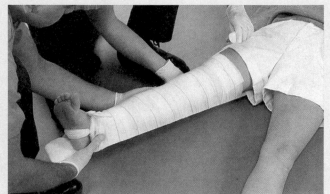

Secure, distal to proximal.

NOTE: Reassess distal pulse and nerve function. Elevate the injured limb, care for shock, and continue to administer a high concentration of oxygen.

SCAN 10–9 THE EXTREMITIES—SELECT MECHANISMS OF INJURY

MECHANISM OF INJURY—

The force that produced the injury, its intensity and direction, and the area of the body that is affected.

DIRECT FORCE—

Any bone or joint can be injured by the direct force produced in a fall, striking an object, or being struck by an object.

DOWNWARD BLOW –
Clavicule
and
Scapula

LATERAL BLOW –
Clavicule
Scapula
and
Humerus

FORCED FLEXION
OR
HYPEREXTENSION –
Elbow
Wrist
Fingers
Femur
Knee
Foot

TWISTING FORCE –
Hip
Femur
Knee
Leg bones
Ankle
Shoulder
Elbow
Forearm
Wrist

INDIRECT
FORCE –
Pelvis
Hip
Knee
Leg bones
Shoulder
Humerus
Elbow
Forearm bones

LATERAL BLOW –
Knee
Hip
Femur
(Very forceful)

Injuries to the Ankle and Foot

Symptoms and Signs

It is often difficult to distinguish between fractures and sprains to the foot or ankle. Pain and swelling characterize both injuries.

Emergency Care

Long splints, extending from above the knee to beyond the foot, can be used. However, soft splinting is an effective, rapid method and is recommended for most patients (Figure 10–12). To soft splint, you should:

1. Assess distal pulse and nerve function.
2. Stabilize the limb.
3. Remove the patient's shoe if possible, but only if it removes easily and can be done with no movement to the ankle.
4. Lift the limb, but *do not* apply traction.
5. Place three cravats under the ankle.
6. Place a pillow, lengthwise under the ankle, on top of the cravats. The pillow should extend 6 inches beyond the foot.
7. Gently lower the limb onto the pillow and stabilize by tying the cravats.
8. Adjust the cravats so that they are at the top of the pillow, midway, and at the heel.
9. Tie the pillow to the ankle and foot, distal to proximal.
10. Tie a fourth cravat at the arch of the foot.
11. Elevate with a second pillow.
12. Reassess distal pulse and nerve function.
13. Care for shock if needed. If there are no other injuries, and no symptoms or signs of shock, oxygen is usually not administered. Some EMS Systems now recommend that oxygen be provided at a high concentration for all patients who may have any possible fractures.

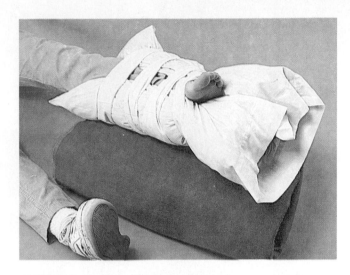

FIGURE 10–12. Pillow splinting an injured ankle.

NOTE: Take care not to change the position of the ankle if there is a distal pulse.

SUMMARY

Each lower extremity consists of the femur, patella, fibula, tibia, tarsals, metatarsals, and phalanges. Each femur joins with the pelvis.

There are some SPECIAL SIGNS you need to know:

- Pelvic pain when you compress the patient's hips = pelvic fracture.
- Pelvic injury with patient's foot turning outward = pelvic fracture.
- Lower limb rotates outward = possible anterior hip dislocation, hip fracture, or pelvic fracture.
- Lower limb rotates inward and knee and hip are bent = possible posterior hip dislocation or hip fracture.

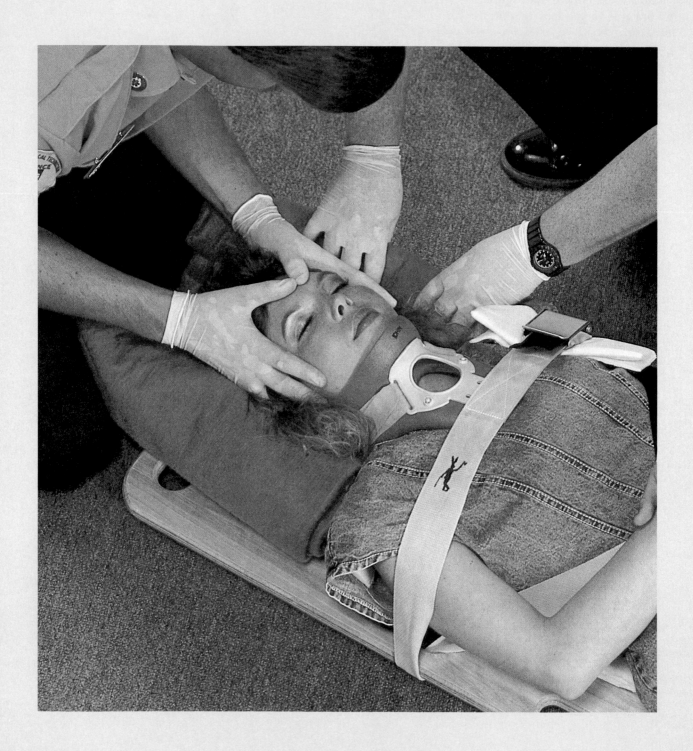

Injuries III:
The skull and spine

OBJECTIVES   As an EMT, you should be able to:

1. Define *axial skeleton*. (p. 296)
2. Distinguish between cranium and face. (p. 296)
3. Define *suture*, *cranial floor*, *temporal bone*, *mandible*, *maxillae*, and *temporomandibular joint*. (pp. 296–297)
4. Name and label the FIVE major divisions of the spinal column. (p. 297)
5. Define *central nervous system*. (p. 297)
6. Define *open head injury*, *closed head injury*, *direct brain injury*, and *indirect brain injury*. (p. 299)
7. List the basic symptoms and signs of possible skull fracture, facial fracture, and brain injury. (pp. 300–302)
8. List, step by step, the care for injury to the cranium and for injury to the facial bones. (pp. 302–305)
9. List the steps for caring for a fracture or dislocation of the mandible. (p. 306)
10. Describe how to remove a helmet from an injured patient. (p. 306)
11. List the types of injuries to the spine and relate these injuries to mechanisms of injury. (p. 306)
12. State how to determine possible spinal injury in the conscious patient. (p. 309)
13. State how to determine possible spinal injury in the unconscious patient. (pp. 310–311)
14. Describe how to apply a rigid cervical or extrication collar. (pp. 313–316)
15. Describe and compare the four-rescuer and the two-rescuer log roll for transferring a patient to a long spine board. (pp. 317–319)
16. Describe how a patient should be secured to a long spine board. (pp. 318–319)
17. Describe, step by step, how to secure a patient to a short spine board and remove him from a vehicle. (pp. 321–323); describe how to apply a vest-style extrication device (pp. 323–324)

SKILLS   As an EMT, you should be able to:

1. Apply patient assessment techniques to detect possible:

• Cranial fractures
• Facial fractures

- Brain injury
- Spinal injury

2. Provide emergency care for patients with possible fractured skulls or facial injuries.
3. Provide emergency care for patients with possible brain injury.
4. Apply an extrication collar and transfer and secure a patient to a long spine board.
5. Apply an extrication collar and a short spine board or extrication device to a patient found in a vehicle or confined space and move the patient to a long spine board.

TERMS you may be using for the first time:

Central Nervous System – the brain and spinal cord.

Concussion – mild closed head injury without detectable damage to the brain. Complete recovery is usually expected.

Epidural Hematoma (ep-i-DU-ral he-mah-TOH-mah) – formed when blood from ruptured vessels flows between the meninges and the cranial bones.

Extrication Collar – a rigid device applied around the neck to help immobilize the head and neck.

Intracerebral Hematoma (in-trah-SER-e-bral he-mah-TOH-mah) – formed when blood from ruptured vessels pools within the brain.

Malar (MA-lar) or **Zygomatic** (zi-go-MAT-ik) **Bone** – the cheek bone.

Mandible (MAN-di-bl) – the lower jaw bone.

Maxillae (mak-SIL-e) – the two fused bones forming the upper jaw.

Meninges (me-NIN-jez) – the three-layered membrane that surrounds the brain and spinal cord.

Temporal (TEM-po-ral) **Bones** – two bones that form part of the lateral walls of the skull and the floor of the cranial cavity. There is a right and a left temporal bone.

Temporomandibular (TEM-po-ro-man-DIB-u-lar) **Joint** – the movable joint formed between mandible and temporal bone.

Spinous Processes – the bony extensions of the posterior vertebrae.

Subdural Hematoma (sub-DU-ral he-mah-TOH-mah) – formed when blood from ruptured vessels flows between the brain and the meninges.

Suture – where two bones of the skull articulate (join) to form an immovable joint.

THE AXIAL SKELETON

In Chapter 9, we divided the skeleton into two subdivisions: the *axial skeleton* and the *appendicular skeleton*. The axial skeleton (Figure 11–1) is composed of the skull, the **vertebral** (VER-te-bral) **column** or spinal column, the ribs, and the sternum. It makes up the longitudinal axis of the human body.

In this chapter, we will consider the skull, the vertebral column, and the close relationship of the axial skeleton to the nervous system. The soft tissues of the head and neck will be covered in Chapter 12. The ribs, sternum, and the remaining structures of the chest will be discussed in Chapter 13.

The Skull

The skull is made up of the **cranium** (KRAY-ni-um) and the **facial bones.** The cranial bones are fused together to form immovable joints. The point at which two bones of the cranium articulate (join together) is known as a **suture.**

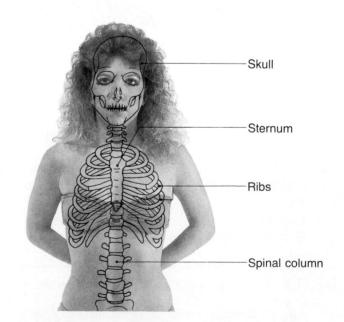

Skull

Sternum

Ribs

Spinal column

FIGURE 11–1. The axial skeleton.

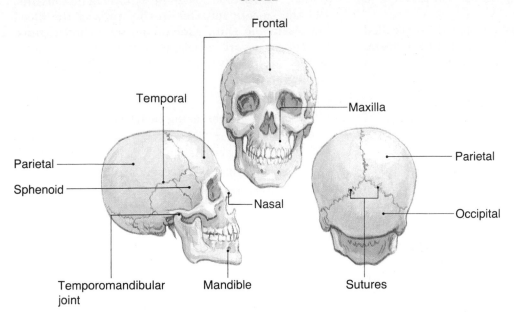

SKULL

Frontal

Temporal

Maxilla

Parietal

Sphenoid

Nasal

Parietal

Occipital

Temporomandibular
joint

Mandible

Sutures

FIGURE 11–2. The bones of the face.

There are 14 irregularly shaped bones forming the face. The facial bones are fused into immovable joints, except for the **mandible** (MAN-di-bl). It joins on each side of the cranium with a **temporal** (TEM-por-al) **bone** to form the **temporomandibular** (TEM-po-ro-man-DIB-u-lar) **joint.** This joint is sometimes referred to as the TM joint.

The upper jaw is made up of two fused bones called the **maxillae** (mak-SIL-e). Each is known as a *maxilla* (mak-SIL-ah). The upper third, or bridge, of the nose contains two **nasal bones.** There is a cheek bone on each side of the skull. The cheek bone can be called the **malar** (MA-lar) or the **zygomatic** (zi-go-MAT-ik) **bone.** The malars and the maxillae form a portion of the **orbits** (sockets) of the eyes.

The Spinal Column

The divisions of the spinal column were presented in Chapter 9. Figure 11–3 serves to review these divisions.

THE NERVOUS SYSTEM

When evaluating a patient for injuries to the head and spine, always consider the possibility of nervous system damage. The same holds true for many types of chest injuries, since the thoracic spine also may have been injured. Of course, injury to the chest can damage the chest nerves.

Anatomically, the nervous system is divided into two systems: (1) the central nervous system

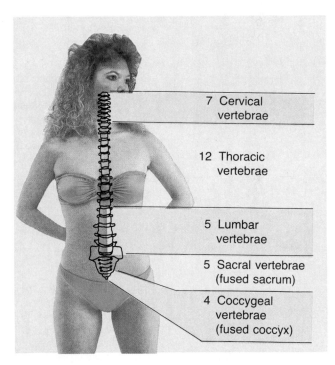

7 Cervical vertebrae

12 Thoracic vertebrae

5 Lumbar vertebrae

5 Sacral vertebrae (fused sacrum)

4 Coccygeal vertebrae (fused coccyx)

FIGURE 11–3. The divisions of the spinal column.

(CNS) and (2) the peripheral nervous system (PNS). The **central nervous system** consists of the brain and the spinal cord. The **peripheral nervous system** includes the nerves that enter and leave the spinal cord and those nerves that travel between the brain and organs without passing through the spinal cord (e.g., the optic nerve between the eye and brain). Messages sent from the body to the brain are carried by sensory nerves. The nerves sending messages from the brain to the muscles and organs are called motor nerves. There are voluntary and involuntary pathways.

The nervous system has a special division called the **autonomic** (aw-toh-NOM-ik) **nervous system.** The motor nerves of this system connect the brain and spinal cord to the heart muscle (myocardium), glands, smooth muscles in the walls of hollow organs, and the smooth muscles in the walls of the blood vessels in the skin, skeletal muscles, and organs. For the most part, messages sent along these motor nerves are involuntary. Autonomic functions include:

• Slowing or increasing heart rate
• Increasing or decreasing the strength of heart contractions
• Constricting blood vessels in the skin
• Constricting or dilating blood vessels in skeletal muscles
• Dilating or constricting blood vessels in the abdominal organs
• Changing bronchial diameter
• Contracting and relaxing the urinary bladder
• Dilating or constricting the pupils of the eye
• Increasing or decreasing the secretion of saliva and digestive juices.

Any injury that interferes with or stops a given autonomic function can be life threatening.

The brain is the master organ of life, the center of consciousness, self-awareness, and thought. It controls basic functions, including breathing, and to some degree, heart activity. Messages from all over the body are received by the brain, which decides how to respond to changing conditions both inside and outside the body. The brain sends messages to the muscles so that we can move, or to a particular organ so that it will carry out a desired function. Any major skull injury can cause damage to the brain, causing vital body functions to fail.

The spinal cord is a relay between most of the body and the brain. A large number of the messages to and from the brain are sent through the spinal cord. Damage to the cord can isolate a part of the body from the brain. Function of this part can be lost, possibly forever.

Reflexes allow us to react quickly to such things as pain and excessive heat, without the brain having to send orders. The spinal cord is the center of reflex activity. Damage to the cord can destroy reflex function in certain areas of the body.

The healing power of the brain and nerve tissue is limited. Once this tissue is damaged to a certain extent, function is lost and cannot be restored. As an EMT, your initial care will often prevent additional damage to the brain, spinal cord, and major nerves of the body.

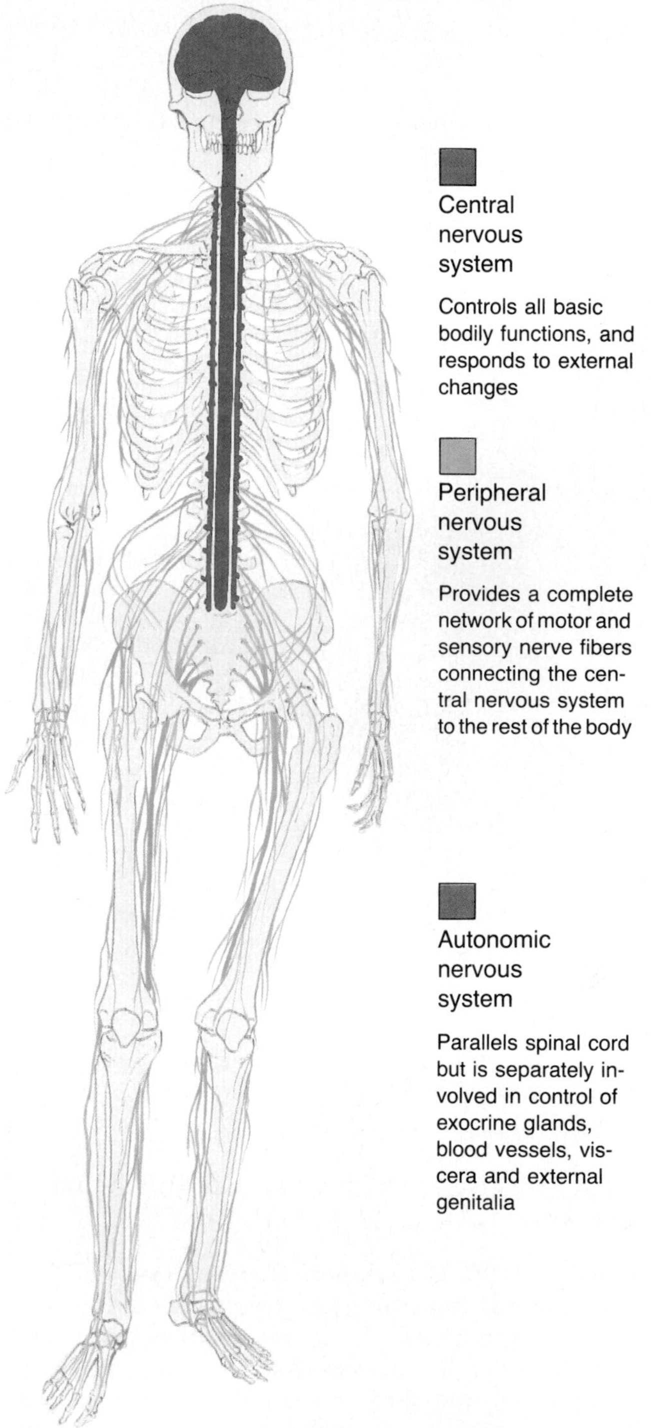

■ Central nervous system

Controls all basic bodily functions, and responds to external changes

■ Peripheral nervous system

Provides a complete network of motor and sensory nerve fibers connecting the central nervous system to the rest of the body

■ Autonomic nervous system

Parallels spinal cord but is separately involved in control of exocrine glands, blood vessels, viscera and external genitalia

FIGURE 11–4.   Anatomy of the nervous system.

INJURIES TO THE SKULL AND BRAIN

NOTE: Indications of possible injury to the skull or brain should alert you to the strong possibility of cervical spine injury.

Types of Injuries

Skull injuries include fractures to the cranium and fractures to the face. If severe enough, these injuries can include direct and indirect injuries to the brain. In addition, there can be cuts to the scalp and other soft tissue injuries as covered in Chapters 8 and 12.

A practical classification of injuries to the skull corresponds to the classification of fractures and wounds, namely, either open or closed. However, the words "open" and "closed" refer to the skull bones. When the bones of the cranium are fractured, if the dura is broken, the patient has an **open head injury.** In a closed head injury, there may be a laceration of the scalp; however, if the cranium is intact, or free of fractures, the term **closed head injury** is used.

There are four major types of skull fractures. A *linear skull fracture* is a thin line crack in the cranium. A *comminuted* (KOM-i-nu-ted) *skull fracture* has cracks radiating out from the center of the point of impact. A *depressed skull fracture* is one in which bone fragments are separated from the skull and driven inward by the object that struck the head. Fractures to the cranial floor are called *basal skull fractures*. Analysis by a physician is needed to detect these fractures; however, clear or bloody fluids in the nose and ears suggests a basal skull fracture.

Sometimes the term *penetrated skull* will be used as a fifth type of skull fracture. This is actually a type of injury, not a type of fracture. It can be caused by bullets, knife blades, or some other object penetrating the cranial bones. A penetrated skull injury may produce any or all of the four types of skull fracture.

Facial fractures are usually produced by an impact, as when a child is struck in the face by a baseball bat or when someone is thrown against the windshield during a motor vehicle crash. These fractures can be so simple that they go undetected, or they may produce serious, grotesque injuries. Of primary concern is the state of the patient's airway. Bone fragments may lodge in the back of the throat, causing airway obstruction. Blood, blood clots, and dislodged teeth also may cause partial or total airway obstruction. Facial fractures are often associated with fractures of the cranial floor.

Brain injuries can be classified as direct or indirect. *Direct* injuries can occur in open head injuries, with the brain being lacerated, punctured, or bruised by the broken bones of the skull, by bone fragments, or by foreign objects.

In cases of closed head injuries and certain types of open head injuries, damage to the brain can be *indirect*. The shock of impact is transferred to the brain. Like any other mass of tissue, the brain swells when it is injured. This swelling is serious since there is little room for expansion within the cranium. Indirect injuries to the brain include:

- **Concussion**—A concussion may be so mild that the patient is unaware of the injury. When a person strikes his head in a fall, or is struck by a blunt object, a certain amount of the force is transferred through the skull to the brain. Usually there is no detectable damage to the brain and the patient may or may not become unconscious. Most patients with a concussion will feel a little "groggy" after receiving a blow to the head. Headache is common. If there is a loss of consciousness, it usually lasts only a short time and does not tend to recur. Some loss of memory (**amnesia**) of the events surrounding the accident is fairly common. Long-term memory loss associated with concussion is rare.

- **Contusion**—A bruised brain can occur with closed head injuries, when the force of the blow is great enough to rupture blood vessels found on the surface of, or deep within, the brain. Since there is little space for the brain to move before striking the walls of the cranial cavity, this bruise or contusion often takes place on the side of the brain *opposite* the point of impact.

With time, as you practice emergency care, you will hear of or care for a patient with a **subdural hematoma** (sub-DU-ral he-mah-TO-mah) (Figure 11–6). When the brain is bruised, lacerated, or punctured, blood from ruptured vessels can flow between the brain and its protective covering, the **meninges** (me-NIN-jez). The thick outer layer of the meninges is known as the *dura mater*. A subdural hematoma is situated between the dura mater and the brain.

Often, this bleeding is a slow venous flow. Even when the bleeding stops, the hematoma will continue to grow in size as it absorbs tissue fluids. Since there is no room for expansion in the cranium, severe pres-

CONCUSSION

- Mild injury usually with no detectable brain damage
- Usually no loss of consciousness
- Headache, grogginess, and short term memory loss common

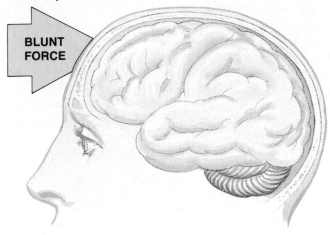

CONTUSION

- Unconsciousness or decreased level of consciousness
- Bruising or rupturing of brain tissue and vessels at any of these levels:

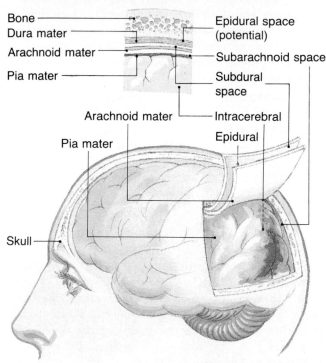

FIGURE 11–5. Closed head injuries.

sure can be placed on the brain. Death can occur if vital brain centers are damaged. This type of hematoma may occur rapidly or take a prolonged period of time to develop.

Two other types of hematomas are related to head injuries (see Figure 11–6). The **epidural** (ep-i-DU-ral) **hematoma** occurs when blood flows between the meninges and the cranial bones (above the dura). Most of this flow is profuse arterial bleeding, causing a true emergency. This type of hematoma is often associated with severe blows to the temples, in front of and just above the ears. The patient will at first be unconscious, followed by a fully conscious period (the lucid interval), only to suffer a second loss of consciousness.

An **intracerebral** (in-trah-SER-e-bral) **hematoma** occurs when blood pools within the brain itself, pushing tissues against the bones of the cranium. This can cause a stroke. Depending on the severity of injury, the time from injury to true emergency can vary greatly. Death can occur before transport.

Lacerations can occur to the brain as a result of penetrating and perforating wounds of the cranium. Not only is there the problem of direct injury, but there may also be severe indirect injury due to hematoma formation.

Symptoms and Signs of Skull Injury

NOTE: If you have reason to believe there is injury to the skull, you must assume possible cervical spine injury.

Skull Fracture

Visible bone fragments and perhaps even bits of brain tissue are the most obvious signs of skull fracture, but the majority of skull fractures do not produce these signs (Figure 11–7). You should consider the possibility of a skull fracture whenever you note:

- The patient is unconscious after injury or displays a decreased level of consciousness.
- An injury that has produced a deep laceration or severe bruise to the scalp or forehead. *Do not* probe into the wound or separate the wound opening to determine wound depth.
- Any severe pain or swelling at the site of a head injury. Pain may be a symptom of skull injury. *Do not* palpate the injury site.
- Deformity of the skull. Are there depressions in the cranium, large swellings ("goose eggs") or anything that looks unusual about the shape of the cranium?
- Any bruise or swelling behind the ear (Battle's sign). This is a late sign.
- Unequal pupils.
- Black eyes or discoloration of the soft tissues under both eyes (raccoon's eyes). This is usually a delayed finding.

Dura

Dura

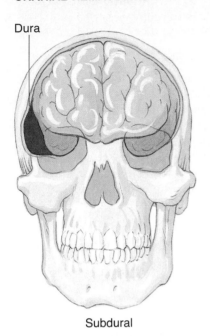

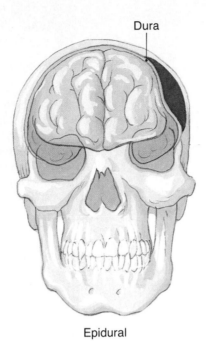

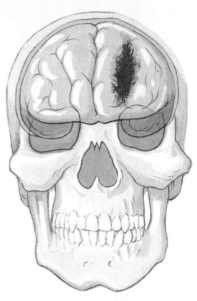

Subdural

Epidural

Intracerebral

FIGURE 11–6. Hematomas within the cranium.

- One eye appears to be sunken.
- Bleeding from the ears and/or the nose.
- Clear fluid flowing from the ears and/or the nose. This could be **cerebrospinal** (ser-e-bro-SPI-nal) **fluid,** also called CSF. This fluid surrounds the brain and spinal cord. It cannot come out through the ears or nose unless the cranium has been fractured.

If fluids coming from the ears or nose are bloody, you will not be able to tell if they contain cerebrospinal fluid unless you gently absorb some fluid onto a gauze dressing and watch the clear fluid separate out from the spot of blood ("targeting" or "halo test"). This test is not always reliable.

Facial Fractures

Consider the possibility of facial fractures when you note:

- Blood in the airway
- Facial deformities
- False face bone movements (e.g., the movement of the upper jaw bones)
- Black eyes or discoloration below the eyes
- A swollen lower jaw, poor jaw function, or poor alignment of teeth
- Teeth that are loose or have been knocked out, or broken dentures

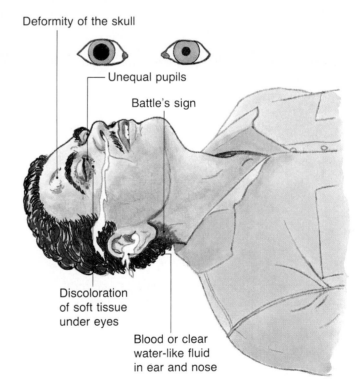

Deformity of the skull

Unequal pupils

Battle's sign

Discoloration of soft tissue under eyes

Blood or clear water-like fluid in ear and nose

FIGURE 11–7. Signs of skull fracture.

- Large facial bruises
- Any other indications of a severe blow to the face

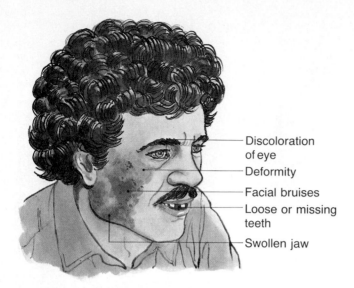

Discoloration of eye

Deformity

Facial bruises

Loose or missing teeth

Swollen jaw

FIGURE 11–8. **Signs of facial fracture.**

Symptoms and Signs of Brain Injury

In cases of head injury, you should consider the possibility of a brain injury if you note:

- Pain, ranging from a headache to severe discomfort
- Loss of consciousness, altered states of consciousness, or amnesia
- Confusion, usually increasing as time passes
- Personality changes, ranging from irritable to irrational behavior (major sign)
- Blood pressure may be elevated while the pulse rate decreases (bleeding inside the skull).
- Respirations may change patterns, becoming labored, then rapid, and then stopping for a few seconds.
- Temperature may increase (late sign due to inflammation, infection, or damage to temperature-regulating centers).
- Unequal and/or unresponsive pupils
- Vision disturbed in one or both eyes
- Hearing may be impaired, or ringing in ears may be present
- Equilibrium—patient may be unable to stand still with eyes closed or stumbles when attempting to walk (*do not* test for this)
- Vomiting (often forceful—projectile vomiting)
- Paralysis (often to one side of the body)
- Any signs of a skull fracture

- Any head injury when the patient displays a deterioration of vital signs

NOTE: Shock is not a sign of head injury.

With so many factors to consider, the mechanism of injury and the location of the injury site become very important when trying to determine if there is possible brain damage. **Some of the symptoms and signs of brain injury can cause untrained personnel to assume that a brain injury patient is merely intoxicated or abusing other drugs.** Never assume intoxication or drug abuse.

CARE FOR HEAD INJURIES

Injuries to the Cranium

The following procedures apply to patients with or without possible brain damage.

When caring for patients with injuries to the cranium, you should assume that neck or spinal injuries also exist and:

1. Ensure an open airway—Careful handling is essential since there may be associated spinal injury. For such cases, the American Heart Association guidelines call for the use of the jaw-thrust. If there are open injuries to the skull, or if skull fracture is obvious, always use the jaw-thrust technique.
2. Maintain an open airway—Monitor the conscious patient for changes in breathing. For the unconscious patient, an oropharyngeal or nasal airway should be inserted. This must be done *without* hyperextending the neck. Have suctioning equipment ready for immediate use.
3. Provide resuscitative measures if needed.
4. Keep the patient at rest. This can be a critical factor.
5. Control bleeding—Do not apply pressure if the injury site shows bone fragments or depression of the bone or if the brain is exposed. *Do not* attempt to stop the flow of blood or cerebrospinal fluid from the ears or the nose. If the skull is fractured, you may increase intracranial pressure and may also increase the risk of infection. Use a loose gauze dressing (see p. 340).
6. Administer oxygen—This is critical should

there be brain damage. Deliver as high a concentration of oxygen as possible.

7. Monitor vital signs.

8. Talk to the conscious patient. Ask him questions so that he will have to concentrate. This procedure will help you to detect changes in the patient's level of consciousness.

9. Dress and bandage open wounds, stabilizing any penetrating objects (*do not* remove any objects or fragments of bone).

10. Manage the patient for shock if present—Avoid overheating.

11. Elevate the head slightly if there is no evidence of shock.

12. Provide emotional support.

13. Position the patient properly and be prepared for vomiting.

NOTE: Some EMS Systems have adopted a special protocol for hyperventilating patients with a head injury. This protocol requires the EMT to deliver oxygen-assisted ventilations (bag-valve-mask or positive pressure) at the rate of 25+ per minute rather than the usual 12 ventilations per minute. This procedure is called "hyperventilating the patient." The hyperventilation may reduce brain tissue swelling.

WARNING: If an unconscious patient regains consciousness, only to lose consciousness again, you *must* report this to the emergency department staff. This is a strong indication of possible life-threatening brain injury.

ALL patients having head injury or suspected brain damage must be carefully monitored during transport. Have suction available at all times. Be prepared in case the patient has a seizure (see p. 406). Keep a constant watch over the patient. What you observe and report can have a great bearing on the initial actions taken by the emergency department staff.

Part of the Champion Sacco trauma score discussed in Chapter 3 was the *Glasgow Coma Scale.* Many EMS Systems use this scale to record data on patients with possible head and brain injury. The scale is shown in Table 11–1. When using this scale, remember—

1. Note if there are eye injuries or injuries to the face that prevent the patient from opening the eyes. If the injuries are more than minor ones, do not ask the patient to open his eyes.

Table 11–1. THE GLASGOW COMA SCALE

Eye opening	Spontaneous	4
	To voice	3
	To pain	2
	None	1
Verbal response	Oriented	5
	Confused	4
	Inappropriate words	3
	Incomprehensible words	2
	None	1
Motor response	Obeys command	6
	Localizes pain	5
	Withdraws from pain	4
	Flexion from pain	3
	Extension from pain	2
	None	1

Glasgow Coma Scale Points: TOTAL =

Reduction of Glasgow Coma Scale points for use in a trauma score:

$$14 - 15 = 5 \quad 5 - 7 = 2$$
$$11 - 13 = 4 \quad 3 - 4 = 1$$
$$8 - 10 = 3$$

NOTE: There are updated variations of this scale. Use the scale provided by your EMS System. See Chapter 3 (pp. 76, 78) for more information.

2. Spontaneous eye opening means that the patient has the eyes open without you having to do anything. If his eyes are closed, then you should say, "Open your eyes" to see if the patient will obey this command. Try a normal level of voice. If this fails, shout the command. Should the patient's eyes remain closed, apply an accepted painful stimulus (e.g., pinch a toe, scratch the palm or sole, rub the sternum).

3. When evaluating the patient's verbal responses, use the following:

   • Oriented—The patient, once aroused, can tell you who he is, where he is, and the year and month.

   • Confused—The patient cannot answer the above questions, but he can speak in phrases and sentences.

   • Inappropriate words—The patient says or shouts a word or several words at a time. Usually this requires physical stimulation. The words do not fit the situation or a particular question. Often, the patient curses.

   • Incomprehensible sounds—The patient responds with mumbling, moans, or groans.

   • No verbal response—Repeated stimulation, verbal and physical, does not cause the patient to speak or make any sounds.

4. The following are the criteria used to evaluate motor response:

- Obeys command—The patient must be able to understand your instruction and carry out the request. For example, you can ask (when appropriate) for the patient to hold up two fingers.
- Localizes pain—Should the patient fail to respond to your commands, apply pressure to one of the nail beds for 5 seconds or firm pressure to the sternum. Note if the patient attempts to remove your hand. *Do not* apply pressure over an injury site. *Do not* apply pressure to the sternum if the patient is experiencing difficult breathing.
- Withdraws—after painful stimulation. Note if the elbow flexes, he moves slowly, there is the appearance of stiffness, he holds his forearm and hand against the body, or if the limbs on one side of the body appear to be paralyzed (hemiplegic position).
- Extension Response—after painful stimulation. Note if the legs and arms extend, there is apparent stiffness with these moves, and if there is an internal rotation of the shoulder and forearm.

Since a number of observations concerning neurologic condition have to be made at relatively close intervals, many ambulances are provided with locally designed neurologic observation forms. An example of the information contained on many local forms is shown in Figure 11–9. Proper use of these forms will allow you to provide emergency department personnel with an accurate record of your observations. If your EMS System does not use a specialized form, you should use the AVPU approach described in Chapter 3 (p. 83).

Positioning the Patient with Cranial Injury

Proper patient positioning is important in caring for patients with head injuries. Conscious patients with apparently minor closed head injuries and *absolutely no signs of neck or spinal injuries* can be positioned in one of two ways:

1. Upper body elevated—Elevate the entire upper body or slant the entire body to a head elevated position (Figure 11–10). *Do not* simply elevate the patient's head at the neck. To do so may partially obstruct the airway. Placing the patient's upper body at an angle gives better control should the patient vomit.

NEUROLOGICAL ASSESSMENT FORM			
TIME	INITIAL ASSESS-MENT _____		
CONSCIOUS	YES/NO	YES/NO	YES/NO
ORIENTED	YES/NO	YES/NO	YES/NO
RESPONSIVE TO VOICE	YES/NO	YES/NO	YES/NO
RESPONSIVE TO COMMAND	YES/NO	YES/NO	YES/NO
TALKS	YES/NO	YES/NO	YES/NO
REACTS TO PAIN	YES/NO/NA	YES/NO/NA	YES/NO/NA
ABILITY TO MOVE • LEFT LEG • RIGHT LEG • LEFT ARM • RIGHT ARM			
PUPILS • REACTIVITY • SIZE	L | R	L | R	L | R

FIGURE 11–9. Neurologic observations form.

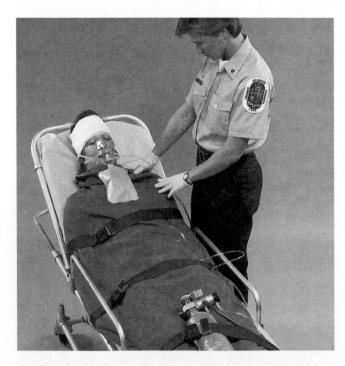

FIGURE 11–10. Head-elevated position for conscious patients with minor closed head injury and no signs of spinal injury.

2. Supine—Some systems have adopted a positioning that places the patient flat on his back. They believe that there is little risk of intracranial pressure buildup in this position and that it helps prevent shock. If you use this positioning, you *must* have suction equipment ready and monitor continuously for vomiting.

If you are not certain as to the severity of the patient's injuries, if there is evidence of cervical spine injury, or if the patient with a head injury is unconscious, then special positioning is required, as well as a rigid cervical or extrication collar and long spine board. Blood and mucus must drain freely, and if the patient vomits (as brain-injured patients are likely to do), the vomitus must not be allowed to cause an airway obstruction or be aspirated. Provide careful support to the entire body, but in such a manner that will not require repositioning in case of sudden vomiting. Some patients with a head injury will vomit without warning. Many vomit without first experiencing nausea.

Cranial Injuries with Impaled Objects

If there is an object impaled in the patient's cranium or face, *do not* remove it. Instead, stabilize the object in place with bulky dressings. This, plus care in handling, minimizes accidental movement of the object during the remainder of care and transport. The exception to this stabilization procedure occurs when the object is impaled in the soft tissues of the cheek and has entered the oral cavity. Care for such cases is presented in Chapter 12.

In some situations you may be confronted with a patient whose skull has been impaled by a long object. This can make transporting of the patient impossible until the object is cut or shortened. Pad around the object with bulky dressings, then carefully (and rigidly) stabilize the object on both sides of where the cut will be made. Cutting should be done with a tool that will not cause the object to move or vibrate when it is finally severed. Often, a hand hacksaw with a fine tooth blade is the best tool to use because it can be carefully controlled. In any case in which you may have to cut a long impaled object, call and seek advice from the emergency department physician.

Facial Fractures

When confronted with a patient having possible facial fractures, your principal concerns are to keep the airway open and to stop profuse bleeding. Direct pressure is the usual method used to control bleed-

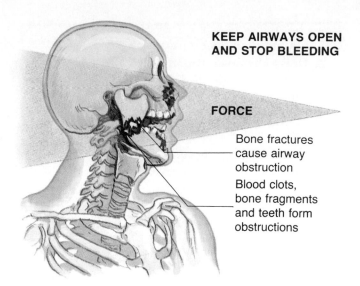

KEEP AIRWAYS OPEN AND STOP BLEEDING

FORCE

Bone fractures cause airway obstruction

Blood clots, bone fragments and teeth form obstructions

FIGURE 11–11. Potential complications from facial fractures.

ing, but care must be exercised not to apply pressure directly over a probable fracture site.

During care at the scene and in transport, positioning for drainage is essential. If the patient is unconscious, or if there are indications of possible facial fractures, application of an extrication or rigid collar is recommended. Such patients must be transported with support provided for the entire spine. This means that you will have to immobilize the spine by securing the patient to a long spine board. The patient and board may need to be rotated to allow for drainage. If both sides of the face are injured, a supine position with suction may be used.

Injuries to the Mandible

The mandible is subject to fracture and dislocation. The symptoms and signs for these injuries include:

- Pain
- Discoloration
- Swelling
- Facial distortion
- Loss of use of the lower jaw or difficulty with speech
- Malocclusion—the improper alignment of the upper and lower teeth when the jaw is closed (*do not* test for this).
- Bleeding around teeth

The care is the same for both fractures and dislocations. To provide care, you should:

1. Maintain an open airway.
2. Dress any open wounds.
3. Apply a cervical or extrication collar if indicated.
4. Properly position the patient.
5. Care for shock.
6. Provide a high concentration of oxygen.
7. Transport, monitoring vital signs.

Care for Patients Wearing Helmets

Helmets are worn in many sporting events and by many motorcycle riders. Facial, neck, and spinal injury care may call for the removal of the helmet. The helmet should not prevent you from reaching the patient's mouth or nose if resuscitation efforts are needed. Protection shields can be lifted, and face guards can be cut away. If the face guard is to be cut, one EMT must steady the patient's head and neck with manual stabilization (see p. 313). The other EMT should place *protective coverings* (towels or folded blankets) directly over the patient's face and anterior neck. This EMT can now use a bolt cutter or other such suitable device to remove the face guard.

Do not attempt to remove a helmet if doing so causes increased pain, or the helmet proves difficult to remove, unless a possible airway obstruction or pulmonary resuscitation must be provided.*

When a helmet must be removed, it is a *two-rescuer* situation. After fully explaining to the patient what you are going to do, the procedure is as follows:

1. EMT 1 is positioned at the top of the patient's head and maintains manual stabilization (p. 313) with a hand on the lower jaw. The construction of the helmet may require stabilization to be applied with the fingers, while the rest of the hand is placed on the side of the helmet.
2. EMT 2 opens, cuts, or removes the chin strap, then places one hand on the patient's chin and, using the other hand, applies stabilization at the occipital region.
3. EMT 1 can now release manual stabilization and slowly remove the helmet. The lower sides of the helmet will have to be gently pulled out to clear the ears. Eyeglasses will have to be removed.

* Follow your local protocols. Some EMS systems call for helmet removal in all cases to allow for proper securing of the patient to a long spine board.

4. EMT 1, after removing the helmet, reestablishes manual stabilization and maintains an open airway by using the jaw-thrust.
5. EMT 2 can release manual stabilization and apply an extrication collar. The patient should then be secured to a long spine board.

NOTE: This method has not been adopted by all EMS Systems. Your instructor will inform you of local policies.

INJURIES TO THE SPINE

Types of Injuries

Injuries to the spine must always be considered when you find serious injury to the body. Remember that spinal injury can be associated with head, neck, and back injuries. Do not overlook the possibility of spinal injury when dealing with chest, abdominal, and pelvic injuries. Even injuries to the upper and lower extremities can be associated with forces intense enough to also produce spinal injury. Remember, you must always do a *complete* patient survey except for special situations. Failure to do so will reduce your chances of detecting possible spinal injury.

Injuries to the spinal column include:

- Fractures, with and without bone displacement
- Dislocations
- Ligament sprains
- Disk injury, including compression

The vertebral column may be injured without damage to the spinal cord or spinal nerves. For example, a fractured coccyx is below the level of the spinal cord. Ligament sprains are relatively simple injuries. However, when displaced fractures and dislocations occur, the cord, disk, and spinal nerves may be severely injured. Serious contusions and lacerations, accompanied by pressure-producing swelling, can take place. The entire column can become unstable, leading to cord compression that may produce paralysis or death.

Mechanisms of Injury

NOTE: There is a simple rule you can follow. If there is any soft tissue damage to the head, face,

METHODS FOR HELMET REMOVAL

1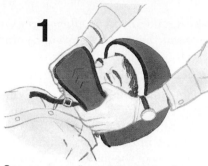

One rescuer applies stabilization by placing his hands on each side of the helmet with the fingers on the patient's mandible. This position prevents slippage if the strap is loose.

2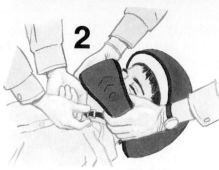

A second rescuer cuts or loosens the strap at the D-Rings while maintaining stabilization.

3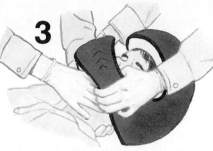

A second rescuer places one hand on the mandible at the angle, the thumb on one side, the long and index fingers on the other. With his other hand, he holds the occipital region. This maneuver transfers the stabilization responsibility to the second rescuer.

4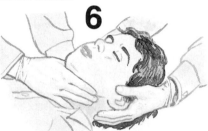

The rescuer at the top removes the helmet.
Three factors should be kept in mind.
(a) The helmet is egg-shaped and therefore must be expanded laterally to clear the ears.
(b) If the helmet provides full facial coverage, glasses must be removed first.
(c) If the helmet provides full facial coverage, the nose will impede removal. To clear the nose, the helmet must be tilted backward and raised over it.

5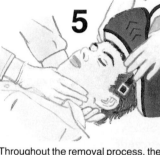

Throughout the removal process, the second rescuer maintains in-line stabilization from below in order to prevent head tilt.

6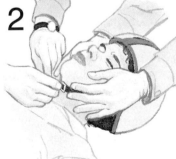

After the helmet has been removed, the rescuer at the top replaces his hands on either side of the patient's head with his palms over the ears, taking over stabilization.

Summary:
The helmet must be maneuvered over the nose and ears while the head and neck are held rigid.
(a) Stabilization is applied from above.
(b) Stabilization is transferred below with pressure on the jaw and occiput.
(c) The helmet is removed.
(d) Stabilization is re-established from above.

7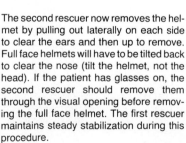

Stabilization is maintained from above until a cervical collar and a spine board are in place.

ALTERNATE METHOD

1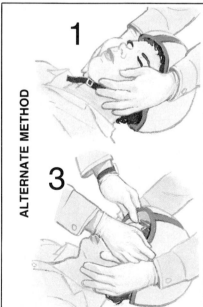

The first rescuer positions himself above or behind the patient and places his hands on each side of the neck at the base of the skull, he applies steady stabilization with the neck in a neutral position. He may use his thumbs to perform a jaw thrust while doing this.

2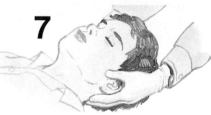

The second rescuer positions himself over or to the side of the patient and removes or cuts the chin strap.

3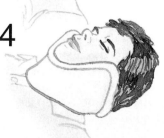

The second rescuer now removes the helmet by pulling out laterally on each side to clear the ears and then up to remove. Full face helmets will have to be tilted back to clear the nose (tilt the helmet, not the head). If the patient has glasses on, the second rescuer should remove them through the visual opening before removing the full face helmet. The first rescuer maintains steady stabilization during this procedure.

4

The second rescuer now applies a suitable cervical immobilization device, and the patient is secured to a long board.

FIGURE 11–12. Helmet removal from injured patient. (From John E. Campbell, M.D., and Alabama Chapter, American College of Emergency Physicians, *BTLS Basic Prehospital Trauma Care,* The Brady Company, 1988.)

or neck due to a sudden deceleration injury (e.g., being thrown against a dashboard), then assume that there is cervical spine injury. Any blunt trauma above the clavicles also may damage the cervical spine.

Some parts of the spine are more susceptible to injury than others. Because they are somewhat splinted by the attached ribs, the segments of the thoracic spine are not usually damaged except in the most violent accidents or in gunshot wounds. The pelvic-sacral spine articulation helps to protect the sacrum in the same way. On the other hand, the cervical and lumbar vertebrae are susceptible to injury because they are not supported by other bony structures. The cervical spine can be damaged in "whiplash" accidents, and the lumbar spine can become injured when a person tries to lift a heavy load improperly.

A common injury in vehicle accidents is "whiplash." When one vehicle strikes another vehicle or a fixed object head on, the neck can whip quickly back and forth. This neck movement may exceed the normal range of motion. Virtually the same thing occurs when a vehicle is struck from behind.

A fall can produce spinal injury as the victim strikes his head on an object, the ground, or the floor. The force generated during a fall may be enough to fracture, crush, or dislocate vertebrae. Cases of needless disability have been reported when the head injuries were noted and cared for but spinal injuries were overlooked.

Many sporting activities can lead to accidents that can cause spinal injury. Sledding and skiing accidents can hurl a person into trees or other fixed objects, twisting or compressing the spinal column in the process. In many of these accidents, there may not be serious open wounds and the extremities may not be fractured, yet spinal injury has occurred. The body of the victim is usually covered by bulky clothing, leaving no obvious signs of injury for the untrained rescuer. As a result, improper care may be rendered as the victim is placed on a stretcher without adequate examination and immobilization.

Diving board and diving accidents often produce injury to the cervical spine. For example, when the victim strikes the board, the side or bottom of the pool, or an underwater object, the head can be severely forced beyond its normal limits of motion. Cervical vertebrae may be fractured or dislocated, ligaments may be severely sprained, and the spinal cord may be compressed or otherwise traumatized in the cervical region and at other spots along the cord.

Football and other contact sports can cause accidents severe enough to produce possible spinal in-

jury. Whenever the game involves player contact or falling to the ground, be on the alert for spinal injury.

REMEMBER: Any violent accident and any falling accident can produce spinal injury. The most common causes of spinal cord injury are motor vehicle accidents, fractured spines in the elderly (often due to falls), diving accidents, and gunshot wounds. You must do a complete survey of the patient. You should assume that all unconscious trauma patients have spinal injury. Whenever you are in doubt, assume that there are spinal injuries and immobilize the head, neck, and spine.

Determining Possible Spinal Injury

REMEMBER: Any unconscious patient who is the victim of an accident *must* be assumed to have spinal injury.

Spinal injuries can be difficult to detect. Your chances of finding possible spinal injury will increase if you:

1. Consider the mechanism of injury—Is the accident the type that can produce spinal injury? Serious falls, motor vehicle accidents, diving accidents, and cave-ins often cause spinal damage.
2. Observe the position (posturing) of the pa-

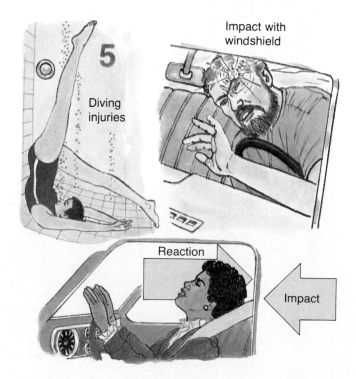

FIGURE 11–13. Mechanisms of neck injury.

tient—The patient in a supine position may have his arms stretched out above the head.

3. Question the patient and bystanders about the accident—They may be able to report something that is not obvious.

4. Conduct a head-to-toe examination
   • Are there injuries that you can associate with spinal injuries? Facial injury, head wounds and fractures, neck wounds, blunt trauma to the back or chest, pelvic fractures, hip dislocations, and penetrating wounds of the neck or trunk indicate a mechanism of injury that may have produced damage to the spine.
   • Are there symptoms and signs indicating possible spinal injury?
   • Does a neurologic survey indicate any problem with nerve function?

5. Monitor the patient to note any changes associated with spinal injury—Numbness and tingling in the extremities may begin, or paralysis may occur.

Symptoms and Signs of Spinal Injury

Indications of possible spinal injury include:

• PAIN WITHOUT MOVEMENT—The pain is not always constant and may occur anywhere from the top of the head to the buttocks. Pain in the leg is common for certain types of injury to the lower spinal cord and vertebral column. Other painful injuries can mask out this symptom.

• PAIN WITH MOVEMENT—The patient normally tries to lie perfectly still to prevent pain on movement. You should not request the patient to move just to determine if pain is present. However, if the patient complains of pain in the neck or back experienced with voluntary movements, you *must* consider this to be a symptom of possible spinal injury. Pain with movement in apparently uninjured shoulders and legs is a good indicator of possible spinal injury.

• TENDERNESS—Gentle palpation of the injury site, when accessible, may reveal point tenderness.

• DEFORMITY—The removal of clothing to check the back for deformity is not recommended. OBVIOUS SPINAL DEFORMITIES ARE RARE. If you note a gap between the spinous processes of the vertebrae or if you can feel a broken spinous process, you *must* consider the patient to have serious spinal injuries.

• IMPAIRED BREATHING—Neck injury can impair nerve function to the chest muscles. Watch the patient breathe. If there is only a slight movement of the abdomen, with little or no movement of the chest, it is safe to assume that the patient is breathing with the diaphragm alone (diaphragmatic breathing). Panting due to respiratory insufficiency may develop.

• PRIAPISM—The persistent erection of the penis is a reliable sign of spinal injury affecting nerves to the external genitalia.

• CHARACTERISTIC POSITIONING (POSTURING) OF THE ARMS—In some cases of spinal injury, motor nerve pathways to the muscles that extend the arm can be interrupted, but those that lead to the muscles that bend the elbow and lift the arm remain functional. The patient may be found on his back, with the arms extended above the head which may indicate a cervical spine injury.

• INVOLUNTARY LOSS OF BOWEL AND BLADDER CONTROL

• NERVE IMPAIRMENT TO THE EXTREMITIES—The patient may have loss of use, weakness, numbness, tingling, or loss of feeling in the upper and/or lower extremities. PARALYSIS OF THE EXTREMITIES IS PROBABLY THE MOST RELIABLE SIGN OF SPINAL INJURY IN CONSCIOUS PATIENTS.

• SEVERE SHOCK—This may occur even when there are no indications of external or internal bleeding. It can be caused by the failure of the nervous system to control the diameter of blood vessels (neurogenic shock).

NOTE: Paralysis, pain, pain on movement, and tenderness anywhere along the spine are reliable indicators of possible spinal injury in the conscious patient. If these are present, you have sufficient reason to immobilize the patient before proceeding with the survey. If immediate immobilization is not possible, use extreme care in handling the patient. In the field, it is not possible to rule out spinal injury even in cases in which the patient has no pain and is able to move his limbs. The *mechanism of injury* alone may be the deciding factor.

The elements of patient assessment that apply to spinal injuries are reviewed in Scan 11–1.

SCAN 11–1 ASSESSING PATIENTS FOR SPINAL INJURIES

Symptoms and Signs

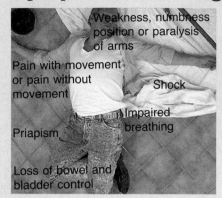

Weakness, numbness position or paralysis of arms

Pain with movement or pain without movement

Shock

Impaired breathing

Priapism

Loss of bowel and bladder control

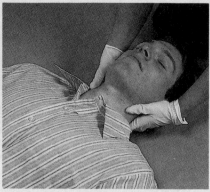

Point cervical tenderness and deformity

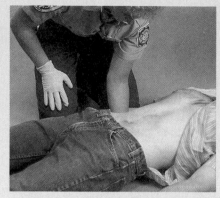

Point spinal column tenderness and deformity

Conscious—Lower Extremities Assessment

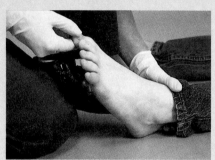

Touch toe

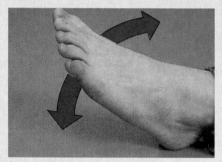

Foot wave

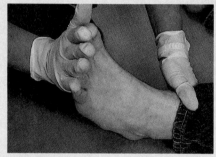

Foot push

RESULTS: If the patient can perform these tasks, there is little chance of severe injury to the cord anywhere along its length, however, immobilizing the spine is called for since this test does not rule out all types of injuries, including vertebral fractures. If the tests can only be performed to a limited degree and with pain, there may be pressure somewhere along the cord. When a patient is not able to perform any of the tests, you must assume that there is spinal injury damage.

Conscious—Upper Extremities Assessment

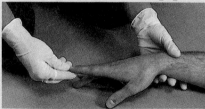

Touch finger

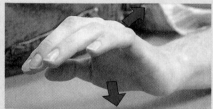

Hand wave

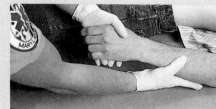

Hand squeeze

RESULTS: Performance of all tests indicates little chance of damage in the cervical area but does not rule out all possibilities. Limited performance and pain—pressure on cord in cervical area. Failure to perform any test and negative lower extremity results—assume severe cord injury in neck.

UNCONSCIOUS PATIENTS: Test the responses to painful stimuli (pinching) applied to the distal limb. If removal of shoes may aggravate existing injuries, apply the stimuli to the skin around the ankles.

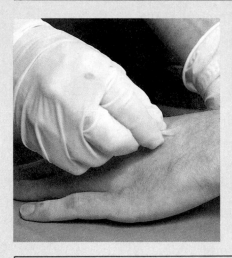

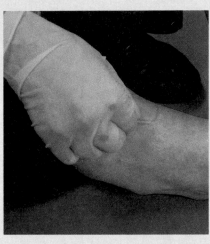

REMEMBER
It is difficult to survey the unconscious patient with accuracy. A deeply unconscious patient will not pull back from a painful stimulus. Should the mechanism of injury indicate possible spinal damage, or if the trauma patient is unconscious, assume that spinal injury is present.

RESULTS: Slight pulling back of foot—cord usually intact. No foot reaction—possible damage anywhere along the cord. Hand or finger reaction—usually no damage to cervical cord. No hand or finger reaction—possible damage to the cervical cord.

Summary of Observations and Conclusions

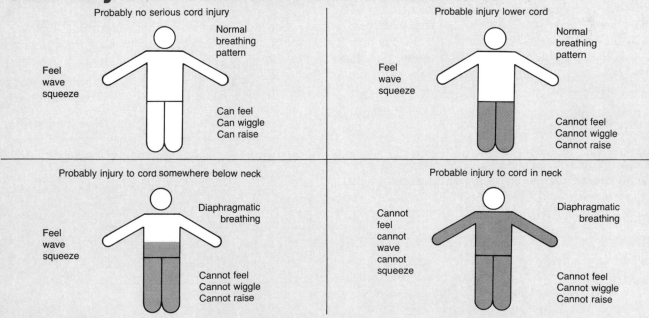

Probably no serious cord injury
Normal breathing pattern
Feel wave squeeze
Can feel
Can wiggle
Can raise

Probable injury lower cord
Normal breathing pattern
Feel wave squeeze
Cannot feel
Cannot wiggle
Cannot raise

Probably injury to cord somewhere below neck
Diaphragmatic breathing
Feel wave squeeze
Cannot feel
Cannot wiggle
Cannot raise

Probable injury to cord in neck
Diaphragmatic breathing
Cannot feel
cannot wave
cannot squeeze
Cannot feel
Cannot wiggle
Cannot raise

WARNING: If the patient is unconscious or the mechanism of injury indicates possible spinal injury, assume that spinal injury is present.

CARE FOR SPINAL INJURIES

Regardless of where the apparent spinal injury is located on the cord, care is the same. For all patients with possible spinal injury, and for all accident victims when there is doubt as to the extent of injury, you should:

1. Provide manual stabilization for the head and neck.
2. Apply an extrication or rigid collar and continue to maintain manual stabilization.
3. Secure the patient on a long spine board.
4. Administer oxygen in high concentration. Edema to the cord may impair oxygen delivery to the cord. When this occurs, cellular death can take place.

In some cases, it will be necessary to secure the patient to a short spine board or similar device prior to securing him to a long spine board. This is the case for patients found seated in motor vehicles and for patients found in locations where physical use of a long board is too restricted or impossible. Additional procedures to follow for difficult to reach patients, including those found in automobiles, will be covered later in Chapter 23. The orthopedic stretcher will be presented at that time. For now, master the skills of the extrication collar, the long spine board, and the short spine board.

Application of an Extrication Collar and Long Spine Board

The techniques for applying an extrication collar and placing and securing a patient on a long spine board are presented in Scans 11–2 and 11–3. Before you study the Scans, consider the following:

1. Always reassure the patient. Having an extrication collar applied and being strapped to a spine board can be a frightening experience. When appropriate, explain the procedures to the patient.
2. Make certain that you have completed an accurate primary survey and you have cared for all life-threatening problems.
3. Use the mechanism of injury, state of consciousness, and a secondary survey to determine the need for an extrication collar and spine board.
4. Always apply a rigid collar when you believe that spinal injury is a possibility.
   - Make certain that you assess the patient's neck prior to placing the collar. Take special care to look for tracheal deviation and distended jugular veins.
   - You must measure the collar to be certain that it is the correct size for the patient. A large patient may not be able to wear a large collar. A small patient with a long neck may need your largest collar. The front width of the collar should fit between the point of the chin and the chest at the suprasternal (jugular) notch. Once in place, the collar should rest on the clavicles and support the lower jaw.
   - Remove necklaces and earrings before applying the collar.
   - Keep the head in the anatomical position when applying manual stabilization and the collar. Be certain to keep the patient's hair out of the way.
   - Maintain manual stabilization while the collar is secured, and continue to manually immobilize the head and neck until the patient is secured to a long spine board.
5. When a patient is secured to a long spine board, the order of ties goes from chest to foot and the head is to be secured last, using 3-inch tape or a cravat. The tape usually offers more support, especially if the patient and board are to be tilted to allow for drainage. However, blood on the patient's skin and hair may make using tape impractical. You should learn both methods. Do not tape or tie the cravats across the patient's eyes.
6. Additional immobilization for the head and neck can be provided with *light* sandbags filled with foam, a Bashaw or other commercial device, blanket rolls, or similar objects or devices.
7. Always manage the patient for shock and administer a high concentration of oxygen.

REMEMBER: If there is any doubt in your mind as to the condition of an injured patient's spine because of the lack of obvious symptoms and signs, RIGIDLY IMMOBILIZE him and transport as though you know for sure that damage to the spinal cord has occurred.

SCAN 11–2 SPINAL INJURIES—RIGID COLLARS

Extrication and Rigid Collars

Rigid cervical and extrication collars are applied to protect the cervical spine. **Do not** apply a soft collar.

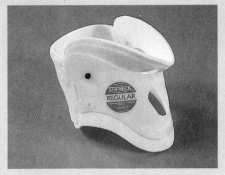

STIFNECK™–Rigid extrication

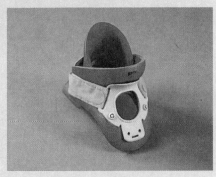

PHILADELPHIA CERVICAL COLLAR™

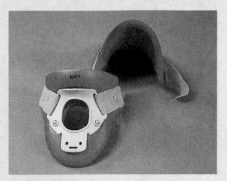

PHILADELPHIA CERVICAL COLLAR™–Opened

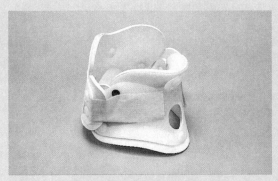

NEC-LOC™–Rigid extrication

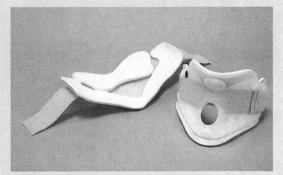

NEC-LOC™–Opened

Applying Manual Stabilization

1

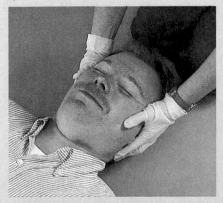

Properly position both hands.

Do not apply traction to the head and neck, or pull and twist the head. You are trying to stabilize the head and neck.

2

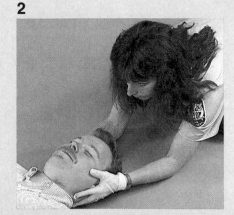

Maintain stabilization—keep head in neutral alignment.

(Scan continues on next page)

Stifneck™ Collar—Seated Patient

1

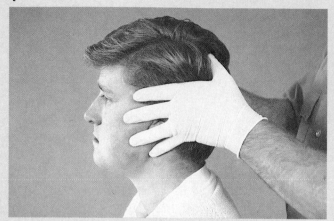

Stabilize the head and neck from the rear.

2

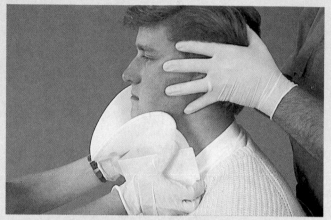

Properly angle the collar for placement.

3

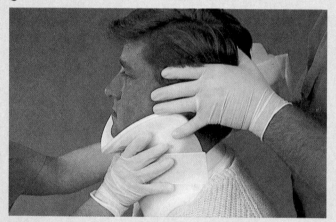

Position the collar bottom.

4

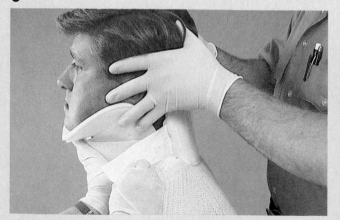

Set collar in place around neck.

5

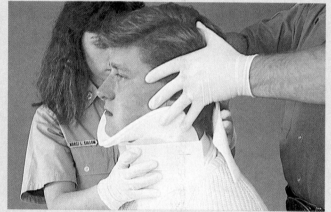

Secure the collar.

6

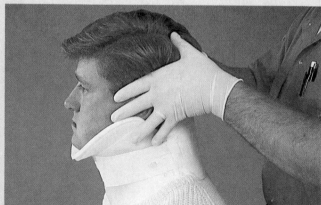

Spread fingers and maintain support.

Stifneck™ Collar—Supine Position

1

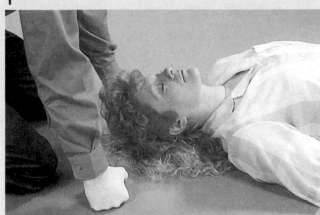

Kneel at patient's head.

2

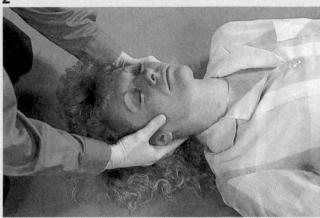

Stabilize the head and neck.

3

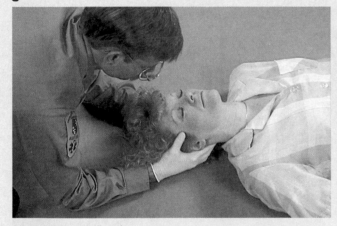

Maintain stabilization.

4

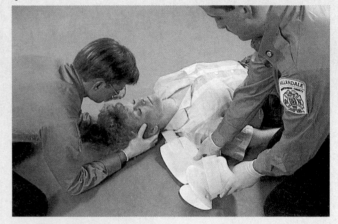

Set collar in place.

5

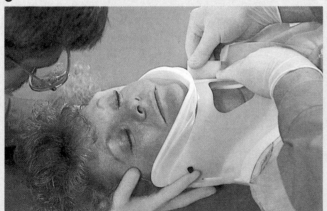

Secure collar.

6

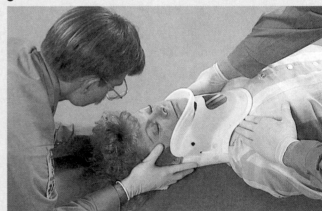

Continue to stabilize.

(Scan continues on next page)

Other Rigid Collars

| NEC-LOC COLLAR™ | PHILADELPHIA CERVICAL COLLAR™ |

1

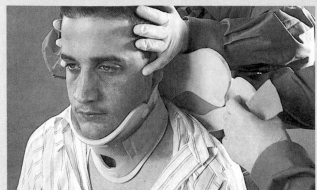

Hold the collar firmly in place (when practical to do so, hold with the thumbs).

1

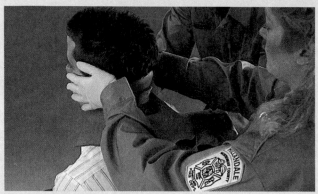

Place or slide the rear piece on the back of the neck.

2

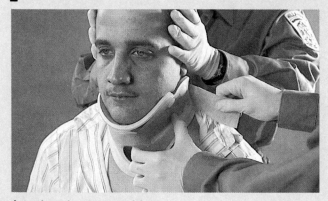

Attach strip on one side.

2

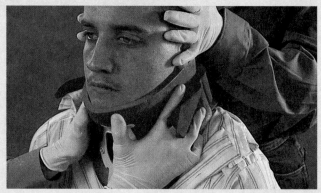

Slide the front up the chest. Seat the chin.

3

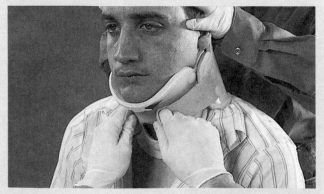

Attach strip on the other side and, if necessary, readjust to align properly.

3

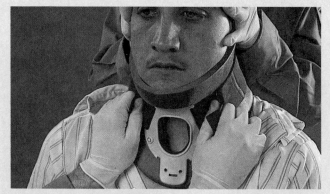

Attach the velcro fasteners.

SCAN 11–3 SPINAL INJURIES—THE LOG ROLL AND THE LONG SPINE BOARD

The Four-Rescuer Log Roll

1

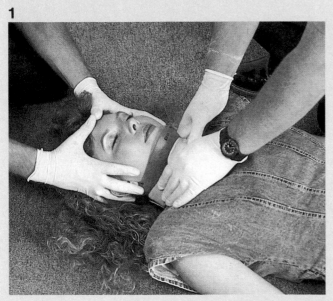

Activity around the patient is restricted. EMT 1 applies manual stabilization and the airway is opened by the jaw-thrust. EMT 2 places a rigid or extrication cervical collar around the patient's neck. EMT 1 maintains manual stabilization.

2

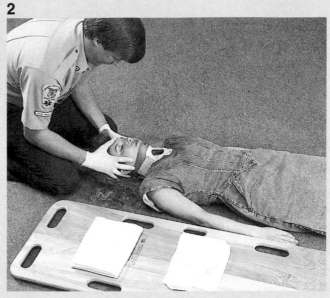

When possible, slide the board under the patient. If not, the board is placed parallel to the patient. When possible, padding is provided at the level of the neck, waist, knees, and ankles to help fill voids between the patient's body and the board.

3

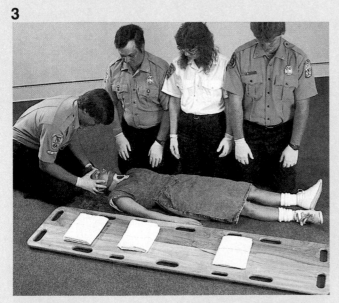

Three rescuers kneel at the patient's side opposite the board, leaving room to roll the patient toward them. Place one rescuer at the shoulder, one at the waist, and one at the knee. EMT 1 continues to stabilize head.

4

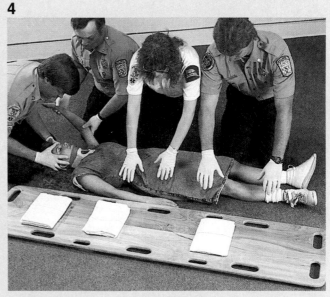

EMT 1 controls the move. The shoulder-level rescuer is directed to extend the patient's arm over the head on the side onto which the patient will be rolled.

(Scan continues on next page)

5

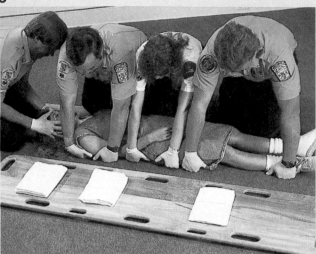

EMT 1 orders the rescuers to reach across the patient and take proper hand placements prior to the roll.

- The shoulder-level rescuer places one hand under the patient's shoulder and the other hand under the patient's upper arm.
- The waist-level rescuer places one hand on the patient's waist and the other hand under the patient's buttocks.
- The knee-level rescuer places one hand under the patient's lower thigh and the other hand under the midcalf.

6

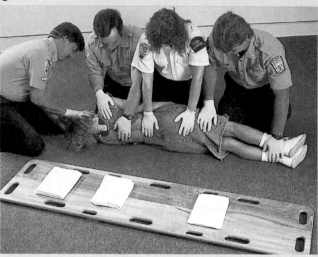

EMT 1 maintains manual stabilization to the head and neck. He directs the others to roll the patient, moving the patient as a unit.

7

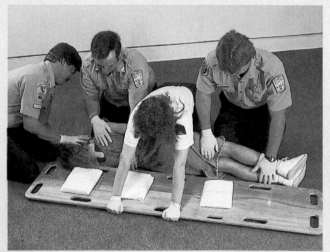

EMT 1 directs the waist-level rescuer to free hand to adjust the pads, grip the spine board, and pull it into position against the patient. (This can be done by fifth rescuer.)

8

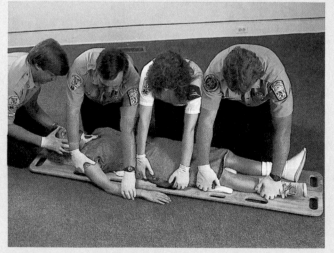

EMT 1 orders the rescuers to roll the patient onto the board.

9

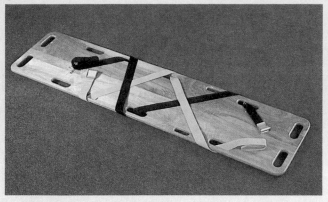

One strap is laced A-D-E. The other is laced B-C-F. Buckle A to B, E to F.

10

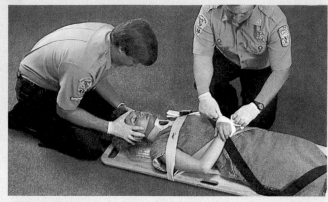

Patient's body is secured to board, wrists are loosely tied together.

11

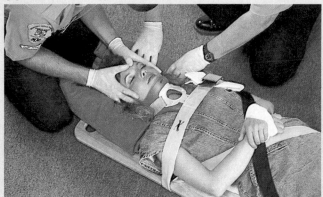

Center ten-inch wide blanket roll under head. Roll ends toward patient's head. Commercial stabilizing devices may be used in place of the blanket.

12

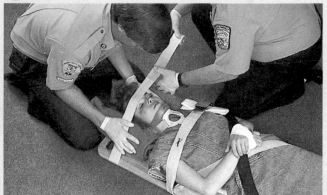

Use tape to secure forehead to long spine board.

13

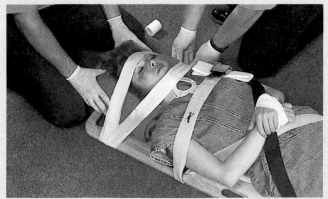

Complete the process of securing the head and neck to the long spine board using tape.

14

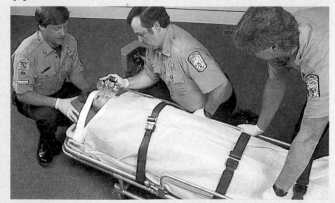

Transfer patient and board as unit.

(Scan continues on next page)

Two-Rescuer Log Roll

NOTE: Use extreme care. This method should be only used when dangers at the scene may threaten patient and rescuers.

A

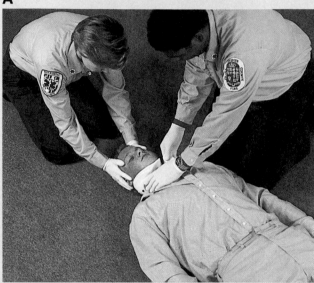

EMT 1 maintains an open airway and manual stabilization while EMT 2 applies an extrication collar.

B

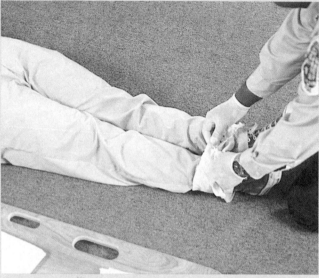

EMT 1 stabilizes head while EMT 2 pads board and places it close to the patient. Cravats are tied around the patient's feet and calves.

C

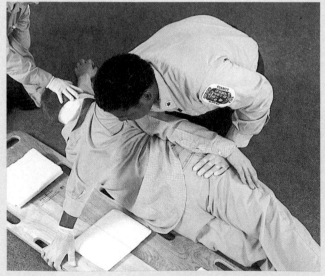

EMT 2 extends the patient's arm over the head and kneels at the patient's hips. EMT 1 orders the roll. Roll patient as a unit. After completing roll, EMT 2 pulls the board against the patient's back.

D

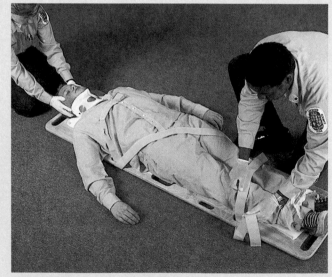

The patient is gently rolled onto the board. He is secured to the board in the usual manner. His hands are loosely tied together.

NOTE: Some authorities recommend securing the patient's head first when placing him on a long spine board. Since the patient may shift as straps are applied, possibly aggravating existing injuries, the "head last" protocol is shown in this text.

Application of the Short Spine Board

All unconscious trauma patients and all patients with possible spinal injuries should be rigidly immobilized. Patients found in a seated position, like those found in some motor vehicle accidents, and patients who have to be moved to a seated position before they can be extricated and moved, should be secured to a short spine board or similar device and then transferred to a long spine board. Before the short board can be used, an extrication or rigid collar *must* be applied. *Manual stabilization* has to be done before and during the application of the collar. Manual stabilization is continued after the collar is secured. This stabilization should continue until the patient is secured to the long spine board.

The procedure for applying a *short spine board* is shown in Scan 11–4. This procedure calls for securing the torso first and the head last. Such an approach offers greater stability in maintaining board position throughout the strapping process and may help prevent compression of the cervical spine. If the patient has suffered abdominal injuries or displays diaphragmatic breathing that prevents adequate securing of the torso, it may be necessary to secure the head first. Torso straps will still be needed to secure the board, but care must be taken so as not to interfere with breathing.

There are seven special warnings that must always be considered when applying a short board to the patient:

1. **WARNING:** Any assessment or reassessment of the back, scapulae, arms, or clavicles must be done before the board is placed against the patient. Assessment is not possible once the board is placed.

2. **WARNING:** The board should be angled to fit between the arms of the rescuer who is stabilizing the head. You *must* push the spine board as far down into the seat as possible. If you do not, the board may shift and the patient's cervical spine may compress during application of the board. To provide full cervical support, the top of the board should be level with the top of the patient's head. The uppermost holes must be level with the patient's shoulders. The base of the board should not extend past the coccyx.

3. **WARNING:** Never place a chin cup or chin strap on the patient. Such devices may pre-

vent the patient from opening his mouth if he has to vomit.

4. **WARNING:** When applying the first strap to secure the torso, you *must not* apply the strap too tightly. This could cause abdominal injury, aggravate existing abdominal injury, or limit respirations for the diaphragmatic breathing patient.

5. **WARNING:** Some short spine boards have buckles with release mechanisms that can be accidentally activated during patient transfer operations. This is especially true of "quick-release" buckles. These buckles must be taped closed after the final adjustment of the straps.

6. **WARNING:** *Do not* allow the buckles to be placed midsternum. Such a placement will interfere with proper hand placement should CPR become necessary.

7. **WARNING:** *Do not* pad between the collar and the board. To do so will create a pivot point that may cause the hyperextension of the cervical spine when the head is secured. Instead, padding should be placed at the occipital region, but only enough to fill any void. This will help keep the head in a *neutral* position.

The placement of straps for the short spine board is a little complex (Figure 11–14). The first

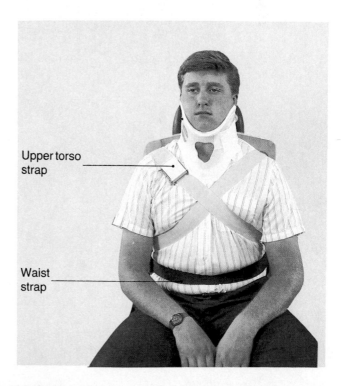

Upper torso strap

Waist strap

FIGURE 11–14. Torso strap placement.

SCAN 11–4 APPLYING A SHORT SPINE BOARD

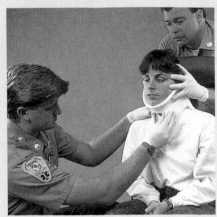

1 Stabilize head and neck . . . apply manual stabilization. Secure extrication or rigid collar.

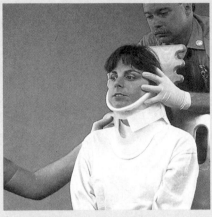

2 Position board behind patient, as far down into seat as possible. You may have to reposition patient.

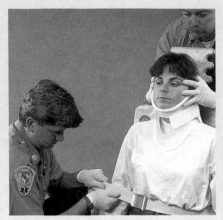

3 Secure the lower torso strap.

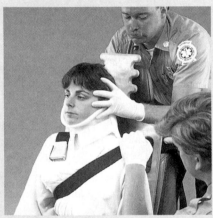

4 Cross the chest with the upper torso strap.

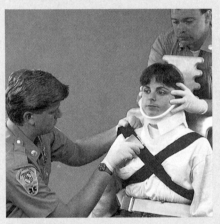

5 Recross the chest and buckle.

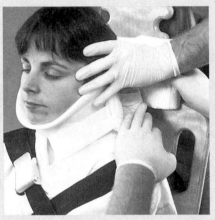

6 Fill voids between patient and board.

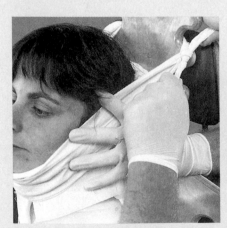

7 Secure the neck and lower head with 3-inch wide cravat. Pass through upper notches and tie.

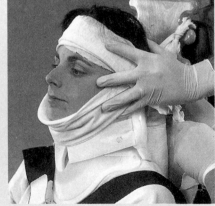

8 Secure the upper head with cravat. Pass through lower notches and tie.

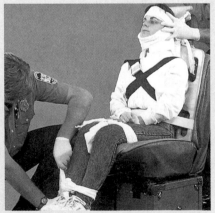

9 Loosely tie together the patient's wrists. Pad between the knees and tie together thighs and ankles.

strap, used to secure the torso and hold the board at the proper height is applied as follows:

1. The strap is taken behind the board and its free end is passed through slot D, from back to front.
2. This free end is pulled across the face of the board and taken through slot B, from front to rear.
3. The strap is pulled until its buckle can be centered over the patient's midline.
4. The strap is buckled, taking care not to apply too much pressure to the abdomen.

The strap for the upper torso is placed as follows (Figure 11–15):

1. Place the buckle below the right clavicle.
2. Pass the free end through slot A.
3. Take the belt behind the board and pass it down through slot B (top A through bottom B).
4. Cross the patient's chest and pass the free end through slot C.
5. Pull the belt down along the back of the board and pass it from back to front through slot D.

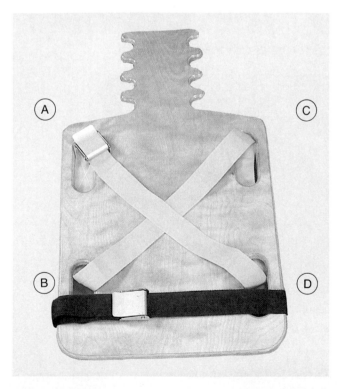

FIGURE 11–15. The upper torso belt and waist belt.

6. Cross the patient's chest and buckle. Before tightening the belt to remove any slack, place a thin pad under the buckle.

The Extrication Device

A number of commercial vest-style extrication devices are available. These devices help to immobilize and ease the task of lifting and moving the patient. You should use the devices approved by your EMS system.

A vest-style extrication device is an example of a flexible piece of equipment useful for immobilizing patients with possible injury to the cervical spine. This device can be used when the patient is found seated in a bucket seat, a short compact car seat, a seat with a contoured back, or in a confined space. It is also useful when the short spine board cannot be inserted into a car because of obstructions.

The use of an extrication device eliminates many of the problems caused by the board's straps and buckles. The device will immobilize the patient's head without the use of a confining chin strap.

SUMMARY

The skull is made up of the cranium and the face. The vertebral column is connected to the skull. That portion of the spine running through the neck is called the cervical spine. The ribs are attached to the thoracic spine. The midback contains the lumbar spine, while the sacral spine and coccyx are lower back structures. The skull, spinal column, sternum, and ribs form the axial skeleton.

The brain is protected by the skull. The spinal column protects the spinal cord. The brain and spinal cord are part of the central nervous system.

Injuries to the skull include open head and closed head injuries. If the cranium remains intact, the injury is classified as a closed head injury.

Open head injuries involve fractures of the cranium (skull fractures). There can be direct injury to the brain in open head injuries. Closed head injuries include indirect injuries to the brain, such as concussions and contusions.

Skull fractures may be obvious or difficult to detect. Always look for wounds to the head, deformity of the skull, bruises behind the ear, discolorations around the eyes, sunken eyes, unequal pupils, and bloody or clear fluids flowing from the ears and/or nose.

Brain injury can occur with head injuries. Look for signs of skull fracture, a decrease in the level

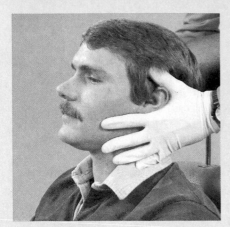

1 Stabilize head and neck.

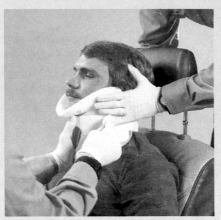

2 Apply a rigid collar.

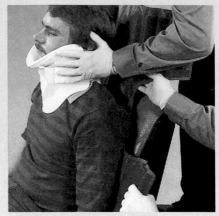

3 Slip device behind patient. Center patient within device.

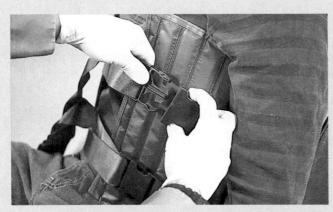

4 Fasten bottom and then the middle chest straps.

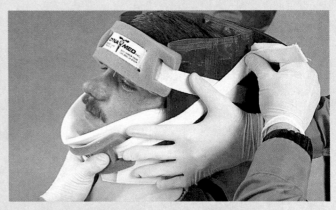

5 Secure head with Velcro head straps.

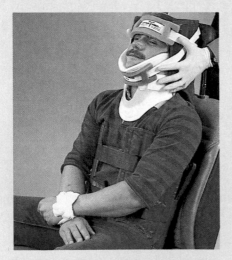

6 Tie hands together.

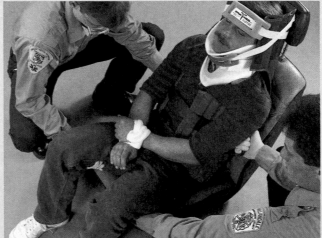

7 Lift the patient using the handles. Lock hands under thigh.

NOTE: Once the patient is extricated, the upper chest strap can be loosened if the patient is uncomfortable when breathing or displays signs of difficult or inadequate breathing.

of consciousness, confusion, unequal pupils, and paralysis.

When caring for a patient with injuries to the cranium, you should maintain an open airway using the jaw-thrust technique. Provide resuscitative procedures, if needed. Keep the patient at rest and talk to him. Control bleeding, but avoid pressure over the site of a fracture. *Do not* remove impaled objects, bone fragments, or any other objects from skull wounds.

Facial fractures often cause airway obstruction. You should maintain an open airway using the jaw-thrust technique.

Neck and spinal injuries can be very serious. The secondary survey is very important in detecting signs of possible spinal injuries. Always look for weakness, numbness, loss of feeling, pain, or paralysis to the limbs of a patient. Remember that you will have to pinch the feet and hands of the unconscious patient. Assume that the unconscious trauma patient has spinal injuries.

You must follow certain rules when caring for a patient who may have neck or spinal injuries. ALWAYS consider the unconscious trauma patient to have neck or spinal injuries. APPLY MANUAL STABILIZATION FOR THE HEAD AND NECK, PLACE AN EXTRICATION COLLAR, AND SECURE THE PATIENT TO A LONG SPINE BOARD. Do your best to immobilize the patient's head and neck and as much of the patient's body as possible. Continuously monitor the patient.

All patients with spinal and head injuries should be managed for shock and receive a high concentration of oxygen.

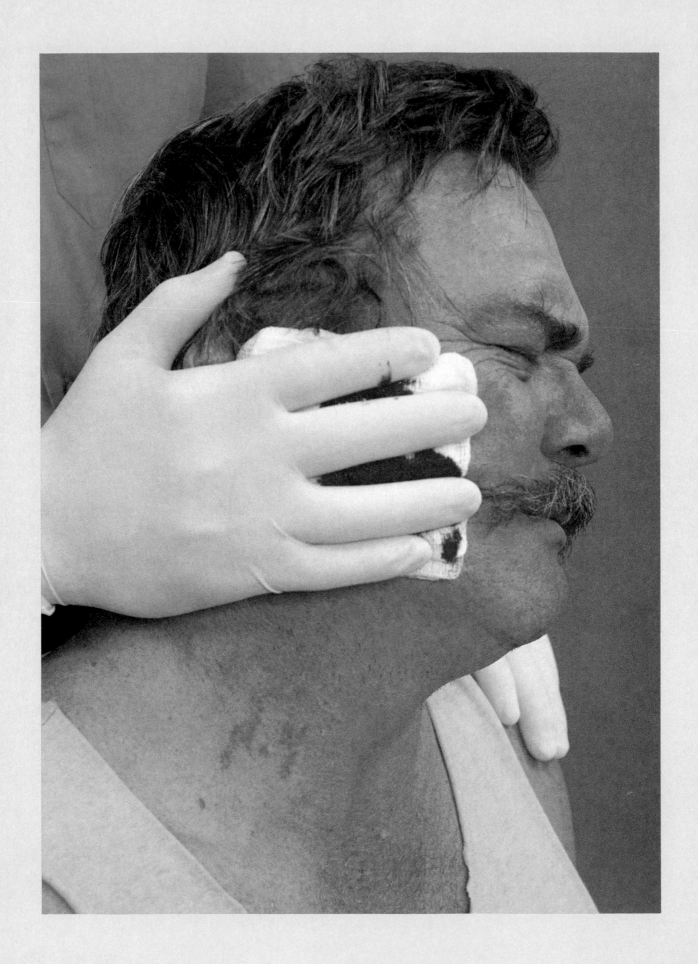

Injuries III:
Soft tissue injuries of the head and neck

WARNING: Avoid direct contact with patient blood and body fluids.

OBJECTIVES   As an EMT, you should be able to:

1. List the procedures for the emergency care of scalp wounds. (pp. 328–329)

2. List the procedures for the emergency care of facial wounds. (pp. 329-330)

3. Describe, step by step, the emergency care for a patient with an object impaled in the cheek. (p. 331)

4. Cite the procedures of care for cuts, burns, and foreign objects in the eye. (pp. 333–337)

5. List the special care procedures for an object impaled in the eye. (p. 336)

6. Describe, step by step, the procedures for removing each of the four types of contact lenses. (pp. 337–339)

7. Describe the basic care for injuries to the external ear and what to do if you suspect internal injury. (pp. 340–341)

8. Describe the emergency care procedures for nosebleeds and nonfracture injuries to the nose. (pp. 341–342)

9. Describe the basic emergency care for injuries to the mouth. (pp. 342–343)

10. List at least FOUR signs of blunt injury to the neck. (p. 344)

11. Contrast the procedures used to control arterial bleeding from the neck to those used to control venous bleeding from the neck. (pp. 344–345)

SKILLS   As an EMT, you should be able to:

1. Assess for and determine types of soft tissue injuries.

2. Control bleeding and apply the proper dressing and bandage for a given injury to the scalp, face, eye, ear, nose, mouth, and neck.

3. Demonstrate the special emergency care procedures for:

- Impaled object in the eye
- Severe bleeding from a neck vein
- Severe bleeding from a neck artery
- Impaled object in the cheek
- Saving avulsed body parts

Cornea (KOR-ne-ah) – the transparent covering over the iris and pupil of the eye.

Epistaxis (ep-e-STAK-sis) – a nosebleed.

External Auditory Canal – the opening of the external ear and pathway to the middle ear.

Iris – the colored portion of the anterior eye that adjusts the size of the pupil.

Jugular (JUG-u-lar) **Veins** – the major neck veins that return blood from the head and face to the heart.

Pinna (PIN-nah) – the external ear; also called the *auricle* (AW-re-kl).

Sclera (SKLE-rah) – the "whites of the eyes."

Sympathetic Eye Movement – the coordinated movement of both eyes in the same direction. If one eye moves, the other eye will carry out the same movement, even if it is covered or the eyelid is shut.

Tympanic (tim-PAN-ik) **Membrane** – the eardrum.

NOTE: Many new anatomical terms are used in this section. Those found in bold type should be used in communications.

INJURIES TO THE SOFT TISSUES OF THE HEAD

NOTE: Any injury above the clavicles may produce injury to the cervical spine. If the patient is unconscious, or the mechanism of injury may produce spinal injuries, assume that the patient has a spinal injury and treat accordingly. Any time a patient suffers a soft tissue injury to the head or neck and has serious blood loss or shows unstable or poor vital signs, care for shock and administer a high concentration of oxygen. Be alert for airway problems.

Injuries to the Scalp and Face

Of the many blood vessels in the scalp and face, quite a few are close to the skin surface. Wounds may bleed profusely even though a major vessel has not been severed. A minor laceration may initially have profuse bleeding. Usually, clotting is rapid and control is not a major problem. However, if an artery is cut, bleeding may be quickly fatal if no effort is made to control the flow of blood. Severe trauma to the face also may produce skull fractures and possible airway obstruction. Many patients with head injuries also have neck injuries that may involve the spinal cord.

Most soft tissue injuries of the scalp and face can be managed as you would any other soft tissue injury. There are three major EXCEPTIONS to the standard procedure:

1. *Do not* attempt to clear or clean the surface of a scalp wound. To do so may cause additional bleeding and can cause great harm to the patient if there are skull fractures present.

2. *Do not* apply finger pressure to the wound in an effort to control bleeding. Since there may be fractures to the skull, you will have to avoid any pressure that may force free bone edges or fragments into the brain.

3. *Do* remove objects that are impaled in the cheek if they penetrate the cheek and exit into the oral cavity.

Care of Scalp Wounds

Contamination occurs with every scalp wound. The hair may mat over the wound site. Foreign objects, such as glass fragments, pieces of metal, or bits of soil, may be on the wound surface and in the wound itself. Dressing the wound will help prevent additional contamination. To care for a scalp wound (Figure 12–1):

1. *Do not* clear the wound surface. *Do not* try to clean the wound. Wiping actions or the irrigation with water could cause objects to be driven through breaks in the skull and contaminate the brain. Large pieces of loose gravel, dirt, or glass may have to be carefully picked from the hair to allow for safe dressing and bandaging.

2. Control bleeding with a sterile dressing carefully held in place with gentle pressure. Avoid finger pressure if there is any indication that the skull is fractured.

3. Strips of adhesive bandage do not work well

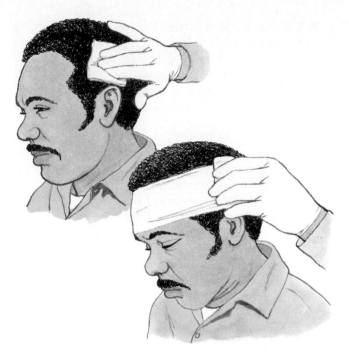

FIGURE 12–1. Caring for scalp wounds. Apply a sterile dressing, and then bandage.

in cases of scalp injury. Self-adherent roller bandage or gauze can be wrapped around the patient's head in order to hold the dressing in place. Remember that bleeding is to be controlled before a dressing is bandaged in place.

WARNING: *Do not* lift or attempt to wrap the patient's head if there are any signs of spinal injury or the mechanism of injury indicates a possible spinal injury.

4. Keep the patient's head and shoulders raised to help control bleeding, provided that the patient survey, degree of trauma, and mechanism of injury do not indicate possible spinal injury, or injury to the chest or abdomen. *Do not* put the unconscious trauma patient into a head-raised position. This position may aggravate spinal injuries. Also, the patient may vomit and aspirate the vomitus.

An effective way to hold a dressing on a scalp wound without applying excessive pressure is to use a triangular bandage.

Care of Facial Wounds

When treating a patient with facial injuries, keep in mind that there is likely to be a breathing problem associated with the wound and there also may be

injury to the neck and spine, especially the cervical spine. Make certain that you monitor the patient to ensure an open airway.

Check the patient's mouth for foreign matter as you assess the extent of oral cavity damage. Use your gloved fingers to carefully sweep the inside of the person's mouth clean of broken dentures and teeth, gum, vomitus, or other obstructions (PROTECT YOUR FINGERS!). Look to see if an external injury to the cheek may have perforated the cheek wall, thus opening into the oral cavity.

If bleeding is profuse, suction away blood, mucus, and vomitus. Position the patient in the lateral recumbent position, with the head tilted back and turned so the mouth tilts downward. **Should you suspect injury to the cervical spine, immobilize the patient's head, neck, and spine before moving him to a position for drainage** (see Chapter 11). Continue to suction the patient as needed.

Start artificial ventilation or CPR as required. Reposition the patient so that basic life support measures will be most effective. When injuries allow, a pocket face mask with a one-way valve or bag-valve-mask unit may have to be used to ventilate the patient. An airway adjunct will have to be inserted for all unconscious patients with head injury; as long as the patient is unconscious, this airway can be left in.

When caring for patients with facial injuries, you should:

1. Ensure an open and clear airway, taking care to protect possible neck and spinal injuries.

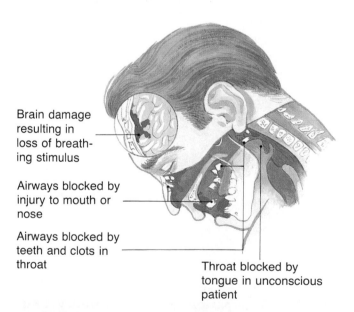

Brain damage resulting in loss of breathing stimulus

Airways blocked by injury to mouth or nose

Airways blocked by teeth and clots in throat

Throat blocked by tongue in unconscious patient

FIGURE 12–2. Injury-related breathing problems.

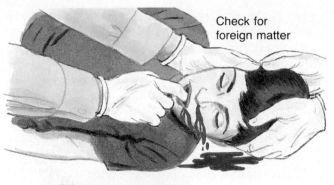

Check for foreign matter

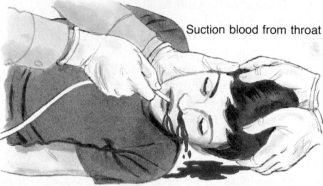

Suction blood from throat

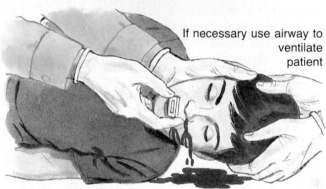

If necessary use airway to ventilate patient

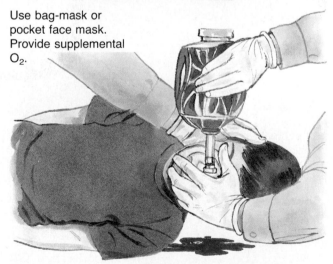

Use bag-mask or pocket face mask. Provide supplemental O₂.

FIGURE 12–3. Correcting a breathing problem for a patient with facial injury (*and with no suspected spinal injury*).

2. Control bleeding by direct pressure on the wound, but use only enough pressure to stop the flow of blood. Remember, there may be facial fractures that are not obvious.
3. Apply a dressing and bandage.

You may need to use pressure point techniques to control bleeding. The temporal artery pressure point sites are useful (see Chapter 7), but be careful not to apply pressure over possible fractures.

If blood vessels, nerves, tendons, or muscles have been exposed, they must be kept from drying out. Even a standard gauze dressing will offer some protection and is the choice of many EMS Systems. A sterile dressing, moistened with normal sterile saline (a commercial salt water solution) can be used to dress this type of open wound. You must be certain that the saline used is from a labeled, sterile source that has not been previously opened.

Partially avulsed facial skin can be returned to its normal position and dressings can be applied. Some systems use a sterile saline or water wash of the wound before repositioning the flap. Your instructor will tell you if this is done in your area. Fully avulsed skin should be wrapped and secured in a dry dressing (or in a moist sterile dressing if

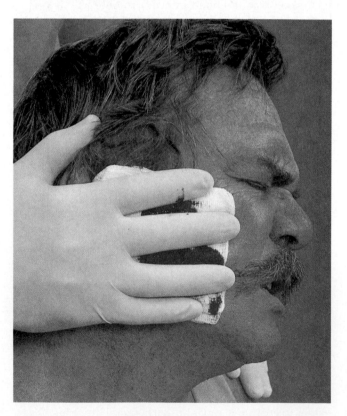

FIGURE 12–4. Care of soft tissue facial injury.

allowed), covered with or bagged in plastic, labeled, kept cool, and transported with the patient.

A dangerous situation exists when the cheek has been penetrated by a foreign object. First, the object may go into the oral cavity and immediately become a possible airway obstruction, or it may stay impaled in the wall to work its way free and enter the oral cavity later. Second, when the cheek wall is perforated, bleeding into the mouth and throat may be profuse and interfere with breathing, or it may make the patient nauseated and induce vomiting. Simple external wound care will not stop the flow of blood into the mouth.

If you find a patient with an object impaled in the cheek, you should:

---

1. Gently examine both the external cheek and the inside of the mouth. Use your penlight and look into the patient's mouth. If need be, *carefully* use your gloved fingers to probe the inside cheek to determine if the object has passed through the cheek wall. This is best done with a dressing pad being used to protect your fingers.

2. If you find perforation, carefully REMOVE THE IMPALED OBJECT by pulling it out in the direction that it entered the cheek. If this cannot be done easily, leave the object in place. *Do not* twist the object.

3. Make certain that you position the patient's head to allow for drainage (the possibility of spinal injuries may require you to immobilize the neck). Keep in mind that an object penetrating the cheek wall also may have broken teeth or dentures, creating the potential danger for airway obstruction.

4. Once the object is removed, pack the inside of the cheek with rolled gauze between the cheek wall and the teeth. This also should be done in cases in which the perforating object cannot be removed. If this is the case, make sure that you stabilize the object on the external side of the cheek wall.

5. If the extent of injuries allow, keep the patient positioned to permit drainage. Provide suctioning as required. A lateral recumbent placement may be necessary during transport.

6. Dress the outside of the wound using a pressure dressing and bandage or apply a sterile dressing and use direct pressure to control the bleeding.

---

7. Provide oxygen and care for shock. You may have to use a nasal cannula if constant suctioning is required. If any dressing materials are placed in the patient's mouth, use of standard face masks can be dangerous unless you leave 3 to 4 inches of the dressing outside of the patient's mouth.

WARNING: Anytime you place something into a patient's mouth, you have taken on added responsibility for the patient. It is possible for objects such as rolled gauze to become airway obstructions. Should the patient vomit, objects in the mouth may trap vomitus, which may be aspirated by the patient. This usually does not happen, but the possibility exists. It is best to leave 3 to 4 inches of the dressing material outside the patient's mouth to allow for easy removal and so that it is visible to the next care provider. Keep a close watch on any patient with anything placed into the mouth. Remember, too, that a conscious patient may be able to monitor the dressings in his mouth, but he may not stay conscious.

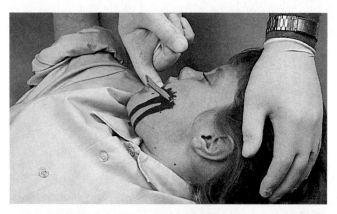

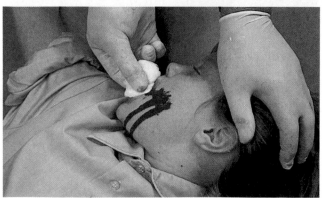

FIGURE 12–5. Procedure for removing an object impaled in the cheek.

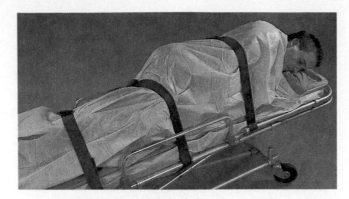

FIGURE 12–6. Transporting the conscious facial injury patient.

Transportation of a Patient with Facial Injuries

Some facial injuries are relatively minor and require no special positioning of the patient. Since respiratory difficulty is often associated with this type of injury, the patient may be transported in the lateral recumbent position with the head low or tilted to aid drainage. If there are indications of spinal and/or neck injuries, fully immobilize the patient using a cervical collar and long spine board. Continuous suctioning may be required. When the facial soft tissues are injured, there may be underlying facial bone fractures. Take care to transport the patient so that no unnecessary pressure is placed on facial injury sites. Monitor the patient and be alert for airway problems.

Injuries to the Eyes

Before considering the various types of eye injuries and their appropriate care, it is important to know the major structures of the eye and how it functions.

Structure and Function of the Eye

The eye is a globular structure, situated in a bony depression of the skull called the **orbit.** Each orbit is made up of parts of the bones of the forehead, temple, and upper jaw. Any serious blow to these bones may transfer the trauma to the eyes. The typical eye is almost one inch in diameter, with over 80% of the globe hidden within the orbit.

The white of the eye is the **sclera** (SKLE-rah). This is a semirigid capsule of fibrous tissue that helps to maintain the shape of the globe and contains the fluids found inside the eye.

The colored portion of the external eye is the **iris,** which has an adjustable opening called the **pupil.** In dim light, the pupil dilates to allow more light to enter the eye, while in bright light, it con-

stricts and restricts the amount of light entering the eye. Over the iris and pupil lies a clear portion of the sclera called the **cornea** (KOR-ne-ah). This structure protects the iris and pupil and helps to keep fluids inside the eye. In addition, the cornea is highly involved with the eye's function of focusing light.

A thin delicate membrane called the **conjunctiva** (kon-junk-TI-vah) covers the sclera, the cornea, and the undersurfaces of the eyelids. When irritated, its tiny blood vessels become swollen with blood, giving the eye a "bloodshot" or pink appearance. This is a sign of the condition known as conjunctivitis.

The internal eye is divided into an anterior cavity and a posterior cavity. The anterior cavity exists between the cornea and the lens. The **lens** is located behind the iris and pupil. This cavity is filled with a clear, watery fluid known as **aqueous** (A-kwe-us) **humor.** In some penetrating eye injuries, this fluid will leak from the eye, but with time and proper care, the body can replace it. The entire posterior cavity is located behind the lens. It is filled with a transparent jelly like substance called the **vitreous** (VIT-re-us) **humor.** This substance is very important in maintaining the shape and length of the globe. Normal lens function takes place with a certain amount of pressure exerted on it by the vitreous humor. This gel *cannot* be replaced, and it cannot be restored by the body.

Light rays are bent when they pass through the cornea and the aqueous humor. This begins the focusing process. As light passes through the lens, muscular action can change the shape of the lens to allow the light to be focused on the retina. During this process, the image is inverted so that it focuses on the **retina** upside down (the brain will revert the image so that everything is seen in an upright position). The cells of the retina convert light into electrical impulses that are conducted through the optic nerve to the vision center of the brain. This is found at the back of the head in the **occipital** (ok-SIP-i-tal) **lobe** of the brain.

The eye is protected by the orbital bones and the eyelids. The inner surface of the eyelids and the surface of the eye are protected and moistened by tears produced by the **lacrimal** (LAK-re-mal) **gland** (tear gland). Each time the eye blinks, the eyelids glide over the exposed surface, sweeping it clean of dust and other irritants. Tears are drained away through a lacrimal duct, located in the medial corner of the eye, at the junction of the eyelids. This duct leads into the nasal cavity.

REMEMBER: It is important to keep the eyelids of an unconscious patient closed. An unconscious person has no involuntary blinking action to sweep tears across the exposed portions of the eyes. An

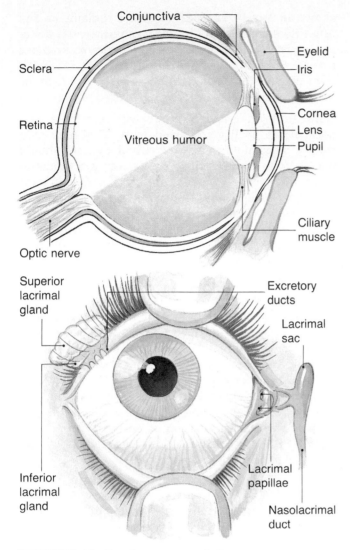

Conjunctiva
Eyelid
Iris
Sclera
Cornea
Lens
Pupil
Retina
Vitreous humor
Ciliary
muscle
Optic nerve
Superior
lacrimal
gland
Excretory
ducts
Lacrimal
sac
Inferior
lacrimal
gland
Lacrimal
papillae
Nasolacrimal
duct

FIGURE 12–7. Anatomy of the eye.

unprotected eye will dry out quickly and become damaged. This damage may be permanent. If the patient's eyes will not stay closed, place sterile dressings moistened with sterile saline over both eyes and bandage these dressings in place.

Types of Eye Injury

Commonly seen eye injuries include:

- *Foreign objects*—Usually the patient complains of feeling the object and shows redness of the eye ("bloodshot"). The eye often waters heavily with tears. These tears may feel slippery.
- *Contusions*—These are closed wound injuries. There may or may not be damage to the eyelids. The patient usually complains of pain. If the patient says that he is having trouble seeing out of the injured eye, or if he reports double vision, then the damage

may be very serious. The eye may appear reddened or swollen. Look at the iris. If it is not easily visible, or if you see blood between the cornea and the iris, the patient should be transported to a medical facility as soon as possible. If other injuries permit, position the patient in a semiseated position to help lower the pressure in the eye.

- *Abrasions*—Minor scratches to the surface of the eye can be caused by foreign objects. These types of scratches are usually invisible. Look for major scratches on the cornea. The cornea should appear clear, smooth, and wet. *Do not* touch the cornea or try to remove any foreign matter. The patient will probably be more comfortable if he keeps both eyes shut.
- *Lacerations*—Look for cuts in the eyelids and the sclera. Consider a lacerated sclera to be a serious situation since a deep cut may allow vitreous humor to escape.
- *Puncture wounds*—Look for punctures, including eyelid perforations. Since the sclera tends to close itself on open wounds, a puncture may appear as an abrasion. You must consider the mechanism of injury and, when possible, gather information by interviewing the patient and/or bystanders. Any puncture wound to the eye must be considered serious. Take great care to look for embedded and impaled objects.
- *Burns*—The patient and bystanders often are the source of information to tell you of a burn to the eyes. The scene also may give clues. Look for highly irritated or damaged tissues, including singed eyebrows or eyelashes. Burns to the eyelids indicate that there may be burns to the eyes.
- *Avulsions*—Look to see if the eyelids are torn or torn away and if the eyeball protrudes or is pulled from its socket.

WARNING: Injury to the eye may mean that there are other head injuries, including brain damage. There also may be injuries to the cervical spine. Assume there are serious head injuries if there are any indications of fractures around the orbit; the sclera is red due to bleeding; one or both eyes cannot be moved; one pupil is larger than the other; both pupils are unresponsive; one or both eyes protrude; or the eyes cross or turn in different directions.

Emergency Care for Eye Injuries

When caring for a patient with eye injuries, you will have to cover *both* eyes, even if only one eye is injured. Remember that when one eye sees something and moves, the other eye duplicates this movement. This action is called **sympathetic eye movement.** Explain to the patient why you must cover both eyes and maintain voice and touch contact with him to reduce his anxiety. If the patient is unconscious or has a low state of awareness, have someone attend to him at all times. This will help calm his fears should he regain consciousness or full awareness.

Foreign Objects Some EMS Systems do not recommend that you wash a patient's eyes unless you are dealing with the problem of chemicals in the eye. Irrigation should not delay transport. Follow your local protocols in terms of the procedure and time spent at the scene. Even for cases in which debris is successfully washed from the eye, transport will be required. The patient must be seen by a physician or qualified eye care specialist. If you are permitted to wash objects from the eye, be certain that the globe of the eye has not been deeply lacerated or penetrated. The steps for washing the eye are

shown in Figure 12–8. If an object remains on the inner lid surface and will not wash away, use a sterile, moist applicator or gauze pad to *carefully remove this foreign body. NEVER ATTEMPT TO REMOVE AN OBJECT ON THE CORNEA. Do not try to probe into the eye socket or remove embedded objects.*

Contusions Some patients will request a cold pack or ice pack for bruised eyes. This may help relieve discomfort; however, this procedure should not be done if the patient shows any symptoms or signs of serious eye or head injury. You do not want to increase the risk of additional contamination or cause rapid changes in circulation in the area of the injury. A cold pack will rapidly constrict blood vessels at and around the injury site. If cold is applied, *do not* use pressure.

Abrasions and Lacerations If the eyelid is bleeding, *do not* apply a pressure dressing unless you are certain that there are no lacerations to the globe of the eye. Should the globe also have an open wound, cover the bleeding lid with loose dressings to aid clotting and prevent additional contamination. Remember to cover both eyes.

In cases where there are no open wounds to the eyelid but the globe of the eye is bleeding or shows any other indication of an open wound, DO NOT APPLY PRESSURE. Use loose dressings. Remember to cover both eyes.

REMEMBER: The jelly-like vitreous humor can be squeezed from an open eye wound. This substance cannot be replaced. Loss of vitreous humor may result in blindness.

An alternate method of care for a lacerated eyeball is similar to the care rendered for impaled objects in the eye. This method also is recommended for avulsed eyes. To provide care, you should:

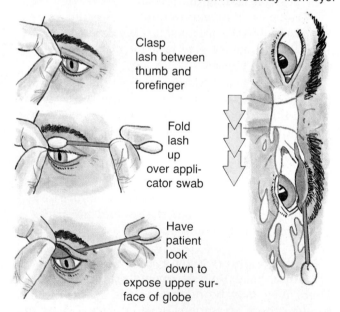

Use sterile water to wash eye, letting water drain down and away from eye.

Clasp lash between thumb and forefinger

Fold lash up over applicator swab

Have patient look down to expose upper surface of globe

FIGURE 12–8. Washing a foreign object from the eye. Clasp the upper lash between your thumb and forefinger. Fold the lash up over the applicator swab. Have patient look down to expose upper surface of globe. Use sterile water (or saline) to wash eye, applying water at the medial corner of the eye socket.

1. Close the injured eye.
2. Place folded 4 × 4's or a "donut ring" around the eye (Figure 12–9). The dressings or ring must not touch the injured globe or lid.
3. Place a non-styrofoam disposable cup over the donut.
4. Set several gauze pads over the uninjured eye.
5. The donut ring, gauze pads, and cup are held in place by self-adherent roller bandage. Have someone stabilize the cup and ring while you apply the bandage.

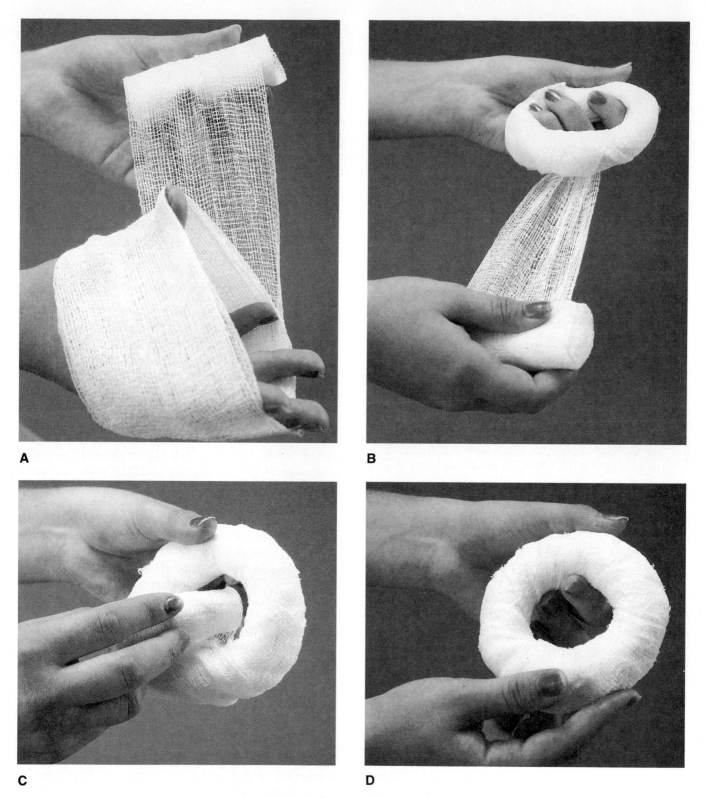

**FIGURE 12–9.   Preparing a donut ring. A. Wrap 2-inch roll around
fingers and thumb seven or eight times. B. Adjust diameter by spread
of fingers. C and D. Wrap rest of roll, alternating between hole and
bandage ring, working around the ring. NOTE: DONUT RINGS
SHOULD BE MADE IN ADVANCE.**

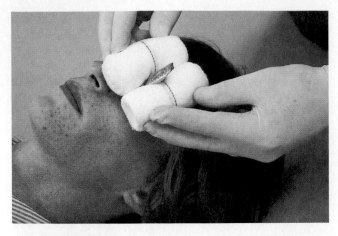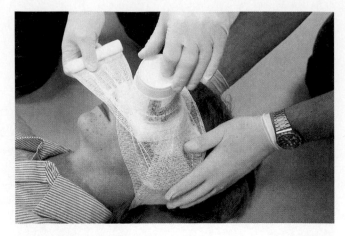

FIGURE 12–10. Managing a patient with an object impaled in the eye.

Puncture Wounds   Use loose dressings for puncture wounds with no impaled objects. If you find an object impaled in the eye, you should:

1. Place a roll of 3-inch gauze bandage on either side of the object, along the vertical axis of the head. These rolls should be placed so that they stabilize the object.
2. Fit a disposable drinking cup (do not use styrofoam) or paper cone over the impaled object and allow it to come to rest on the dressing rolls. *Do not* allow it to touch the object. This will offer rigid protection and will call attention to the patient's problem.
3. Have another rescuer stabilize the dressings and cup while you secure them in place with self-adherent roller bandage or with a wrapping of gauze. *Do not* secure the bandage over top of the cup.
4. The uninjured eye should be dressed and bandaged to reduce eye movements.
5. Provide oxygen and care for shock.
6. Continue to reassure the patient and provide emotional support.

An *alternative* to the above method calls for the rescuer to make a thick dressing with several layers of sterile gauze pads or multitrauma dressings. A hole is cut in the center of this pad, approximately the size of the impaled object. The rescuer then carefully passes this dressing over the impaled object and positions the pad so that the impaled object is centered in the opening. The rest of the procedure remains the same as previously described. If your EMS System has you use this technique, remember that you must take great care not to touch the object as the dressing is set in place.

Burns   Burns to the eyes can be caused by chemicals, heat, or light.

Chemical Burns.   Turn the patient's head to the side so that you can flush the eyes with a steady stream of water. The pour should be from the medial (nasal) corner across the globe to the lateral corner. Use sterile water if it is available; otherwise, use tap water. For patients wearing contact lenses, remove the lenses while washing the eyes (see p. 337). Some EMS Systems are very specific on the time of the wash; however, the safest policy is to wash the eyes for 20 minutes or until transfer is made to the medical facility.

For most chemical burns, it is best to start the wash as soon as possible and continue to irrigate the patient's eyes during transport to the medical facility. This will prevent transport delay and allow the patient to receive specialized care much sooner. If the ambulance does not carry equipment for eye irrigation, use the rubber bulb syringe in the obstetric kit or an IV of normal saline, using the tube for irrigation. When this bulb is used, control the flow so that it gently washes the eye. After washing, close the eyelid and apply a loose sterile dressing.

Heat Burns.   In many cases, only the eyelids will be burned. *Do not* attempt to inspect the eyes if the eyelids are burned. With the patient's eyelids closed, apply a loose, moist dressing.

Light Burns.   Light injuries can be caused by a strong source of light or an ultraviolet light source. Light burns commonly occur from the flash of an arc welder or by the extreme brightness of the sun as it is reflected off sand or snow. These burns are generally very painful, with many patients saying that it feels as if there is sand in the eyes. The onset is usually slow, often taking several hours after exposure before symptoms develop. To make the patient more comfortable, close his eyelids and apply

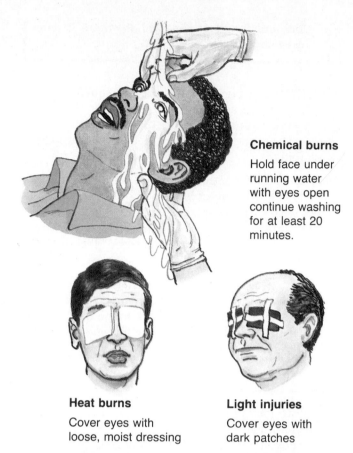

Chemical burns

Hold face under running water with eyes open continue washing for at least 20 minutes.

Heat burns

Cover eyes with loose, moist dressing

Light injuries

Cover eyes with dark patches

FIGURE 12–11. Managing burns to the eyes.

dark patches over both eyes. If you do not have dark patches, apply a pad of dressings followed with a layer of opaque (light-blocking) material such as dark plastic. Instruct the patient not to rub his eyes.

Avulsions　　An avulsed eye is an eye pulled from its socket. This is a very rare occurrence. *Do not* try to force the eye back in. Care for an avulsed eye the same as you would a lacerated eyeball (folded 4 × 4's or donut ring and rigid shield) or as you would an impaled object in the eye. Some EMS Systems allow the initial dressing pads to be moistened with sterile water or saline, especially if transport is delayed or will take a long time to accomplish. When a donut ring is used, it is usually not moistened. Prior to its application, a sterile moist dressing may be added as per local protocol.

　　Lacerated and "torn" eyelids should be carefully covered with dressing materials. When the eyelid is torn off completely, the loose fragment should be recovered after proper wound care is completed on the remaining lid. Standard care is provided for the avulsed part, and it is kept cool and transported with the patient. Your EMS System's protocol may require that the part be placed in sterile dressings that have been soaked in sterile saline.

Removing Contact Lenses

Care of eye injuries can be complicated by the presence of contact lenses (e.g., chemical burns). In some cases, when transport is delayed or will take a long time, the patient's contact lenses may be removed to avoid drying of the eyes and possible abrasive damage to the cornea. Most of the time, the lenses are left in place rather than delay the transport of an unconscious patient.

　　It is not recommended that you remove contact lenses if there is obvious injury to the eye. To do so may cause additional damage. Some EMS Systems have guidelines as to *when* you can remove contact lenses. Be certain to follow the guidelines established in your area. Whenever you observe that a patient is wearing contact lenses, always report this fact to the medical facility staff.

　　Caring for patients wearing contact lenses is not as rare as you may think. Always ask the conscious patient if he or she is wearing contact lenses. Four types of contact lenses are widely prescribed, including the hard corneal, soft lens (flexible), extended wear, and scleral lens.

- *Hard contact lenses* are in wide use, even though soft lenses have become the most popular type of contact lens. When in place, this hard lens covers the cornea. It will appear to cover the entire iris. The typical size is about 0.3 inch in diameter (about the size of a shirt button).
- *Soft contact lenses* (flexible lenses) are very popular. A flexible lens is slightly larger than a dime (about 0.5 inch in diameter), covering the entire cornea and part of the sclera.
- *Extended wear lenses* or "perma lenses" are long-term wear lenses. They are gaining in popularity with the general public and also are worn by many postoperative cataract patients. In the field, you will not be able to distinguish these lenses from soft contact lenses.
- *Scleral lenses* are the least common contact lenses. They are about the size of a quarter, covering the cornea and a large portion of the sclera.

To remove hard corneal lenses, you should:

1. With gloved hands, position one thumb on the upper eyelid and one thumb on the lower eyelid. Keep your thumbs near the margin (edge) of each lid.
2. Separate the eyelids and look for the lens

over the cornea. The lens should slide easily with a gentle movement of the lids. If the lens is not directly over the cornea, slide it to that position with an appropriate movement of the eyelids.

3. Once the lens is over the cornea, open the eyelids further so that the margins of the lids are beyond the top and bottom edges of the lens (Figure 12–12). Maintain this opening.

4. Press both eyelids gently but firmly on the globe of the eye and move the lower eyelid to a position barely touching the edge of the lens.

5. Bring the upper eyelid margin close to the upper edge of the lens, keeping both lids pressed on the globe.

6. Press slightly harder on the lower lid, to move it underneath the bottom edge of the lens. This action should cause the lens to tip outward from the eye.

7. When the lens has tipped slightly, begin to move the eyelids together. The lens should

slide out between the eyelids where it can be removed.

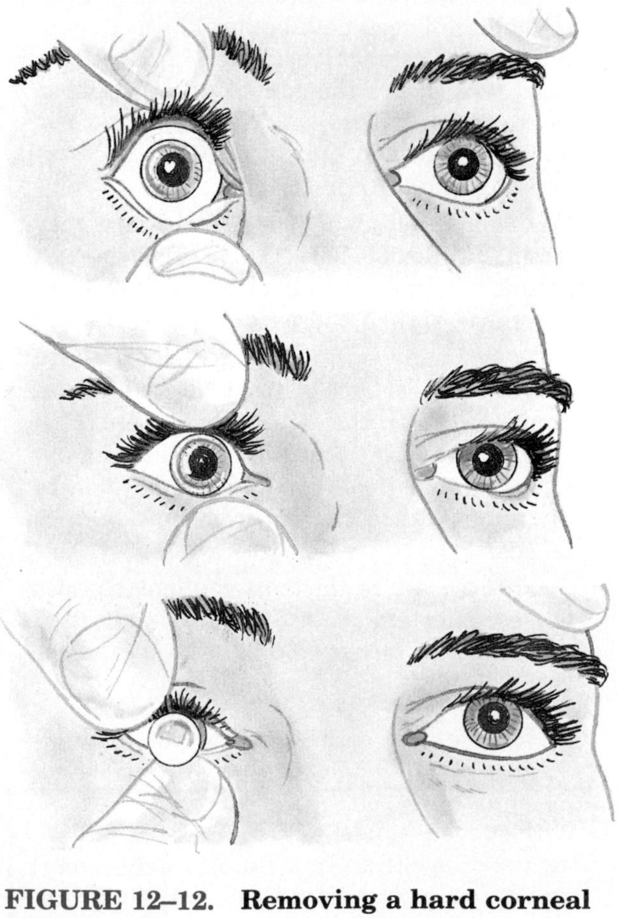

REMEMBER: Never use force in removing a contact lens. If you see the lens but cannot remove it, gently slide it onto the sclera. The lens can remain there with greater safety until more experienced help is available.

NOTE: Special suction cups are available for the removal of hard contact lenses. They should be moistened with saline or sterile water before being brought into contact with the lens. The use of these cups is not recommended in cases of lacerated or chemically burned eyes.

As a general rule, unless there are chemical burns, soft contact lenses are not removed in an the prehospital setting. They are made of a special material that can be left in place for several hours. If you must remove a flexible contact lens, you should:

1. With gloved hands, pull down on the lower eyelid, using your middle finger. Place your index fingertip on the lower edge of the lens.
2. Slide the lens down onto the sclera.
3. Compress the lens slightly between the thumb and index finger, using this pinching motion to cause the lens to double up.
4. Remove the lens from the eye.

NOTE: Some ambulances carry irrigating solutions to add to the eye before attempting to remove soft

FIGURE 12–12. **Removing a hard corneal contact lens.**

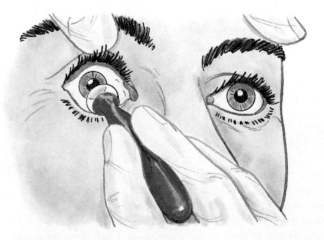

FIGURE 12–13. **Using a moistened suction cup to remove a hard contact lens.**

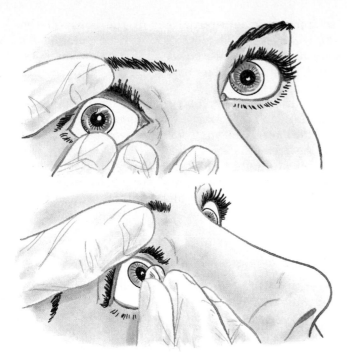

FIGURE 12–14. Removing flexible contact lenses.

contact lenses. Such solutions should not be used if the eye is injured, particularly in cases of deep lacerations. Follow your local guidelines.

To remove scleral lenses, you should:

1. With gloved hands, position the index finger on the lower eyelid near the margin.
2. Slowly and carefully press the eyelid down until the bottom edge of the lens becomes visible. This requires more pressure than for the smaller corneal lenses. Be careful to avoid excessive pressure.
3. Maintaining gentle but firm pressure on the eyelid, move your finger in a lateral direction to pull the eyelid taut.
4. The eyelid margin should slide under the lower edge of the lens, lifting the lens to a position where it can be grasped.

After the contact lenses have been removed, place them in a container with a little water or saline and label the container with the patient's name. Soft lenses are best placed in normal saline. The patient may have a contact lens case with him. Use this case when possible, making certain that it is labeled with the patient's name and the right and left lenses are placed in their correct compartments.

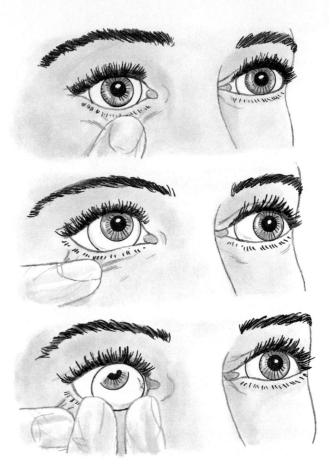

FIGURE 12–15. Removing a scleral lens.

For additional information, request a contact emergency care and instruction packet from the American Optometric Association, 243 N. Lindbergh Blvd., St. Louis, MO 63141.

Injuries to the Ears

Injuries to the ear may go undetected by the EMT, or if detected they may be disregarded or treated lightly. Noting injury to the ear is very important since such an injury may be a sign of a more serious head injury. In addition, the internal structures of the ear may be damaged, leading to deafness and serious problems of balance.

Structure and Function of the Ears

The ear is actually two important organs housed in one anatomical structure (Figure 12–16). One is the mechanism for *hearing,* in which sound waves are converted into nerve impulses. The other is a major part of our *system of balance,* keeping track of head positioning and motion.

The ear is divided into three parts: (1) the exter-

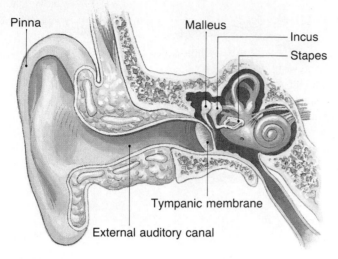

FIGURE 12–16. Anatomy of the ear.

nal ear, (2) the middle ear, and (3) the internal ear. Most of the ear's structures are hidden from view, housed in the temporal bone.

The most prominent structure of the *external ear* is the **pinna** (PIN-nah) or **auricle** (AW-re-kl). Its shape is maintained by cartilage. The opening and canal that run from the pinna into the skull are called the **external auditory canal** (also called the external acoustic meatus, me-A-tus). This canal ends at the eardrum, known as the **tympanic** (tim-PAN-ik) **membrane.**

On the other side of the eardrum lies the *middle ear,* an air-filled chamber that connects with the nasal cavity by way of the **internal auditory canal** (eustachian tube). The middle ear contains three small bones, connected together to stretch from the drum to the inner ear. The *inner ear* is a maze of fluid-filled chambers (hollowed out bone). Sound waves cause the eardrum to vibrate. These vibrations, carried by the middle ear bones to the inner ear, cause the fluids to vibrate and stimulate special nerve endings. These nerves send impulses to the auditory center of the brain to be interpreted as specific sounds.

The inner ear also has receptors that react to the motion of fluids each time the head and body change positions. Impulses are sent to the brain so that body adjustments can be made to maintain balance.

Types of Ear Injuries

All three parts of the ear can be injured. Contusions and crushing injuries to ear cartilage are closed wounds of the ear. Lacerations, abrasions, and avulsions occur to the external ear. Rupture of the eardrum is considered an external injury. You will not be able to tell if middle and inner ear structures are damaged or if the symptoms and signs indicate

an injury to the internal ear or the bones of the skull. Specific care procedures can be followed for external ear injuries, but the rest of the ear, if injured, must be cared for as if there is a skull fracture (see Chapter 11).

Patients may complain of ringing in the ears, internal ear pain, excessive wetness in their ears, and dizziness. You may observe blood or clear fluid coming from the ears or a loss of balance as the patient attempts to reposition himself. Remember, ALL of these symptoms and signs may indicate a skull fracture. Clear or bloody fluids coming from the ear *must* be considered to be a sign of possible skull fracture.

Emergency Care for Ear Injuries

Abrasions and Lacerations Apply a sterile dressing, and bandage (Figure 12–17).

Tears Apply bulky dressings so that the torn ear rests between layers of dressing. Bandage in place.

Avulsions Apply bulky dressings and bandage in place. If the avulsed part can be retrieved, it is to receive the same care as any other avulsed part, to be kept cool, and to be transported with the patient.

Bleeding from the Ears *Do not* pack the external ear canal. To do so may cause additional injury and serious problems if there is a skull fracture. Loosely apply dressings to the external ear and bandage in place.

Clear Fluids Draining from the Ears *Do not* remove any impaled objects. *Do not* pack the external ear canal. Apply loose sterile external dressings. Bandage the dressings in place.

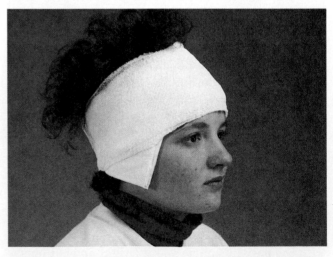

FIGURE 12–17. For external injuries to the ear, apply a dressing and bandage in place.

"Clogged" Ear and Objects in the Ear When a patient complains of a clogged ear, this may be an indication that there is damage to the eardrum, fluids are in the middle ear, or foreign objects are in the ear canal. DO NOT PROBE INTO THE EARS. Prevent the patient from hitting the side of his head in an effort to free objects from the canal.

Injuries to the Nose

Structure and Function of the Nose

The nasal cavity is divided into two chambers, right and left. Separating these two chambers is the **nasal septum.** It is made of cartilage that can be broken easily when struck by a blunt object. This can complicate soft tissue injury assessment and care. The nasal bones, located between the eyes, can also be broken. Too often, assessment of the nose is made only in terms of the skin and the internal soft tissues.

We inhale primarily through the nose. Airway obstruction in the nasal cavity can occur with facial injury. Even though the mouth may be clear, blood and mucus released from nasal injuries can flow from the nose into the throat to cause a major airway obstruction. An open airway is your first priority in emergency care.

Types of Nasal Injuries

Injury can take place to the external nose and the internal nose (nasal cavity). Contusions, abrasions, lacerations, puncture wounds, and avulsions can occur to the soft tissues of the nose. In addition, the

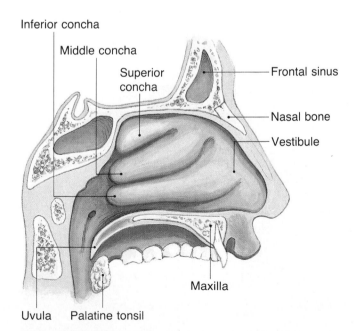

Inferior concha
Middle concha
Superior concha
Frontal sinus
Nasal bone
Vestibule
Maxilla
Uvula   Palatine tonsil

FIGURE 12–18. Anatomy of the nose.

EMT may have to treat problems caused by foreign objects in the nose.

When you see damage to the soft tissues of the nose, realize that other tissues also may be injured. The nasal septum or the nasal bones also may be damaged, increasing the chances of airway obstruction. The bones of the upper jaw, the **maxillae,** and the lower jaw bone, the **mandible,** may be fractured. The blow causing nasal damage may cause posterior head injuries in cases where the head is forced back against some kind of hard object. Neck injuries also can be associated with nasal injuries.

Emergency Care of Nasal Soft Tissue Injuries

Nasal injuries indicate the possibility of injury to the cervical spine. If the nasal injury patient is unconscious or if the mechanism of injury or symptoms and signs indicate possible spinal injury, assume there are spinal injuries and treat accordingly. Most of the care provided for nasal injuries is usually conservative, directed toward maintaining an open airway, controlling bleeding, and positioning the patient so that blood does not drain into the throat.

Abrasions, Lacerations, and Punctures Control bleeding, apply a sterile dressing, then bandage in place.

Avulsions Return attached flaps to their normal position, then apply a pressure dressing and bandage. Fully avulsed flaps of skin and any avulsed portions of the external nose (usually the tip) should be recovered and cared for the same as any avulsed part. It should be kept cool and transported with the patient.

Foreign Objects If the object protrudes, *do not* pull it free. It may have penetrated the septum or tissues high in the nose. Transport the patient without disturbing the object. If the object cannot be seen, *do not* probe for it. Have the patient gently blow his nose, keeping both nostrils open. Do not allow the patient to blow forcefully. If the object cannot be dislodged easily in this manner, transport the patient to a medical facility. *Do not* have the patient blow his nose if he is bleeding from the nostrils or has recently controlled a nosebleed.

Nosebleeds The medical term for a nosebleed is **epistaxis** (ep-e-STAK-sis). In cases in which there are no signs or symptoms of skull fracture, have the patient assume a seated position, leaning slightly forward. This position will provide better drainage for blood and mucus. If the patient is injured in such a way that a seated position is not practical, lay the patient back with the head elevated slightly, or simply turn the head to one side. Should the pa-

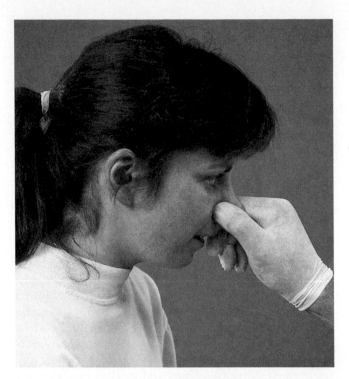

FIGURE 12–19.   Managing a simple nosebleed.

tient be unconscious, or if there are any indications of possible spinal damage, you will have to immobilize the neck and spine before positioning the patient for drainage. Suctioning may be required to keep the airway open.

When the patient can do so, have him pinch his nostrils shut to control bleeding. If the patient cannot do this, you will have to do so, or have a bystander (gloved hand) help to allow you to attend to other patients. Pressure should be applied for at least 5 minutes. Pinching the nostrils is the simplest method and almost always yields the desired results. *Do not* pack the patient's nostrils.

WARNING: If there is clear fluid coming from the nose or ears (halo sign), clear fluid in the ears, or a mix of blood and clear fluids draining from the nose or ears, the patient probably has a skull fracture. In this case, *do not* pinch the nostrils shut or attempt to stop the flow in any way.

Keep in mind that *all* nosebleeds are not the result of injuries related to accidents. High blood pressure can cause nosebleeds. So, too, can infections and excessive sneezing. Such cases are usually easy to treat. Patients with bleeding disorders can have nosebleeds. Sometimes this type of bleeding can be difficult to control. Trauma-induced nosebleeds can range from minor to very serious. Often, the patient will swallow blood and vomit. Prolonged profuse nasal bleeding can cause a patient to develop shock.

Injuries to the Mouth

Injury to the soft tissues of the mouth generally results from blunt trauma, as when the lips are forcefully compressed against the teeth. Common injuries to the mouth include lacerations of the lips, inner cheek wall, or tongue. Avulsions of the lips and tongue can also occur. Often associated with soft tissue damage in the mouth is damage to the teeth or dental appliances. An open airway and proper drainage must be maintained throughout the care of the patient.

Emergency Care for Oral Injuries

Lacerated Lip or Gum   Control bleeding by placing a rolled or folded dressing between the lip and gum. If bleeding is profuse, position the patient to allow for drainage. Monitor so the patient does not swallow the dressing.

Lacerated or Avulsed Tongue   *Do not* pack the mouth with dressings. Position the patient for drainage. If the tongue is fully avulsed (extremely rare), save and wrap the avulsed part and transport with the patient. Although rare, you may find a portion of fully avulsed tissue still in the patient's mouth. You must remove this tissue, provide the standard care for an avulsed part, keep it cool, and transport the part with the patient.

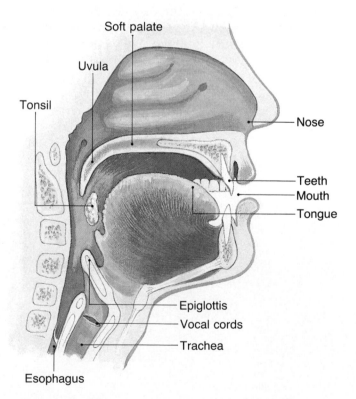

FIGURE 12–20.   Anatomy of the mouth.

Avulsed Lip Control bleeding with a pressure dressing and position for drainage. Do not bandage across the mouth. Save, wrap, label, and transport any fully avulsed tissues, keeping the part cool.

Lacerated or Perforated Inner Cheek External pressure dressings will not control bleeding in the case of perforations. Rolled dressings placed between the wound and the teeth, should be used for perforations and lacerations. The patient must be positioned for drainage. Monitor the patient to prevent him from swallowing dressing materials.

Dental Injuries

Problems involving teeth and dental appliances often occur with soft tissue injuries to the mouth. Search for and remove any completely dislodged teeth, crowns, and bridges. Remove loose dentures and the parts of broken dentures. Transport any dental appliance you remove, broken or intact, with the patient.

Be alert for adult patients with a unilateral partial appliance known as a Nesbit (commonly called a "spider"). This is typically a one- or two-tooth partial that is held in place at four points. Individuals have been known to swallow such devices. If you find one in the mouth of an injured or an unconscious patient, remove it. You must take care not to drop the appliance down the patient's throat. When practical, position the patient with his head turned to the same side as the Nesbit. To avoid the problems caused by blood, mucus, and saliva, grasp the Nesbit with a piece of gauze dressing. Your hands should be gloved. Transport the device with the patient.

Take great care in searching for dislodged teeth. There will be bleeding from the socket of a dislodged tooth. To control this bleeding, have the conscious patient bite down on a pad of gauze placed over the socket. In the case of the unconscious patient, you may have to place gauze into the socket. The less you disrupt the tissues of the socket, the better the chances a dentist will have to replace the avulsed tooth. *Do not* try to insert cotton packets into the socket.

Any avulsed tooth should be wrapped in moist dressings and transported with the patient. The tooth also can be kept moist by placing it in milk. *Do not* rub the tooth in order to clean it: doing so will destroy microscopic structures needed to replant the tooth. Inform the emergency department staff that you have the avulsed tooth. The sooner a dentist or oral surgeon can replant the tooth, the better the chances of success. Best results are seen if the procedure is carried out within 30 minutes of the accident.

INJURIES TO THE SOFT TISSUES OF THE NECK

Injuries to the soft tissues of the neck can be classified as *blunt* or *sharp*. Either type of injury can be so serious a life-threatening emergency that only immediate surgical intervention can save the patient.

Any injury to the neck must be considered to be serious until proven otherwise. The neck contains many vital structures, including the cervical portion of the spinal cord, the larynx and part of the trachea, a portion of the esophagus, the carotid arteries, and the **jugular** (JUG-u-lar) **veins** (Figure 12–21).

Blunt Injuries

Blunt injuries to the neck can occur in a variety of accident situations. In a head-on vehicular accident, the driver may pitch forward and strike his neck against the steering wheel. Passengers often strike their necks on projections of the dashboard. The violent movements produced during an accident can throw persons around inside the vehicle. Passengers may strike their necks on arm rests, seatbacks, and objects being carried in the passenger compartment. However, you should realize that a person may receive a serious neck injury in nothing more than a simple fall should he strike his neck on some object.

Regardless of the cause, the major problem faced in blunt trauma to the neck is usually the collapse of the larynx or the trachea or swelling of their tissues, which creates a blocked airway. These

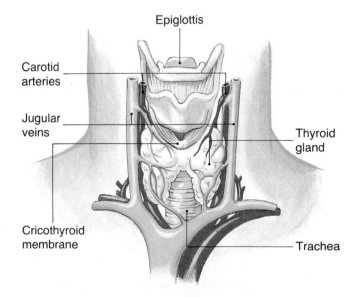

FIGURE 12–21. **The anatomy of the neck.**

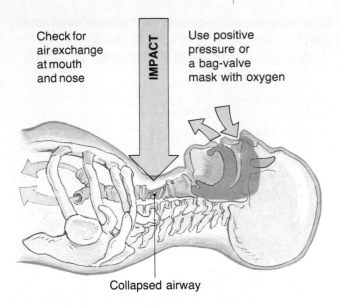

Check for
air exchange
at mouth
and nose

IMPACT

Use positive
pressure or
a bag-valve
mask with oxygen

Collapsed airway

FIGURE 12–22. **Blunt injuries to the neck.**

are both rigid structures containing cartilage. Once they collapse or are crushed, they cannot spring back to their original shape and resume normal function. When such severe injury occurs to the neck, spinal injury also must be assumed to be present.

Signs and Symptoms

For cases of blunt injury to the soft tissues of the neck, assess for:

- Loss of voice or hoarseness
- Signs of airway obstruction when the mouth and nose are clear and no foreign body can be dislodged from the airway
- Contusions on or depressions in the neck
- Deformities of the neck
- Air or crackling sensations under the skin. This is known as subcutaneous emphysema, the result of air leaking into the soft tissues of the neck.

Emergency Care

If the injury is mild, ensure an open airway, manually stabilize the head and neck, care for shock, administer a high concentration of oxygen, and apply cold packs to the site.

For serious blunt trauma injury to the neck, manually stabilize the head and neck, apply a cervical collar, immobilize on a long spine board, and transport the patient to a medical facility without delay; emergency surgery may be needed to open

the airway. Keep the patient calm and ask that he try to breathe slowly, if possible. Administer oxygen, using a bag-valve-mask unit or other form of ventilation-assisted device if air must be forced past an obstruction. Cold packs should be applied to the injury site to reduce swelling.

REMEMBER: If the accident was serious enough to produce a blunt injury to the neck, it may have produced serious injury to the cervical spine. If basic life support measures must begin before immobilizing the neck, *extreme care* must be taken to move the patient's head no more than absolutely necessary. Aggravation of cervical spine injuries can lead to permanent paralysis or death.

Sharp Injuries

The carotid arteries and the jugular veins pass through the neck, relatively close to the body's surface. Sharp injuries to these vessels can produce catastrophic bleeding. Arterial bleeding will be profuse, with bright red blood spurting from the wound site. Venous bleeding can be profuse with dark red to maroon-colored blood flowing steadily from the wound.

Emergency Care—Severed Neck Artery

1. Manage arterial bleeding with direct pressure.
2. Administer a high concentration of oxygen.
3. Care for shock.
4. Transport immediately.

NOTE: Bleeding from neck arteries is very difficult to control. Some EMS Systems have now adopted

For bleeding from a vein, seal wound and tape seal in place

For bleeding from an artery, control bleeding by direct pressure on artery

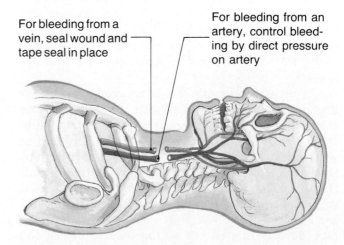

FIGURE 12–23. **Sharp injuries to the neck.**

the technique described below for both arterial and venous neck bleeding.

Emergency Care—Severed Neck Vein

Bleeding from a large neck vein usually cannot be controlled by direct pressure. Sometimes a large bulky dressing and firm hand pressure will control bleeding, but usually the ends of the veins pull away from the wound site and bleed freely. In addition to the loss of blood, there may be the problem of air being sucked into the vein and carried to the heart as an air embolism. This is usually fatal.

To control bleeding from a neck vein, you should apply an occlusive dressing. The problem with this procedure has always been bandaging the dressing in place. The blood on the skin and flowing from the wound prevents the effective use of tape as a bandage. Note that this procedure allows for pressure to be applied over the site and usually above and below the injury.

SUMMARY

The basic rules of open and closed injury care learned in Chapter 8 apply to specific areas of the head and neck. You must know care procedures in an exact step by step fashion, so no attempt will be made to quickly review each procedure. Specific care procedures require you to remember certain rules and exceptions to rules. For example:

SCALP WOUNDS—*Do not* try to clear the surface of the scalp and *do not* apply finger pressure if there is any chance of skull fracture. Control bleeding with a dressing held in place by roller bandage, or apply a triangular bandage.

FACIAL WOUNDS—Maintain the airway, control bleeding, and dress and bandage the wound. *Position for drainage.* Remember, you can remove impaled objects from the cheek, provided that the object has passed through the cheek wall into the oral cavity.

EYE WOUNDS—You need to remember:
- *Do not* apply direct pressure to a lacerated eyeball.
- *Do not* attempt to remove foreign materials from the cornea.

- *Do not* remove impaled objects. Stabilize the object with a donut ring or folded 4 × 4's, cover with a rigid shield (e.g., paper cup), and bandage both in place.
- *Do not* try to replace an avulsed (extruded) eyeball. Manage as you would a lacerated eye or object impaled in the eye.
- *Do not* open the eyes of a patient with burns to the eyelids.
- Close the eyes of unconscious patients.
- If done in your EMS System, wash foreign objects from the eyes if there are no serious lacerations or puncture wounds.
- Manage burns by washing the patient's eyes with flowing water. For the wash to be effective, you must hold the eyelids open. The safest procedure is to wash the eyes for 20 minutes or until the patient is transported to the medical facility.
- When you must cover a patient's injured eye, cover both eyes to reduce sympathetic movements.

EAR WOUNDS—*Do not* probe into the external ear canal and *do not* pack the canal with dressing or cotton. For lacerations and bleeding, apply dressings and bandage. Save avulsed parts using standard procedures, keep the parts cool, and transport with the patient.

NOSE INJURIES—*Maintain an open airway. Do not* pack the nostrils. Bleeding from the nose (epistaxis) is best controlled by pinching the nostrils shut. Provide for proper drainage away from the throat. Avulsed parts are cared for using the standard procedures approved by your EMS system (e.g., dry versus moist).

INJURY TO THE MOUTH—*Maintain an open airway and allow for drainage. Do not* pack the mouth with dressing materials. If dressings are placed between cheek and gum, keep alert so they are not swallowed. It is best to leave 3 or 4 inches of dressing material outside the patient's mouth. Save all avulsed parts, including teeth. Avulsed teeth should be transported wrapped in moist dressings.

NECK WOUNDS—A neck wound indicates *possible spinal injury.* Manage arterial bleeding with pressure dressings. Venous bleeding from the neck may require the application of a bulky dressing and direct pressure. Manage serious venous bleeding with an occlusive dressing.

SCAN 12–1 SEVERED NECK VEINS— OCCLUSIVE DRESSING

1

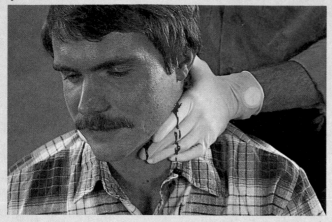

Do not delay! Place your gloved palm over the wound.

Dressing must be heavy plastic . . . sized to be no more than 2″ larger in diameter than site.

2

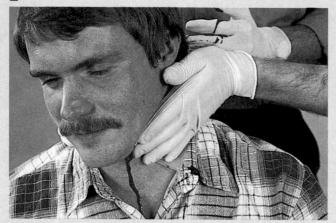

Occlusive dressing is placed over wound site.

3

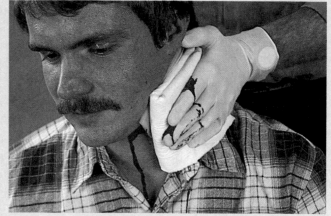

A roll of gauze is placed over the dressing.

4

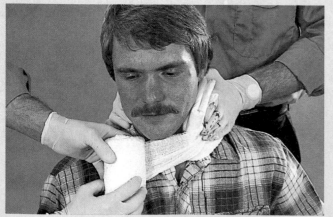

Start a figure-eight . . . bringing bandage over dressing.

5

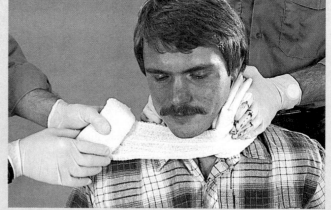

Cross over the shoulder . . .

NOTE: For demonstration purposes, patient is upright.

6

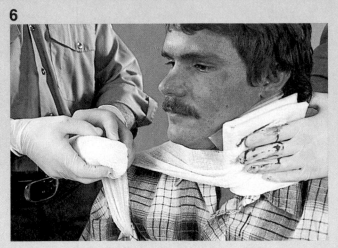

Bring bandage under the armpit . . .

7

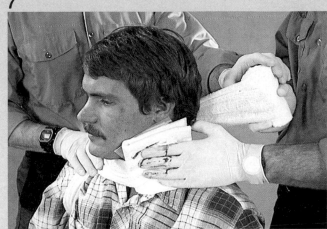

Cross back over shoulder and anchor several times to cover entire dressing.

8

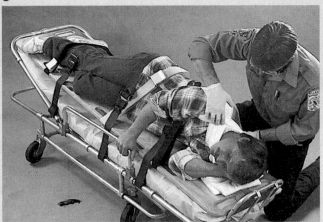

Place the patient on left side, tilting body to raise feet (Trendelenburg position)

9

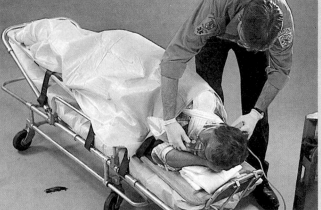

Care for shock and continue to administer a high concentration of oxygen.

Placing the patient on the left side in the Trendelenburg position will trap air emboli in the right atrium. Do not simply raise the legs. Tilt the entire body by 15 degrees.

NOTE: Bandaging should control bleeding without restricting breathing.

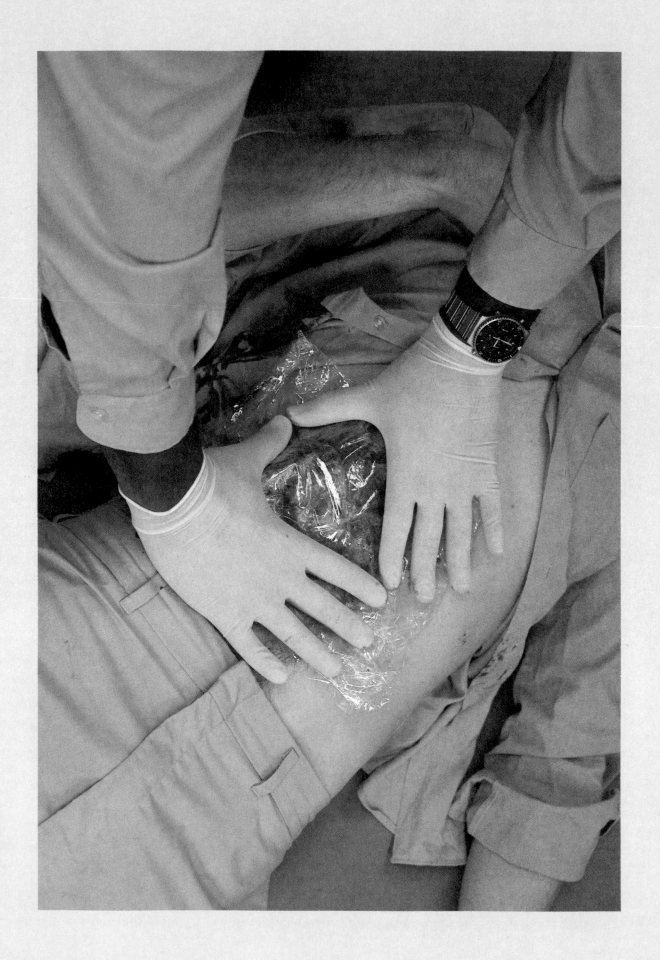

Injuries IV:
The chest, abdomen, and genitalia

OBJECTIVES   As an EMT, you should be able to:

1. Use anatomical terms to define the chest. (pp. 240–242)
2. List the types of nonpenetrating soft tissue injuries to the chest and the care for each type of injury. (pp. 350–351)
3. Classify chest injuries and describe the general symptoms and signs associated with open and closed chest wounds. (pp. 351–352)
4. Describe how to determine and care for possible pneumothorax, objects impaled in the chest, possible rib fractures, and flail chest. (pp. 352–358)

5. List and describe the common complications associated with injuries to the chest. (pp. 358–360)
6. List the major signs of abdominal injury and the symptoms associated with closed abdominal injury. (p. 361)
7. State the procedures used to care for open and closed abdominal injury. (pp. 362–363)
8. Describe the basic care for injuries to the genitalia. (pp. 363–366)
9. Describe the basic care for a patient with an inguinal hernia. (p. 366)

SKILLS   As an EMT, you should be able to:

1. Control bleeding and apply the proper dressing and bandage for a given open soft tissue injury to the chest, abdomen, pelvis, and genitalia.
2. Apply patient assessment techniques to detect possible:
   • Blunt trauma to the chest
   • Fractured ribs
   • Flail chest

• Pneumothorax
• Tension pneumothorax
• Open abdominal injury
• Closed abdominal injury
3. Care for patients with flail chest, including the steps needed to correct paradoxical movement of the flailed section.

4. Care for pneumothorax and correct the problems of tension pneumothorax associated with this care.

5. Detect possible hemothorax, pneumothorax, hemopneumothorax, cardiac tamponade, traumatic asphyxia, and tension pneumothorax.

6. Provide basic EMT-level care for complications due to injuries to the chest.

7. Provide care for both open and closed abdominal injury.

8. Provide care for the major injuries to the genitalia.

TERMS you may be using for the first time:

Eviscerate (e-VIS-er-ate) – usually applies to the intestine or other internal organ protruding through an incision or wound in the abdomen. (See also Chapter 8.)

Flail Chest – injury in which usually three or more consecutive ribs on the same side of the chest are fractured, each in at least two locations. A flail chest also can occur when the sternum is fractured loose from its attachments with the ribs. This is sometimes referred to as a flailed sternum.

Genitalia (jen-i-TAL-le-ah) – the external reproductive system.

Hiatal (hi-A-tal) **Hernia** – occurs when part of the stomach bulges upward through the opening that allows the esophagus to pass through the diaphragm. The opening is the hiatus (hi-A-tus).

Inguinal (IN-gwin-al) **Canal** – the passageway from the scrotum into the pelvic cavity that carries the blood vessels, nerves, and cord of the testis.

Inguinal (IN-gwin-al) **Hernia** – or "rupture" a soft tissue injury in which the lining of the abdomino-pelvic cavity ruptures and the intestine protrudes through the opening into the inguinal canal.

Paradoxical Movement – movement of a flailed section in the opposite direction to the rest of the chest during respirations.

Pneumothorax (NU-mo-THO-raks) – condition resulting when air enters the thoracic cavity and is trapped in the pleural space.

Subcutaneous (SUB-ku-TA-ne-us) **Emphysema** (EM-fi-SEE-mah) – air under the skin. This is observed most frequently when a lung is punctured and air escapes into the surrounding tissues of the thorax.

Sucking Chest Wound – an open wound to the chest that draws air from the atmosphere into the chest cavity. This is a form of pneumothorax.

Tension Pneumothorax – condition in which air escapes from a punctured lung and is trapped in the thoracic cavity (pleural space). In some cases, the air may enter through a sucking chest wound and be trapped as the wound seals itself shut. This may produce rapid death.

Traumatic Asphyxia – a group of symptoms and signs associated with sudden severe compression of the chest. This is sometimes classified as acute thoracic compression syndrome.

INJURIES TO THE CHEST

The basic anatomy of the chest was presented in Chapter 9. Whenever you are assessing chest injuries, keep in mind that there may be injuries to the heart, great blood vessels, lungs, trachea, liver, gallbladder, stomach, and spleen. Remember that there is a posterior portion of the thoracic cavity. Back injuries may involve chest structures, including the ribs, lungs, and heart.

Types of Chest Injuries

The chest can be injured in a number of ways, including:

- *Blunt Trauma*—A blow to the chest can fracture the ribs, the sternum, and the costal cartilages. Whole sections of the chest may collapse. With severe blunt trauma, the lungs and airway can be damaged and the heart may be seriously injured.

- *Penetrating Objects*—Bullets, knives, pieces of metal or glass, steel rods, pipes, and various other objects can penetrate the chest wall, damaging internal organs and impairing respiration.

- *Compression*—This is a severe form of blunt trauma in which the chest is rapidly com-

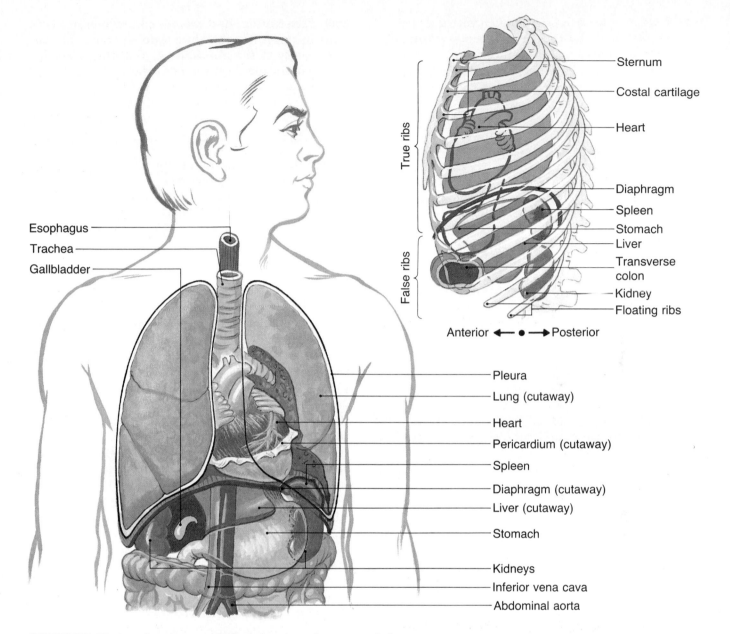

Esophagus
Trachea
Gallbladder

Sternum
Costal cartilage
Heart
True ribs
Diaphragm
Spleen
Stomach
Liver
Transverse colon
False ribs
Kidney
Floating ribs

Anterior ← ● → Posterior

Pleura
Lung (cutaway)
Heart
Pericardium (cutaway)
Spleen
Diaphragm (cutaway)
Liver (cutaway)
Stomach
Kidneys
Inferior vena cava
Abdominal aorta

FIGURE 13–1. Anatomy of the chest and upper abdomen.

pressed, as when the driver of a motor vehicle pitches forward after a head-on collision and strikes his chest on the steering column. The heart can be severely squeezed, the lungs can be ruptured, and the sternum and ribs can be fractured.

Injuries to the chest also may injure the lungs, heart, or great blood vessels. Basic cardiac life support may be the only course of action for the EMT. However, there are other care procedures that can undoubtedly help save the patient's life.

Chest injuries can be classified as OPEN or CLOSED.

Open—When the skin is broken, the patient has an open wound. However, most people use the term *open chest wound* to mean that the chest wall is penetrated, as, for example, by a bullet or a knife blade. An object can pass through the wall from the outside, or a fractured and displaced rib can penetrate the chest wall from within. The heart, lungs, and great vessels can be injured at the same time the chest wall is penetrated. It may be difficult to tell if the chest cavity has been penetrated by looking at the wound. *Do not* open the wound to determine its depth. Specific symptoms and signs will indicate possible open chest injury (see p. 352).

• *Closed*—The skin is not broken with a closed chest injury, leading many people to think that the damage done is not serious. Such injuries, sustained through blunt trauma and compression injuries, can cause contusions and lacerations of the heart, lungs, and great vessels.

General Symptoms and Signs of Chest Injury

An obvious wound is the most reliable sign of chest injury. When there is no such wound, check for the following:

• Pain at the injury site
• Painful breathing
• Difficult breathing
• Indications of developing shock, including rapid and weak pulse, indicating shock from blood loss or respiratory shock; low blood pressure; and cyanosis, indicating oxygen deficiency
• Coughing up bright red, frothy blood, indicating a possible punctured lung
• Distended neck veins
• Tracheal deviation—the trachea is pushed off to the uninjured side
• Failure of the chest wall to expand and contract normally—look closely for unequal chest movements
• Pain on compression of the lateral chest wall
• Subcutaneous emphysema (SUB-ku-TA-ne-us EM-fi-SEE-mah)—air has escaped from a puncture in the airway or the lung and has invaded the tissues of the thorax and neck. The patient may report "crackling" sensations under the skin, or you may feel this by placing your fingers over the injury site.
• Unequal air entry

Note how the above may be determined from a complete and proper patient assessment.

Specific Open Chest Wounds

Puncture Wounds

Puncture wounds can range from minor to life threatening. The object producing the wound may remain impaled in the chest, or the wound may be completely open. Penetrating chest wounds occur when an object tears or punctures the chest wall, opening the thoracic cavity to the atmosphere. You must consider ALL penetrating chest wounds to be life threatening. If there is an exit wound, then penetration is easy to determine. Otherwise, you will be able to tell if a puncture wound is a penetrating wound by noting:

• A severe chest wound in which the chest wall is torn or punctured.
• A sucking sound may be made each time the patient inhales. These wounds are sometimes called "sucking" chest wounds.
• The patient coughs up red, frothy blood.

Pneumothorax

Pneumothorax (NU-mo-THO-raks) occurs when the pleural sac is punctured and air enters the thoracic cavity (Figure 13–2). The air can come through the external wound opening, or it may come out of a punctured lung. In pneumothorax, the lung collapses. The term *sucking chest wound* is used when the thoracic cavity is open to the atmosphere. Each time the patient breathes, air can be sucked into the opening. There may or may not be a characteristic sucking sound, especially when the lung completely collapses.

This patient will develop severe **dyspnea** (difficult breathing) and he may be gasping for air. The delicate pressure balance within the thoracic cavity is destroyed and the lung on the injured side collapses.

The object penetrating the chest wall may have seriously damaged a lung, major blood vessel, or the heart itself. This type of injury is a TRUE EMERGENCY that requires immediate initial care and transport to a medical facility as soon as possible.

Care for Open Pneumothorax

1. Maintain an open airway. Provide basic life support if necessary.
2. Seal the open chest wound as quickly as possible. If need be, use your gloved hand. *Do not* delay sealing the wound to find an occlusive dressing.
3. Apply an occlusive dressing to seal the wound (Figure 13–3). When possible, the occlusive dressing should be at least two inches wider than the wound. If there is an exit wound in the chest you will have to apply an occlusive dressing over this wound also.

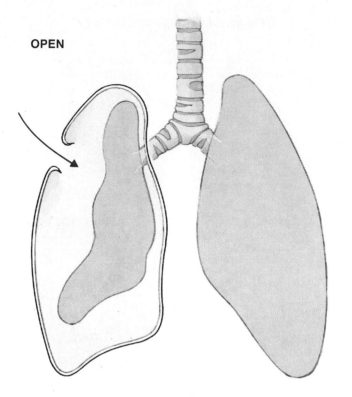

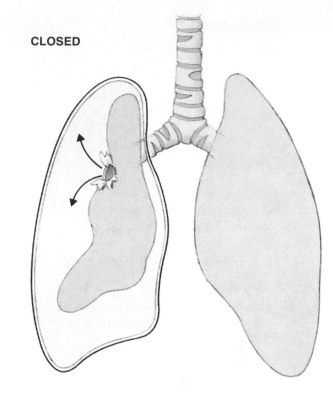

FIGURE 13–2.   Pneumothorax.

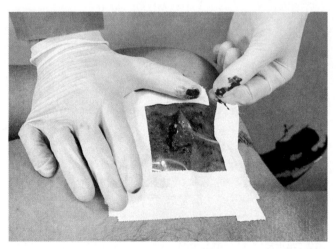

A

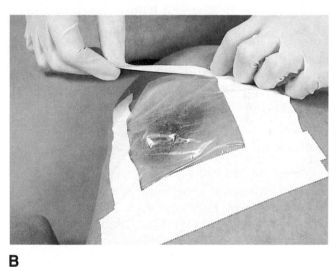

B

FIGURE 13–3.   Applying an occlusive dressing for an open pneumothorax: A. Flutter valve. B. Traditional approach.

There are two methods now in use. The newer approach calls for taping the occlusive dressing in place, leaving a corner of the dressing unsealed to relieve pressure in the thoracic cavity (see Figure 13–5). As the patient inhales, the dressing will seal the wound. During exhalation, the free corner acts as a flutter valve to release air that is trapped in the thoracic cavity.

The traditional procedure calls for sealing all four edges with tape. The last edge should be sealed when the patient forcefully exhales. If the seal is effective, respirations will be partially stabilized.

If blood or perspiration prevents taping, place thick dressings, trauma pads, or a sanitary napkin over the occlusive dressing and hold in place with cravats tied around the patient's chest.

4. Administer a high concentration of oxygen.

5. Care for shock.

6. Transport as soon as possible. Unless other injuries prevent you from doing so, keep the patient positioned on the injured side.

7. Monitor the patient, making certain that the airway is open. Be prepared to suction blood from the oral cavity. Call ahead to alert the emergency department staff.

NOTE: Household plastic wrap is not thick enough to make an effective occlusive dressing for open chest wounds. If no other source of an occlusive dressing is available, this wrap can be used, but it must be folded several times to be of the proper thickness. Even then, it may fail. Most ambulances carry sterile disposable items that are wrapped in plastic. The inside surface of the plastic is sterile. If you do not have an occlusive dressing, use one of these wrappers or an IV bag. If there is no other choice, aluminum foil can be used to make the seal.

A complication can develop with an open pneumothorax that has been managed with the application of a sealed occlusive dressing. This complication is called **tension pneumothorax.*** If a patient has a penetrating chest wound with a punctured lung, air will enter the thoracic cavity through the open wound in the chest wall and through the opening in the lung (Figure 13–4). If you seal off the chest wall opening, air will still flow from the punctured lung into the cavity with each breath. The air will not be able to escape and pressure will build in the cavity. The signs of tension pneumothorax include:

- Increasing respiratory difficulty
- Indications of developing shock, including rapid, weak pulse; cyanosis; and low blood pressure due to decreased cardiac output
- Distended neck veins
- Tracheal deviation to the uninjured side
- Uneven chest wall movement
- Reduction of breathing sounds heard in the affected side of the chest

If you seal a sucking chest wound with an occlusive dressing and find that the patient worsens rap-

* This condition also can occur if an open chest wound with a punctured lung seals itself or seals around an impaled object, or if the patient has a punctured or damaged lung with no open chest wound.

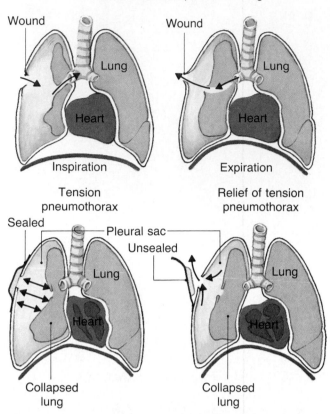

Pneumothorax with punctured lung

FIGURE 13–4. Tension pneumothorax may be a complication of open chest wound care.

idly, then you will have to lift a corner of the seal to let air escape and close the seal before the patient exhales. The patient should respond almost immediately as pressure is released around the heart, great blood vessels, and uninjured lung. Reseal the wound and monitor the patient. You may have to unseal and reseal the wound again, continuing this process throughout care and transport.

Tension pneumothorax is the reason why many medical authorities are calling for the newer procedure of care requiring a corner of the occlusive dressing to be left *unsealed*. The pressure buildup is released through the flutter valve (Figure 13–5).

REMEMBER: Whenever you apply an occlusive dressing to a patient with pneumothorax, stay alert for tension pneumothorax. If you use a flutter valve, you still must monitor the patient for this condition. The free corner of the dressing may stick to the chest

On inspiration, dressing seals
wound, preventing air entry

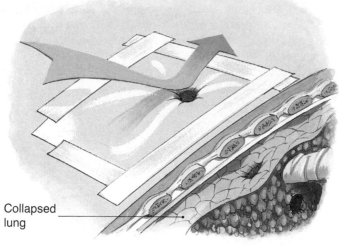

Collapsed
lung

Expiration allows trapped air to escape
through untaped section of dressing

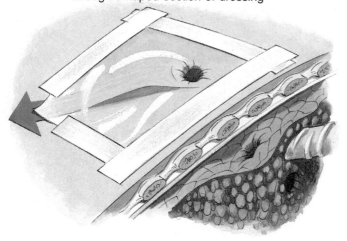

FIGURE 13–5. Creating a flutter valve to relieve tension pneumothorax.

or the dressing may be drawn into the wound causing the valve to fail.

Impaled Objects

As discussed in Chapter 8, an impaled object should be left in place. The object must be stabilized with bulky dressings or pads (Figure 13–6). You should use tape to hold all dressings and pads in place. If tape proves to be ineffective due to blood or sweat on the patient's skin, hold the dressings and pads in place with wide cravats. These should be tied at the patient's side but not over wound sites. Do not lay the patient on the side containing the impaled

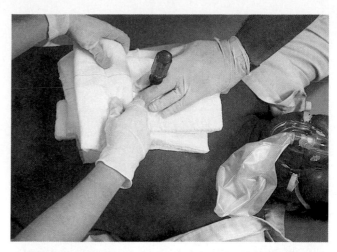

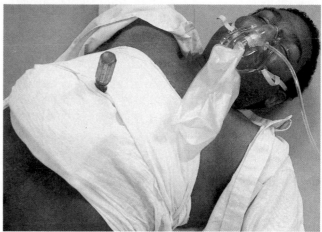

FIGURE 13–6. Stabilizing and dressing an object impaled in the chest.

object and make certain that nothing touches the impaled object during transport.

Specific Closed Chest Injuries

Closed chest injuries include rib fractures, flail chest, and compression injuries.

Rib Fractures

Rib fractures usually result from blunt trauma or compression. Often, you will not know for sure if a rib is fractured; however, some ribs are more susceptible to injury than others. The upper four pairs of ribs are rarely fractured because they are protected by the structures of the shoulder girdle. The fifth through tenth pairs of ribs are the ones most commonly fractured. The freedom of movement found in the "floating" ribs often prevents them from being fractured.

A conscious, coherent person with fractured ribs can usually point out the exact injury site. Seldom is there any deformity associated with the injury. The symptoms and signs of fractured ribs include:

- Pain at the site of the fracture, with increased pain on moving and breathing
- Tenderness over the site of the fracture
- Shallow breathing, usually due to the pain associated with respiratory movements of the chest
- Sometimes the patient will report a crackling sensation (subcutaneous emphysema) at or near the site of fracture. You may be able to feel this by placing your fingertips over the injury site. This indicates a complication in the form of a pneumothorax.
- Characteristic stance, with the patient leaning toward the injured side and holding his hand over the fracture site (self-splinting).

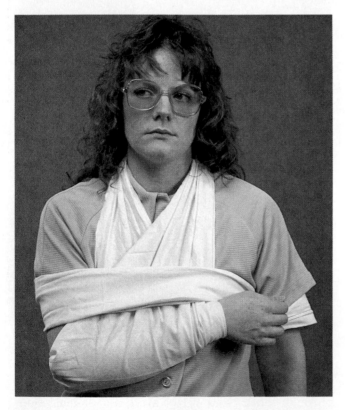

FIGURE 13–7. Care for fractured ribs. Apply sling and swathe to hold the arm against the chest.

Care of Fractured Ribs   Always render care for possible fractured ribs. You will probably help reduce the patient's pain, and you will provide protection for his lungs and the blood vessels that are located between the ribs (intercostal arteries and veins). You will not be able to determine if the patient's injuries are limited to a "simple rib fracture."

To provide care for possible fractured ribs: Place the forearm of the injured side in a sling across the patient's chest. A swathe can be applied to support the arm.

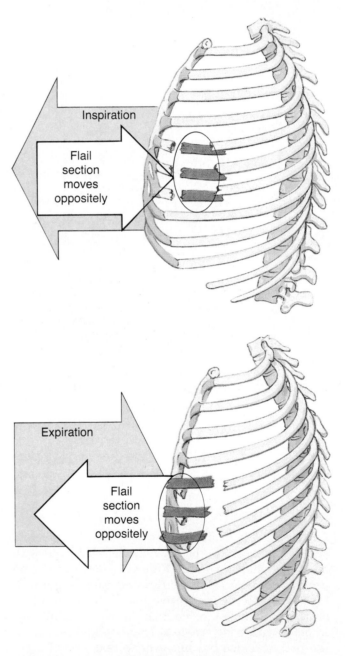

FIGURE 13–8. Paradoxical motion.

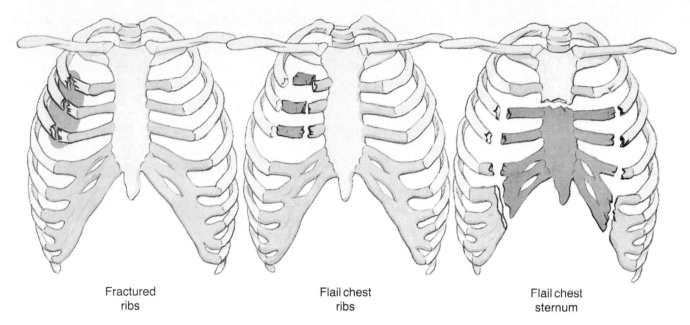

Fractured
ribs

Flail chest
ribs

Flail chest
sternum

FIGURE 13–9. **Rib fractures and flail chest.**

NOTE: EMTs apply a sling and swathe for patients with possible rib fractures. In a few localities, no action other than positioning for comfort and transport is done for possible rib fractures.

Flail Chest

Flail chest usually occurs when *three* or more consecutive ribs on the same side of the chest are fractured, each in at least *two* places. This produces a section of chest wall that is unstable and will move independently of the rest of the chest wall. Often, this movement is in the opposite direction to the rest of the chest wall. This is known as **paradoxical motion** (sometimes incorrectly called paradoxical respirations). The same problem occurs when the sternum is broken away from its cartilage attachments with the ribs. Both of these conditions are called **flail chest.** EMTs see flail chest most often at motor vehicle accidents, usually caused by the patient being forced against the vehicle's steering wheel. The flail section usually occurs to the lateral chest wall or the sternum. Forceful blows to the back also may cause a flail chest, with damage usually being done to the lateral chest walls.

The symptoms and signs of flail chest include:

• The symptoms and signs of fractured ribs. These are usually more pronounced with flail chest.

• The failure of a section of the chest wall to move with the rest of the chest when the patient is breathing. Typically, paradoxical motion is observed.

• The symptoms and signs of shock will develop.

Care for Flail Chest   You must try to hold the flail section in place. Do not attempt to bind, strap, or tape the injured section of ribs or the loose sternum. Instead, stabilize the flailed section. To care for the flail chest patient, you should:

1. Carefully locate the edges of the flail section by gently feeling the injury site.
2. Apply a thick pad of dressings over the site. This pad should be several inches thick. A small pillow can be used in place of the pad of dressings or other low-weight items can also be used, depending on the location of the flailed section and the position of the patient.
3. Use large strips of tape to hold the pad in place. (Place the tape as shown in Figure 13–10.) The tension on the tape bears down on the pad, which in turn depresses the flail section. If tape will not hold, place the patient on injured side.

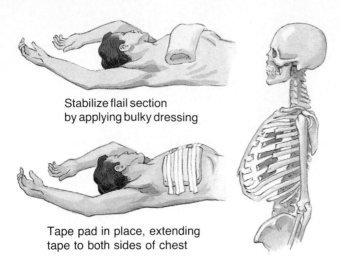

Stabilize flail section
by applying bulky dressing

Tape pad in place, extending
tape to both sides of chest

FIGURE 13–10.   Care for flail chest.

4. Administer a high concentration of oxygen. Assisted ventilation may be necessary.
5. Care for shock.
6. Monitor the patient, taking extra care to look for signs of heart, lung, or abdominal organ injury.
7. Transport as soon as possible with the patient in a semi-reclined position. If the patient cannot tolerate this position, gently place him on the injured side. This will help the flailed section move with the rest of the chest and reduce rubbing together of the broken ends of the ribs. The patient will be more comfortable and will be able to breathe more easily.

WARNING: ALL cases of flail chest are very serious emergencies and must be viewed as life threatening. Even the patient who appears stabilized may rapidly develop severe respiratory problems and shock. Often the severity of other internal injuries is not immediately noticed. Closely monitor the flail chest patient.

Complications of Chest Injuries

The lungs, heart, and great vessels can be injured in accidents involving the chest.

Hemothorax and Hemopneumothorax

In *hemothorax,* lacerations within the thoracic cavity can be produced by penetrating objects or fractured ribs. Blood will flow into the pleural space, the lung may collapse, and the heart may be forced against the uninjured lung.

Hemopneumothorax is a combination of air and blood, usually producing the same results: a collapsed lung and pressure on the heart and uninjured lung.

These two complications usually present the same symptoms and signs as pneumothorax (Figure 13–11). The patient may cough up frothy red blood or flecks of blood may appear on the lips.

Cardiac Tamponade

Cardiac tamponade occurs when a penetrating or blunt injury to the heart causes blood to flow into the surrounding pericardial sac. This unyielding sac fills with blood and compresses the chambers of the

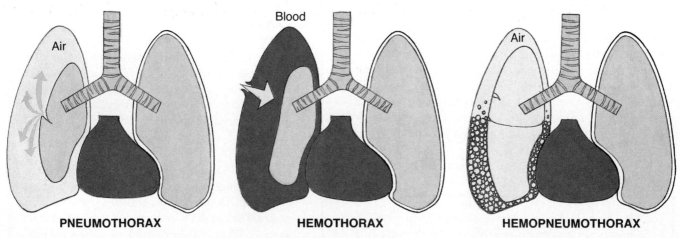

PNEUMOTHORAX   HEMOTHORAX   HEMOPNEUMOTHORAX

FIGURE 13–11.   Conditions produced by chest injuries.

heart to a point where they will no longer fill adequately, backing up blood into the veins. The patient's neck veins will distend, the pulse will become very weak, sweating will be profuse, and successive blood pressure measurements will show systolic and diastolic readings that approach each other (systolic falling, diastolic rising or remaining the same) as the patient's condition deteriorates.

The difference in pressure between systolic and diastolic readings is called **pulse pressure.** If a patient with a chest injury shows a steadily decreasing pulse pressure, this is a reliable sign of serious injury in the thoracic cavity. A pulse pressure below 15 mmHg is critical, indicating an immediate life-threatening emergency. This is a true emergency. Administer a high concentration of oxygen, immobolize if indicated, and transport immediately.

Traumatic Asphyxia

Traumatic asphyxia is one aspect of what is known as acute thoracic compression syndrome. It is not a condition but a group of symptoms and signs that can be associated with sudden compression of the chest, and in some cases the abdomen. When this occurs, the sternum exerts severe pressure on the heart, forcing blood out of the right atrium up into the jugular veins in the neck. The symptoms and signs of traumatic asphyxia are shown in Figure 13–12. THIS IS A TRUE EMERGENCY, requiring immediate transport. Artificial ventilation with 100% oxygen provided through positive pressure is probably the only way to keep the patient alive during transport. When subcutaneous emphysema is present, a bag-valve-mask unit with supplemental oxygen (O_2 reservoir) is probably a better choice. It will provide adequate ventilation with less chance of harming the patient. (Follow local protocols.)

Tension Pneumothorax

Tension pneumothorax can arise in two ways. We have discussed the problem of air escaping from a punctured lung into the thoracic cavity with no exit for this air due to the application of an occlusive dressing. It is possible for a patient to have a closed chest injury in which a lung is punctured (e.g., by a fractured rib). Air will build up within the closed thoracic cavity, quickly impairing heart and lung function. THIS IS A TRUE EMERGENCY. Such patients need immediate advanced medical care. You will have to provide 100% oxygen (bag-valve-mask assist) and transport immediately. Positive pressure

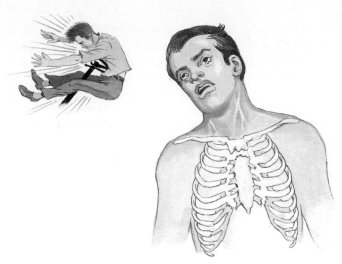

- Distended neck veins
- Head, neck and shoulders appear dark blue or purple
- Eyes may be bloodshot and bulging
- Tongue and lips may appear swollen and cyanotic
- Chest deformity may be present

FIGURE 13–12. Symptoms and signs of traumatic asphyxia.

may be required if the pressure in the thoracic cavity becomes too great for normal lung activity; however, seek a physician's advice since positive pressure may worsen a patient who has tension pneumothorax.

The signs of tension pneumothorax include increasing respiratory difficulty, a weak pulse, cyanosis, and low blood pressure noted due to the decrease in cardiac output. Breath sounds may be abnormal (unilaterally decreased) and air entry will be unequal. The veins of the neck may appear distended, and the trachea may be deviated to the uninjured side (late sign).

Spontaneous Pneumothorax

Spontaneous pneumothorax is usually a medical problem seen when a weakened section of the lung ruptures and releases air into the thoracic cavity (see Chapter 14, Section One). Breath sounds will usually be decreased on the injured side. This condition is almost never life threatening, but it can become tension pneumothorax and require the same basic care.

NOTE: Except for flail chest, sucking chest wounds, and tension pneumothorax caused by an occlusive dressing, there is little the EMT can do for major complications occurring with chest injuries. Provide immediate transport and continued administration of 100% oxygen. It may be necessary to assist ventilations with a bag-valve-mask unit. Use positive pressure when needed. This may be all that you can do. If basic life support measures are provided, often requiring artificial ventilation with oxygen, you may be able to keep the patient alive until more advanced medical procedures can be delivered by the staff of the medical facility.

WARNING: The use of positive pressure on patients with closed chest injuries requires approval by local medical control. Too great a pressure may cause a tension pneumothorax to develop or rapidly worsen an existing case of tension pneumothorax. Some EMS Systems have decided that the bag-valve-mask unit with supplemental oxygen (with O_2 reservoir) is more advisable than oxygen powered breathing devices. Follow local guidelines.

INJURIES TO THE ABDOMEN

The more you know about the structures of the abdomen and their positioning, the better able you will be to evaluate injuries in this region. Referred pain often occurs in the abdomen. This means that pain may be felt in an area other than the site of injury. Damage to the appendix through disease or injury may be expressed as pain around the umbilicus. Injury or disease of the gallbladder may be felt as pain on the back of the right shoulder (see p. 407).

In Chapter 2, the structures of the abdomen were presented and related to the abdominal quadrants. Study this section of Chapter 2 again so that you can look at someone and know the approximate position for each major organ and gland, relating these structures to the abdominal quadrants.

The abdominal organs can be classified as hollow and solid. The hollow organs are:

- *Stomach*—where the initial chemical breakdown of foods begins, producing a semisolid substance called **chyme** (kIm).
- *Small Intestine*—where chemical digestion is completed and absorption of foods take place.
- *Large Intestine*—where the collection and removal of the wastes from digestion occurs. The large intestine includes the colon, rectum, and anus.
- *Appendix*—hollow fingerlike tube located at the beginning of the large intestine. It has no proven function.

- *Gallbladder*—a pear-shaped reservoir for bile, located on the posterior undersurface of the liver.

The solid organs are:

- *Liver*—a large, multifunctional gland in the right upper quadrant, protected by the lower ribs. Its dome-shaped top presses against the diaphragm. Extremely vascular, the liver is a delicate gland that can be easily torn by blunt impact or cut by penetrating objects. The resultant bleeding can be massive and quickly fatal. Injury may release bile into the abdominal cavity causing a severe reaction. The liver is essential to life.
- *Spleen*—a highly vascular organ located behind the stomach and protected by the lower ribs on the left side of the body. The spleen is involved with blood storage and the removal of old blood cells. It is prone to rupture as a result of blunt trauma to the abdomen.
- *Pancreas*—an elongated, flat triangular gland located behind the stomach. It is involved with producing digestive juices and insulin. Serious injury to the pancreas is not common in accidents, but damage is seen in cases of kicking injuries, impacts with steering wheels, stabbings, and gunshot wounds. When injured, as in abdominal gunshot wounds, the pancreas can bleed profusely and release digestive juices into the abdomen. The pancreas is essential to life.

As you consider the names, functions, and locations of the organs and glands in the abdominal cavity, do not forget that this region has many blood vessels and nerves. In addition to these structures, there are many sensitive membranes in the cavity. A large, fat-filled membrane attaches to the stomach and spreads downward like an apron over top of the intestine. It is called the *greater omentum* (o-MEN-tum) and may be seen as a yellowish, spongy tissue pushing out through open abdominal wounds. The small and large intestines are attached to the posterior wall of the cavity by a membrane called the *mesentary* (MES-en-ter-e). This membrane is rich with blood vessels. A penetrating object may slide off the intestine, then lacerate many of the mesenteric blood vessels. All these membranes are part of the major membrane that lines the abdominal cavity and covers the abdominal organs, the *peritoneum* (per-i-toe-NE-um). This membrane is very susceptible to serious infection when the abdomen is opened or the intestines rupture. If bile or other digestive juices, partially digested foods, or free blood comes into contact with the peritoneum, a reaction of severe pain and abdominal wall muscle spasms usually occurs (peritonitis).

Types of Abdominal Injuries

Abdominal injuries can be *open* or *closed,* with closed injury usually due to blunt trauma. Internal bleeding can be severe if organs and major blood vessels are lacerated or ruptured. Very serious and painful reactions can occur when the hollow organs are ruptured and their contents leak into the abdominal cavity.

Penetrating wounds to the abdomen can be caused by objects such as knives, ice picks, arrows, and the broken glass and twisted metal of vehicular and structural accidents. Very serious perforating wounds can be caused by bullets (Figure 13–13), even when the bullet is of low caliber (small). Although some persons believe otherwise, gunshot wounds without exit wounds can cause as serious abdominal damage as those with exit wounds. Another misconception about bullet wounds is the ease with which internal damage can be assessed. Any projectile entering the body can be deflected, or it can explode and send out pieces in many directions. Do not believe that only the structures directly under the entrance wound have been injured. Also, keep in mind that the pathway of a bullet between entrance wound and exit wound is seldom a straight line.

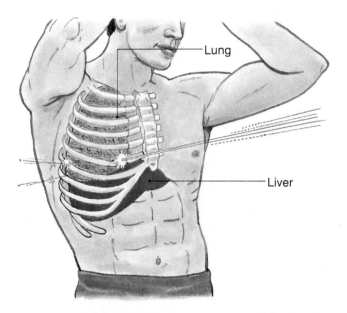

FIGURE 13–13. The damage done by gunshot wounds cannot be fully assessed in field emergency care.

Complicating the problem even more is the fact that penetrating abdominal wounds can be associated with wounds in *adjacent areas* of the body. For example, a bullet can enter the thoracic cavity, pierce the diaphragm, and cause widespread damage in the abdomen. A complete patient survey is essential in determining the probable extent of injuries.

REMEMBER: *Always* check for an exit wound.

Symptoms and Signs of Abdominal Injury

The symptoms of abdominal injury can include:

- Pain, often starting as mild pain then rapidly becoming intolerable
- Cramps
- Nausea
- Weakness
- Thirst

The signs of abdominal injury can include:

- Indications of developing shock, including restlessness, delayed capillary refill, rapid shallow breathing, a rapid pulse, and low blood pressure (sometimes patients with abdominal injury who are in extreme pain show an initial elevated blood pressure)
- Obvious lacerations and puncture wounds to the abdomen
- Lacerations and puncture wounds to the pelvis and middle and lower back or chest wounds near the diaphragm
- Coughing up or vomiting blood—the vomitus may contain a substance that looks like coffee grounds (partially digested blood)
- Indications of blunt trauma, such as a large bruised area or an intense bruise on the abdomen
- Rigid and/or tender abdomen
- The patient tries to protect the abdomen (guarded abdomen)
- The patient tries to lie very still, with the legs drawn up in an effort to reduce the tension on the abdominal muscles

In Chapter 3, the methods used for palpating the abdomen were described (see p. 99). Remember to assess the patient for abdominal rigidity (firmness), tenderness, and distention.

Emergency Care for Abdominal Injuries

Care for *open* abdominal wounds by:

1. Controlling external bleeding and dressing all open wounds
2. Laying the patient on the back, with the legs flexed to reduce pain by relaxing abdominal muscles
3. Caring for shock and constantly monitoring vital signs (anti-shock garments may be required)
4. Being alert for vomiting
5. Being certain not to touch or try to replace any eviscerated (e-VIS-er-a-ted) or exposed organs. Apply a sterile dressing moistened with sterile saline. Place this dressing directly over the wound site before you apply an occlusive dressing. Cover such organs with an occlusive dressing (or plastic wrap) and maintain warmth by placing dressings or a lint-free towel over top of the occlusive dressing.
6. *Not* removing any impaled objects. Stabilize any impaled objects with bulky dressings that are bandaged in place.
7. Administering a high concentration of oxygen and caring for shock as soon as possible. Give nothing to the patient by mouth. This may induce vomiting or pass through open wounds in the esophagus or stomach and

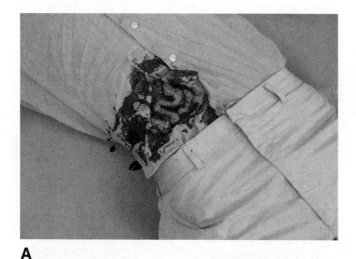

A

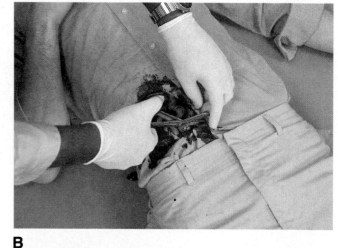

B

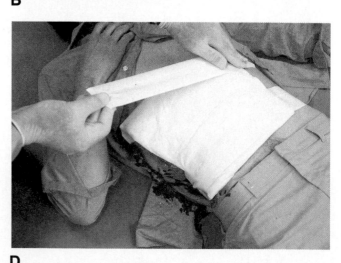

C

D

FIGURE 13–14. **A. Open abdominal wound with evisceration. B. Cut away clothing from wound. C. Apply an occlusive dressing. D. Cover occlusive dressing to maintain warmth.** *Note:* **A saline-soaked dressing can be applied before the occlusive dressing.**

enter the abdominal cavity. Stay alert for vomiting.

8. Transporting as soon as possible, continuing to monitor vital signs.

NOTE: Aluminum foil occlusive dressings have been found to cut eviscerated abdominal organs.

To care for *closed* abdominal injuries, you should:

1. Place the patient on his back with the legs flexed at the knees.
2. Administer a high concentration of oxygen.
3. Care for shock.
4. Apply PASG if indicated.
5. Keep alert for vomiting, making certain that the airway remains open.
6. Transport as soon as possible, administering oxygen and giving nothing by mouth. Monitor the patient's vital signs.

If the patient has symptoms suggestive of heart attacks, serious respiratory disorders, and serious abdominal injuries and digestive disorders, you should assume that the patient has more serious problems and care for shock and transport him as soon as possible.

INJURIES TO THE PELVIS AND GROIN

The major structures housed in the pelvis include the urinary bladder, the end portions of the large intestine (including the rectum), and the internal reproductive organs. These structures are reasonably well protected, but they can be injured by intense blunt trauma, crushing injuries of the pelvis, the movement of fractured pelvic bones, and gunshot wounds and other penetrating injuries.

Injuries to the Urinary System

The urinary system (Figure 13–15) includes the *kidneys*, which filter out wastes from the bloodstream and make urine; the *ureters* (u-RE-ters), with one

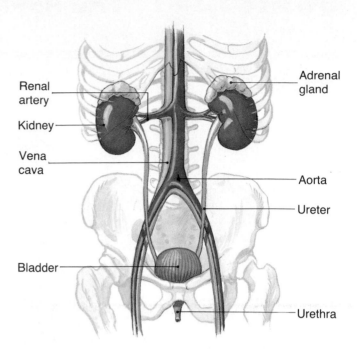

FIGURE 13–15. The urinary system.

connecting each kidney to the urinary bladder; the *urinary bladder*, which serves as a reservoir for urine; and the *urethra* (u-RE-thrah), through which urine is expelled from the bladder.

The kidneys are not abdominal or pelvic organs. They are located behind the abdominal cavity (retroperitoneal). Severe blows to the back or abdomen can cause kidney damage. Kidney damage is not found by the EMT, even after a complete and proper patient survey. Likewise, damage to the urinary bladder, although severe, may not be evident to the EMT. The pain experienced by the patient cannot be *specifically* said to be from the kidneys or the bladder.

NOTE: Consider back or flank pain following blunt trauma to be an indication of possible spinal injury and kidney damage. If the patient has blood in his urine, assume that there are serious problems within the urinary system. Management is the same as for a combination of spinal injury and internal abdominal organ injuries. In any trauma case, blood in the urethra must be considered to be an indication of a fractured pelvis.

Injuries to the Reproductive System

Injury can occur to both the external and the internal reproductive organs (Scan 13–1). The external reproductive organs are often referred to as the **external genitalia** (jen-i-TA-le-ah). More injuries occur to these structures than to the internal reproductive

SCAN 13–1 THE REPRODUCTIVE SYSTEM

MALE REPRODUCTIVE SYSTEM

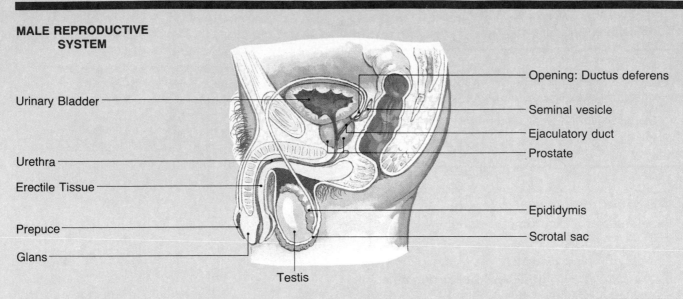

Urinary Bladder

Urethra

Erectile Tissue

Prepuce

Glans

Testis

Opening: Ductus deferens

Seminal vesicle

Ejaculatory duct

Prostate

Epididymis

Scrotal sac

STRUCTURE	INJURY	CARE
Scrotum (SKRO-tum) surrounds and protects the testes	Blunt trauma	Padded ice pack, transport.
	Lacerations and avulsions (rare)	Direct pressure, dressing, and triangular bandage applied like diaper. Keep avulsed parts moist, wrapped, and cool.
Testes (TES-tez) produce sperm cells and male hormone	Blunt trauma Lacerations and avulsions (rare)	Same as scrotum Same as scrotum
Spermatic (sper-MAT-ic) cords: suspend testes, contain blood vessels, nerves and vas deferens (vas DEF-er-en's) which transport sperm	Blunt trauma Lacerations (rare)	Same as scrotum Same as scrotum
Prostate (PROS-tat) gland: produces seminal fluids	Rare, usually gunshot wounds	Pressure dressing, treat for shock, oxygen, apply PASG when appropriate
Seminal vesicles: store seminal fluids	Rare, usually gunshot wounds	Same as prostate
Penis Erectile organ containing the urethra	Blunt trauma Lacerations and avulsions (also called amputation), self-mutilation	Same as scrotum Same as scrotum
	Blunt trauma of the erect penis (known as ''fracture'')	Padded ice pack and transport

**FEMALE REPRODUCTIVE
     SYSTEM**

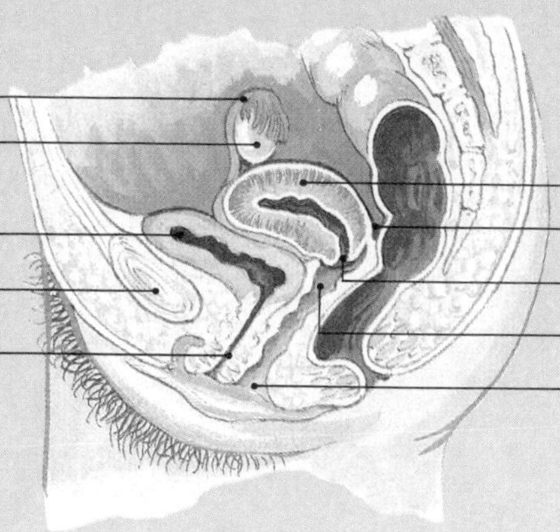

Fallopian (uterine) tube
Ovary

Bladder
Pubis
Urethra

Uterus
Pouch of Douglas
Cervix
Fornix
Vagina

STRUCTURE	INJURY	CARE
Vulva (VUL-vah); external genitalia	Blunt trauma	Padded ice pack, transport.
	Lacerations and avulsions	Sanitary napkin and triangular bandage applied like diaper. Keep avulsed parts moist, wrapped, and cool.
Vagina (birth canal)	Lacerations (seen in rape, self-mutilation cases, abortion attempts)	External application of sanitary napkin and triangular bandage.
Uterus (U-ter-us) womb for the developing baby (fetus)	Rupture due to extreme blunt trauma or crushing injury	Unable to tell in field that specific organ is injured. Vaginal bleeding is often profuse. Treat as internal injury with internal bleeding; apply sanitary napkin and triangular dressing over vaginal opening. This is a **true emergency.** Apply PASG garment when appropriate.
	Lacerations (rare), usually due to gunshot or stab wound, abortion attempts	Treat as penetrating or perforating wound. Vaginal bleeding may or may not be seen. Apply PASG when appropriate.
Oviducts (O-vi-dukt's) or fallopian (fah-LO-pe-an) tubes: carry egg (ovum) from the ovary to the uterus	Lacerations (rare), usually due to gunshot wound	Treat as penetrating or perforating wound. Vaginal bleeding is usually not seen. Apply PASG when appropriate.
Ovaries (O-vah-re's) produce female hormones and ova (O-vah) or eggs	Lacerations and puncture wounds (rare), usually due to gunshot or stab wounds	Treat as penetrating or perforating wound. Associated vaginal bleeding is not likely. Apply PASG when appropriate.

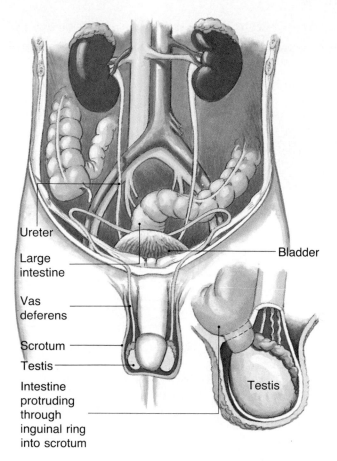

Ureter
Large intestine
Vas deferens
Scrotum
Testis
Intestine protruding through inguinal ring into scrotum
Bladder
Testis

FIGURE 13–16. An inguinal hernia.

organs, because of the protection offered by the bones of the pelvis. However, because of the location of the external reproductive organs, injuries are not common.

NOTE: Inappropriate management of genital injuries can be embarrassing to the patient. Approach the problem in a professional manner. Decide on a course of action and then act with authority as a member of the professional health care team. Timid, hesitant movements will only add to the patient's embarrassment. Explain what you are going to do and why, then provide care with no hesitation. Protect the patient from the stares of onlookers. When emergency care measures are completed, cover the patient with a sheet.

Inguinal Hernia

Commonly called a "rupture," the **inguinal** (IN-gwin-al) **hernia** occurs when abdominal membranes and part of the intestine bulge through due to a defect in the abdominal wall.

Since the blood supply to the intestine can be shut off due to constriction (strangulated hernia), transport is required for all hernia patients. Patient positioning is important to reduce pain. Basically,

let the patient assume a position that feels most comfortable. For the patient with an inguinal hernia, suggest that he try lying on his back. Next, try to tilt the patient's body slightly so that he is in a head-low position. Should the pain remain too severe for the patient, try placing a pillow under his knees. If pain is still intense, have the patient turn over onto his stomach and assume a knee-chest position by drawing the knees up until they rest against the chest. Keep in mind that the most favorable position for the patient may not be possible during transport to ensure patient safety.

SUMMARY

Injuries to the chest can include soft tissue injuries, fractured ribs, flail chest, spinal injuries, lung injuries, and heart injuries.

Many chest wounds are obvious; nevertheless, ALWAYS assess the patient for pain at the injury site, painful or difficult breathing, indications of developing shock, the coughing up of bright red, frothy blood, distended neck veins, tracheal deviation, abnormal or unequal chest movements, pain on lateral compression, subcutaneous emphysema, and unequal air entry.

If pain and tenderness at the site indicate rib fractures, place the forearm of the injured side across the chest and secure a sling and swathe. If rib or sternum movements indicate flail chest (paradoxical movements), apply a thick pad or bulky dressing over the site and tape or tie into place.

An object impaled in the chest should not be removed. Stabilize the object with pads and tape or tie the pads into place.

Air in the pleural space is known as pneumothorax. Wounds that have penetrated the chest wall ("sucking" chest wounds) require you to apply an occlusive dressing. Stay alert for tension pneumothorax. If the patient worsens after applying the occlusive dressing, loosen one sealed edge. If there is pressure from air escaping through a punctured lung, the patient should show immediate improvement, if tension pneumothorax is the problem.

The complications associated with chest injuries often involve the heart and lungs. Care for shock, administer 100% oxygen (assist with a bag-valve-mask or use positive pressure if appropriate), and transport immediately. Be ready to resuscitate.

When caring for abdominal injuries, look for the signs of abdominal injury (including bruises) and internal bleeding. Note if the patient's abdomen is rigid or tender and if the patient is guarding his abdomen. Care for shock, provide oxygen, and be alert for vomiting. Flex the patient's legs to help reduce pain in cases of closed injury. When indicated, apply anti-shock garments. Wounds that have opened the abdominal cavity require the application of an occlusive dressing to prevent the loss of moisture and to reduce contamination. This dressing should be covered with a folded towel or bulky dressings to prevent heat loss.

NOTE: Your EMS System may require that a sterile dressing soaked with saline be applied before the occlusive dressing for patients who have wounds that have opened the abdomen.

Injuries to the genitalia require you to conduct your examination and provide care in the strictest professional manner. Control bleeding by direct pressure and obey the general rules for open wound care. Remember that a sanitary napkin serves well as a bulky dressing and that a triangular bandage can be applied like a diaper.

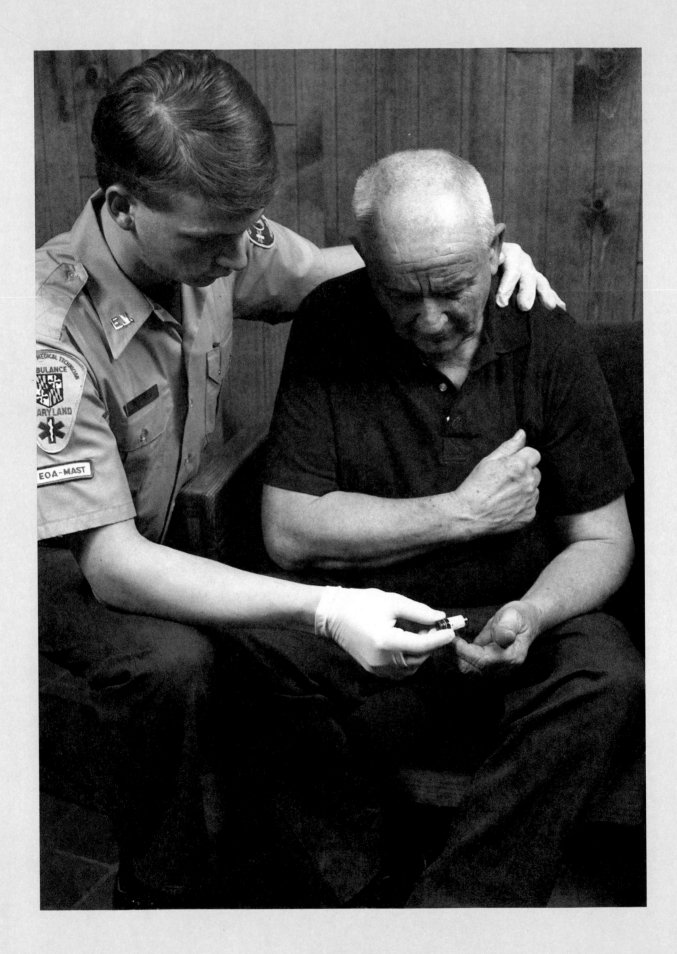

14

Medical Emergencies

SECTION ONE

OBJECTIVES As an EMT, you should be able to:

1. Define *medical emergency*. (p. 371)
2. List the major diagnostic symptoms and signs associated with medical emergencies. (pp. 372–373)
3. Define *poison* and state the *four* ways in which a poison can enter the body. (pp. 373–374)
4. Define *poison control center* and describe the role of such centers when you are providing emergency care for a poisoning patient. (p. 374)
5. List the symptoms and signs of ingested poisoning and describe the emergency care for patients who have ingested a poison, plus any exceptions to these procedures. (pp. 375–377)
6. List the symptoms and signs of inhaled poisoning and describe the emergency care for patients who have inhaled a poison. (pp. 377–378)
7. List the symptoms and signs of absorbed poisoning and describe the emergency care for patients who have absorbed a poison. (p. 378)
8. List the symptoms and signs of an injected poisoning (toxin) and describe the emergency care for patients who have been injected with a toxin. (pp. 379–381 and p. 385)

9. List the symptoms and signs of snakebite and describe the emergency care for patients who have been bitten by a snake. (pp. 380–381)
10. List the symptoms and signs of poisoning caused by marine life forms and describe the care for stings and punctures. (p. 385)
11. Relate coronary artery disease to specific changes in arterial walls. (pp. 386–387)
12. Compare and contrast the symptoms and signs of angina pectoris and acute myocardial infarction. (pp. 389–391)
13. List the emergency care procedures for angina pectoris. (p. 389)
14. List the emergency care procedures for possible acute myocardial infarction. (pp. 390–391)
15. Define *congestive heart failure* and explain its symptoms and signs in terms of this definition. (pp. 392–393)
16. Describe the emergency care for possible congestive heart failure. (pp. 392–393)
17. List the symptoms and signs of stroke. (p. 394)
18. Describe the emergency care provided for stroke. (p. 395)

19. Define *dyspnea* and relate this term to respiratory distress. (p. 394 and p. 396)
20. List the symptoms and signs of respiratory distress. (p. 396)
21. Compare and contrast emphysema and chronic bronchitis in terms of symptoms and signs. (p. 397)
22. Describe the emergency care procedures for chronic obstructive pulmonary disease. (pp. 397–398)
23. List the symptoms and signs of asthma. (p. 398)
24. Describe the emergency care procedures for asthma. (p. 398)
25. Describe the emergency care procedures for hyperventilation. (p. 399)
26. Define *spontaneous pneumothorax* and describe the care for this condition. (p. 399)

SKILLS   As an EMT, you should be able to:

1. Assess a patient for medical emergencies.
2. Evaluate obvious cases of ingested, inhaled, absorbed, and injected poisons (toxins).
3. Contact your local poison control center and provide them with the patient information they require.
4. Receive and carry out instructions given by a poison control center.
5. Provide the proper care for adults and children who are poisoning victims, including the correct use of syrup of ipecac and activated charcoal (where allowed by law).
6. Evaluate when a patient is the victim of snakebite and provide prompt and efficient emergency care.
7. Evaluate when a patient is the victim of a marine life form poisoning and provide prompt and efficient emergency care.

8. Assess patients for:
   • Disorders of the heart
   • Stroke
   • Respiratory distress, including hyperventilation
   • Chronic obstructive pulmonary disease
9. Provide emergency care for possible angina pectoris, acute myocardial infarction, and congestive heart failure.
10. Provide emergency care for possible stroke.
11. Provide emergency care for possible chronic obstructive pulmonary disease, asthma, and hyperventilation.
12. Promptly and efficiently deliver oxygen to patients having medical emergencies.

TERMS   you may be using for the first time:

Acute – a medical problem with a sudden onset. Usually, the symptoms are severe and the critical stage of the problem is reached quickly.

Acute Myocardial Infarction (AMI) – occurs when a portion of myocardium dies when deprived of oxygenated blood.

Aneurysm (AN-u-riz'm) – the dilation of a weakened section of an arterial wall.

Angina Pectoris (AN-ji-nah PEK-to-ris) – the sudden pain occurring when a portion of the myocardium is not receiving enough oxygenated blood.

Aphasia (ah-FAY-zhe-ah) – the complete loss or impairment of speech usually associated with a stroke or brain lesion.

Apnea (ap-NE-ah) – the cessation of breathing.

Arteriosclerosis (ar-TE-re-o-skle-RO-sis) – "hardening of the arteries" caused by calcium deposits.

Ascites (a-SI-tez) – the accumulation of excessive fluids.

Asphyxia (as-FIK-si-ah) – suffocation. The loss of consciousness will quickly develop because too little oxygen is reaching the brain. The functions of the brain, heart, and lungs will cease.

Atherosclerosis (ATH-er-o-skle-RO-sis) – a build up of fatty deposits and other particles on the inner wall of an artery. This buildup is called plaque. Calcium may deposit in the plaque, causing the wall to become hard and rigid.

Cerebrovascular Accident (CVA) – a stroke; the blockage or rupture of a major blood vessel supplying the brain.

Chronic – a medical problem that is consistently present over a long period of time.

Congestive Heart Failure (CHF) – the failure of the heart to pump efficiently, leading to excessive blood or fluids in the lungs, the body, or both.

Coronary (KOR-o-nar-e) **Artery** – a blood vessel that supplies the muscle of the heart (myocardium).

Coronary Artery Disease (CAD) – the narrowing of a coronary artery brought about by atherosclerosis. Occlusion (blockage) occurs in many cases.

Diaphoresis (DI-ah-fo-RE-sis) – profuse perspiration. The patient is said to be *diaphoretic* (DI-ah-fo-RET-ik).

Dyspnea (disp-NE-ah) – difficult breathing.

Episodic – a medical problem that affects the patient at irregular intervals.

Hypersensitivity – extremely sensitive.

Hyperventilation – a temporary condition of rapid, deep breathing.

Myocardium (mi-o-KAR-de-um) – heart muscle.

Occlusion – blockage, as in the blockage of an artery.

Poison – any solid, liquid, or gaseous chemical that can harm the body by altering cell structure or functions.

Pulmonary Edema (PUL-mo-nar-e e-DE-mah) – when the pulmonary vessels are engorged with blood and the alveoli contain excess fluids and foam. This may be associated with congestive heart failure.

Rale (rAl) – an abnormal breathing sound that can be heard in the lungs. It is usually associated with fluids or mucus building up in the lungs (fluid overload). A crackling or gravelly sound can be heard with a stethoscope. The sound can be imitated by rubbing the hair behind your ears.

Spontaneous Pneumothorax (NU-mo-tho-raks) – a closed pneumothorax that is not directly associated with trauma. Air enters the thoracic cavity through an opening in the weakened wall of a lung. The lung partially or completely collapses.

Syrup of Ipecac – a compound used to induce vomiting in appropriate cases involving conscious poisoning victims.

Venom – a poison (toxin) produced by living organisms such as certain snakes, spiders, and marine life forms.

WHAT ARE MEDICAL EMERGENCIES?

In the basic level EMT course there is much emphasis placed on injury. However, the EMT also is expected to provide care for medical emergencies. These are problems that the layperson would call illness or sickness. In emergency care, a medical emergency occurs as a result of one of the following factors:

- A defect in the structure or function of an organ or organ system. This can be present at birth (**congenital**) or acquired during life. Heart disease is an example.
- A disease caused by an infectious organism such as a bacterium or a virus. An example of this would be bacterial meningitis.
- The effect of a harmful substance, such as a poison or a drug.

Medical emergencies do not include any problems caused by trauma, nor do they include problems that are primarily psychological or emotional. The problems related to trauma have been studied in preceding chapters and will be completed in the environmental emergencies chapter. Psychological and emotional emergencies are given a special heading in emergency care. These will be covered in Chapter 19.

Environmental and medical emergencies overlap when we start to consider the effect of harmful substances. A patient's severe reaction to a wasp sting and the development of anaphylactic shock (see p. 207) would be an example. Poisonings are usually environmentally induced emergencies; yet the medical problems faced are the concern of the EMT in primary care. Substance abuse presents as a medical emergency, closely linked to special patient management and psychological emergencies.

As an EMT, you will have to be familiar with:

- Cardiovascular emergencies—including heart attack and stroke
- Respiratory emergencies—including respiratory distress, emphysema, and asthma

- Diabetes—including the problems associated with its management
- Disorders and diseases of the brain—including convulsive disorders such as epilepsy
- Abdominal distress—including the abdominal disorders and diseases classified as acute (sudden onset) abdominal distress
- Communicable diseases—including the major bacterial and viral illnesses of our society
- Poisonings—including ingested, inhaled, absorbed, and injected chemicals, snakebites, and marine life form poisonings
- Substance abuse—including alcohol abuse and withdrawal and the abuse and withdrawal associated with both licit and illicit drugs

Medical problems can be **chronic,** consistently present over a long period of time. Diabetes and bronchitis are examples of medical problems that are chronic. As an EMT, your care for chronic medical problems will be required in cases that have suddenly turned worse or when complications have quickly changed the patient's condition. These types of medical emergencies will require you to provide some very basic emergency care measures and to transport the patient. Other medical problems can be **episodic,** affecting the patient at irregular intervals and leaving him unaffected at other times. The patient expects problems, but the onset may not be predictable.

The unknown medical problem faces the EMT when the patient has an acute medical problem, occurring for the first time. **Acute** refers to a sudden onset with the rapid development of severe symptoms, as when a heart attack occurs without warning or an abdominal inflammation suddenly produces severe pain. Carefully gathering and evaluating symptoms and signs will be your only way to be certain that you are dealing with a specific acute medical emergency.

Problems of evaluating and providing care for medical emergencies may arise at the accident scene. Always remember that a medical emergency requiring immediate EMT-level care can be hidden because of injuries suffered at an accident. A patient having a heart attack or stroke or a patient having trouble managing his diabetes may fall and injure himself. Caring for the injury and letting the medical emergency go undetected can lead to serious, life-threatening problems for the patient. This is another reason why you must conduct a proper patient assessment.

The stress of an accident may set off both known and unknown medical problems. A heart attack, stroke, or seizure may occur at an accident scene. A complete patient assessment and the monitoring of vital signs may be the only way you can be prepared for such events.

Evaluating Medical Emergencies

Interviews with the patient and other individuals at the medical emergency scene may be the primary way of obtaining information. The patient, family, neighbors, or fellow workers may be able to alert you to a known medical problem. In some cases, a medical identification device may prove to be the major factor in determining what could be wrong with the patient. For acute cases, what the patient tells you and what you determine from the physical examination will probably be your only sources of information.

WARNING: Some patients experiencing a medical emergency will deny that they are having a problem. In rare cases, the family or friends will support this denial. Gaining patient and bystander confidence may help you reduce the patient's denial. If the signs evaluated in the assessment point the way to a medical emergency, even if the symptoms are not there to support the finding, assume that there is a medical emergency and seek the necessary consent to begin care and to transport.

The patient's relevant medical history and the symptoms and signs gathered and evaluated during the patient assessment are critical in determining the nature of the medical emergency. Keep in mind that you have been developing an understanding of illness and disease since childhood. In many cases, you can tell someone is probably ill. You cannot make a diagnosis, but you can draw certain conclusions. You are aware that pain, aches, fever, nausea, vomiting and other such indicators point to illness. Take this previous knowledge and apply it through the discipline of the patient survey.

The symptoms gathered from the patient, combined with certain signs may lead you to determine what possible type of medical emergency is causing problems for the patient. You will have to pay strict attention to:

- Pain, anywhere in the body
- Feelings of "temperature" or fever and chills
- A tight feeling in the chest
- An upset stomach
- Unusual bowel or bladder habits
- Unusual thirst or hunger
- An odd taste in the mouth

- "Burning" sensations
- Dizziness or feelings of faintness
- Numbness or tingling sensations
- The inability to move a body part or restricted movements

Important signs are collected during the patient survey including:

- Altered states of consciousness
- Pulse rate and character—remember that a pulse rate above 100 or below 50 beats per minute usually indicates a true emergency for the adult patient.
- Breathing rate and character—a true emergency exists in the adult patient when respirations are over 30 or below 10 per minute.
- Skin temperature, condition, and color
- Pupil size, equality, and response
- Color of the lips, tongue, nailbeds, ear lobes, or sclerae (scleras)
- Breath odors
- Abdominal tenderness, distention, or rigidity
- Muscular activities—spasms and paralysis
- Bleeding or discharges from the body

REMEMBER: If anything about the patient's general state of health appears to be unusual, assume that there is a medical emergency. If the patient has atypical vital signs (not what is typically expected), assume that there is a medical emergency. Consider all patient complaints relating to the way he feels to be valid. If the patient says he is not feeling "normal" in any way, assume that there is a medical emergency. Your role as an EMT is not to diagnose but to assess the patient, provide the proper initial care appropriate for a certain set of symptoms and signs, and transport the patient to the appropriate medical facility so that a physician will have the opportunity to make a diagnosis and provide needed care.

POISONING

A **poison** is any chemical that can harm the body. Associated with this damage are symptoms and signs that indicate the patient is having a medical emergency. In the United States, there are more than one million cases of poisoning annually. Although some of these cases are the results of murder or suicide attempts, most are accidental. These accidents usually involve common substances such as medications, petroleum products, cosmetics, and pesticides. In fact, a surprisingly large percentage of chemicals in everyday use contain substances that are poisonous if misused.

We usually think of poisons as being some kind of liquid or solid chemical that has been ingested by the poisoning victim. This is often the case, but keep in mind that many living organisms are capable of poisoning humans. Certain snakes, lizards, spiders, scorpions, insects, and some fish and marine life forms produce poisons called **venoms.** Usually, these venoms are injected into victims by a bite or sting. Poisonous plants such as poison ivy contain substances that cause reactions when they come into contact with the skin. There are also mushrooms and other common plants that can be poisonous if eaten. These include some varieties of house plants, including the rubber plant and certain parts of holiday ornamentals such as mistletoe and holly berries. Bacterial contaminants in food may produce **toxins**

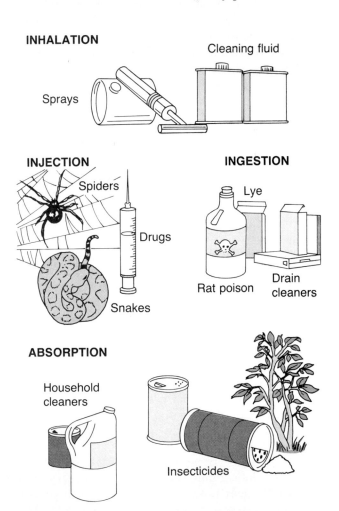

FIGURE 14–1. How poisons enter the body.

(poisons), some of which can cause a deadly disease (e.g., botulism).

Poisons can be taken into the body by way of ingestion, inhalation, absorption (through the unbroken skin), and injection (through tissues and the bloodstream) (Figure 14–1). A great number of substances can be considered to be poisons, with different people reacting differently to various poisons. As odd as it may seem, what may be a dangerous poison for one person may have little effect on another person. For most poisonous substances, the reaction is far more serious in children and the elderly.

Once in the body, poisons can do damage in a variety of ways. A poison may act as a corrosive or irritant, destroying skin and other body tissues. A poisonous gas can act as a suffocating agent, displacing oxygen in the air. Some poisons are **systemic poisons,** causing harm to the entire body or to an entire body system. These poisons can critically depress or overstimulate the central nervous system, cause vomiting and diarrhea, prevent red blood cells from carrying oxygen, or interfere with the normal biochemical processes in the body. The actual effect and extent of damage rendered by a poison is dependent on the nature of the poison, on its concentration, and sometimes on how it enters the body. These factors vary in importance depending on the victim's age, weight, and general health.

Types of Poisons

Ingested poisons can include many common household and industrial chemicals, medications, improperly prepared foods, plant materials, petroleum products, and agricultural products made specifically to control rodents, weeds, insects, and crop diseases (Table 14–1).

Inhaled poisons take the form of gases, vapors, and sprays. Again, many of these substances are in common use in the home, industry, and agriculture. Such poisons include carbon monoxide (from car exhaust, wood burning stoves, and furnaces), ammonia, chlorine, the gases produced from volatile liquid chemicals (including many industrial solvents), and insect sprays.

Absorbed poisons may or may not damage the skin. However, most are corrosives or irritants that will injure the skin and then be slowly absorbed into body tissues and the bloodstream. Included in this group are many of the insecticides and agricultural chemicals in common use. At first, corrosive chemicals may damage only the skin, but their activity usually does not stop there. They will continue to damage tissues and then be absorbed by the body, possibly causing widespread damage. Contact with

a variety of plant materials and certain forms of marine life can damage the skin and possibly be absorbed into tissues under the skin.

Injected poisons (toxins) come from a number of sources. Insects, spiders, snakes, and certain marine forms are able to inject venoms into the body. The poison may be a drug or caustic chemical self-administered by way of a hypodermic needle. Unusual industrial accidents also can be a source of poisons being injected into the body. Caustics, acids, and industrial solvents may be forced into the body in cases of open wounds.

Poison Control Centers

The emergency care of patients in poisoning cases presents special problems for the EMT. Symptoms and signs can vary greatly. Some poisons produce a characteristic set of symptoms and signs very quickly, while others are slow to appear. Those poisons that act almost immediately usually produce obvious signs, and the particular poison or its container is often still at hand. Slow-acting poisons can produce effects that mimic an infectious disease or some other medical emergency.

There will be times when you will not know the substance that caused the poisoning. In some of these cases, an expert may be able to tell, based on the combination of certain symptoms and signs. Even when you know the source of the poison, correct emergency care procedures may still be in question. The ideas about proper care keep changing as more research is done on poisoning. This constant change makes it impossible to print guides and charts for poison control and care that will be up to date when you use them. Even the information printed on labels of chemical containers may no longer be accurate at the time of the poisoning. All these factors mean that the proper emergency care techniques are best selected when based on expert opinion.

To overcome these problems, a network of **poison control centers** has been established throughout the country. In *most localities*, a poison control center can be reached 24 hours a day. The staff through local EMS protocols and on-line medical direction can tell you what should be done for most cases. You must know the telephone number for the center serving your area. Make certain to carry this number with you at *all* times.

So that you may best help the poison control center staff, note and report any containers at the scene of the poisoning. Let them know if the patient has vomited and describe the vomitus. When possible, quickly gather information from the patient or from bystanders before you call the center. An accurate description of symptoms and signs may be

Table 14–1. COMMON POISONS

Poison	Helpful Symptoms and Signs	Poison	Helpful Symptoms and Signs
ACETAMINOPHEN	Nausea, vomiting, heavy perspiration. The victim is usually a child.	IODINE	Upset stomach and vomiting. If a starchy meal has been eaten, the vomitus may appear blue.
ACIDS	Burns on or around the lips. Burning in mouth, throat, and stomach, often followed by heavy vomiting.	METALS (copper, lead, mercury, zinc)	Metallic taste in mouth, with nausea and abdominal pains. Vomiting may occur. Stools may be bloody or dark.
ALKALIS (ammonia, bleaches, detergents, lye, washing soda, certain fertilizers)	Check to see if mouth membranes appear white and swollen. There may be a "soapy" appearance in the mouth. Abdominal pain is usually present. Vomiting may occur, often full of blood and mucus.	PETROLEUM PRODUCTS (some deodorizers, heating fuel, diesel fuels, gasoline, kerosene, lighter fluid, lubricating oil, naphtha, rust remover, transmission fluid)	Note characteristic odors on patient's breath, on clothing, or in vomitus.
ARSENIC (rat poisons)	"Garlic breath," with burning in the mouth, throat, and stomach. Abdominal pain can be severe. Vomiting is common.	PHOSPHORUS	Abdominal pain and vomiting. Vomitus may be phosphorescent.
ASPIRIN	Delayed reactions, including ringing in the ears, rapid and deep breathing, dry skin, and restlessness.	PLANTS—Contact (poison ivy, poison oak, poison sumac)	Swollen, itchy areas on the skin, with quickly forming "blister-like" lesions.
CHLOROFORM	Slow, shallow breathing with chloroform odor on breath. Pupils are dilated and fixed.	PLANTS—Ingested (azalea, castor bean, elderberry, foxglove, holly berries, lily of the valley, mistletoe berries, mountain laurel, mushrooms and toadstools, nightshade, oleander, rhododendron, rhubarb, rubber plant, some wild cherries)	Difficult to detect, ranging from nausea to coma. Always question in cases of apparent child poisoning.
CORROSIVE AGENTS (disinfectants, drain cleaners, household acids, iodine, pine oil, turpentine, toilet bowl cleaners, styptic pencil, water softeners, strong acids)	(See Acids)		
FOOD POISONING	Difficult to detect since symptoms and signs vary greatly. Usually, you will note abdominal pain, nausea and vomiting, gas and loud, frequent bowel sounds, and diarrhea.	STRYCHNINE (rat poisons)	The face, jaw, and neck will stiffen. Strong convulsions occur quickly after ingesting.

needed before the poison control center staff can tell you and the on-line medical direction what needs to be done for the patient.

Many people have the impression that the poison control center should be called only for cases of ingested poisonings. The center's staff can provide you with valuable care information for all types of poisoning.

NOTE: Learning how to evaluate the effects of some poisons takes experience. Many can be learned through careful study. Your community may have special poisoning problems. Not every community is exposed to rattlesnakes, jellyfish, or powerful agricultural chemicals. Many EMS Systems have compiled lists of special poisoning problems specific for their areas. Check to see if this has been done for the area in which you will be an EMT.

Emergency Care for Poisoning

Ingested Poisons

WARNING: Providing mouth-to-mouth ventilations in cases of ingested poisoning may be hazardous to the rescuer. Use a pocket face mask with one-way valve, bag-valve-mask unit with supplemental oxygen, or positive pressure ventilation to avoid danger.

You must gather information quickly in cases of possible ingested poisoning. If possible, do so while you are making a primary survey. Note any *containers* that may contain poisonous substances. See if there is any *vomitus*. Check if there are any substances on the patient's clothes or if the clothing indicates the nature of the patient's work (e.g., farmer, miner). Can the *scene* be associated with certain types of poisonings? Question the patient and any bystanders. If the patient is a child, be on the alert for poisonous plant materials. These are commonly the source of poisoning when children "play house" or have "tea parties." Any poisoning related to plant materials requires immediate transport with care provided while en route. It is critical to reach a physician as soon as possible since there are *no antidotes* for many plant poisons.

The symptoms and signs for ingested poisons can include any or all of the following:

- Burns or stains around the patient's mouth
- Unusual breath odors, body odors, or odors on the patient's clothing or at the scene.
- Abnormal breathing
- Abnormal pulse rate and character
- Sweating—often in the form of *diaphoresis* (DI-ah-fo-RE-sis), that is, profuse perspiration
- Dilated or constricted pupils
- Excessive tear formation
- Excessive salivation or foaming at the mouth
- Pain in the mouth or throat, or painful swallowing
- Abdominal pain
- Abdominal tenderness, sometimes with distention
- Nausea
- Retching, vomiting
- Diarrhea
- Convulsive seizures
- Altered states of consciousness
- Any of the signs of shock

To provide the proper emergency care, call the on-line medical command and the *poison control center*. You should follow the directions given to you by your medical control. In most cases of ingested poisoning, emergency care will consist of diluting the poison in the patient's stomach using one or two glasses of water or milk, and then inducing the patient to vomit. *Never* attempt to dilute the poison or induce vomiting if the patient is not fully alert.

NOTE: Transport should not be delayed while you wait for the patient to vomit.

The directions given to you by the poison control center and the on-line medical command may vary depending on the patient. For example, you will probably not be directed to induce vomiting if the patient is pregnant, has a history of heart or esophagus disease, has had a seizure related to the poisoning, or has taken an overdose of a drug that helps prevent vomiting (antiemetics).

WARNING: *Do not* induce vomiting if the patient is not fully conscious or if the source of the poison is a strong acid, alkali (including plant products such as strychnine), or a petroleum product.* Vomiting of such substances can cause severe damage to the esophagus and other tissues and will usually cause the patient to aspirate the vomitus. When the vomitus contains petroleum products, it is often aspirated, causing a severe, often lethal pneumonia. Examples of these substances are oven cleaners, drain cleaners, toilet bowl cleaners, lye, ammonia, bleaches, kerosene, and gasoline. Always check for burns around the patient's mouth and the odor of petroleum products on the breath.

For CONSCIOUS patients, the typical procedures for care include:

---

1. Maintain an open airway.
2. CALL THE POISON CONTROL CENTER. If directed by your medical command . . .
3. Dilute the poison by having the patient drink one or two glasses of water or milk unless otherwise directed by a physician and poison control center. *Do not* give anything by mouth if the patient is having convulsions.
4. Induce vomiting by giving the patient syrup of ipecac followed by water in accordance with local protocol. Not all EMS Systems allow their EMTs to administer syrup of ipecac. Be certain that you follow your local guidelines.

---

* Some poison control centers now recommend that vomiting be induced for cases of petroleum product poisoning if care can be initiated *soon* after the ingesting of the product. The word "soon" is in question, with some authorities saying that it means no more than 10 minutes after ingesting. Follow the directions of your local medical command and poison control center.

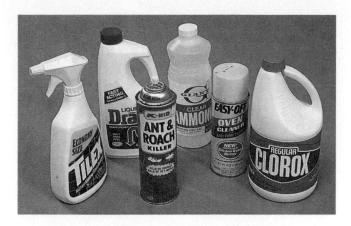

FIGURE 14–2. **If the patient has taken certain poisons, vomiting is usually not induced.**

5. Position the patient to prevent aspiration of vomitus and transport IMMEDIATELY. Place the patient in a semireclined position and monitor closely for vomiting. If he becomes unconscious, place him in a lateral recumbent position to help prevent aspiration of vomitus.

6. If transport is delayed, contact medical command and the poison control center for additional instructions.

7. Save all vomitus and transport it with the patient.

NOTE: Instead of inducing vomiting, you may be directed to give the patient activated charcoal mixed vigorously into water. If you are directed to induce vomiting and then give charcoal, give the patient ipecac and water, followed by charcoal and water after the patient has vomited in accordance with local guidelines.

When possible, transport the poisoned patient as soon as possible, calling your medical command and the poison control center en route. Actions to dilute the poison and to induce vomiting are carried out during transport. Treat the patient for shock and administer oxygen as soon as it is practical to do so. Be prepared for vomiting, even after you have successfully induced vomiting with syrup of ipecac. Keep the patient in the lateral recumbent position to provide better drainage to minimize the risk of aspiration. Transport without delay is *critical* if the poisoned patient is unconscious.

Inhaled Poisons

WARNING: If you suspect a patient has inhaled poison, approach the scene with care. Do only what you have been trained to do and go only where your protective equipment will allow you to safely go. You must be safe while you are gaining access to the patient and while you are providing care. If the source of the poison is an industrial compound (e.g., chlorine or ammonia), care at the uncontrolled scene cannot be rendered unless you use protective clothing and breathing apparatus. Make certain that your entire body is protected. Move the patient from the scene as quickly as possible. Again, do *only* what you have been trained to do.

Gather information from the patient and bystanders without delay. Note if there are any indications of inhaled poisons, including broken or breached containers, distinctive odors, signs of fire or smoke, and poor ventilation. Possible sources of the poison can be automobile exhaust, stoves, charcoal grills, fire, industrial solvents, and spray cans.

The symptoms and signs of inhaled poisons vary depending on the source of the poison. They include:

- Unconsciousness or altered states of behavior (depression or euphoria)
- Shortness of breath
- Coughing
- Rapid or slow pulse rate
- Eyes may appear to be irritated, or the patient may complain of burning eyes.
- The patient may complain of burning sensations in the mouth, nose, throat, or chest.
- Burning or itching (often complaints are made about the underarms, groin, and moist areas of the body)
- Severe headaches
- Nausea and vomiting
- Changes in skin color (usually cyanosis)
- Spray paint or other substances may be found on the patient's face

Carbon monoxide poisoning is a common problem, usually associated with motor vehicle exhaust and fire suppression activities. The number of cases has increased recently because of the carbon monoxide that can accumulate from the use of improperly vented wood burning stoves* and the unvented use of charcoal for heating and indoor cooking. Since carbon monoxide is an odorless and tasteless gas,

---

* Oil, gasoline, gas, and coal-burning furnaces and stoves also generate carbon monoxide.

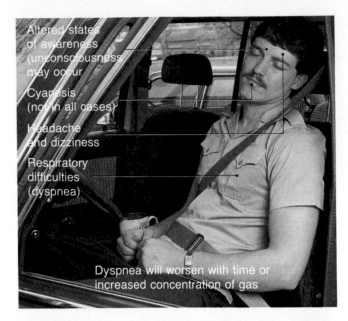

Altered states
of awareness
(unconsciousness
may occur

Cyanosis
(not in all cases)

Headache
and dizziness

Respiratory
difficulties
(dyspnea)

Dyspnea will worsen with time or
increased concentration of gas

FIGURE 14–3. Carbon monoxide poisoning.

you will not be able to directly detect its presence without special equipment. Look for indications of possible carbon monoxide poisoning, including wood-burning stoves, doors that lead to a garage or bedrooms above a garage where a vehicle has been kept running, closed garage doors where motor repair work is in progress, and any evidence that suggests that the patient has spent a long period of time sitting in an idling motor vehicle. If they are at the scene, ask family members and those who live or work nearby to determine if they have headaches, dizziness, or nausea.

When inhaled, carbon monoxide will combine with hemoglobin (much more rapidly than oxygen) to prevent the normal carrying of oxygen by the red blood cells. Long exposure, even to low levels of the gas, can cause dramatic effects. Most patients initially develop a headache and dizziness. They soon experience some difficulty with breathing that worsens with time or the exposure to higher concentrations of the gas. Cyanosis may appear. In time, the patient will suffer a loss of consciousness. Death may occur as hypoxia becomes more severe.

NOTE: The cherry red skin color that is associated with carbon monoxide poisoning is a rare, late sign. This coloration usually develops after death.

Other possible sources of inhaled poisons include chlorine gas (often from swimming pool chemicals), ammonia (often released from household cleaners), spray agricultural chemicals and pesticides, and carbon dioxide (from industrial sources). The most common signs are difficult breathing and dizziness.

The basic field emergency care for inhaled poisoning is to:

1. Remove the patient from the source of the inhaled poison.
2. Maintain an open airway.
3. Provide needed basic life support measures.
4. Administer a high concentration of oxygen. When possible, deliver this oxygen by nonrebreathing mask.
5. Place the patient in the lateral recumbent position.
6. Transport as soon as possible.
7. Access on-line medical direction.

It may be necessary to remove contaminated clothing from the patient. Take care to avoid touching this clothing since the chemical may cause skin burns. Since some poisonous gases condense into liquids, you may have to care for the patient's chemical burns (see p. 464). Transport the patient as soon as possible, administering a high concentration of oxygen. If the patient is unconscious ensure an open airway, place him in a lateral recumbent position to reduce the chances of the aspiration of vomitus.

REMEMBER: Unless you are trained to enter a scene having poisonous gases and have the proper equipment, *do not* try to provide care for a patient in a poisonous atmosphere.

Absorbed Poisons

Absorbed poisons usually irritate or damage the skin. A poison can be absorbed with little or no damage done to the skin, but such cases are very rare. The patient, bystanders, and what you observe at the scene will help you to determine if you are dealing with a case of absorbed poisoning. In the vast majority of cases, absorbed poisoning will be detected because of skin reactions related to chemicals or plants at the scene.

The symptoms and signs of absorbed poisoning include any or all of the following:

- Skin reactions (from mild irritations to chemical burns)
- Itching
- Irritation of the eyes
- Headache
- Increased relative skin temperature
- Abnormal pulse and/or respiration rates
- Anaphylactic shock (rare)

Emergency care for absorbed poisoning includes moving the patient from the source of the poison and using water to immediately flood all the areas of the patient's body that have been exposed to the poison.* After the initial washing with water, remove all contaminated clothing (including shoes, jewelry, and watches) and wash the affected areas of the patient's skin a second time (the poison control center and on-line medical command may direct you to use soap and water for this wash). More specific directions for various chemical burns will be covered in Chapter 17. Be on the alert for anaphylactic shock. Remember, this is a true emergency requiring immediate transport.

NOTE: You are responsible for any clothing or jewelry removed from the patient.

Injected Toxins

Insect stings, spider bites, and snakebites are typical sources of injected toxins. Commonly seen are reactions to the stings of wasps, hornets, bees, ants, and scorpions. The bites of the black widow and brown recluse ("fiddleback") spiders also can produce medical emergencies. Insect stings and bites are rarely dangerous; however, 5% of the population will have an allergic reaction to the venom and a few people may develop shock. Those who are *hypersensitive* develop severe anaphylactic shock that is quickly life threatening.

As an EMT, you are not expected to be able to classify insects and spiders as to their genus and species. Proper identification of these organisms is best left to experts. If the problem has been caused by a creature that is known locally and is not normally dangerous (such as bees, wasps, and puss caterpillars), the major concern will be anaphylactic shock. If this does not appear to be a problem, care is usually simple. However, if the cause of the bite or sting is unknown, or the organism is unknown, the patient should be seen by a physician. Do not try to classify spiders and scorpions. Your best course of action is to call the emergency department or take the patient to a medical facility and let experts decide on the proper treatment for the patient. If the dead organism is at the scene, be sure it is dead. Even if you are certain the organism is dead, do not touch it with your hands. Transport the dead organism (in a sealed container) along with the patient.

Poisons also can be injected into the body by way of a hypodermic needle. Drug overdose and drug contamination can produce serious medical emergencies. This will be covered in Section Two of this chapter.

* Dry chemicals should be brushed from the skin before washing.

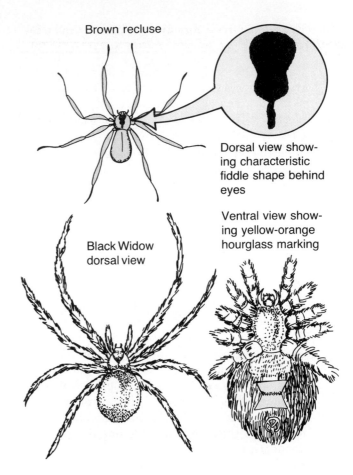

Brown recluse

Dorsal view showing characteristic fiddle shape behind eyes

Ventral view showing yellow-orange hourglass marking

Black Widow dorsal view

FIGURE 14–4. Poisonous spiders.

Gather information from the patient bystanders, and the scene. The symptoms and signs of injected poisoning can include:

- Altered states of awareness
- Noticeable stings or bites on the skin
- Puncture marks (especially note the fingers, forearms, toes, and legs)
- Blotchy skin (mottled skin)
- Localized pain or itching
- Numbness in a limb or body part
- Burning sensations at the site followed by pain spreading throughout the limb
- Swelling or blistering at the site
- Weakness or collapse
- Difficult breathing and abnormal pulse rate
- Headache and dizziness
- Nausea and vomiting
- Muscle cramps, chest tightening, joint pains
- Excessive saliva formation, profuse sweating
- Anaphylactic shock

Emergency care for injected poisons includes:

1. Calling the on-line medical command and the local poison control center—This can be skipped if the organism is known and your EMS System has a specific protocol for care.
2. Treating for shock—This is done even if the patient does not present any of the signs of shock.
3. Scraping away bee and wasp stingers and venom sacs—*Do not* pull out stingers. To do so may inject another dose of venom. Instead, scrape them from the patient's skin. Carefully scrape the site using a blade or a card.
4. Removing jewelry from any affected limbs.
5. If an extremity is the site of the sting, place a constriction band above and below the site. This is done to slow the spread of venom in the lymphatic vessels and superficial veins. The band should be made of ¾ to 1½ inch wide soft rubber. It should be placed about 2 inches from the wound (do not place the band around a joint). The band must be loose enough so that you can slide one finger underneath it.
6. Placing a covered ice bag or cold pack over the bitten or stung area.*
7. Keep the limb immobilized.

Some patients sensitive to stings or bites carry medication to help prevent anaphylactic shock. Help all such patients to take their medications. Your EMT course may include training in how to administer injectable medications for cases when the patient cannot do so for himself. This is a serious legal question. Make certain that you follow local policies.

REMEMBER: Be certain to look for medical identification devices.

Snakebites

Snakebites require special care. Nearly 50,000 people in the United States are bitten by snakes each year. Over 8,000 of these cases involve poisonous snakes, with fewer than ten deaths being reported anually.† The symptoms and signs of poisoning may take several hours to develop. Very few people die

* Applying cold is part of many EMS System protocols; however, the current trend is not to use cold for any injected poison.
† In the United States, more people die each year from bee and wasp stings than from snakebites.

of snakebite. If death does result, it is usually not a rapidly occurring event unless anaphylactic shock develops. Most victims who will die survive at least one to two days.

In the United States, there are two types of poisonous snakes, *pit vipers* and *neurotoxic* (nerve poisons) *snakes*. Rattlesnakes, cottonmouths, and copperheads are pit vipers. The coral snake is a neurotoxic snake. The bite from a diamondback rattler or coral snake is considered very serious. Since each person reacts differently to snakebites, you should consider the bite from any known poisonous snake to be a serious emergency. Staying calm and keeping the patient calm and at rest is critical. There is time to transport the patient.

Unless you are dealing with a known species of local snake that is not considered poisonous, consider all snakebites to be from poisonous snakes. The patient or bystanders may say that the snake was not poisonous. They could be mistaken. If the dead or captured snake is at the scene, your role as an EMT is not to identify the snake, but to provide care and to transport the dead snake (in a sealed container) along with the patient. Arrange for separate transport of a live specimen. Do not attempt to transport a live snake in the ambulance.

Should you see the live, uncaptured snake, take great care or you may be its next victim. When possible, note its size and colorations. Getting close enough to look for details of the eyes or for a pit between the eye and mouth is foolish. How you classify a snake, be it dead or alive, will probably have little to do with subsequent care. The medical center staff will arrange to have an expert classify captured or dead specimens and they have protocols to determine care if the snake has not been captured. Unless you are an expert in capturing snakes, do not try to catch the snake. Never delay care and transport in order to capture the snake.

The symptoms and signs of snakebite may include:

- A noticeable bite on the skin—This may appear as nothing more than a discoloration.
- Pain and swelling in the area of the bite—This may be slow to develop, from 30 minutes to several hours.
- Rapid pulse and labored breathing
- Progressive general weakness
- Vision problems (dim or blurred)
- Nausea and vomiting
- Convulsions
- Drowsiness or unconsciousness

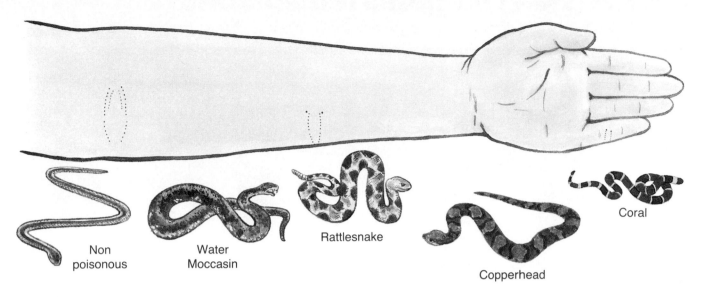

Non poisonous

Water Moccasin

Rattlesnake

Copperhead

Coral

FIGURE 14–5. Venomous snakes and their bites.

The emergency care for snakebite includes:

1. Keep the patient calm.
2. Treat for shock; conserve body heat.
3. Contact your on-line medical command and the poison control center.
4. Locate the fang marks and clean this site with soap and water. There may be only one fang mark.
5. Remove any rings, bracelets, or other constricting items on the bitten extremity.
6. Keep any bitten extremities immobilized—the application of a splint will help. Try to keep the bite at the level of the heart or, when this is not possible, below the level of the heart.
7. Apply a light constricting band above and below the wound. This is to restrict the flow of lymph, not the flow of blood. The coral snake is a small-mouthed creature that is usually able to bite a finger or a toe. If the patient was bitten by a coral snake, apply one band above the site.
8. Transport the patient, carefully monitoring vital signs.

Apply a constricting band above and below the fang marks. Each band should be about two inches from the wound, but *never* place one band on each side of a joint, such as above and below the knee. If the bite is to a finger, one band can be applied to the wrist of the affected extremity. This is the typical site for coral snake bites due to their small mouths. The constricting bands should be from a snakebite kit or made of ¾ to 1 ½ inch wide soft rubber. If only one band is available, place it above the wound (between the wound and the heart). If no bands are available, use a handkerchief.

The constricting bands should be snug but not tight enough to cut off venous circulation. Do not place them so that they cut off arterial flow. Monitor for a pulse at the wrist or ankle depending on the extremity involved. Check to be certain that tissue swelling has not caused the constricting bands to become too tight.

Do not place an ice bag or cold pack on the bite unless you are directed to do so by a physician. Do not cut into the bite and suction or squeeze unless you are directed to do so by a physician. *Never* suck the venom from the wound using your mouth. Instead, use a suction cup. Suctioning is seldom done

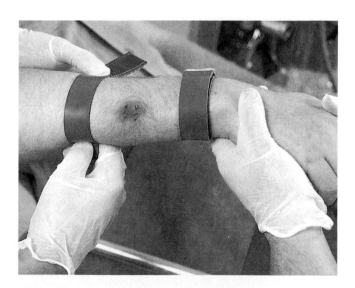

FIGURE 14–6. Care for snakebite.

SCAN 14—1A INGESTED POISONS

1

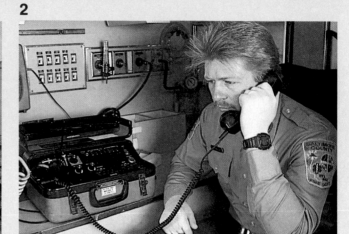

Quickly gather information and transport immediately.

2

Call medical command and poison control while en route.

3

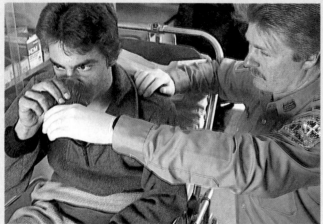

If directed, dilute the poison with water.

4

If directed, induce vomiting with syrup of ipecac and water.

5

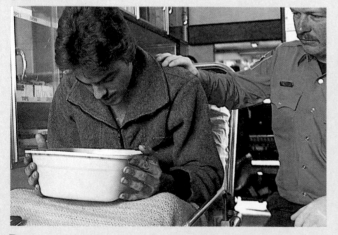

Position for vomiting, and save all vomitus

6

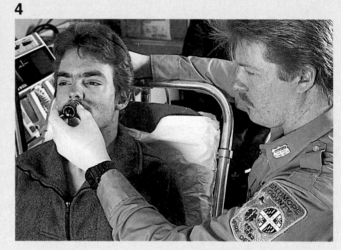

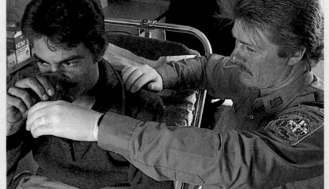

If directed, give activated charcoal and water.

SCAN 14-1B INHALED POISONS

WARNING: Protect yourself . . . do only what you have been trained to do and what your equipment allows.

1

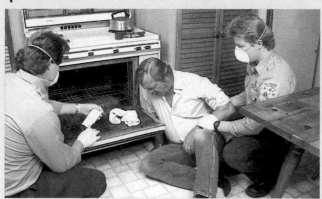

Remove patient from source.

2

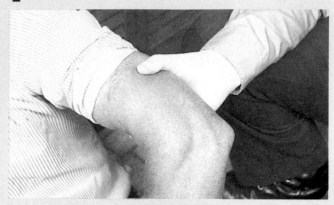

Avoid touching contaminated clothing.

3

REMEMBER: It is critical to establish and maintain an open airway.

4

CAUTION: Stay alert for vomiting. Properly position the patient and have suctioning equipment ready for use.

5

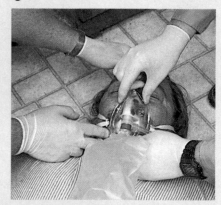

Administer oxygen.

6

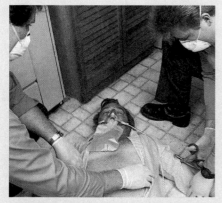

Remove contaminated clothing

7

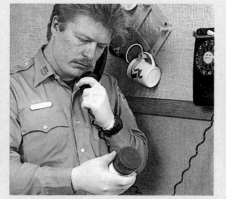

Call medical command and poison control . . . Follow directions.

8

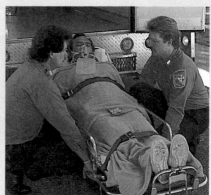

Transport as soon as possible.

NOTE: Masks shown on EMTs are used to filter large particulate matter. They will not protect the airway in a dangerous atmosphere.

(Scan continues on next page)

SCAN 14—1C ABSORBED POISONS

1

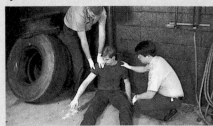

Remove patient from source or source from patient.

2

If appropriate . . . wash or brush patient.

3

Remove contaminated clothing and articles

4

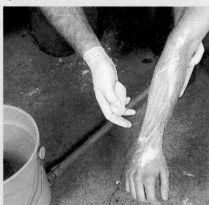

If appropriate . . . wash with soap and water.

5

Transport as soon as possible.

Injected Toxins (not snakebite)

1

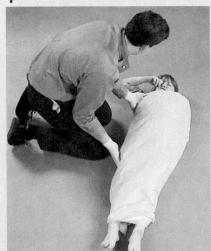

Care for shock. Call medical command and poison control.

2

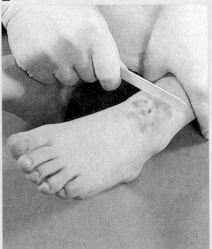

Scrape away stinger and venum sac. Apply constricting bands.

3

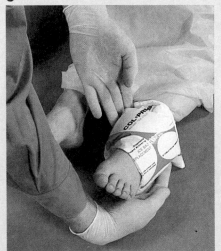

Apply cold to site . . . ready for transport.

by EMTs. When done, it is for pit viper bites that have occurred within 30 minutes of initial care. Suctioning is not recommended for coral snake bites.

Poisoning from Marine Life Forms

Poisoning from marine life forms can occur from improperly prepared seafood, eating poisonous organisms, and stings and punctures. Patients who have ingested spoiled, contaminated, or infested seafood may develop anaphylactic shock. They should receive the same care as any patient in anaphylactic shock. During care, you must be prepared for vomiting. Most patients will show the signs of food poisoning. The care for seafood poisoning is the same as for all other food poisonings.

It is extremely rare for someone in the United States to eat a poisonous variety of marine life. Creatures such as puffer fish and paralytic shellfish are not readily available. For all cases of suspected poisoning due to ingestion, call your on-line medical command and the poison control center. Be prepared for vomiting, convulsions, and respiratory arrest.

Venomous marine life forms producing sting injuries include the jellyfish, the sea nettle, the Portuguese man-of-war, coral, the sea anemone, and the hydra. For most victims, the sting produces pain with few complications. Some patients may show allergic reactions and possibly develop anaphylactic shock. These cases require the same care as rendered for anaphylactic shock. Stings to the face, especially those near or on the lip or eye, require a physician's attention.

Puncture wounds occur when someone steps on or grabs a stingray, sea urchin, spiny catfish, or other form of spiny marine animal. Although it is true that soaking the wound in hot water for 30 minutes will break down the venom, you should not delay transport. Puncture wounds must be treated by a physician and the patient may need an antitetanus inoculation. Remember, the patient could react to the venom by developing anaphylactic shock.

DISORDERS OF THE CARDIOVASCULAR SYSTEM

Cardiovascular diseases are major health problems in the United States. A large percentage of the medical emergencies seen by EMTs deal with such problems as heart attacks, strokes, heart failure, or some other disorder of the cardiovascular system. Before beginning this segment of the chapter, let us review the basics of the cardiovascular system (Figure 14–7):

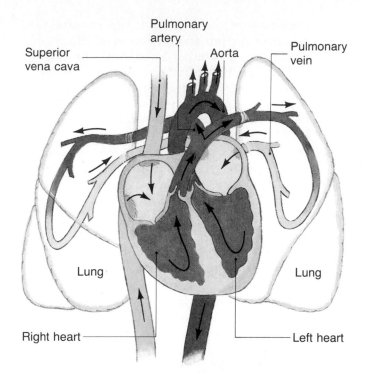

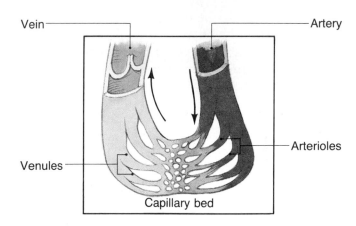

FIGURE 14–7. Anatomy of the cardiovascular system.

- The heart is a cone-shaped, hollow organ, roughly the size of the individual's clenched fist.
- The superior surface of the heart is the base, while the inferior point is known as the apex.
- The heart is located in the midportion of the thoracic cavity. The base of the heart is directly behind the sternum, at about the level of the third rib. The lower portion of the heart extends from behind the sternum into the lower left chest. The apex terminates between the fifth and sixth ribs.
- The heart is vertically divided down the middle by a septum; thus, there is a right side and a left side of the heart.

- Each side of the heart has two chambers, an upper atrium and a lower ventricle. The right atrium receives blood from the body and the right ventricle sends blood to the lungs. Blood returning from the lungs enters the left atrium, to be sent to the left ventricle and pumped out into systemic (the entire body) circulation.
- One-way valves control the direction of blood flow in the heart. They are located between atria and ventricles and in the great arteries that leave the ventricles.
- Heart contraction is initiated by the heart's pacemaker located in the right atrium. Control is by way of electrical impulses sent from the cardiac control center of the brain. Epinephrine (adrenalin) released into the bloodstream also affects heart action.
- Blood leaves the heart by way of arteries. These turn into smaller vessels known as arterioles. The arterioles lead into the capillary beds where exchange between the blood and the tissues takes place. Venules take blood from the capillaries to the veins. Blood returns to the heart by way of the veins.
- The circulation of blood between the heart and the lungs is the pulmonary circuit. The circulation of blood pumped from the heart, out to the body, and returned to the heart is the systemic circuit.

To better understand cardiovascular disease, you must know two additional terms. The heart has its own set of blood vessels to supply its tissues with oxygen and nutrients and to remove carbon dioxide and other wastes. This is the **coronary** (KOR-o-nar-e) **system** (Figure 14–8). Of chief concern in heart disease are the *coronary arteries*. The muscle of the heart is the **myocardium** (mi-o-KAR-de-um). The health of the myocardium and the amount of oxygenated blood reaching this tissue are of great importance in heart disease.

The Nature of Cardiovascular Diseases

Most of the cardiovascular emergencies covered in this section are caused, directly or indirectly, by changes taking place in the inner walls of arteries. These arteries can be part of the systemic circulatory system, the pulmonary circulatory system, or the coronary system. Two conditions, **atherosclerosis** (ATH-er-o-skle-RO-sis) and **arteriosclerosis** (ar-TE-re-o-skle-RO-sis), are involved in the changes found in these artery walls.

Atherosclerosis is a buildup of fatty deposits on the inner walls of arteries (Figure 14–9). This buildup causes a narrowing of the inner vessel diameter, restricting the flow of blood. Fats and other particles combine to form this deposit known as **plaque.** As time passes, calcium can be deposited

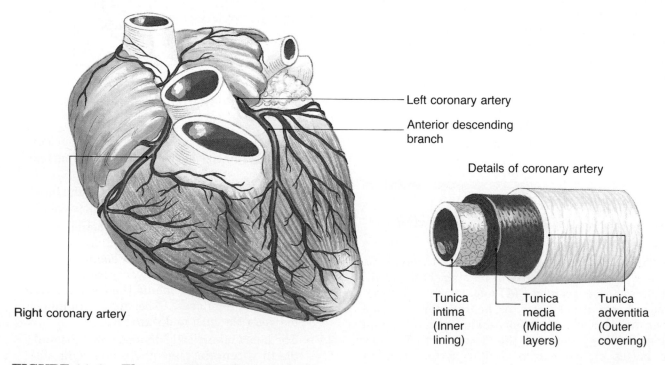

Left coronary artery

Anterior descending branch

Details of coronary artery

Right coronary artery

Tunica intima (Inner lining)   Tunica media (Middle layers)   Tunica adventitia (Outer covering)

FIGURE 14–8. The coronary artery system.

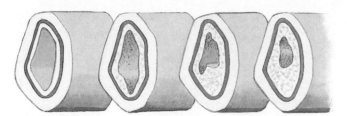

FIGURE 14–9. Atherosclerosis, the process of plaque formation.

at the site of the plaque, causing the area to harden. In arteriosclerosis, the artery wall becomes hard and stiff due to calcium deposits. This "hardening of the arteries" causes the vessel to lose its elastic nature, changing blood flow and increasing blood pressure.

Throughout the entire process of both atherosclerosis and arteriosclerosis, the amount of blood passing through the artery is restricted. The rough surface formed in the artery can lead to blood clots being formed, causing increased narrowing or occlusion (blockage) of the artery. The clot and debris from the plaque form a **thrombus** (THROM-bus). These thrombi can reach a size where they **occlude** (cut off) blood flow completely or they may break loose to become **emboli** (EM-bo-li) and move to occlude the flow of blood somewhere in a smaller artery. In cases of partial or complete blockage, the tissues beyond the point of blockage will be starved of oxygen and may die. If this blockage involves a large area of the heart or brain, the results may be quickly fatal (Figure 14–10).

Another cause of cardiovascular system disorder stems from weakened sections in the arterial

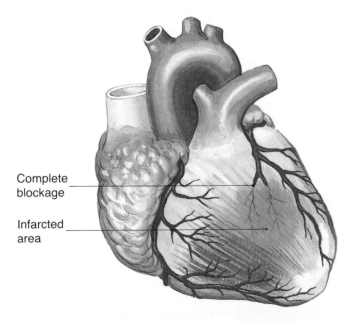

Complete blockage

Infarcted area

FIGURE 14–10. The relationship of arterial disease and heart disease.

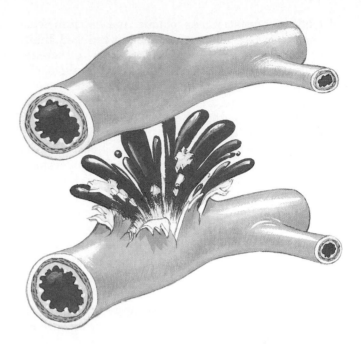

FIGURE 14–11. Formation and rupture of an aneurysm. A weakened area in the wall of an artery will tend to balloon out, forming a sac-like aneurysm, which may eventually burst.

walls. Each weak spot that begins to dilate is known as an **aneurysm** (AN-u-riz′m). This weakening can be related to other arterial diseases, or it can exist independently. When a weakened section of an artery bursts, there can be rapid, life-threatening internal bleeding (Figure 14–11). Tissues beyond the rupture can be damaged by the cut-off of oxygenated blood. Tissues around the site often can be damaged by the pressure exerted on them by the blood pouring from the artery. If a major artery ruptures, death from shock can occur very quickly. When an artery in the brain ruptures, a severe form of stroke occurs. The severity is dependent on the site of the stroke and the amount of blood loss.

Disorders of the Heart

Coronary Artery Disease

Physical and emotional stress cause the heart to work harder. For this to happen, the myocardium must receive more oxygenated blood than usual. This presents no problem when the heart and its coronary vessels are normal. However, when coronary vessels are diseased, their ability to carry blood is reduced. Since the blood supply to the heart is reduced, so is the oxygen supply, and the myocardium becomes starved for oxygen. The processes of arteriosclerosis and atherosclerosis cause the narrowing or **occlusion** of the coronary vessels, leading to this state of oxygen starvation. As plaque and calcium form on the inner arterial wall, elasticity is reduced, limiting the vessel's ability to dilate in order to increase the blood flow to the heart muscle. Should a clot block off a vessel or should a vessel burst (rare), the patient is placed in an immediate life-threatening crisis. Usually, it is the effect on the myocardium due to partial blockage of a coronary artery that shows itself as the first indication of heart disease.

Factors identified as contributors to coronary artery disease (CAD) include sex (male), hypertension, smoking, family history of coronary disease, diabetes, race (white), excessive saturated fat intake, high cholesterol level in the blood, stressful occupation or environment, a sedentary (lack of exercise) existence, obesity, heavy or muscular build, and excessive sugar intake. An aggressive competitive personality may be a factor, but recent research indicates this may not be as important as once believed.

Most patients with coronary artery disease exhibit many of the above factors.

In the majority of cardiac-related medical emergencies, it is the reduced blood supply to the myocardium that produces the emergency that requires EMS assistance and care.

Angina Pectoris

When the heart muscle has to work harder because of physical or emotional stress, healthy coronary arteries dilate to supply the myocardium with more oxygenated blood. As these vessels are narrowed by coronary artery disease, the supply of oxygenated blood cannot meet the increased demand, even for a few seconds. The restriction of blood flow is so severe that the patient's heart will not provide the oxygen required. Even the administration of oxygen will not solve the problem by itself. In some patients, a severe pain develops as myocardial tissue becomes oxygen starved. This pain is angina pectoris (AN-ji-nah PEK-to-ris) or, literally, a pain in the chest (Figure 14–12).

The pain of an angina attack generally diminishes and disappears when the physical or emotional stress ends. Seldom does this painful attack last longer than 3 to 5 *minutes*. As the heart rate returns to normal, the supply of blood moving through the diseased coronary arteries can meet the decreased demand. This means that rest is indicated for a person experiencing an angina attack.

Some patients have an unstable angina that occurs even when there is no physical or emotional stress to cause an attack. Usually, this fact will be made known during the patient interview.

Nitroglycerin tablets, paste, or patches are prescribed for persons subject to angina attacks caused by coronary artery disease. For example, at the onset

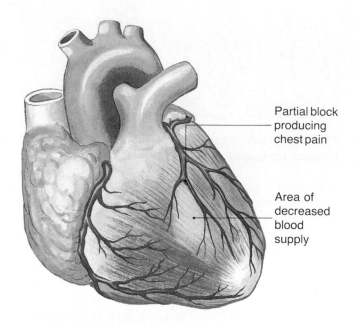

Partial block producing chest pain

Area of decreased blood supply

FIGURE 14–12. Angina pectoris produces pain in the chest that may be similar to that of a heart attack.

of an episode, the patient places a tablet under the tongue, allowing the medicine to enter the bloodstream quickly. Nitroglycerin works to dilate blood vessels, including the coronary arteries. In turn, blood pressure is reduced, as is the myocardial workload. Emergency medical personnel can help angina patients to take their medication, as well as to place them in a restful position and provide emotional support. You should administer oxygen to the angina patient. *Transport* the patient, even if the pain disappears. The patient should not take his nitroglycerin if the systolic blood pressure is below 90 mmHg. Discuss with medical control.

NOTE: If a patient has taken three nitroglycerin tablets over a 10-minute period and has rested during this period and still has no relief from pain, you must assume the patient is having a heart attack (see p. 392).

A complete guide to symptoms, signs, and emergency care for angina pectoris is provided in Scan 14–2.

Acute Myocardial Infarction

Acute myocardial infarction (AMI) is the condition in which a portion of the myocardium dies as a result of oxygen starvation. This is brought on by the narrowing or occlusion of the coronary artery that supplies the region with blood. Rarely, the interruption of blood flow to the myocardium may be due to the rupturing of a coronary artery.

SCAN 14—2 ANGINA PECTORIS

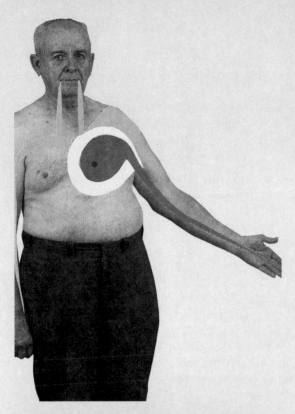

SYMPTOMS AND SIGNS may include:
- Early symptoms are often mistaken for indigestion
- As an attack worsens, pain originates behind the sternum and radiates to . . .
  - Either or both of the upper extremities (usually the left) with pain radiating to the shoulder, arm, and elbow. In some cases, the pain may extend down the limb to the little finger.
  - The neck, jaws, and teeth
  - The upper back
  - The superior, medial abdomen
  The pain may not originate under the sternum. Some patients have pain only in the jaw or the teeth.
- Shortness of breath
- Nausea
- Pain lasts throughout the attack and is not influenced by movement, breathing, or coughing.
- Pain usually lasts three to five minutes
- Patient usually remains still
- Pain diminishes when physical or emotional stress ends or when nitroglycerin is taken

Additional signs may include sweating, increased pulse rate, and, on rare occasions, a shock-level blood pressure. Patients who have taken repeated dosages of nitroglycerin may have low blood pressure as a result of blood vessel dilation.

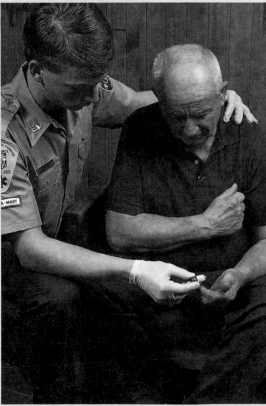

EMERGENCY CARE
- Provide emotional support—keep the patient calm and reassured
- Supply oxygen at a high flow rate as soon as possible
- Place the patient in a restful, comfortable position
- Find out if patient takes nitroglycerin and when last dose was taken and how much was taken over what period of time
- Contact medical facility and let them know:
  1. You have a patient with chest pain
  2. When last medicated
  3. Patient's vital signs and history
- Assist the patient with prescribed dose of medication (nitroglycerin) if systolic blood pressure is above 90 mm Hg
- Provide "quiet" transport and continue to monitor vital signs

SCAN 14–3 ACUTE MYOCARDIAL INFARCTION (AMI)

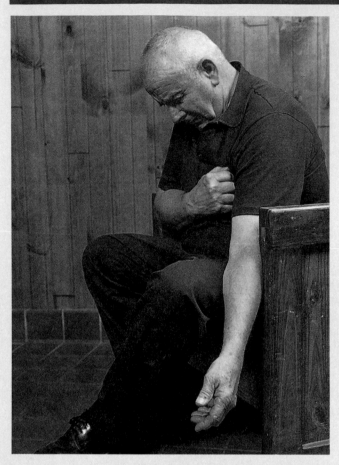

SYMPTOMS AND SIGNS MAY INCLUDE:

Respiratory:

- Dyspnea—shallow or deep respirations
- Cough that produces sputum

Behavioral:

- Anxiety, irritability, inability to concentrate
- Depression
- Feeling of impending doom
- Mild delirium, personality changes
- Fainting
- Occasional thrashing about and clutching of the chest

Circulatory:

- Signs of shock
- Increased pulse rate, sometimes irregular
- Some patients may have a slowed pulse rate
- Reduced blood pressure in 50% of the patients
  Normal blood pressure in 25% of patients
  Increased blood pressure in 25% of patients

Pain:

- 15% to 20% are painless ("silent") attacks
- Marked discomfort that continues when at rest rather than a sharp or throbbing pain
- Usually not alleviated by nitroglycerin
- May last 30 minutes to several hours
- Originates under sternum and may radiate to arms, neck, or jaw.

An Ami Can Lead to:

- Mechanical heart failure with pulmonary edema
- Shock (usually within 24 hours)
- Congestive heart failure (immediately, or up to a week or more later)
- Cardiac arrest (40% die before they reach the hospital)

Distinguishing between Angina and AMI

ANGINA PECTORIS

- Pain follows exertion or stress.
- Pain is relieved by rest.
- Pain is usually relived by nitroglycerin (if not relieved after three doses in ten minutes, assume AMI).
- Pain usually lasts three to five minutes.
- Arrhythmias usually are not associated.
- Blood pressure is usually not affected.
- Short-termed diaphoresis may be present.

AMI

- Pain is often related to stress or exertion but may occur when at rest.
- Rest usually does not relieve pain.
- Nitroglycerin may relieve pain.
- Pain lasts 30 minutes to several hours.
- Arrhythmias are often associated.
- Blood pressure is often reduced, but many patients have "normal" blood pressure.
- Diaphoresis is usually present.

AMI—Emergency Care

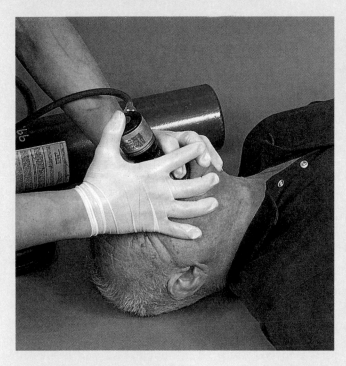
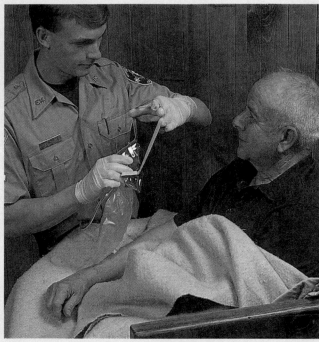

FOR THE UNCONSCIOUS PATIENT:

- Establish and maintain an airway.
- Provide pulmonary resuscitation or CPR if needed. If respiratory or cardiac arrest develops, deliver oxygen with a bag-valve-mask unit or a demand valve resuscitator.
- Administer high concentration of oxygen.
- Loosen restrictive clothing.
- Conserve body heat, but do not allow overheating.
- Transport immediately—quiet transport.
- Monitor vital signs.

FOR THE CONSCIOUS PATIENT:

- Keep the patient calm and still—*do not* allow patient to move himself to the ambulance stretcher.
- Take history and determine vital signs.
- Help patient with medication.
- Administer high concentration of oxygen.
- Conserve body heat.
- Transport as soon as possible in a semi-reclined or sitting position. Provide quiet transport.
- Monitor vital signs during transport.

Emergency care may be complicated by many factors. If the patient is conscious, his irritability, restlessness, and feeling of impending doom may make him uncooperative and unwilling to settle down, even though it is vital that he do so. Many AMI patients will resist the placement of a face mask for oxygen delivery. If he resists after an explanation of the importance of oxygen, use a nasal cannula at 6 liters/minute. Provide needed oxygen, but do not upset the patient.

WARNING!
TREAT ALL SUSPECTED ANGINA AND AMI PATIENTS AS IF THEY ARE HAVING AMIs.

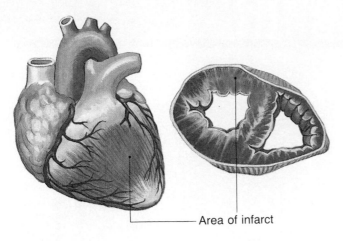

— Area of infarct

FIGURE 14–13. Cross section of a myocardial infarction.

The American Heart Association reports nearly 1.2 million cases of AMI in the United States each year. About 980,000 deaths annually are the result of cardiovascular disease. A major factor in heart disease is *sudden death,* a cardiac arrest that occurs within two hours of the onset of symptoms. Each year, approximately 400,000 people experience this sudden death away from hospitals. Nearly 25% of these individuals have no previous history of cardiac problems. Cardiologists believe that many of these sudden death victims could be saved if they received prompt and efficient care in the early warning stages or CPR immediately upon onset of cardiac arrest. Thus, it is vital that EMTs be able to recognize a possible AMI and to furnish appropriate care from the first contact to transfer to the medical facility.

A variety of factors can cause an AMI. Coronary artery disease in the form of atherosclerosis is usually the underlying reason for the incident. However, for some patients, factors often regarded as harmless may be responsible for setting off the heart attack. These factors include unusual exertion, severe emotional distress, and/or unrelieved fatigue. These patients may have an undetected, preexisting disturbance in heart rate and rhythm known as **arrhythmia** (ar-RITH-me-ah), undetected coronary artery disease, or prolonged chronic problems with respiration.

The complications from AMI are both common and dangerous. It is estimated that 85% to 90% of all AMI victims experience some sort of arrhythmia. Some of the arrhythmias associated with AMI may be lethal. Arrhythmias often associated with AMI include:

- *Asystole* (a-SIS-to-le)—cardiac standstill
- *Ventricular fibrillation* (ven-TRIK-u-lar fi-bre-LAY-shun) — when the ventricles no

longer beat with a full, steady, symmetrical pattern. Instead of a forceful contraction, there is a "quivering" of the heart muscle.

- *Atrial fibrillation or atrial flutter* —a highly irregular, inefficient atrial contraction. Atrial fibrillation is common in elderly patients and does not always indicate the potential for an AMI.
- *Bradycardia* (bra-de-KAR-de-ah)—when the heart rate is below 60 beats per minute.
- *Tachycardia* (tak-e-KAR-de-ah)—when the heart rate climbs above 100 beats per minute.

Another common complication seen with AMI is **mechanical pump failure,** or the inability of the heart to function normally due to damaged tissues. This can lead to cardiac arrest, cardiogenic shock (11%), pulmonary edema (fluids "backing up" in the lungs) and edema of other body organs (congestive heart failure, 60%), and cell death in various regions of the body due to oxygen starvation. About 4% of all AMI victims develop aneurysms in the ventricles that also can lead to mechanical pump failure or lethal arrhythmias. Nearly 2% of AMI patients suffer *cardiac rupture* as the dead tissue area of the myocardium bursts open. You will not be able to detect this in the field. Even though resuscitative measures are not usually effective for such patients, you must provide basic cardiac life support.

Scan 14–3 presents the symptoms, signs, and care for AMI. Note that there is a comparison of angina pectoris and AMI. As an EMT, you should be able to recall the major differences between the two as you evaluate a possible heart patient. When in doubt, treat as if there is an AMI. Transport all patients with indications of angina or possible AMI.

REMEMBER: Transportation of a patient with a heart condition must be carried out in a thoughtful, calm, and careful fashion. A high-speed ride with siren wailing is likely to increase the patient's fear and apprehension, placing additional stress on the heart. Conceivably, the patient's condition could worsen and he could die due to the complications brought about by improper methods used in transport.

Congestive Heart Failure

Congestive heart failure (CHF) may be brought on by an AMI , diseased heart valves, hypertension, or some form of obstructive pulmonary disease such as emphysema. This condition is often a complication of AMI, occurring several days after the heart attack.

The problem arises when a damaged or weakened heart cannot pump a sufficient amount of blood to maintain proper circulation throughout the body. It typically starts as **left heart failure,** related to damage in the left ventricle. Blood becomes "backed up," first in the pulmonary vessels and finally in the systemic vessels. **Pulmonary edema** occurs when fluids build up in the microscopic alveoli of the lungs. Poor respiratory exchange leads to shortness of breath (**dyspnea**—disp-NE-ah), with noisy and labored respirations. Crackling or gravelly sounds known as rales can be heard with the stethoscope.* Some patients cough up blood-tinged sputum from their lungs.

Left heart failure, if untreated, commonly causes **right heart failure,** as edema of the liver, spleen, and lower extremities develops. The abdomen may become noticeably distended by fluids. This is a condition known as **ascites** (a-SI-tez), the accumulation of fluids. In most cases of pulmonary edema, rales are heard with the stethoscope (see p. 106).

The symptoms and signs of congestive heart failure (Figure 14–14) can include:

- Tachycardia (rapid pulse, 100 beats per minute or above)
- Dyspnea (shortness of breath)—usually no chest pains
- Normal or elevated blood pressure
- Cyanosis
- Diaphoresis or cool and clammy skin
- Pulmonary edema with rales, sometimes coughing up of frothy white or pink sputum
- Anxiety or confusion due to poor oxygen/carbon dioxide exchange
- Edema of lower extremities
- Enlarged liver and spleen, with abdominal distention (develop late)
- Engorged pulsating neck veins (develop late)

Note that the patient will probably wish to remain in a seated or semireclined position. This should be encouraged since it allows for less labored respiration. Keep the patient calm, and conserve body heat. Whereas some AMI patients will fight a face mask, the "oxygen hungry" patients with congestive heart failure often accept oxygen therapy without difficulty. Some will resist taking the mask, while others will complain once it is in place.

Give a high concentration of oxygen unless the patient's problem is emphysema, chronic bronchitis, or an unclassified form of chronic obstructive pulmo-

---

* The sound known as a rale can be imitated by rolling the hair behind your ears with the thumb and forefinger.

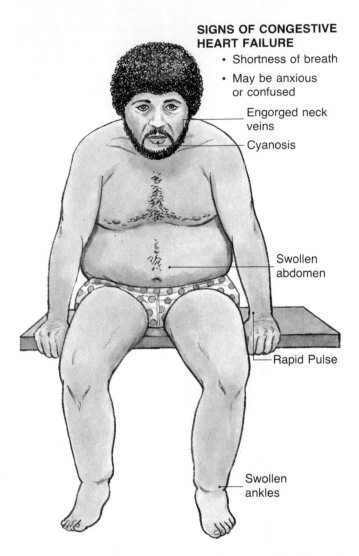

SIGNS OF CONGESTIVE HEART FAILURE
- Shortness of breath
- May be anxious or confused
- Engorged neck veins
- Cyanosis
- Swollen abdomen
- Rapid Pulse
- Swollen ankles

FIGURE 14–14. The signs of congestive heart failure.

nary disease (COPD) rather than congestive heart failure. For these patients, 24% oxygen delivered by Venturi mask is recommended. If the patient fears the mask, a nasal cannula can be used for short transport. It is best to call the emergency department physician for recommendations as to the flow rate of the oxygen. Some patients can only tolerate several liters per minute. Remember, never withhold oxygen from a patient who may be developing shock. (See Chapter 6 for more information on oxygen delivery to COPD patients and the problems created by hypoxic drive.)

Cardiac Pacemakers

Many people have had cardiac pacemakers surgically implanted to keep the heart beating at a steady, efficient rate. These devices replace the heart's own natural pacemaker when it becomes defective or damaged.

On occasion, you may find a patient with a cardiac pacemaker with the symptoms and signs of an AMI, angina pectoris, or congestive heart failure. The pacemaker will not prevent someone from having any of these problems. Care will be the same as for any patient displaying these symptoms and signs. Transport all angina pectoris patients having a pacemaker. Remember, as an EMT, you do not have the training or equipment necessary to evaluate the pacemaker in terms of efficiency and proper function.

Even though it would be a rare happening, you may respond to find a patient suffering a medical emergency due to a pacemaker malfunction. This is a serious emergency and requires *immediate transport*. You cannot evaluate or repair the device. Indications of pacemaker problems include a very slow pulse rate (below 50, possibly going as low as 35 beats per minute), often regular, but at times irregular. The patient almost certainly will be faint, dizzy, or very weak. Usually the patient will have a low blood pressure.

Coronary Artery Bypass Patients

The coronary artery bypass has become a relatively common procedure in cardiac surgery. Should you find a patient who has had this surgery, or an unconscious patient with a midline surgical scar on the chest, provide care as you would for any patient with the same symptoms and signs. Treat the AMI patient with a bypass as you would any patient with an AMI. If cardiac arrest occurs, provide CPR in the same prompt, efficient manner.

Stroke

Often thought of as a disorder of the brain, a stroke or **cerebrovascular accident (CVA)** is initially a problem of the cardiovascular system. It is the result of damage (accident) to one of the arteries (-vascular) supplying oxygenated blood to the brain (cerebro-). The pathway of blood may be occluded by a clot (thrombis or embolism), a large plaque of fatty deposits, or the compression of the artery by an adjacent tumor or the trauma-induced swelling of tissues. The pathway of blood also can be disrupted by the rupturing of an artery, resulting in cerebral hemorrhaging.

Age and physical condition influence the type of stroke suffered by a patient. This and the various sizes and locations of arteries involved give varied symptoms and signs. Sometimes the patient may have nothing more than a headache when first evaluated. Early transport is indicated, especially if the patient is elderly, has a previous history of stroke, or has chronic heart or pulmonary disease.

When providing emergency care for possible stroke patients, do all that you can to calm and reassure them. Protect any paralyzed limbs and constantly monitor the airway. Transport the patient carefully, avoiding high speed and the use of sirens.

In many cases, you will find it difficult to communicate with the stroke patient because of the presence of **aphasia** (ah-FAY-zhe-ah). This is a partial or complete loss of the ability to use words. The patient may be able to understand you but will not be able to talk, or will have great difficulty with speech. Sometimes, the patient will exhibit a special form of aphasia resulting from the stroke. He will understand you and know what he wants to say, but he will say the wrong words. When this happens, tell the patient not to be frightened. Let him know you understand what is happening. Tell the patient you will rely on gestures and, when possible, on written messages. Always let the patient know when he has been understood.

REMEMBER: The conscious CVA patient may not be able to speak to you; nonetheless, he probably will be able to hear everything that you say and understand what is going on around him. The patient will undoubtedly be frightened, in need of thoughtful and compassionate care.

See Scan 14–4 for the symptoms, signs, and emergency care of stroke patients.

RESPIRATORY SYSTEM DISORDERS

Dyspnea and Respiratory Distress

The term **dyspnea** (disp-NE-ah) means labored or difficult breathing. It is not a primary illness but a condition brought about by a number of medical, traumatic, and environmental causes. This problem can be related to airway obstruction, pulmonary edema, lung diseases, heart conditions, allergic reactions, pneumothorax, and carbon monoxide poisoning just to name a few. In most cases, dyspnea occurs when a disease has caused some kind of direct interference with either the flow of air into and out of the lungs or with the exchange of oxygen and carbon dioxide within the lungs. In the typical dyspnic patient, the problem causing the interference originates in the lungs, as in the case of asthma.

Dyspnea is just one of a series of stages that may be seen in **respiratory distress** (Fig. 14–15).

SCAN 14—4 STROKE—CEREBROVASCULAR ACCIDENT

Causes of Cerebrovascular Accidents—Stroke

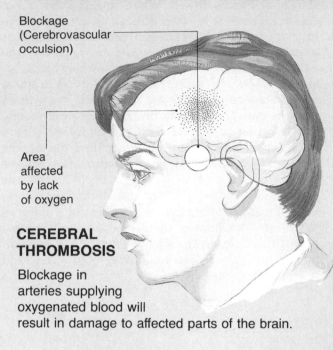

Blockage (Cerebrovascular occulsion)

Area affected by lack of oxygen

CEREBRAL THROMBOSIS

Blockage in arteries supplying oxygenated blood will result in damage to affected parts of the brain.

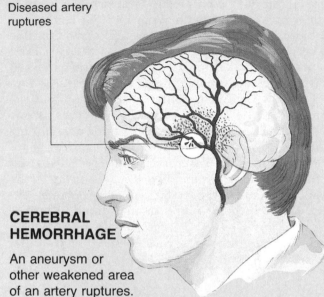

Diseased artery ruptures

CEREBRAL HEMORRHAGE

An aneurysm or other weakened area of an artery ruptures.

This has two effects:
1. An area of the brain is deprived of oxygenated blood.
2. Pooling blood puts increased pressure on the brain, displacing tissue and interfering with function.

Cerebral Hemorrhage is Often Associated with Arteriosclerosis and Hypertension.

SYMPTOMS AND SIGNS OF STROKE

- Headache
- Confusion and/or dizziness
- Loss of function or paralysis of extremities (usually on one side of the body)
- Numbness (usually limited to one side of the body)
- Collapse
- Facial flaccidness and loss of expression (often to one side of the face)
- Impaired speech
- Unequal pupil size
- Impaired vision
- Rapid, full pulse
- Difficult respiration, snoring
- Nausea
- Convulsions
- Coma
- Loss of bladder and bowel control

EMERGENCY CARE OF STROKE PATIENTS

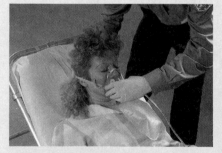

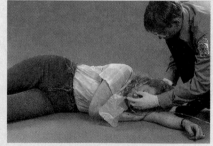

CONSCIOUS PATIENT:

- Ensure an open airway.
- Keep patient calm.
- Administer high concentration of oxygen.
- Monitor vital signs.
- Transport in semi-reclined position.
- Give nothing by mouth.
- Keep warm.
- Sit in front of the patient. Keep eye contact, and speak slowly and clearly.

UNCONSCIOUS PATIENT:

- Maintain open airway.
- Provide high concentration of oxygen.
- Monitor vital signs.
- Transport in lateral recumbent position. Keep affected limbs underneath patient. Use protective padding.

As something occurs to limit air flow or exchange, the patient will begin to increase the rate and depth of respirations. This is followed by dyspnea, in the form of shortness of breath. Hypoxia may follow, resulting from the decreased supply of oxygen. The patient may be gasping for air, cyanotic, and possibly suffering problems with vision. At the same time blood oxygen levels are too low and carbon dioxide levels are on the increase. The respiratory control center is at first stimulated by the increase in blood carbon dioxide, causing the patient to breathe rapidly. With time, this center is depressed and the breathing rate slows. Unless this condition is corrected, the patient will have a cessation of breathing **(apnea).** The patient may go through periods of apnea, regaining his respirations (Cheyne–Stokes respirations), or respiratory arrest may develop. If the apnea is not temporary, the patient will become unconscious. He will exhibit dilated pupils. Respirations will cease and the patient will soon develop cardiac arrest. Basically, the patient will have suffocated **(asphyxia).**

Emergency Care for Respiratory Distress

It is fairly obvious when a person is suffering from respiratory difficulty. The symptoms and signs are shown in Figure 14–15. When the distress is not due to trauma, it is often difficult to determine the exact medical or environmental problem. An efficient patient interview is very important. Question the patient, family members, fellow workers, and bystanders. Do not accept responses using medical terms. Someone may tell you the patient has asthma when he really has chronic bronchitis or emphysema. The information gained from the interview should be weighed with the signs determined during the physical examination. Medical identification devices and the prescription medicines being taken by the patient also can serve as sources of information. Do not try to determine what the medications indicate, but relay the names of the drugs to the emergency department physician. This must be done immediately if the patient has taken the medications and is still in distress.

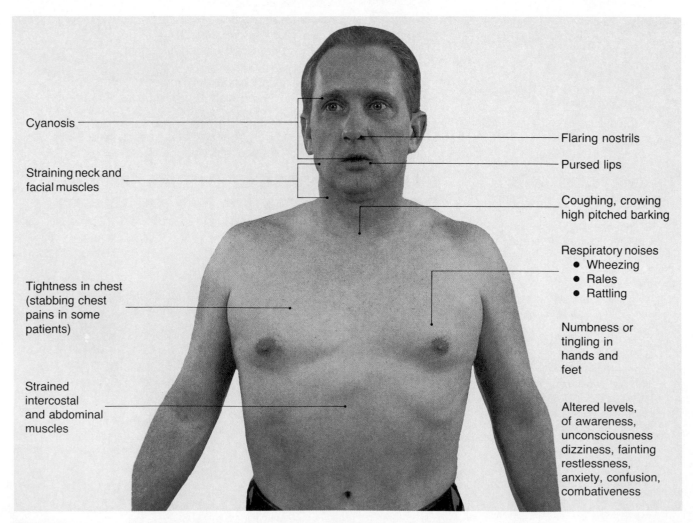

Cyanosis

Straining neck and facial muscles

Tightness in chest (stabbing chest pains in some patients)

Strained intercostal and abdominal muscles

Flaring nostrils

Pursed lips

Coughing, crowing high pitched barking

Respiratory noises
- Wheezing
- Rales
- Rattling

Numbness or tingling in hands and feet

Altered levels, of awareness, unconsciousness dizziness, fainting restlessness, anxiety, confusion, combativeness

FIGURE 14–15. The symptoms and signs of respiratory distress.

Once the medical problem is known, a specific course of action can be taken. If the reason for the respiratory distress cannot be determined, you must ensure an open airway, treat for shock, and transport the patient. The majority of patients who are having respiratory problems will benefit from as high a concentration as possible, or at least they will not be harmed by its delivery. Providing 100% oxygen may be dangerous for some patients (e.g., some COPD patients). Many EMS Systems start the patient on 24% oxygen by Venturi mask and radio the emergency department physician to ask if the concentration and method of delivery should be changed. If a high concentration of oxygen is needed because of severe hypoxia or the development of shock, the EMTs should be prepared to use a bag-valve-mask unit or positive-pressure ventilation.

Some patients fight the mask, believing that it will interfere with their breathing. Explain to them that they will receive more oxygen if they wear the mask. If they still refuse, try using a nasal cannula.

Chronic Obstructive Pulmonary Disease

Chronic obstructive pulmonary disease (COPD) includes *chronic bronchitis, emphysema, black lung,* and many undetermined respiratory illnesses that cause the patient problems like those seen in emphysema. Chronic bronchitis can be seen in children and teenagers; however, COPD is mainly a problem of middle-aged or older patients. This may be due to the long-term reactions of tissues in the respiratory tract to smoking, allergens, chemicals, air pollutants, or repeated infections.

Chronic bronchitis and emphysema are compared in Figure 14–16. In chronic bronchitis, the bronchiole lining is inflamed. Excess mucus is formed and released. The cells in the bronchioles that normally clear away accumulations of mucus are not able to do so. The sweeping apparatus on these cells, the cilia, have become paralyzed.

The typical *chronic bronchitis* patient will be an older person, usually a current or past heavy smoker. The symptoms and signs of chronic bronchitis include:

- Persistent cough
- Shortness of breath, with the tendency to tire easily
- Tightness in chest
- Periods of dizziness in some cases
- Cyanosis, edema of the lower extremities, and the patient's desire to sit upright at all times occur in advanced cases.

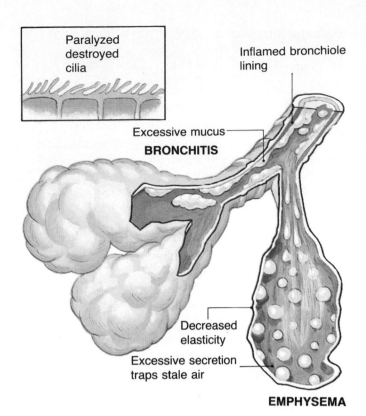

FIGURE 14–16. Chronic bronchitis and emphysema are chronic obstructive pulmonary diseases.

In *emphysema,* the walls of the alveoli and bronchioles break down, greatly reducing the surface area for respiratory exchange. The lungs begin to lose elasticity, and the alveoli and bronchioles secrete excess mucus. These factors combine to allow stale air to be trapped in the lungs, reducing the effectiveness of normal breathing efforts.

The typical emphysema patient is usually an older person who is a current or past heavy smoker or has been exposed to industrial smoke and gases. The symptoms and signs of emphysema can include:

- Patient often has past history of respiratory problems or respiratory allergies
- Signs that are the same as chronic bronchitis
- Patients with advanced cases have:
  Rapid pulse, occasionally irregular
  Breathing in puffs through pursed lips
  Blood pressure usually normal
  Barrel-chest appearance
  Wheezing

The emergency care is essentially the same for both bronchitis and emphysema:

1. Ensure an open airway.
2. Monitor vital signs.

3. Allow the patient to assume the most comfortable position (usually sitting or semi-seated).

4. Loosen any restrictive garments.

5. Keep the patient warm but not overheated.

6. Do all you can to reduce stress.

7. Administer oxygen as soon as possible, at 24% by Venturi mask or nasal cannula, unless the COPD patient is in serious distress. Follow local guidelines . . . usually 100% oxygen at 2 to 5 liters per minute to deliver 24%. Be prepared to use the bag-valve-mask or positive pressure. If the patient develops a more serious respiratory problem or has a possible heart attack or stroke, is developing shock, or has respiratory distress not related to the COPD, a higher concentration can be delivered (see below).

8. Transport as soon as possible.

9. Encourage coughing when necessary.

Take great care in administering oxygen to the COPD patient. A high flow rate of oxygen will increase the blood concentration of oxygen, but it will not lower the carbon dioxide levels. This could cause the patient to reduce his breathing efforts too soon and develop respiratory arrest (see hypoxic drive in Chapter 6, p. 175). If you cannot reach a physician and the patient is in severe respiratory distress and not responding to oxygen, transport immediately, change to a mask that will deliver a higher concentration of oxygen, and slowly increase the flow. This increase should be in small increments. Be very cautious, since the increase in oxygen may lead to respiratory arrest. If the patient dramatically slows his breathing, remind him to breathe. Should the patient lose consciousness, be prepared to assist with respirations using a bag-valve-mask unit and oxygen or a demand valve. Be prepared for respiratory arrest. Realize that respiratory arrest will be easier to care for than the cardiac arrest that may develop from severe hypoxia. Do not decrease the oxygen delivered once you start administering it.

Asthma

Seen in young and old patients alike, asthma is an episodic disease. This is far different from chronic bronchitis and emphysema, both of which *continually* afflict the patient. Between episodes, the asthmatic patient can lead an essentially normal life. When an asthma attack occurs it may be triggered by an allergic reaction to something inhaled, swallowed, or injected into the body. Attacks can be precipitated by insect stings, air pollutants, infection, strenuous exercise, or emotional stress.

When an asthma attack occurs, the small bronchioles that lead to the air sacs of the lungs become narrowed because of contractions of the smooth muscles that make up the airway. To complicate matters, there is an overproduction of thick mucus. The combined effects of the contractions and the mucus cause the small passages to practically close down, severely restricting air flow. The air flow is mainly restricted in one direction. When the patient inhales, the expanding lungs exert an outward force, increasing the diameter of the airway allowing air to flow into the lungs. During exhalation, the opposite occurs and the stale air becomes trapped in the lungs. This requires the patient to forcefully exhale the air, producing the characteristic wheezing sounds associated with asthma.

The patient having an asthmatic attack will not usually have chest pain. There will usually be an increased pulse rate, as high as 120 to 130 beats per minute. The rhythm of the pulse will be normal. There will be no doubt that the patient is having difficulty with expirations. Wheezing sounds can be frequently heard without a stethoscope. He will be tense and anxious and obviously frightened. The veins in the neck may distend and "stick out." He may hunch his shoulders and pull up his chest wall in an attempt to breathe. Other signs include cyanosis and coughing.

To provide care, you should:

1. Try to reassure and calm the patient.

2. Assist the patient in taking any prescribed asthma medications.

3. Help the patient position himself so that he feels most comfortable.

4. Provide oxygen, humidified if possible. Many guidelines call for starting the patient on 24% oxygen.

5. Transport—oxygen may only provide temporary relief.

WARNING: All cases of asthma must be taken seriously since asthma can be fatal. In addition to the serious respiratory distress brought about by asthma, additional problems may develop. The asthma attack may have been set off by an allergen. Anaphylactic shock could develop. This must be considered a possibility any time you are caring for an asthma patient. Bronchospasms may occur before the patient develops anaphylactic shock.

Some patients develop prolonged asthma attacks that are life threatening **(status asthmaticus).** These patients can move only a small amount of air. For such patients, the chest is distended, the pulse rate is rapid, and breathing is obviously labored. So little air may be moved that the breathing sounds associated with asthma may not be heard. The patient should be given humidified oxygen the same as all asthma patients. Transport must be initiated immediately. Ventilation assists from a demand valve may prove harmful since dry oxygen can cause thick mucus secretions that may add to the airway obstruction. Follow local protocols.

Hyperventilation

A patient who is hyperventilating patient breathes too rapidly and too deeply. Often fear or stress will trigger the attack. Some patients will have chest pain or other symptoms resembling an impending heart attack. A few patients report a tingling sensation in the upper extremity and may display a cramping of the fingers. The patient may tell you that he has attacks of hyperventilation. Even with this information, you should stay alert for changes in vital signs. The patient's problem in the past *may* have been simple hyperventilation, but this time it could be something more serious.

In most cases, the hyperventilating patient will not be cyanotic. This is a reliable clue that helps you to rule out severe respiratory distress.

The carbon dioxide level in the blood of a hyperventilating patient is too low. Having the hyperventilating patient breathe into a paper bag (not plastic) increases the carbon dioxide level in

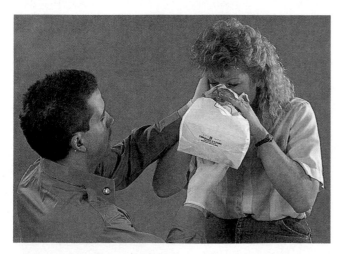

FIGURE 14–17. Have the simple hyperventilating patient rebreathe into a paper bag. Cover both the mouth and nose.

the blood, bringing it closer to normal (Figure 14–17). In some cases, there may very well be a more serious medical problem. Transport the patient, monitoring vital signs. You may not have to provide oxygen unless there are signs of oxygen deficiency or you are ordered to do so by a physician. Oxygen will not worsen the patient's condition. **Some EMS Systems recommend that oxygen be provided in case a more serious problem exists, usually with the approval of the emergency department physician.**

NOTE: Hyperventilation is not only a condition, it can also be a sign. Patients with respiratory distress or AMIs may also show hyperventilation. You must assess all hyperventilating patients. Remember that cyanosis usually indicates a problem more serious than the condition of hyperventilation. If the breathing is rapid, but shallow rather than deep, then the patient is not hyperventilating. Rapid, shallow breathing (tachypnea) must be considered to be a sign of more serious medical problems.

Spontaneous Pneumothorax

Most cases of pneumothorax are associated with chest injuries (see Chapter 13). In rare cases, a weakened area of the lung ruptures and releases air into the thoracic cavity. This is known as **spontaneous pneumothorax.** It is most frequently seen as a problem in young, thin adult males. The condition can be the result of congenital weakness, weakened scar tissue from previous injury or surgery, or certain types of lung cancer. When air enters the pleural space and sometimes the thoracic cavity, the lung will collapse. Tension pneumothorax may result. This condition develops as the pressure in the cavity increases and pushes the collapsed lung against the heart and the undamaged lung. This is a true emergency that may rapidly lead to death.

Patients with spontaneous pneumothorax will exhibit dyspnea. They often will report a sharp pain in the chest prior to the dyspnea. Care requires providing oxygen and immediate transport. If tension pneumothorax develops, the patient will continue to have dyspnea and will develop a weak and rapid pulse, low blood pressure, and uneven air entry into the lungs. The neck veins will become distended and bulge outward. The trachea may deviate to the side opposite the ruptured lung, and areas of the chest wall may bulge between the ribs and superior to the clavicles.

Cases of tension pneumothorax require immediate transport and the administration of a high concentration of oxygen.

SUMMARY

For specific care procedures, review the scans and lists provided in this chapter.

A chronic illness is one that is constantly present over a long period of time. Some medical problems are episodic, only affecting the patient at irregular intervals. When a medical problem has a sudden onset, it is said to be acute.

Detecting medical problems depends on a proper patient assessment, including patient and bystander interviews, looking for medical identification devices, taking vital signs, and conducting a physical examination. You must gather symptoms and signs and relate these to possible medical problems.

If you are dealing with a possible poisoning, always look for evidence at the scene that may indicate poisoning and the nature of the poison. In conjunction with your on-line medical command, learn to make use of your local poison control center.

There is a wide variety of symptoms and signs associated with ingested poisons. Always look for burns or stains around the patient's mouth and note any odd breath odors. Expect unusual breathing, pulse rate, and sweating. Abdominal pain, nausea, and vomiting are common. Be sure to save all vomitus.

Inhaled poisons can cause shortness of breath or coughing. Often, the patient will have irritated eyes, rapid or slow pulse rate, and changes in skin color.

Absorbed poisons usually irritate or damage the skin. Look for irritated eyes.

Venoms sometimes cause pain and swelling at the site. Difficult breathing and abnormal pulse rate are often seen.

In ALL cases of poisoning, contact your on-line medical command and local poison control center. For conscious patients, you will usually be directed to dilute ingested poisons with water or milk. The next step will probably be to induce vomiting with syrup of ipecac and water or as directed by the on-line medical command. Transport the patient as soon as possible, positioned to reduce the chances of aspiration of vomitus. Charcoal and water may be given when vomiting is not called for or after vomiting has occurred.

WARNING: *Do not* induce vomiting if the patient is not alert or if the poison is a strong acid, alkali, or petroleum product. Follow directions of on-line medical command and your local poison control center.

In cases of inhaled poisons, make certain that you are safe, then remove the patient from the source.

Provide basic life support measures as needed. It may be necessary to remove contaminated clothing.

Remove the patient from the source of absorbed poisons and flood with water all body areas that have come into contact with the poison. Remove contaminated clothing and jewelry. Continue to flood the exposed areas of the patient's skin, or wash with soap and water.

When managing injected toxins other than snakebite, provide care for shock, scrape away stingers and venom sacs, and place a covered ice bag or cold pack over the stung area (if ordered to do so). In some EMS systems, the protocol requires a constricting band to be placed above and below the site if an extremity is involved.

For snakebite, you should keep the patient calm, clean the site, and keep any bitten extremities immobilized. DO NOT APPLY COLD TO THE AFFECTED AREA. Provide care for shock. Apply a constricting band above and below the wound site but never on both sides of a joint. Bites of a coral snake require one constricting band placed above the wound since the bite is on the hand or foot. The snake's mouth is too small to bite elsewhere.

Most cardiovascular emergencies can be related to changes in arterial walls. Atherosclerosis is the buildup of fatty deposits to form plaque on the inner wall of an artery. When calcium deposits form, arteriosclerosis has occurred. Both can occlude an artery. This can take place in a coronary artery, leading to coronary artery disease. This disease is associated with smoking, hypertension, poor diet, stressful living, and lack of exercise.

Angina pectoris is a condition in which the patient suffers chest pain during emotional or physical stress. This pain indicates that an area of the myocardium is not receiving an adequate supply of oxygenated blood. The pain usually lasts from 3 to 5 minutes but may last longer. It is often relieved by rest and administration of nitroglycerin. Administer oxygen and transport the patient.

Acute myocardial infarction (AMI) occurs when an area of the myocardium dies because it has not received enough oxygenated blood. The patient will usually have chest pains that do not go away after rest. The pain may last several minutes or longer. He may have difficult breathing, increased pulse rate, and a reduced blood pressure in some cases. Many patients will develop an elevated blood pressure. The patient will be anxious and depressed and will have feelings of impending doom. Maintain an open airway, keep the patient calm, administer oxygen, help him take medications, treat for shock, and transport as soon as possible.

Avoid the use of sirens and excessive speed during transport according to local protocol.

Congestive heart failure is usually related to

a damaged or weakened heart that can no longer maintain proper circulation. Blood is "backed up" into pulmonary, then systemic, vessels. Fluids are forced from the blood into the tissues. In left-sided heart failure, pulmonary edema brings about dyspnea (difficult, labored breathing). Rales can sometimes be heard. Right-sided heart failure produces distension of the neck veins, edema of the liver, spleen, and lower extremities. Ascites, or an abdomen distended by fluids, may develop.

Allow the congestive heart failure patient to place himself in a comfortable position, keep him calm, and conserve body heat. Unless the patient suffers from COPD, administer a high concentration of oxygen. If he has COPD, deliver no higher than 24% oxygen by Venturi mask, unless there is a possible heart attack or stroke, developing shock, or respiratory distress that is not COPD related. For such patients, provide the oxygen needed. Transport as soon as possible.

A patient with a cardiac pacemaker can still suffer angina pectoris, AMI, or congestive heart failure. Do not try to evaluate the efficiency of the pacemaker. Treat as you would any patient having the same problem and transport. The same holds true for a patient who has had a coronary artery bypass.

A stroke or cerebrovascular accident (CVA) is caused by occlusion or rupturing of an artery supplying the brain. The conscious patient will usually be confused and have a headache, loss of extremity function (often to one side only), facial flaccidity, impaired speech, unequal pupil size, impaired vision, and a rapid and full pulse. Often the patient will have dyspnea and nausea. The patient may become comatose.

If the stroke patient is conscious, maintain an open airway, keep him calm, administer oxygen, and transport in a semireclined position. Do the same for the unconscious patient, but transport him in a lateral recumbent position, with the affected limbs padded and placed under the body.

Administer a high concentration of oxygen to a patient with respiratory distress, unless he has chronic bronchitis, emphysema, or some other form of COPD. The COPD patient should receive 24% oxygen by Venturi mask, unless there is a possible heart attack or stroke, developing shock, or respiratory distress that is not COPD related. For such patients, provide the oxygen needed.

Reassure and calm the asthma patient, assisting him with medications. Transport all asthmatic patients; oxygen may provide only temporary relief.

Simple hyperventilation, as a condition and not a sign of more serious problems, can be cared for by having the patient breathe into a paper bag. Rapid, shallow breathing must always be considered to be a sign of more serious medical problems than simple hyperventilation.

Spontaneous pneumothorax requires immediate transport and the administering of oxygen. Tension pneumothorax may occur where the collapsed lung pushes against the heart and the undamaged lung. This is a true emergency requiring immediate transport and administration of oxygen. Positive pressure may be required but can cause injury to the patient. Follow the directions provided by a physician.

SECTION TWO

OBJECTIVES As an EMT, you should be able to:

1. Compare and contrast diabetic coma (diabetic ketoacidosis) and insulin shock (hypoglycemia) in terms of symptoms, signs, and emergency care. (p. 405)

2. Describe what occurs during each phase of a convulsive seizure and relate specific emergency care procedures to each phase. (p. 404 and pp. 406–407)

3. List the general symptoms and signs associated with acute abdominal distress. (p. 408)

4. Describe the emergency care procedures for acute abdomen. (p. 408)

5. List the general symptoms and signs of an infectious disease. (p. 408)

6. List how communicable diseases may be transmitted. (p. 410)

7. Describe the basic procedures for:
   - Protecting yourself from communicable diseases. (pp. 409–410)
   - Making the ambulance ready after transporting a patient with a possible communicable disease. (p. 409)

8. Describe the special problems faced when dealing with a patient under the influence of alcohol. (p. 411)

9. Describe the symptoms and signs of alcohol abuse and alcohol withdrawal. (p. 411)

10. Summarize the emergency care provided for the alcohol abuse patient. (pp. 411–412)
11. Define *uppers*, *downers*, *hallucinogens*, *narcotics*, and *volatile chemicals*. (p. 412)
12. Describe in general a patient under the

influence of each of the above substances. Include a description of drug withdrawal. (pp. 412–414)
13. Summarize the emergency care provided for substance abuse patients. (pp. 414–415)

SKILLS As an EMT, you should be able to:

1. Determine if a patient is having a medical emergency.
2. Assess patients for:
   • Diabetic emergencies
   • Convulsive seizures
   • Acute abdomen
   • Possible infectious disease
3. Provide emergency care for diabetic coma and insulin shock patients.
4. Provide emergency care for all three phases of a convulsive seizure.
5. Provide emergency care for an acute abdomen patient.
6. Provide emergency care for patients who have possible infectious diseases.

7. Protect yourself from communicable diseases.
8. Ready an ambulance for the next run after transporting a patient with a possible communicable disease.
9. Provide the prompt and efficient delivery of oxygen for patients having medical emergencies.
10. Determine if a patient is having a medical emergency or if he has abused alcohol or drugs.
11. Provide emergency care for patients under the influence of alcohol or drugs and for patients suffering alcohol or drug withdrawal.

TERMS you may be using for the first time:

Acute Abdomen – inflammation in the abdominal cavity producing intense pain.

Convulsion (kun-VUL-shun) – the violent, involuntary contraction of skeletal muscles.

Delerium Tremens (DTs) – a severe reaction that can be part of alcohol withdrawal. The patient's hands tremble, hallucinations may occur, the patient displays atypical (unusual) behavior, and convulsion may take place. Severe alcohol withdrawal with the DTs frequently leads to death.

Diabetic Coma – a condition that begins with the buildup of the sugar glucose in the blood (hyperglycemia) when enough insulin is not available to allow the body's cells to take up this sugar. If an adequate supply of sugar is not available to the brain cells, the patient will suffer a loss of consciousness. If allowed to go untreated, death will occur.

Downers – depressants such as barbiturates that depress the central nervous system to relax the user.

Epilepsy (EP-i-LEP-see) – an episodic medical disorder of sudden onset characterized by attacks of unconsciousness, with or without convulsions.

Hallucinogens – mind-affecting or altering drugs

that act on the central nervous system to produce excitement and distortion of stimuli from the environment.

Insulin Shock – a condition that occurs to the diabetic when there is a sudden drop in the level of blood sugar (severe hypoglycemia).

Narcotics – a class of drugs that affect the nervous system and change many normal body activities. Their legal use is for the relief of pain. Illicit use is to produce an intense state of relaxation.

Seizure (SE-zher) – a sudden attack, usually related to brain malfunctions that can be the result of diseased or injured brain tissues. The more severe forms produce violent muscle contractions called *convulsions*.

Uppers – stimulants such as amphetamines that affect the central nervous system to excite the user.

Volatile Chemicals – vaporizing compounds, such as cleaning fluid, that are breathed in by the abuser to produce a "high."

Withdrawal – referring to alcohol or drug withdrawal, in which the patient's body acts severely when deprived of the abused substance.

DIABETES MELLITUS

The cells of the body need *glucose* as a source of energy. More complex sugars are converted into this simple sugar, which is then absorbed into the bloodstream. This blood sugar cannot simply pass from the bloodstream into the body's cells. To enter the cells, **insulin** must be present. Without insulin the cells can be surrounded by glucose and still starve for this sugar (Figure 14.2–1). When sugar intake and insulin are balanced, the body can effectively use sugar as an energy source. If, for some reason, insulin production decreases, the glucose cannot be used by the cells. This glucose remains in circulation, increasing in concentration as more sugars are di-

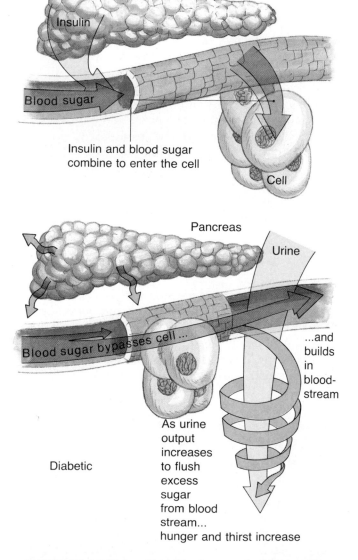

FIGURE 14.2–1. Insulin is needed for cells to take up sugar.

gested by the person who is now experiencing feelings of great hunger. The level of blood sugar climbs, eventually to be spilled over into the urine. The urine output of the body increases in an effort to rid the body of excess sugar in the blood.

The condition brought about by decreased insulin production is known as **diabetes mellitus** or sugar diabetes. The person suffering from this condition is a diabetic. There are two major classifications of diabetes mellitus. **Type I** or insulin-dependent diabetes occurs in individuals with little or no ability to produce and secrete insulin from the pancreas. This type of diabetes has been called *juvenile diabetes* since it tends to begin in childhood.

Type II or noninsulin-dependent diabetes occurs in individuals who have the ability to produce insulin but are unable to develop enough or use the insulin needed for survival. This disorder usually develops in adults and has been called *maturity-onset diabetes*.

Diabetes is seen more often in older people. There are at least 5 million diabetics in the United States. The danger of undetected and untreated diabetes is severe. As the condition develops, the diabetic can become weak and show a loss of weight even though he has increased his sugar and fat intake. He will take in large quantities of water to offset the loss of fluids through excessive urination. Acids and ketones (compounds that are in the same class as those used to make fingernail polish remover) begin to concentrate in the blood. This can cause coma and lead to death.

There is no cure for diabetes; it can only be controlled. Some patients can do this by strictly following medically supervised diets. About 30% must take daily doses of insulin. Therefore, there are two possible sources of problems for the diabetic who is taking insulin: an overuse or an underuse of insulin. Either can prove to be life threatening.

Diabetic Coma and Insulin Shock

Diabetic coma results from a decreased or absent insulin supply. Enough insulin is not being produced by the body or the person is not taking effective dosages of insulin. The body attempts to overcome the lack of sugar in the cells by using other foodstuffs for energy, notably stored fats. However, fats are not an efficient alternative to glucose and the waste products of their utilization greatly increase the acidity of the blood **(acidosis).** If allowed to go untreated, acidosis and the loss of fluids brought on by the high level of glucose in the blood eventually lead to diabetic coma.

Insulin shock occurs when there is too much insulin in the blood. Typically, this is caused when the diabetic:

- Takes too much insulin
- Has reduced sugar intake by not eating, causing an excess of insulin in the blood
- Has overexercised or overexerted himself, thus using sugars faster than normal

In any case, sugar rapidly leaves the blood and enters the cells. Not enough sugar remains for the brain, leading to unconsciousness. Permanent brain damage can occur quickly if the sugar is not replenished. Insulin shock can cause greater damage more quickly than diabetic coma.

The terms *diabetic coma* and *insulin shock* are most commonly used in EMT-level emergency care. Diabetic coma is the end result of severe **hyperglycemia** (HI-per-gli-SE-me-ah), or too much sugar in the blood. Physicians consider diabetic coma to be part of *diabetic ketoacidosis* (KE-to-as-i-DO-sis), which occurs when the body breaks down too many fats in an effort to obtain fuel compounds. As the term *coma* implies, the diabetic patient with severe hyperglycemia has not developed diabetic coma until unconsciousness occurs. However, since this is a complex diagnosis and uses many medical concepts that are not part of an EMT's training, most EMS Systems have their EMTs use the term *diabetic coma*.

Insulin shock is part of a severe case of **hypoglycemia** (HI-po-gli-SE-me-ah), or too little sugar in the blood. If any of the symptoms and signs for insulin shock that are described in Scan 14.2–1 can be detected for a diabetic patient, you are to consider the patient to have developed insulin shock.

Care for Diabetic Emergencies

Many students find that they confuse diabetic coma and insulin shock. For this reason, the signs, symptoms, and procedures for care are presented side by side on Scan 14.2–1. Note that diabetic coma usually has a slower onset, while insulin shock tends to come on suddenly. This is because some sugar still reaches the brain in hyperglycemic states. When insulin shock occurs, the hypoglycemia is so severe that it is possible that no sugar is reaching the brain. Seizures may occur. Diabetic coma patients have dry, warm skin and a rapid, weak pulse. Insulin shock patients have moist skin, often cold and "clammy." Their pulse beat is full and rapid. The diabetic coma patient often has acetone breath while the insulin shock patient does not. Continue to make the comparison for yourself.

As you consider evaluating the patient, keep in mind that many diabetic coma patients and some insulin shock patients will appear to be intoxicated. Always suspect a diabetic problem in cases that seem to involve no more than intoxication. Keep in mind that the patient intoxicated on alcohol may also be a diabetic, with the alcohol breath covering over the acetone smell characteristic of diabetic coma. The alcoholic diabetic is a good candidate for emergency care because he tends to neglect taking insulin during the course of prolonged drinking and usually has a low blood sugar level.

Whenever you are in doubt as to whether a *conscious patient* is suffering from diabetic coma or insulin shock, *give the patient* instant glucose or glucose and orange juice and treat for insulin shock. The "glucose for everyone" policy is correct for conscious patients since diabetic coma patients will not be hurt by what you do provided they are transported. Insulin shock patients need sugar, as soon as possible. Giving anything by mouth to an unconscious patient is a dangerous policy, since it may lead to aspiration. A "sprinkle" of granulated sugar under the tongue is acceptable in some EMS Systems, but no one advocates administering liquids by mouth to the unconscious patient. If you sprinkle sugar, do it from your fingers to avoid an accidental pouring. Provide just enough to be absorbed and keep the patient in a lateral recumbent position.

Whenever you provide sugar, make certain that you are using *sucrose* (table sugar) and not a sugar substitute. Artificial sweeteners will not benefit the patient. Any candy given to the patient must be a sugared candy. If you are giving the conscious patient soda as a sugar source, do not use diet soda.

EPILEPSY AND OTHER CONVULSIVE DISORDERS

In a conscious, healthy individual, muscular movements are usually smooth and coordinated. However, if the normal functions of the brain are upset by injury, infection, or disease, the electrical activity of the brain can become irregular. This irregularity can bring about sudden uncontrolled muscular con-

SCAN 14.2–1 DIABETIC EMERGENCIES

DIABETIC COMA (Hyperglycemia)

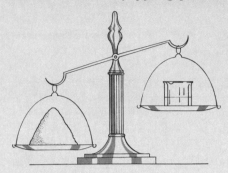

CAUSES:

- The diabetic's condition has not been diagnosed and/or treated.
- The diabetic has not taken his insulin.
- The diabetic has overeaten, flooding the body with a sudden excess of carbohydrates.
- The diabetic suffers an infection that disrupts his glucose/insulin balance.

EMERGENCY CARE:

- Administer a high concentration of oxygen.
- Immediately transport to a medical facility.

SYMPTOMS AND SIGNS:

- Gradual onset of symptoms and signs, over a period of days.
- Patient complains of dry mouth and intense thirst.
- Abdominal pain and vomiting common.
- Gradually increasing restlessness, confusion, followed by stupor.
- Coma, with these signs:
  · Signs of air hunger—deep, sighing respirations
  · Weak, rapid pulse.
  · Dry, red, warm skin.
  · Eyes that appear sunken.
  · Normal or slightly low blood pressure.
  · Breath smells of acetone—sickly sweet, like nail polish remover.

INSULIN SHOCK (Hypoglycemia)

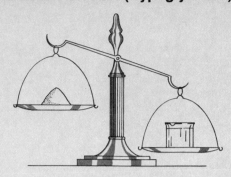

CAUSES:

- The diabetic has taken too much insulin.
- The diabetic has not eaten enough to provide his normal sugar intake.
- The diabetic has overexercised or overexerted himself, thus reducing his blood glucose level.
- The diabetic has vomited a meal.

EMERGENCY CARE:

- Conscious patient—Administer sugar. Granular sugar, honey, lifesaver or other candy placed under the tongue, orange juice, or glu-tose.
- Avoid giving liquids to the unconscious patient; provide "sprinkle" of granulated sugar under tongue.
- Turn head to side or place in lateral recumbent position.
- Provide oxygen.
- Transport to the medical facility

SYMPTOMS AND SIGNS:

- Rapid onset or symptoms and signs, over a period of minutes.
- Dizziness and headache.
- Abnormal hostile or aggressive behavior, which may be diagnosed as acute alcoholic intoxication.
- Fainting, convulsions, and occasionally coma.
- Normal blood pressure.
- Full rapid pulse.
- Patient intensely hungry.
- Skin pale, cold, and clammy; perspiration may be profuse.
- Copious saliva, drooling.

SPECIAL NOTES: DIABETIC COMA AND INSULIN SHOCK

When faced with a patient who may be suffering from one of these conditions:

- Determine if the patient is diabetic. Look for medical alert medallions or information cards; interview patient and family members.
- If the patient is a known or suspected diabetic, and insulin shock cannot be ruled out, assume that it is insulin shock and administer sugar.

Often a patient suffering from either of these conditions may simply appear drunk. Always check for other underlying conditions—such as diabetic complications—when treating someone who appears intoxicated.

tractions (a seizure). Unconsciousness is common to convulsive seizures.

Convulsive seizures may be seen with:

- Epilepsy (grand mal or major seizure)
- CVA (stroke)
- Brain injury
- High fever
- Infection
- Measles, mumps, and other childhood diseases
- Insulin shock
- Eclampsia (see Chapter 16)
- Undetected reasons

A convulsive seizure has three distinct phases:

1. Tonic phase—the body becomes rigid, stiffening for no more than 30 seconds. Breathing may stop, the patient may bite his tongue (rare), and bowel and bladder control could be lost.
2. Clonic phase—the body jerks about violently, usually for no more than 1 or 2 minutes (some can last 5 minutes). The patient may foam at the mouth and drool. His face and lips often become cyanotic.
3. Postictal phase—this begins when convulsions stop. The patient may regain consciousness immediately and enter a state of drowsiness and confusion, or he may remain unconscious for several hours. Headache is common.

Epilepsy

Epilepsy is an **episodic** disease that is chronic. It may result from the effects of scar tissue in the brain following head injury or surgery, a reduced flow of blood to the brain, or a brain tumor. More often than not the cause of a patient's epilepsy remains a mystery.

Epilepsy may cause two forms of seizure: a **grand mal,** or major, seizure characterized by convulsions or a **petit mal,** or minor, seizure that does not produce convulsions. A petit mal seizure may go unnoticed by everyone except the patient and knowledgeable members of his family. A conscientious use of special medications usually allows most epileptics to live normal lives without convulsions of any type.

A person who suffers a grand mal seizure often experiences sudden brain cell activity known as an *aura*. The individual may see bright light or a sudden burst of colors and may also experience the sensation

of certain smells. Whatever the sensation, the person knows that a seizure is coming and will usually let family members or associates know of the coming attack and will then lie down.

Emergency Care for Convulsive Disorders

Emergency care is the same for epilepsy as for the other types of convulsive seizures. The basic emergency care for seizure patients is to:

1. Place the patient on the floor or ground. If possible, position for drainage from the mouth.
2. Loosen restrictive clothing.
3. Protect the patient from injury, but *do not* try to hold the patient still during convulsions.
4. After convulsions have ended, keep the patient at rest, positioned for drainage from the mouth. Some patients become hypoxic during a seizure. Provide oxygen if needed.
5. Take vital signs and monitor respirations closely.
6. Protect the patient from embarrassment by having onlookers give the patient privacy.
7. Transport him to a medical facility, monitoring vital signs.

NOTE: Never place anything in the mouth of a convulsing patient. Many objects can be broken and obstruct the patient's airway.

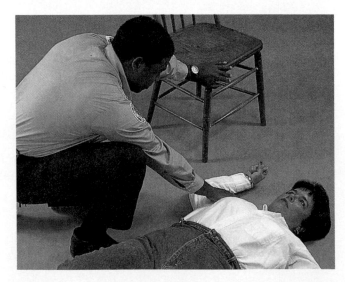

FIGURE 14.2–2. Protect the patient from injury.

Status epilepticus occurs when the patient has two or more seizures without regaining full consciousness. This is a TRUE EMERGENCY requiring immediate high priority transport. Do not try to restrain the patient, even if the convulsions appear to have ended. Oxygen should be administered at the scene and while en route.

ACUTE ABDOMINAL DISTRESS (ACUTE ABDOMEN)

Acute abdominal distress or *acute abdomen* is the sudden onset of severe abdominal pain and discomfort. Many abdominal problems start out as simple "indigestion" in the mind of the patient as he waits for it to "go away." However, when pain does not go away, or it becomes so severe that it frightens the patient and his family, emergency medical services may be called to respond. Sometimes, after arrival at the hospital, it is determined that the cause of the pain is nothing more than indigestion. Other times it may prove to be such problems as:

- Appendicitis
- Intestinal obstruction
- Strangulated hernia (see Chapter 13)
- Inflammation of the gallbladder
- Perforated ulcer
- Kidney stones
- Ectopic pregnancy (see Chapter 16)
- Inflammation of the pancreas
- Inflammation of the abdominal cavity membranes (peritonitis)
- An aneurysm

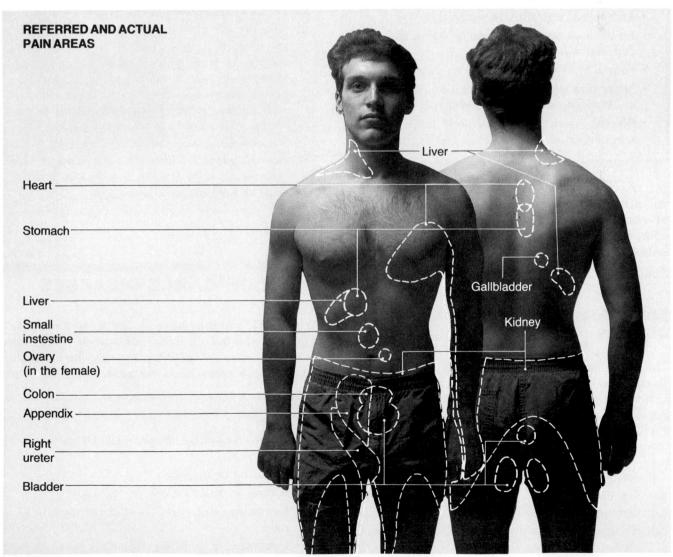

REFERRED AND ACTUAL PAIN AREAS

Liver

Heart

Stomach

Liver

Small instestine

Ovary (in the female)

Colon

Appendix

Right ureter

Bladder

Gallbladder

Kidney

FIGURE 14.2–3. **Patterns of abdominal pain.**

The general symptoms and signs of acute abdomen can include:

- Pain—diffuse (generalized, widespread) (Figure 14.2–3)
- Nausea and vomiting
- Diarrhea or constipation
- Rapid pulse (usually)
- Low blood pressure (sometimes elevated when the patient is in severe pain)
- Rapid and shallow breathing (usually a response to pain)
- Fever
- Distention of the abdomen (may be pronounced)
- Tenderness (local or diffuse)
- Rigid abdomen (can the patient relax the abdomen on command?)
- Abdominal wall muscle guarding
- An obvious protrusion seen or felt in the abdominal wall
- Fear
- Signs of shock (may be severe if there is internal bleeding or a major infection)
- Bleeding from the rectum, blood in the urine, nonmenstrual bleeding from the vagina

As you look for these indicators, consider the patient's overall appearance. Does he appear ill? Is he restless? Does he try to lie perfectly still in an effort to alleviate the pain? Does he try to draw his knees up against his abdomen? Is he reluctant to move? All of these point to acute abdominal distress.

Emergency Care for Acute Abdominal Distress

The symptoms and signs of acute abdominal distress should not be taken lightly. What you do and do not do can be critical for the patient. Do not try to guess the nature of the distress. TRANSPORT THE PATIENT. You should also:

1. Maintain an open airway and be on the alert for vomiting.
2. Provide care for shock.
3. Position the patient face up with the knees flexed, but stay on the alert for vomiting.

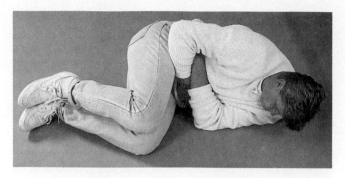

FIGURE 14.2–4. **Posturing that is characteristic of severe abdominal distress.**

4. Reassure the patient . . . do not try to diagnose.
5. Administer oxygen if there is shallow breathing or other indications of respiratory difficulties.
6. Do not give anything to the patient by mouth.
7. Attempt to collect information as to the time of onset, if it was gradual or sudden, the nature of the pain (stabbing, gnawing, sharp), any chills or fevers, any unusual bowel movements (e.g., dark, tarry stools), and if there is any rectal bleeding or blood in the urine. Find out when the patient last ate and what was consumed.
8. Save all vomitus. Since the patient may have a communicable disease, avoid contact with ALL body fluids and discharges.

COMMUNICABLE DISEASES

As an EMT, you may have to care for and transport a patient who has an infectious disease. There may be no indications of infection or it may be noticeable because upon assessment the patient presents with:

- Fever
- Profuse sweating (diaphoresis, DI-ah-fo-RE-sis)
- Vomiting or diarrhea
- A rash or other lesions on the skin
- Headache, stiff neck, chest pain, abdominal pain
- Coughing or sneezing

Your role will be to transport, maintain an open airway, treat for shock, keep the patient warm, and give nothing by mouth. However, your duties go beyond this. If the disease is communicable, you must protect yourself and make certain that no one else using the ambulance or its supplies will contract the disease (Figure 14.2–5).

The typical patient requiring your services because of illness will not cause you to take any unusual steps to protect yourself. You should avoid touching any discharges from the body (wear surgical gloves). You should avoid direct contact with the patient's blood, saliva, urine, stools, or contaminated articles of clothing and bed linens. Use latex gloves that are free of holes, breaks, and tears. Wear goggles if there is any chance of eye contamination. When necessary wear a gown and mask. Use a pocket face mask with a one-way valve or bag-valve-mask unit to deliver artificial ventilations. Do not touch your face in case you have touched something contaminated. Wash your hands and face. Ask the emergency department physician if you need to do anything else or if you need special immunization or antibiotic treatment. Ask to be informed if the patient is diagnosed as communicable. If so, it means that you need to be examined also. Make certain that you

METHODS OF TRANSMISSION

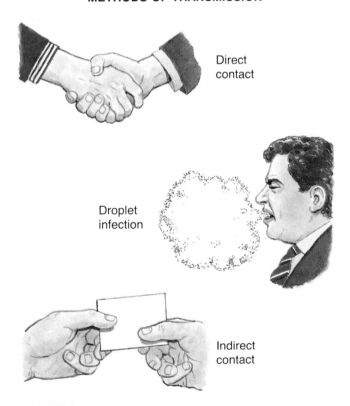

Direct contact

Droplet infection

Indirect contact

FIGURE 14.2–5. How communicable diseases may be transmitted.

follow all local protocols to be sure that others helping at the scene (e.g., first responders, police, fire service personnel) also will be notified.

When in quarters, unload and properly dispose of any contaminated bedding, properly discard all disposable items used by the patient, and clean any nondisposable items used in patient care. This includes disinfecting respiratory equipment and the ambulance cot. Unless directed otherwise, air the ambulance and scrub the patient compartment (see Chapter 26). Always wear rubber gloves.

NOTE: Some systems have disposal of contaminated items done at the hospital.

Remember to care for yourself. Remove and place your clothing in a plastic bag. This clothing should be laundered separately, as soon as possible, using a disinfecting laundry product. Shower thoroughly, using a disinfecting soap. Be certain to clean your fingernails and wash your hair.

If the emergency department physician believes that the patient's disease requires special procedures, you will be informed. You are to follow the directions that are provided by this physician. Make certain that your organization's medical officer is contacted so that there will be proper supervision for the special cleaning of equipment and caring for personnel.

Some EMTs express a fear of contracting an infectious disease. Part of this fear is due to reading the long lists of diseases found in books and magazines designed for laypersons. Some of these diseases are very rare, are difficult to "catch" from simple exposure, or are no longer a problem. For example, malaria is included on many of these lists. Malaria is "caught" by being bitten by an infective mosquito, not by contact with someone who has the disease. Polio is often listed, but its occurrence is now rare in the United States and immunization is available. Smallpox continues to be listed, even though it has been declared eradicated worldwide.

There are some diseases that can cause problems if you have never had them or been immunized specifically against them. Mumps is a good example. The risk is there, even if you wear gloves, a gown, and a mask. Know your own medical history. Have the immunizations recommended by your EMS System.

Because of their coverage in the media and press, and the social problems they bring, diseases related to sexual contact are of concern to many EMTs. Acquired immune deficiency syndrome (AIDS) is a deadly disease; however, those working with AIDS patients express no fear of contracting the disease. The mode of transmission (the way you catch it) for AIDS is known to be sexual contact,

Table 14.2–1. COMMUNICABLE DISEASES

Disease	Mode of Transmission	Incubation Period
Acquired immune deficiency syndrome (AIDS)	Sexual contact, blood or body fluids from someone with AIDS or carrying the virus, drug abusers sharing needles with someone who has or is carrying the virus, infected mothers passing the virus to their unborn children	Unknown
Chickenpox (varicella)	Direct contact. Note: moist crusts are infectious	14 to 16 days
Diphtheria	Person to person by respiratory droplets, or indirectly from contaminated objects	2 to 5 days
German measles (rubella)	Airborne droplets	14 to 21 days
Infectious hepatitis	Contact with objects contaminated by person's feces (including their hands), blood or body fluids	25 to 30 days
Measles (rubeola)	Airborne droplets and secretions from the mouth, nose, and eyes	10 to 12 days
Meningitis (bacterial)	Oral and nasal secretions	2 to 10 days
Mumps	Droplets of saliva or objects contaminated by saliva	14 to 21 days
Pneumonia (bacterial and viral)	Droplets and secretions from mouth and nose	Several days
Scarlet fever (scarlatina)	Nose and throat secretions; pus from ears	Several days
Staphylococcal skin infections	Direct contact with sore, its discharge, or contaminated objects	Several days
Syphilis	Venereal contact: saliva, semen, vaginal discharge, and blood can carry the organism into open cuts	10 days to several months
Tuberculosis (TB)	Respiratory secretions, contaminated objects, organisms on patient's hands	4 to 6 weeks
Typhoid fever	Feces, urine, and contaminated objects	7 to 21 days
Whooping cough (pertussis)	Respiratory secretions and airborne droplets	5 to 21 days

receiving a blood transfusion from a donor having or carrying the agent for AIDS, sharing needles with someone having the disease or carrying the agent, or the passage of the viral agent from mother to unborn child. The viral agent believed responsible for AIDS has been found in saliva, but transmission by contact with the saliva has not been demonstrated. Those working with AIDS patients recommend that you wear gloves and avoid contact with the patient's blood, body fluids, and discharges.

Genital herpes is acquired through sexual contact with someone having genital herpes in its active stage (open lesions or sores). If care for an injury requires you to touch the genitalia of a herpes victim, wear protective gloves. "Fever blisters" on the lips are caused by a different herpes virus. Herpes lesions may occur anywhere on the body. Your best protection from this type of herpes is to wear gloves.

Syphilis can be acquired through sexual contact; however, it also may be transmitted by coming in contact with the patient's blood, saliva, lesions in the mouth, and open cuts. The organism can enter your body through breaks in your skin. If you know the patient has syphilis (which is doubtful), wear protective gloves. Because of the risks of contracting syphilis and infectious hepatitis, it is recommended for EMTs to wear latex gloves when they have open cuts on their hands.

The mode of transmission for gonorrhea is direct sexual contact. You may not contract the disease by being with the patient and delivering care.

The main concern is viral diseases carried in blood, body fluids, and wastes. AIDS and infectious hepatitis are most often mentioned as problems. Other viruses can cause problems or are believed to be the cause of serious diseases. The Epstein–Barr virus (E–B virus) may be the cause of a chronic hepatitis-like infection. Cytomegalovirus (CMV), common in stools, has been associated with coronary artery disease. A virus found in some human blood (HTLV-I) may be the cause of a form of leukemia. Protect yourself! Avoid direct contact with blood and body fluids and wastes.

ALCOHOL AND SUBSTANCE ABUSE

Alcohol Abuse

Even though use of alcohol is socially acceptable when done in moderation, alcohol is still a drug. As with any other drug, abuse can lead to illness, poisoning of the body, antisocial behavior, and even death. As an EMT, you must take a professional approach when caring for a patient under the influence of alcohol. Remember, the patient needs your care and concern. The intoxicated patient is not a joke. There can be serious medical problems or injuries requiring your care. Take special precautions when working with the intoxicated patient. He may attempt to injure himself, bystanders, or even those trying to provide care.

EMS System personnel believe that EMTs should provide care for the patient suffering from alcohol abuse the same as for any other patient. An alcohol problem is not looked on as a crime, but as a disease. To provide proper care, you must determine quickly that the patient's difficulties are caused by alcohol and that it is the *only* problem. Remember, diabetes, epilepsy, head injuries, high fevers, and other *medical problems* may make the patient appear to be intoxicated. If allowed to do so, conduct a primary and secondary survey and an interview. In some cases, the interview will have to depend on bystanders for meaningful results.

When needed, call on the police for assistance so that you can conduct the patient assessment, provide care, and transport the patient. Remember to protect yourself by staying alert for violent behavior.

The signs of alcohol abuse in an intoxicated patient include:

- The odor of alcohol on the patient's breath or clothing. By itself, this is not enough to conclude alcohol abuse. Be certain that this odor is not "acetone breath" as experienced by the diabetic.
- Swaying and an unsteadiness of movement.
- Slurred speech and the inability to carry on a normal conversation. Do not be fooled into thinking that the situation is not serious because the patient jokes or acts humorously.
- A flushed appearance to the face, often with the patient sweating and complaining of being warm.

- Nausea and vomiting or the wish to vomit even when there is no nausea.

The alcoholic patient may not be under the influence of alcohol but suffering from **alcohol withdrawal.** This can be a severe reaction occurring when the patient cannot obtain alcohol, is too sick to drink alcohol, or has decided to quit drinking ("gone on the wagon"). The alcohol withdrawal patient may experience hallucinations and **delirium tremens (DTs).** In some cases, the DTs can be fatal. Upon assessment the patient with DTs may present with:

- Confusion and restlessness
- Atypical behavior, to the point of being "mad" or demonstrating "insane" behavior
- Hallucinations.
- Gross tremor (obvious shaking) of the hands
- Profuse sweating
- Convulsions (common and often very serious)
- The symptoms and signs of shock due to fluid loss (rare). Initially, pulse, respirations, blood pressure, and skin temperature will be elevated.

Note that some of the signs seen in alcohol abuse are similar to those found in medical emergencies. BE CERTAIN that the only problem is alcohol abuse. There may be other signs, such as depressed vital signs, due to the patient's having mixed alcohol and drugs. When interviewing the intoxicated patient or the patient suffering from alcohol withdrawal, do not begin your questioning about the abuse of other substances by asking the patient if he is taking drugs. He may react to this question as if you are gathering evidence of a crime. Ask if any medications have been taken while drinking. If necessary, when you are certain that the patient knows you are concerned about his well-being, you can repeat the question using the word "drugs."

The basic care for the intoxicated patient and the patient suffering alcohol withdrawal consists of:

1. A proper survey and interview to assess any medical emergencies or injuries. Look carefully for fractures and indications of other injuries.
2. Monitoring of vital signs, staying alert for respiratory problems.
3. Talking to the patient in an effort to keep him as alert as possible.

4. Helping the patient during vomiting so that vomitus will not be aspirated.

5. Protecting the patient from self-injury, without the illegal use of restraint. Your instructor will tell you if you may use restraint.

6. Providing care for shock.

7. Staying alert for convulsions.

8. Transporting the patient in a position to allow for drainage should the patient vomit.

NOTE: In some systems, patients under the influence of alcohol who are not suffering from a medical emergency or apparent injury are not transported. They are given over to the police. This may not be wise since as many as 15% of patients having an alcohol-related medical emergency may die unless they receive additional care. In addition to this, the EMTs may have missed a medical problem or injury. *All patients with the DTs must be transported to a medical facility as soon as possible.*

Substance Abuse

Individuals who abuse drugs and other chemical substances should be considered to have an illness. They have the right to professional-level emergency care the same as any patient.

The most common drugs and chemical substances that are abused and may lead to problems requiring an EMS response can be simply classified as **uppers** (stimulants), **downers** (depressants), **narcotics, hallucinogens** (mind-affecting drugs), and **volatile chemicals.** Uppers are stimulants af-

fecting the nervous system to excite the user. Many abusers use these drugs in an attempt to relieve fatigue or to create feelings of well-being. Examples include amphetamines and cocaine. Downers are depressants such as barbiturates and are meant to affect the central nervous system to relax the user. Narcotics affect the nervous system and change many of the normal activities of the body. Often they produce an intense state of relaxation and feelings of well-being. Heroin is a commonly abused narcotic. Hallucinogens such as LSD and PCP are mind-affecting drugs that act on the nervous system to produce an intense state of excitement or a distortion of the user's surroundings. Volatile chemicals can give an initial "rush" and then act as depressants affecting the central nervous system. Cleaning fluid, glue, and solutions used to correct typing mistakes are commonly abused volatile chemicals.

As an EMT, you will not need to know the names of very many abused drugs or their specific reactions. It is far more important for you to be able to detect possible drug abuse at the overdose level and to relate certain signs to certain types of drugs and drug withdrawal. Your care for the drug abuse patient will be basically the same for all drugs and will not change unless you are ordered to do something by a poison control center with on-line medical command. Table 14.2–2 provides some of the names of commonly abused drugs. Do not worry about memorizing this chart. Read it through so that you can place some of the more familiar drugs into categories in terms of drug type.

Signs of Drug and Chemical Substance Abuse

The symptoms and signs of substance abuse, dependency, and overdose can vary from patient to patient,

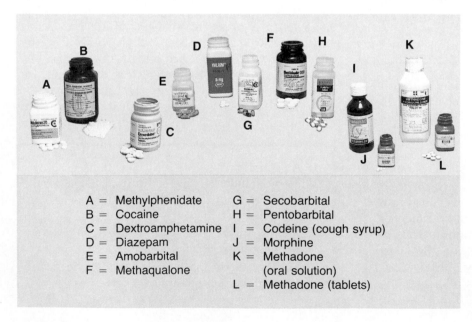

A = Methylphenidate
B = Cocaine
C = Dextroamphetamine
D = Diazepam
E = Amobarbital
F = Methaqualone
G = Secobarbital
H = Pentobarbital
I = Codeine (cough syrup)
J = Morphine
K = Methadone (oral solution)
L = Methadone (tablets)

FIGURE 14.2–6. Abused substances.

Table 14.2–2. COMMONLY ABUSED DRUGS

Uppers	Downers	Narcotics	Mind-Altering Drugs	Volatile Chemicals
AMPHETAMINE (Benzedrine, bennies, pep pills, ups, uppers, cartwheels)	AMOBARBITAL (blue devils, downers, barbs, Amytal)	CODEINE (often in cough syrup)	DMT	AMYL NITRATE (snappers, poppers)
BIPHETAMINE (bam)	BARBITURATES (downers, dolls, barbs, rainbows)	DEMEROL	LSD (acid, sunshine)	BUTYL NITRATE (locker room, rush)
COCAINE (coke, snow, crack)	CHLORAL HYDRATE (knockout drops, Noctec)	DILAUDID	MESCALINE (peyote, mesc)	CLEANING FLUID (carbon tetrachloride)
DESOXYN (black beauties)	ETHCHLORVYNOL (Placidyl)	FENTANYL (Sublimaze)	MORNING GLORY SEEDS	FURNITURE POLISH
DEXTROAMPHETAMINE (dexies, Dexedrine)	GLUTETHIMIDE (Doriden, goofers)	HEROIN ("H," horse, junk, smack, stuff)	PCP (angel dust, hog, peace pills)	GASOLINE
METHAMPHETAMINE (speed, meth, crystal, diet pills, Methedrine)	METHAQUALONE (Quaalude, ludes, Sopor, sopors)	METHADONE (dolly)	PSILOCYBIN (magic mushrooms)	GLUE
METHYLPHENIDATE (Ritalin)	NONBARBITURATE SEDATIVES (various tranquilizers and sleeping pills: Valium or diazepam, Miltown, Equanil, meprobamate, Thorazine, Compazine, Librium or chlordiazepoxide, reserpine, Tranxene or chlorazepate and other benzodiazepines)	MORPHINE	STP (serenity, tranquility, peace)	HAIR SPRAY
PRELUDIN		OPIUM (Op, poppy)	*Nonhallucinogenic Mind-Altering*	NAIL POLISH REMOVER
		MEPERIDINE (Demerol)	HASH	PAINT THINNER
	PARALDEHYDE	PAREGORIC (contains opium)	MARIJUANA (grass, pot, weed, dope)	TYPEWRITING CORRECTION FLUIDS
	PENTOBARBITAL (yellow jackets, barbs, Nembutal)	TYLENOL with Codeine (1,2,3,4)	THC	
	PHENOBARBITAL (goofballs, phennies, barbs)			
	SECOBARBITAL (red devils, barbs, Seconal)			

even for the same drug or chemical. The problem is made more complex by the fact that many substance abusers take more than one drug or chemical at a time. Often, you will have to carefully combine the information gained from the signs, the symptoms, the scene, the bystanders, and the patient in order to be certain that you are dealing with substance abuse. In many cases, you will not be able to determine the substance involved. When questioning the patient and bystanders, you will get better results if you begin by asking if the patient has been taking any medications rather than using the word "drugs." Then, if necessary, ask if the patient has been taking drugs.

Some significant symptoms and signs related to specific drugs include:

- Uppers—Excitement, increased pulse and breathing rates, rapid speech, dry mouth, dilated pupils, sweating, and the complaint of having gone without sleep for long periods. Repeated high doses can produce a "speed run." The patient will be restless, hyperactive, and usually very apprehensive and uncooperative.

- Downers—Sluggish, sleepy patient lacking typical coordination of body and speech. Pulse and breathing rates are low, often to the point of a true emergency.
- Hallucinogens (mind-altering drugs)—Fast pulse rate, dilated pupils, and a flushed face. The patient often "sees" or "hears" things, has little concept of real time, and may not be aware of the true environment. Often what he says makes no sense to the listener. The user may become aggressive or may withdraw.
- Narcotics—Reduced rate of pulse and rate and depth of breathing, often seen with a lowering of skin temperature. The pupils are constricted, often pinpoint in size. The muscles are relaxed and sweating is profuse. The patient is very sleepy and does not wish to do anything. In overdoses, coma is a common event. Respiratory arrest or cardiac arrest may develop rapidly.
- Volatile chemicals—Dazed or showing temporary loss of contact with reality. The patient may develop coma. The linings of the nose and mouth may show swollen membranes. The patient may complain of a "funny numb feeling" or "tingling" inside the head. Changes in heart rhythm can occur. This can lead to death.

When reading the above list, you should have noticed that many of the indications of drug abuse are similar to those for quite a few medical emergencies. As an EMT, you must *never* assume drug abuse occurring by itself. You must be on the alert for medical emergencies, injuries, and combinations of drug abuse problems and other emergencies.

In addition to seeing the effects of long-term drug use and overdose, you will have to deal with cases of severe *drug withdrawal*. As in reactions to drugs, withdrawal varies from patient to patient and from drug to drug. In most cases of drug withdrawal, you may see:

- Shaking
- Anxiety
- Nausea

- Confusion and irritability (sometimes retreating from the persons at the scene)
- Diaphoresis
- Increased pulse and breathing rates

Care for Substance Abuse Patients

When providing care for substance abuse patients, you should make certain that you are safe and identify yourself as an EMT to the patient and bystanders. The procedures for care may require you to:

1. Provide basic life-support measures if required.
2. Call the emergency department and the poison control center in accordance with local policies.
3. Monitor vital signs and be alert for respiratory arrest. Provide oxygen if needed.
4. Talk to the patient to gain his confidence and to help maintain his level of consciousness. Use his name often, maintain eye contact, and speak directly to the patient.
5. Protect the patient from self-injury and attempting to hurt others without using illegal restraint. Your instructor will tell you if you may use restraint.
6. Provide care for shock.
7. Assess closely for signs of fractures and internal injuries.
8. Check carefully for head injuries.
9. Look for gross tissue damage on the extremities resulting from the injection of drugs ("tracks"). Dress and bandage all such sites.
10. Transport the patient as soon as possible, monitoring vital signs, staying alert for convulsions, and being on guard for vomiting that could obstruct the airway.
11. Continue to reassure the patient throughout all phases of care.

WARNING: Many drug abusers may appear calm at first and then become violent as time passes. You are always to be on the alert and be ready to protect yourself. If the patient creates an unsafe scene and you are not a trained law enforcement officer, **GET OUT** and find a safe place until the police arrive. Be extra cautious if you know the patient has been using **PCP.** This drug may cause the patient to lose the understanding of right and wrong. Some PCP abusers will find nothing wrong in killing you! Have police support when dealing with substance abuse patients, especially if you suspect a patient used PCP.

SUMMARY

Diabetes mellitus is usually controlled by diet, or by diet and insulin. When the diabetic patient does not take enough insulin or he takes too much sugar, he becomes hyperglycemic and may develop diabetic coma. The patient will have acetone breath. Transport immediately, provide sugar to the conscious patient if you cannot tell if he is developing diabetic coma or insulin shock.

Insulin shock develops from severe hypoglycemia when the patient takes too much insulin or too little sugar. Provide sugar, but do not give liquids to the unconscious patient (sprinkle granulated sugar under the tongue, if allowed). Transport as soon as possible.

Convulsive seizures, including epilepsy, require you to protect the patient from physical harm and embarrassment. Transport of the patient is the best policy. Status epilepticus is a true emergency requiring immediate transport and the administration of oxygen.

Acute abdomen has many different symptoms and signs, including pain, nausea, vomiting, rapid pulse, and rapid and shallow breathing. Do not try to diagnose the source of the problem. Maintain an open airway, treat for shock, provide oxygen as needed, and transport. Place the patient on his back with the knees flexed. STAY ALERT FOR VOMITING.

A patient may have a communicable disease if he has fever, diaphoresis (profuse sweating), vomiting or diarrhea, a rash or lesions, headache, cough-ing, or sneezing. Non-trauma-related neck, chest, or abdominal pain may also indicate an infectious disease. Transport the patient, treating for shock. Protect yourself from contamination during care and transport. Consult with the emergency department physician and follow his directions for personal care and the disposal, cleaning, and sterilization of equipment and supplies.

Patients suffering from alcohol abuse are to receive the same level of professional care as any other patient. Be certain that the problem is due to alcohol or alcohol withdrawal. There may be another medical problem or injuries. Try to detect the odor of alcohol, slurred speech, swaying and unsteadiness of movement. Find out if the patient is nauseated. Be alert for vomiting. In cases of alcohol withdrawal, look for hand tremors that may indicate DTs. In all cases of alcohol abuse, monitor vital signs and be alert for respiratory arrest.

Drug abuse can show itself in many ways, depending on the drug, the patient, and whether you are dealing with withdrawal or overdose. Withdrawal from most drugs will produce shaking, anxiety, nausea, confusion and irritability, sweating, and increased pulse and breathing rates.

Uppers usually speed up activity, speech, pulse, and breathing and tend to excite the user. Downers do just the opposite. Hallucinogens (mind-altering drugs) increase pulse rate, dilate the pupils, and cause the patient to see or hear things and to lose touch with reality. Narcotics reduce pulse and breathing rates. Pupils of narcotic patients usually will be constricted. The patient may appear sleepy and may not wish to do anything. Volatile chemicals act as depressants, causing the patient to be dazed.

In cases of drug abuse or withdrawal, provide life-support measures as needed. Monitor vital signs and be alert for respiratory arrest. Treat for shock. Remember to provide emotional support to the patient. Remember to consider your own safety and have police support. Be especially careful of patients who may be abusing PCP.

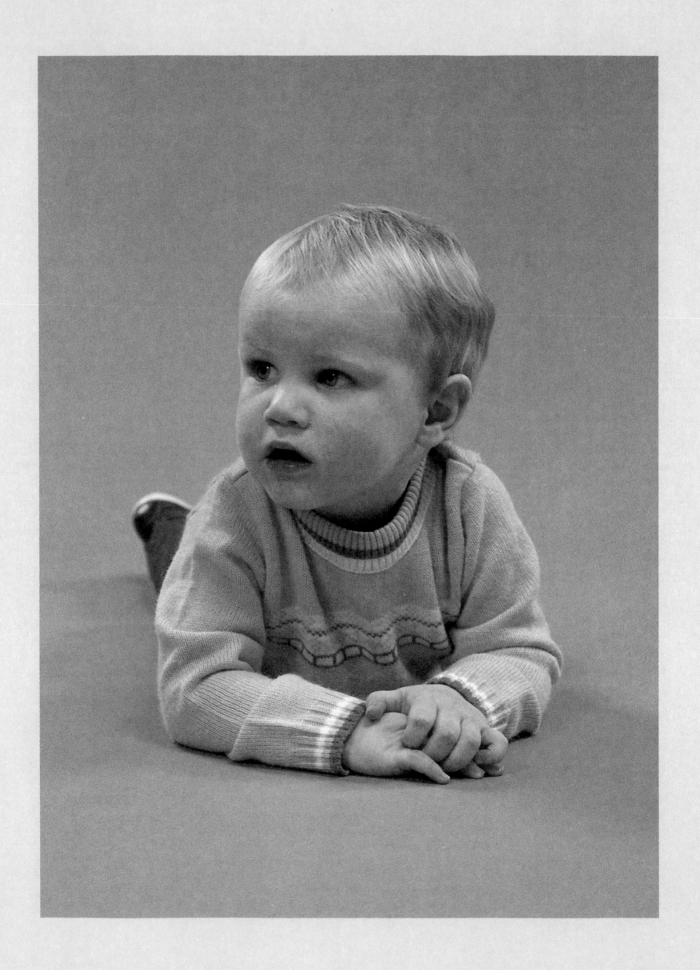

15

Pediatric Emergencies

OBJECTIVES As an EMT, you should be able to:

1. State the age ranges for infant and child. (p. 418)

2. Describe how to conduct a primary survey on an infant and a child. (pp. 420–421)

3. State, step by step, the basic life support procedures for both infant and child patients. (pp. 420–421)

4. Describe the changes made in the interview method used when the patient is a child. (p. 419 and p. 422)

5. List the normal vital signs for the infant and the child patient. (p. 422)

6. List in general what special problems are searched for during the secondary survey when the patient is an infant and when the patient is a child. (p. 423)

7. State the appropriate basic EMT-level care for pediatric emergencies involving:
   • Fever (pp. 428–429)

   • Seizures (p. 429)
   • Respiratory distress (pp. 429–430)
   • Acute abdomen (p. 430)

8. Define *sudden infant death syndrome* (SIDS) and state the EMT's role in a possible SIDS-related infant death. (p. 431)

9. Describe the symptoms and signs associated with bike fork compression injury and state the emergency care for such an injury. (p. 425)

10. State the common burn injuries received by infants and children. (pp. 424–425)

11. Define *child abuse* in terms of the battered child syndrome and sexual assault. (p. 426)

12. List the typical injuries associated with the battered child. (pp. 426–427)

13. State the EMT's role in cases of possible child abuse, including care for possible sexual assault. (p. 427)

1. Determine if a patient is a child or an infant.
2. Conduct a proper primary survey on infants and children.
3. Control your emotions and remain professional during a pediatric emergency.
4. Provide appropriate basic life support for both infants and children.
5. Properly conduct an interview of a child patient.
6. Conduct a secondary survey physical examination on infants and children, detecting atypical vital signs, possible injuries, and indications of possible medical emergencies.
7. Provide prompt and efficient care in cases of injury when the patient is an infant or child.
8. Evaluate infants and children for possible medical emergencies.
9. Provide emotional support to parents in cases of possible sudden infant death syndrome.
10. Act as a professional in cases of possible child abuse.

TERMS   you may be using for the first time:

Apnea – the temporary cessation of breathing.

Bike Fork Compression Injury – an injury usually sustained when the victim's heel is caught in the spokes of the front wheel of a bicycle or tricycle. The foot is driven into the fork of the front wheel, producing crushing injuries to the tissues behind and around the ankle. This same type of injury may involve the rear fork when the accident involves a passenger "riding double."

Child Abuse – assault of the infant or child that produces physical and/or emotional injuries. Sexual assault is included as a form of child abuse.

Croup (Kroop) – the general term for a group of viral infections that produce swelling of the larynx.

Epiglottitis (ep-i-glo-TI-tis) – a bacterial infection causing the swelling of the epiglottis.

Sudden Infant Death Syndrome (SIDS) – an unexplained sudden death of an apparently healthy infant while asleep. Death can usually be related to respiratory arrest.

INFANTS AND CHILDREN— SPECIAL PATIENTS

By definition, an **infant** is anyone younger than 1 year of age. A **child** is anyone from 1 to 8 years of age. In the past, any patient over 8 years of age was to be treated using adult techniques. Even though this may be true in terms of pulmonary resuscitation and CPR, such a statement cannot be made for all aspects of care. Even when exact age guidelines are established, there must be some variations in care based on the size of the patient.

The maturity of the patient can be significant. One hardly expects a 9-year-old child to be able to deal with an emergency in the same fashion as a 14-year-old adolescent. The procedures of the interview and the amount of emotional support required certainly would be different for the two age groups. Add to this the fact that many children and individuals in their early adolescence have been observed to react to crises in a *regressive* manner. This means that a patient who is a mature 10-year-old may act more like a 6-year-old in an emergency. Care for the patient must be applied as needed by the individual in the particular situation.

The concept of adolescent medicine is a fairly new one. The lower limits of systolic blood pressure used to indicate the onset of shock cannot be the same for a 12-year-old and a 17-year-old patient. One cannot apply children's blood volumes to the 14-year-old. In most cases, adult blood volumes cannot be applied to the 14-year-old patient either. Such factors require you to judge the individual in terms of body size and apparent emotional and physical maturity.

Your own reactions to a pediatric emergency make infants and children special patients. A broken bone is a broken bone, and a bleeding wound is a bleeding wound. The principles of basic emergency care are essentially the same, regardless of the age of the injured patient. Yet we all react more intensely to the cries of children. We want to immediately stop the suffering and correct all problems. Those in emergency medicine must control their emotions so as not to be overwhelmed by cries of pain, expressions of fear, and the unnerving silence of children who should be crying. There is no doubt that you should be strongly motivated to care for the infant or child patient and that you should want him to "feel better." However, unless you control your emotions as you provide care so that you can be objective and efficient, the care needed to help the child may not be provided. If you let your emotions control your actions, the emotional support and comfort needed by child, family, and bystanders will not be part of the care you provide. Unless you are *calm* and *professional*, the emotional reactions of the patient and others at the scene may become more intense.

Always keep in mind that parents, family, friends, and bystanders at the scene need your support. In fact, unless each individual believes that you are concerned and that you wish to help, you may not be allowed to provide care, or you may be prevented from providing effective care. There is usually little time for long conversations. Identify yourself and show through your *interactions* with the child that you are concerned. The way you provide care shows that you are a well-trained professional.

The Primary Survey and Basic Life Support

Details for the procedures used in the primary survey and basic life support for infants and children were presented in Chapters 3 through 7. Scan 15–1 is provided to remind you of what to do to establish and maintain an open airway, provide pulmonary resuscitation and CPR, control profuse bleeding, and treat for shock.

The Secondary Survey

The Patient Interview

Obviously, you will not be able to interview an infant. If an adult family member is at the scene, this person may be able to provide you with a history of illnesses and injuries. Young children can be interviewed if you take your time and keep your language as simple as possible. If the parents or guardians are at the scene and they are not injured or ill, talk with them, but do not exclude the child. Talking with the parents will help gain the child's confidence. However, if you do not follow this by talking *directly* to the child, you may find the child unwilling to accept your help and the parents losing confidence in your ability to help their child.

All patients have some degree of fear at the emergency scene. Infants and children are usually more fearful than adults because they lack the experience needed in order to understand illness and injury. In addition to this, the infant or child is easily frightened by the unknown. Since so many things are unknowns to a child, it is easy to see why emergencies can be so scary for children. The infant is unclear as to what comprises the world immediately around him. The elements associated with the emergency (e.g., pain, noise, bright lights, cold) often set off a reaction of pure panic on the part of the infant.

A child lacks communication skills. At an emergency, as the child finds he does not understand you, or believes that you do not understand him, a growing fear will develop. If the child is to use the communications skills available to him, he must remain calm. This is part of the care you must provide.

Keep in mind that any problems faced by the child will be intensified if his parents are not at the scene. Children find security by interacting with their parents when facing new problems or emergencies. Asking for his parents may be the child's first priority, even above that of having you help him or relieve his pain.

When you are dealing with a child patient, you should:

- Identify yourself to the child. Keep this very simple. For example, "Hi. My name is Mark. What's yours?"
- Let him know that someone will call his parents.
- If the child has a toy on the scene and wants it, let him have the toy.
- Kneel or sit with the child so as not to tower over him.
- SMILE at the child. This is one sign from an adult that carries a lot of weight with most children.
- Touch the child on the forehead and hold his hand. If the child does not wish to be touched, he will let you know. Do not force the issue; simply smile and provide comfort to the child by way of conversation.
- Do not let the child see scissors, clamps, or other tools and equipment. Many children fear these items, thinking that they will cause pain.

The Primary Survey and Basic Life Support

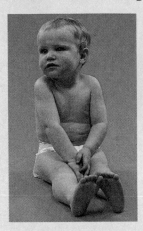

INFANTS

BIRTH TO ONE YEAR

- Act as a professional—control your emotions and facial expressions. This may help reduce fear.
- Protect the head and spine. Remember, head and neck injuries are common because the infant's head is so large and heavy.
- Always ensure an adequate airway. When needed, provide adequate ventilations.
- Remember, even a small loss of blood may lead to shock.

ESTABLISHING UNRESPONSIVENESS: The infant should move or cry gently when gently tapped or shaken.

AIRWAY: Use the head-tilt, chin-lift. (The head-tilt, neck-lift may be needed to provide an adequate airway.)

EVALUATING BREATHING: Use the LOOK, LISTEN, FEEL approach. If the infant is cyanotic or he is struggling to breathe. Immediate transport is recommended.

CLEARING THE AIRWAY:
- Use the mouth-to-mouth and nose or mouth-to-mask technique.
- Provide two adequate breaths.

If there is evidence of airway obstruction requiring action:
- Make certain that you have not overextended or underextended the neck.
- Straddle the infant over your arm face down and with the head lower than the trunk. Support the head by placing your hand around the jaw and chest. Add support by placing your forearm on your thigh.
- Rapidly deliver four back blows using the heel of your free hand. Strike directly between the shoulder blades.
- Place your free hand on the infant's back, sandwiching him between your two hands. Turn the infant over and place his back on your thigh. The head should be lower than the trunk.
- Rapidly deliver four chest thrusts as you would if providing external chest compressions for CPR.
- If the airway remains obstructed, but the patient is conscious, continue backblows and chest thrusts.
- If the airway remains obstructed, but the patient is unconscious, place your thumb into the patient's mouth, over the tongue. Wrap your other fingers around the lower jaw and look for an obstruction.
- Do NOT attempt blind finger sweeps. When removing an obstruction, use your little finger.
- If the patient is unconscious and the obstruction has not been dislodged, provide two breaths and repeat the procedure of back blows and chest thrusts, looking for and removing visible obstructions, and reattempting ventilations.

RESCUE BREATHING:
- Open the airway.
- Use mouth-to-mouth and nose or mouth-to-mask technique
- Provide two adequate breaths, noting the chest rise (take 1 to 1.5 seconds/ventilation).
- If airway is clear and patient is still not breathing, determine if there is a brachial pulse.
- If there is no pulse, provide CPR. Should there be a pulse, but no breathing, provide rescue breathing.

- Deliver one adequate breath every THREE SECONDS.
- Check for a pulse every few minutes.

CPR:
- If patient is unresponsive and not breathing,—
  Open the airway.
  Provide two adequate breaths.
  Look, listen, and feel for breathing. If there is no indication of obstruction, but the patient is unconscius and is not breathing . . .
- Determine if there is a BRACHIAL PULSE. If no pulse and no breathing, provide CPR.
  Apply compressions to the sternum, one finger width below an imaginary line drawn between the nipples.
  Use the tips of two or three fingers.
- Depress the sternum ½ to 1 inch.
- Deliver compressions at a rate of at least 100 per minute.
- Deliver a ventilation, mouth-to-mouth and nose or mouth-to-mask, 1 EVERY 5 COMPRESSIONS ("one, two, three, four, five"-breathe).
- Check for a brachial pulse every few minutes.

BLEEDING:
- Use direct pressure as a primary method.
- When necessary, use elevation, pressure points, or a blood pressure cuff. A tourniquet is a last resort.
- Consider a blood loss of 25 milliliters or more to be very serious.

SHOCK:
- Consider the infant to be in shock if the blood loss is 25 milliliters or greater.
- Consider the infant to be developing shock if the systolic blood pressure is below 70 mmHg. The infant is probably in severe shock if the systolic blood pressure is under 40 mmHg.
- Consider shock to be more severe if there is evidence of dehydration (vomiting, diarrhea, exposure to high temperatures, overheating, high skin temperature).
- Ensure adequate breathing and circulation, and control serious bleeding.
- Administer oxygen per local guidelines.
- Elevate the lower extremities, but avoid placing pressure on the cervical spine and head.
- Prevent the loss of body heat.
- Splint fractures.
- Avoid rough handling.
- Give nothing by mouth.
- Transport as soon as possible, monitoring vital signs.

The Primary Survey and Basic Life Support

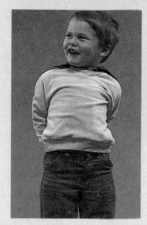

CHILDREN

1 TO 8 YEARS

- Act as a professional—control your emotions and facial expressions. This may help reduce fear.
- Protect the head and spine. A child's head is proportionally large.
- Always ensure an open airway. When needed, provide adequate ventilations.
- Carefully evaluate blood loss.

Caution: The Size and Weight of the Child May Be More Important Than Age.

ESTABLISHING UNRESPONSIVENESS: The child should move or cry when gently tapped or shaken.

AIRWAY: Use the head-tilt, chin-lift or modified jaw-thrust to provide an adequate aireay.

EVALUATING BREATHING: Use the LOOK, LISTEN, FEEL approach. If the child is cyanotic or struggling to breathe, immediate transport is recommended. Should the child be in respiratory arrest, or is cyanotic and failing at attempts to breathe, make certain that the airway is open and clear of obstructions so you can begin rescue breathing efforts.

CLEARING THE AIRWAY:
- Make certain that you have the proper heat-tilt.
- Use the mouth-to-mouth and nose or mouth-to-mask techniques for small children and the mouth-to-mouth technique for large children.
- Provide two adequate breaths. Watch for the child's chest to rise.

If there is evidence of airway obstruction requiring action:
- Rapidly deliver six to ten abdominal thrusts.
- If the airway remains obstructed, but the patient is conscious, continue with sets of abdominal thrusts.
- If the airway remains obstructed, but the patient is unconscious, place the child on his back upon a hard surface. Provide support for his head and back as you move him. Place your thumb into the patient's mouth, over the tongue. Wrap your other fingers around the lower jaw and look for an obstruction. Do NOT attempt blind finger sweeps.
- If the patient is unconscious and the obstruction has not been dislodged, transport immediately, attempting two ventilations and repeating the procedure of abdominal thrusts, looking for and removing visible obstructions, and reattempting to ventilate.

RESCUE BREATHING
- Open the airway without overextending the neck.
- Provide two adequate breaths, noting the chest rise.
- If airway is clear and patient is still not breathing, determine if there is a carotid pulse. If there is no pulse, provide CPR. Should there be a pulse, but no breathing, provide rescue breathing . . .
- Deliver one adequate breath every FOUR SECONDS. Check for a pulse every few minutes.

CPR:
- If the patient is unresponsive and not breathing,
  Open the airway.
  Provide two adequate breaths.
  Look, listen, and feel for breathing. If there is no indication

of obstruction, but the patient is still unconscious and is not breathing.
- Determine if there is a CAROTID PULSE. If no pulse and no breathing, provide CPR.
- Apply compressions to the CPR compression site (locate the same way as you would an adult), using the tips of three fingers if the patient is a small child. For larger children, use the heel of one hand to apply compressions.
- Depress the sternum 1 to 1½ inches.
- Deliver compressions at a rate of 80 to 100 per minute.
- Deliver a ventilation as an adequate breath, mouth-to-mouth and nose or mouth-to-mouth or mouth-to-mask, 1 EVERY 5 COMPRRESSIONS.
- Check for a carotid pulse every few minutes.

BLEEDING:
- Use direct pressure as a primary method.
- When necessary, use elevation, pressure points, or a blood pressure cuff. Use a tourniquet as a last resort.
- Consider a blood loss of 500 milliliters (½ liter or about 1 pint) or more to be very serious.

SHOCK:
No one sign is absolute, but:
- Consider the child to be in severe shock if blood loss is 500 milliliters (about 1 pint) or more.
- Consider the patient to be in shock if the systolic blood pressure is under:
  50 mmHg in pre-school children.
  60 mmHg in children up to age 12.
  70 mmHg in teenagers.
  Any systolic blood pressure below 80 mmHg indicates that the child or adolescent may be developing shock.
- Consider shock to be more severe if there is evidence of dehydration (vomiting, diarrhea, exposure to high temperature, overheating, high skin temperature).
- Ensure adequate breathing and circulation, and control serious bleeding.
- Administer oxygen per local guidelines.
- Evaluate the lower extremities, but avoid placing pressure on the cervical spine and head.
- Prevent loss of body heat.
- Splint fractures.
- Avoid rough handling.
- Give nothing by mouth.
- Transport as soon as possible, monitoring vital signs.

- Let the child see your face and keep eye contact. Speak directly to the child, making a special effort to speak clearly and slowly. Be sure that the child can hear you.
- Stop occasionally to find out if the child understands what you have said or asked. Even if you communicate easily with children, never assume that a child has understood you. Find out if you have been understood by questioning the child periodically.
- Determine as quickly as you can if there are any life-threatening problems and care for them. If there are no problems of this nature, continue the patient survey and interview at a relaxed pace. Fearful children cannot take the pressure of a rapidly paced examination and a lot of "meaningless" questions all being controlled by a stranger.
- Always tell the child what you are going to do as you take vital signs and do a physical examination. Do not try to explain the entire procedure at once. Explain one step, do the procedure, then explain the next step.
- NEVER LIE TO THE CHILD. Tell him when he may feel pain during the physical examination. If he asks if he is sick or hurt, tell him so, but be certain to add that you are there to help and you will not leave. Let the child know that other people also will be helping him.

The Physical Examination

Vital Signs   You will need to determine vital signs for the infant or child patient. Do not tell the child that you are going to "take" his pulse or his blood pressure. Some children will think that you are literally going to take something away from them. Instead, tell the child you need to "check" them. Try to obtain pulse, respirations, and relative skin temperature as you talk to the child patient. This will give you time to gain the child's confidence before trying to measure blood pressure. Be certain to show the child the blood pressure cuff. Let him see the surface of the cuff that will be placed against his arm. This will help dispel fear that the cuff contains needles or other objects that may hurt. Wrap the cuff around an area of your wrist or arm that will accept the small size of the pediatric cuff. Pump the bulb to show that the procedure will not hurt. Tell him that it will feel "tight" for a little while.

Remember that a child is naturally curious, even when experiencing pain. If he expresses an interest in your stethoscope, let him listen. Should he want to operate your penlight, let him do so.

Table 15–1. VITAL SIGNS: INFANTS AND CHILDREN

	Infant	*Children*
PULSE RATE	120 to 150 (birth) 110 (average 6 month old)	Range: 70 to 140 110 (average 1 year old) 95 (2 to 4 years) 90 (5 to 10 years) 85 (10 to 15 years) 75 (15 years +)
BREATHING RATE	30 to 70 (birth) 30 (6 months)	Range: 16 to 44 28 (average 1 year old) 25 (2 to 4 years) 24 (5 to 10 years) 20 (10 to 15 years) 16 to 18 (15 years +)
SYSTOLIC BLOOD PRESSURE	60 to 80 mmHg (birth) 90 mmHg (6 months) (90 mmHg + 2 × age for older than 6 months)	Range: 90 to 150 mmHg 90 (average 1 year old) 100 (2 to 4 years) 100 to 110 (5 to 10 years) 110 (10 to 15 years) 110 to 120 (15 years +)
DIASTOLIC BLOOD PRESSURE	Very serious if below 40 mmHg or above 76 mmHg	Very serious if below 50 or above 76 mmHg for children from 1 to 5 years. Very serious if below 60 or above 86 mmHg for ages 5 to 12. Very serious if below 60 or above 106 mmHg from age 12 to adult

Such activities build a rapport with the child that will reduce his fears and make him more receptive to your care.

Table 15–1 lists the vital signs for infants and children. Remember that a child will have even less understanding than an adult as to why you are doing certain things. Most children will remain confident in what you are doing if you continue to talk with them and keep direct eye contact whenever possible.

Patient Survey   The head-to-toe survey is usually performed as a *toe-to-head survey* on alert infants and small children since they often object to having a stranger attempt to touch them around the head and face. The survey for the older child and the unconscious pediatric patient is conducted in much the same manner as for adult patients. If the parents are at the scene, explain what you are going to do and the importance of the physical examination. Unless there are possible injuries that indicate that the child should not be moved, the child should be held on the mother's or father's lap. Kneel and try to stay at the child's eye level. Explain to the child

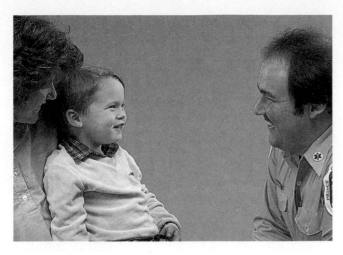

FIGURE 15–1. Keep the child at ease during the examination.

that you are going to ask questions from time to time as you check from the "tips" of his toes to the "top" of his head. Tell the child what you are going to do *before* you do it, making certain to warn him of any possible pain. Simply tell the child that what you do may hurt, but the pain should go away quickly. Let him know that you must do what you are doing so you can help him. Always tell the child that you need his help.

Many EMS squads carry a doll or a stuffed animal to be given to the child during the physical examination. If a toy is to be carried on the ambulance, it must be made of materials that allow for proper sanitizing. Such a toy serves to provide comfort to the child and allows you to explain the survey to the child. You can point to an area on the toy and tell the child this is where you must touch him during the survey. You also can use the toy to explain what you need to do when providing emergency care. This type of one-to-one communication not only helps you and the child, but it also helps to build parent and bystander confidence, letting them know that a professional, compassionate EMT is caring for the child.

Most young children usually suffer no embarrassment when articles of clothing are removed or repositioned during an objective examination. Nonetheless, you should protect the child from the stares of onlookers. Many children around the age of five to eight go through a stage of intense modesty. You may have to keep explaining why you must remove certain articles of clothing. Many parents and day care centers teach children that strangers should not remove their clothing or touch them. The children that you examine may not understand your intentions and may offer a great deal of resistance. Some

children may become upset because they feel you are taking something away from them. Take your time so as not to rush children into accepting all that is happening.

The young adolescent is often worried about the changes occurring to his or her body. This is a new experience for patients and, they may be uncertain if these changes are "normal." Handling the clothing of a teen-age girl can be a little awkward for the male EMT. In most cases, a simple description of the survey will set the patient at ease. However, you should make sure that the parents understand what you are going to do and why it must be done. Whenever possible, conduct the examination in the presence of a female EMT. *Do not* delay patient evaluation and care because you or the patient may be embarrassed. As a professional, you must put such feelings aside and act in a manner that will allow the patient to relax and understand that there is no need for embarrassment.

The survey is done to look for the same signs of injury and illness as in the case of the adult patient. However, you should take special care with the following:

- Head—Remember that an infant has "soft spots" (fontanelles) on the skull. Make certain that you do not apply pressure to these spots. These fontanelles may bulge, naturally, when the infant cries. Many accidents involving infants and children produce head injuries.
- Nose and ears—Blood and clear fluids may be missed during the survey. Look carefully and relate these findings to skull fractures.
- Neck—Cervical spine injuries can occur more easily with pediatric patients since the head is large compared with the rest of the body. In medical emergencies, the neck may be sore, stiff, or swollen.
- Chest—Listen closely for even air entry and the sounds of breathing. Be alert for rales and wheezes.
- Abdomen—Note any rigid or tender areas.
- Pelvis—Be on the alert for rectal bleeding.
- Extremities—You *must* do a neurologic assessment for both infants and children.

The neurologic evaluation often produces special problems. Infants have to be watched carefully to see their responses to your touching, squeezing, and pushing. It is often necessary to treat all infants as if they were unconscious patients, and test them for reaction to painful stimuli. Always note if the conscious infant's or child's eyes look in the direction of your hand or your face as you touch him. Children should follow your movements with their eyes. Notice if the patient stays alert, responds only when you call his name or speak loudly; or lapses quickly into a sleepy state. See if the patient will squeeze your fingers or a ball or other toy. If you reach a point in the evaluation at which you do not think spinal injuries are likely, continue to test the young child's neurologic reactions by simple childhood games such as "peek-a-boo." Holding your hand up to the young child's hand will often lead the patient to compare the size of his hand with yours. In doing so, the child will move his fingers and will press against your hand. If the child does not respond, see if he wants to play "pattycake," or if he wants to hold an object that requires him to use both hands and eyes in coordination. The stethoscope is ideal for this purpose, provided the child shows no fear of the instrument.

Most infants and children can be comforted (consoled) by a parent. Continued irritability is a sign that something may be wrong with the child.

Injuries Common to Children

When providing emergency care for the injured child, always tell him what you are going to do before you do it. Try to make him feel special. Tell the child that he is very brave and has been a big help to you. If the child is crying, let him know that it is all right if he cries and that everybody becomes a little scared when they are hurt.

Carry a brightly colored adhesive bandage and apply this to a suitable dressing. Make a fuss over using this tape only for him, calling it a "battle ribbon," a reward for bravery, or some other special name.

Head Injuries

Again, remember that head injuries are common in accidents involving infants and children. Take special care in noting any signs of such injury. The possibility of cervical spine injury exists whenever a child receives a head injury. If the injury appears to be minor and the parents do not want you to transport the child, warn them that there are often hidden injuries and problems to be considered when a child has an accident. Tell them that it would be best if the child saw a physician.

When the parents still refuse transport after your warnings, contact the hospital for instructions. A child with a possible head injury must be watched for 48 hours. If you are allowed to do so by the medical advisors for your EMS System, tell the parents that they should awaken the child every couple of hours the night of the head injury and check for any indications of problems. If the child is difficult to awaken or if over the next few days he has headaches, clear or bloody fluids in the ears or nose, or vomits, tell them they *must* contact a physician or phone the EMS System (e.g., rescue squad) so the child can be transported IMMEDIATELY to a medical facility. Stress that once any of the signs of head problems appear care *cannot* be delayed. **NOTE:** Have the parents sign a release form.

In addition to noting obvious scalp, cranial, and facial injuries, you should look for:

- Vomiting, typically seen in cases of head injury
- Clear or bloody fluids coming from the nose, ears, or ears and nose
- Drowsiness or the child lapsing into a sleepy state
- Problems with speech, including the inability to talk
- Headache (often delayed)
- Unequal pupils
- Cases in which the child says he is seeing double
- Any convulsion associated with a head injury
- A stiff or sore neck occurring several days after a head injury (possible meningitis . . . transport!)
- Any sign associated with head injury in the adult (e.g., raccoon eye, Battle's sign)

Burns

You should look carefully for burns when caring for young children. They are often the victims of first- and second-degree burns to the hands and face resulting from contact with hot water, steam, cooking utensils, and hot radiators. Transport is necessary to provide proper treatment for the burns and to make certain that the child did not receive any injuries due to smoke or toxic fume inhalation.

If you note that the burn is on both hands or feet, or if you note that the child shows evidence of past burns, transport the child, no matter how minor

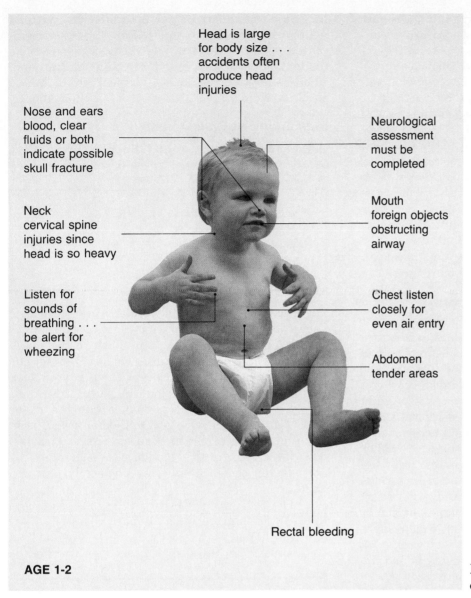

Nose and ears
blood, clear
fluids or both
indicate possible
skull fracture

Head is large
for body size . . .
accidents often
produce head
injuries

Neurological
assessment
must be
completed

Neck
cervical spine
injuries since
head is so heavy

Mouth
foreign objects
obstructing
airway

Listen for
sounds of
breathing . . .
be alert for
wheezing

Chest listen
closely for
even air entry

Abdomen
tender areas

Rectal bleeding

AGE 1-2

FIGURE 15–2. Special survey considerations.

the burn. The emergency department staff may wish to examine the child to determine if he is being abused or if he is developmentally disabled and has not had the benefit of proper medical evaluation.

Bike Fork Compression Injury

Children often ride on the cross bars of bicycles. When the passenger is not careful, the heel of one foot may catch in the spokes of the front wheel. The foot is quickly carried into the fork of the front wheel, where it jams. Bent spokes are usually your first clue of a bike fork compression injury. This injury may occur involving the rear fork if the passenger is riding behind the seat ("riding double").

Expose the injured foot and look for areas of pale or white skin behind the ankle. The tissue has

probably been crushed. Considerable pain usually accompanies this injury. Examine the patient for other possible injuries, looking carefully for fractures to the leg. If there are no apparent leg fractures or dislocations, immobilize the ankle as you would for a fractured ankle, using a folded pillow. Transport the patient to a medical facility.

Trapped Extremities

Children often stick their heads, legs, arms, feet, hands, or fingers into places where they become trapped. In some localities, specially trained personnel from the rescue squad or fire service are called to handle these situations. If you must act in such emergencies, begin by having the child relax. Once this is done, he may be able to slowly free himself or to free himself with your help in guiding the part from the point of entrapment. Lubricating substances can be used to help slide the child free. If nothing else works, you may have to cut away the material that is holding the child. Explain what you are going to do, step by step; then proceed with great caution, making sure that the trapped part is well protected by padding and the rest of the child's body is safe. Delay working if the child becomes upset. It is important that he does not move around or struggle to free himself. Do not chop or tear away obstructions. Careful sawing is usually the best approach. Once the child is freed, conduct a proper patient assessment and care for all injuries. Usually, minor abrasions and lacerations are all that result. The parents should be told to call or see a physician since an anti-tetanus injection may be required.

The Battered Child Syndrome

At one time, people thought child abuse was a rare phenomenon. It now appears as if this problem has been part of our culture and is on the increase. For example, the Commonwealth of Virginia recently reported between 30,000 and 35,000 cases of child abuse annually. Virginia's figures are typical for its population. States that are larger tend to report proportionally higher figures, while those with a smaller population tend to report proportionally lower figures. The problem is thought to be even more serious than the statistics would have you believe. For every battered child seen by an emergency department or family physician, there are apparently many more *unreported cases* who never receive such care.

Many surveys have been conducted to find the number of children classified as "battered." These are the children beaten with fists, hair brushes, straps, electric cords, pool cues, razor straps, bottles, broom handles, baseball bats, pots and pans, and almost any object that can be used as a weapon. Included in this group are children who are intentionally burned by hot water, steam, open flames, cigarettes, and other thermal sources. Battered children include those thrown down steps, pushed out of windows and over railings, and even pushed from moving cars.

The horror grows as we find children who are shot, stabbed, electrocuted, and suffocated. The Bureau of Community Health Services reports 1,000 to 4,000 deaths a year due to child abuse and neglect. At least 300 of these victims are infants. Emergency department physicians indicate on various surveys that 10% of ALL children under 5 years of age are battered children.

Child abusers are mothers, fathers, sisters, brothers, grandparents, stepparents, babysitters, white-collar workers, blue-collar workers, unemployed persons, the rich, and the poor. There is no distinction as to race, creed, or ethnic background. There is no such person as a "typical" child abuser. In other words, ANYONE could be a child abuser.

Indications of Child Abuse

Child abuse can take several different forms, often occurring in combination. These forms include:

- Psychological abuse
- Neglect
- Physical assault
- Sexual assault

A child's psychological problems and pathologic behavior are difficult to trace back to specific abuse. This is not typically a direct problem in the realm of the EMT. What constitutes neglect is a serious legal question. As a child goes without proper food, shelter, clothing, supervision, and love, the effects surely will be seen, but seldom is this the major part of an emergency response. Sexual assault and molestation are problems seen by EMTs. This will be covered later in this section of the chapter. For now, let us consider only the physically battered child.

The best way to describe the types of injuries that can be inflicted in child-abuse cases is to say, "if it can happen to the body, it has been done by a child abuser." In child abuse cases, you will find:

- Bruises, abrasions, lacerations, and incisions of all sizes and forms. These include welts, swollen limbs, split lips, black eyes, and loose or broken teeth. Often the injuries are to the back, legs, and arms. The injuries may be in various stages of healing.
- Broken bones are common, with all types of fractures. Many battered children have multiple fractures, often in various stages of healing, or have fracture-associated complications.
- Head injuries are common, with concussions and skull fractures being reported. Closed head injuries occur to many infants and small children who have been severely shaken.
- Abdominal injuries include ruptured spleens, livers and lungs lacerated by broken

---

ribs, internal bleeding from blunt trauma, and lacerated and avulsed genitalia.

There are times when you will treat an injured child and never think that he has been abused. The child relates well with his parents and there appears to be a strong bond between them. However, there are certain indications that abuse may be occurring in or outside the home, with the family feeling they must not admit to the problem. Be on the alert for the following:

- Repeated responses to provide care for the same child or children in a family.
- Indications of past injuries. This is why you must do a physical examination and why you must remove articles of clothing. Pay special attention to the back and buttocks of the child.
- Poorly healing wounds or improperly healed fractures. It is extremely rare for a child to receive a fracture, be given proper orthopedic care and then show angulations and large "bumps" and "knots" of bone at the "healed" injury site.
- Indications of past burns or fresh bilateral burns. Children seldom put both hands on a hot object or touch the same hot object again (true, some do . . . this is only an indication, not proof). Some types of burns are almost always linked to child abuse, such as cigarette burns to the body and burns to the buttocks and lower extremities that result from the child being dipped in hot water.
- Many different types of injuries to both sides or the front and back of the body. This gains even more importance if the adults on the scene keep insisting that the child "falls a lot."
- Fear on the part of the child to tell you how he was injured. Combine this with the adults on the scene indicating they do not wish to leave you alone with the child, parents who tell conflicting or changing stories, or parents who overwhelm you with their explanations of the cause of the injury.

Pay attention to the adults as you treat the child. Do they have trouble controlling anger? Do you feel that at any moment there may be an emotional explosion? Do any of the adults appear to be in a deep state of depression? Are there indications of alcohol or drug abuse? Do any of the adults speak of suicide or seeking mercy for their unhappy children?

Take note of any parent who refuses to have the child sent to the nearest hospital or to a hospital where the child has been seen many times. This may indicate a fear of the staff remembering or seeing a record of past injuries that indicate possible abuse.

The Role of the EMT

Remember that you are an EMT charged with providing emergency care for an injured child. You are not a physician trained to detect abuse, a police officer, court investigator, judge, or one-person jury. Provide prompt and efficient care, controlling your emotions and holding back any accusations. *Do not* give any indications to the parents or other adults at the scene that you suspect them of child abuse. *Do not* ask the child if he has been abused. To do so when others are around could produce too great a stress for the injured child to handle. Properly assess the patient and provide appropriate care. If you are suspicious about the mechanism of injury, transport the child even though the severity of injury may not warrant such action.

ALWAYS report your suspicions to the emergency department staff in accordance with local policies. Almost every medical facility staff will take action to see if your fears are well founded. If for some reason you do not believe that the medical staff at an institution has taken you seriously or you believe they do not wish to become involved (this would probably never happen), then you *must* report your suspicions to the juvenile authorities of the local police department. This may not be a legal requirement in your state, but it is a professional obligation.

Keep accurate records of possible child abuse. State all your findings, but do not conclude that there is abuse. Draw a picture to indicate the size and location of all the child's injuries. Do *not* assume the cause of an injury (e.g., a cigarette burn). Instead, provide a detailed description of the injury site.

Maintain patient and family confidentiality. You cannot give any details concerning the family that was involved. *Do not* name the child or his family. Report the problem to your superior officer at the squad or service where you work. This will allow for past responses to be checked and future responses to be noted in case a pattern in the family develops to indicate possible abuse. Even when talking to your partner, the hospital staff, and your squad leaders, use the terms *suspicious* and *possible*. Do not call someone a child abuser. If you break confidentiality, you could be sued. Keep in mind that the courts can deal harshly with those who provide patient care and then violate the confidentiality of the patient, the family, and the home. Keep in mind that rumors about abuse may, in the long run, cause mental or physical harm to your child patient.

Sexual Assault

It is not certain as to how many children are victims of sexual molestation and abuse. The problem ranges from adults exposing themselves to children, to adults touching children's genitals or having children touch their genitals, to sexual intercourse, oral sex, or sexual torture. Many of the cases reported are for adults exposing themselves to children. The other extreme, in which there is physical injury done to the child, also is usually reported. The cases in between, especially those receiving emotional injury or minor physical injury, are usually not reported, and therefore are difficult to estimate. However, it is believed that 10% of all boys and 20% of all girls are molested or abused sexually in some way before they reach the age of 18. At least 5% of all child abuse victims are also sexually abused.

In some cases, you may find a child who obviously has been sexually assaulted or has unexplained genital injury. In rare cases, the child may tell you that he was sexually assaulted. When any of these things occur, remain professional and control your emotions. Do not allow the child to become embarrassed. Do not say anything that may make the child believe that he is to blame for the sexual assault (many believe that they are). Tell the child that the people at the hospital will help him and that he is not to be embarrassed.

Provide care as needed. Do not examine the genitalia unless there is obvious injury or the child tells you of a recent injury. Discourage the child from going to the bathroom (for both defecation and urination). Do not have the child wash or change clothes. It is very important that you do not give the patient anything by mouth. Transport the child and report your suspicions to the medical staff, making certain that they understand that you are talking about *possible* sexual assault. As with all cases of child abuse, maintain patient and family confidentiality.

Medical Problems Common to Children

Like adults, children can suffer a variety of medical problems from "belly ache" to heart attack. Although emergency care measures for medical problems are the same for children as for adults, there are a few problems common to childhood that deserve special attention.

Fever

Above-normal body temperature is one of the most important signs of an existing or impending acute illness. Fever usually accompanies such childhood diseases as measles, mumps, chickenpox, mononucleosis, pneumonia, and Reye's syndrome (a serious condition producing a high fever that sometimes follows a recent case of influenza). The fever also may be due to heat stroke or some other noninfectious disease problem. *Never* regard a fever as unimportant. Do not try to diagnose or accept what the parents believe may be the problem. As an EMT, you cannot tell specifically what is wrong with the child or what is likely to happen over the next few hours.

Use *relative skin temperature* as a sign. If the infant or child feels too warm, or if he feels hot, then prepare the patient and transport. If the parents report having taken the child's temperature, or if you work with a squad that takes temperature by thermometer, be aware that a mild fever can quickly turn into a high fever that may indicate a very serious, if not life-threatening problem. Any child 1 to 5 years old with a body temperature (oral measurement) above 103°F *must* be evaluated at the hospital. Any child from 5 to 12 with a body temperature above 102°F *must* be evaluated at the hospital.

NOTE: In most field cases, oral temperature evaluation is not done on a child under 5 years of age. A high relative skin temperature is always enough reason to seek medical opinion.

High temperature can cause seizures (these are called febrile seizures), coma, permanent damage to the central nervous system, or even death. Should you find an infant or child with a high fever:

1. Remove the child's clothing, but do not allow him to be exposed to conditions that may bring on sudden chills. If the child objects, let him or her keep on light clothing or underwear.
2. Cover the child with a towel that has been saturated in tepid water. Some localities allow properly wrapped cold packs to be used for high fever. Before applying these packs, it is best to seek directions from the emergency department physician. Always monitor for shivering and stay alert for developing

Do not: use rubbing alcohol to cool the patient; submerge the child in a tub of cold water; or cover the child with a towel saturated with ice water. It is not the duty of an EMT to administer aspirin or other such fever-reducing compounds. In fact, it is probably illegal for you to do so in your locality.

Seizures

High fever, epilepsy, meningitis, diabetic states, and many other medical problems can bring on seizures. Usually, you will arrive after the convulsion has passed. You should ensure an open airway and be on the alert for vomiting. Interview the patient and any family members and bystanders who saw the convulsion. Ask them if they can tell you how long it lasted and what part of the body was shaking or twitching. Assess the child for symptoms and signs, taking care to note any injuries sustained during the convulsion. All infants and children who have undergone a convulsive seizure require medical evaluation. If the patient has another seizure in your presence, care for the patient the same as you would an adult (see pp. 406–407). The child will be in great need of emotional support.

Respiratory Disorders

All infants and children in respiratory distress or indicating difficult breathing *must* be seen by a physician.

The EMT's primary concern when caring for infants and children with respiratory problems is to establish and maintain an open airway. The basic procedures used to clear an airway of foreign object obstruction are of little use if the cause of obstruction is due to swollen, inflamed tissues. If the patient appears to have a partial obstruction and is breathing adequately, place him in a semiseated position on his parent's lap, cover him for warmth, provide oxygen (a humidified source is best), and transport. Monitor the patient constantly during transport. If the patient does not respond to oxygen or the obstruction is total, basic life support measures must be initiated. The unconscious patient should receive a *properly* sized oropharyngeal airway. **Do not use if epiglottitis is suspected** (see below).

An infant or child can have the same breathing problems as an adult; however, certain additional problems are commonly seen with pediatric patients. These problems include:

- *Croup* (Kroop)—A group of viral illnesses that cause inflammation of the larynx, trachea, and bronchi. It is typically an illness of children 6 months to about 4 years of age. This problem sometimes follows a cold or other respiratory infection. Tissues in the airway (particularly the upper airway) become swollen and restrict the passage of air. The child usually will have a mild fever during the day and some problems with hoarseness. At night, the child's condition will worsen and he will develop a loud "seal bark" cough and difficult breathing. Respiratory distress may develop.

  The croup patient should be placed lying down or in a position he finds to be most comfortable. Oxygen should be administered at a high concentration. When possible, this should be from a humidified source. The patient will probably benefit from vaporized or nebulized water. Do not delay transport unless ordered to do so by the emergency department physician.

- *Epiglottitis* (epi-glo-TI-tis)—This is most commonly caused by a bacterial infection that produces swelling of the epiglottis and partial airway obstruction. The typical patient will be between 3 and 7 years old. There will be a sudden onset of high fever and painful swallowing (the child often will drool to avoid swallowing). The patient will assume a "tripod" position, sitting upright and leaning forward with the chin thrust outward and the mouth wide open in an effort to maintain a wide airway opening. The child will not want to lie down.

  ALL cases of epiglottitis must be considered to be life threatening, no matter how early the detection. *Do not* force the child to lie down. The child *must* be handled gently, since rough handling and stress could lead to a total airway obstruction. Transport the child immediately, sitting on the parent's lap, providing oxygen at a high concentration from a humidified source. Constantly monitor the child and be ready to resuscitate should respiratory arrest occur. DO NOT PLACE ANYTHING INTO THE CHILD'S MOUTH, including a thermometer, tongue blade, or oropharyngeal airway. To do so may set off spasms along the upper airway (laryngospasms) that will totally obstruct the airway.

- *Bronchitis* (brong-KI-tis) and *Bronchiolitis* (BRONG-ke-o-li-tis)—These are airway inflammations below the level of the trachea. The patient may have coughing and fever. Wheezing is sometimes heard.

  The child should be given oxygen from a humidified source and transported. Usually, the patient will be most comfortable in a semisitting or sitting position.

- *Asthma*—Like an adult, a child can have acute asthma attacks and status asthmaticus, showing the same signs, including wheezing. As with the adult, status asthmaticus is a life-threatening condition. Any first case of asthma must be cared for as if anaphylactic shock is a real possibility.

Beware of lay guidelines that imply you can diagnose children's respiratory problems. If croup or epiglottitis are possibilities, immediate transport is required. For all other respiratory problems, gather information as quickly as possible from the primary survey (when appropriate), interviews, and the necessary physical examination. Do not put a tongue blade in the patient's mouth. This may cause airway spasms that could totally obstruct the airway. Do not give the child anything by mouth. This could induce airway spasms or vomiting. Do not attempt to distinguish asthma from other respiratory problems based on respiratory sounds.

Acute Abdomen

Infants and children can develop abdominal pain for a variety of reasons: appendicitis, intestinal influenza, gas pains, indigestion, and bacterial infection of the bowels. You will not be able to tell one problem from another, nor would the basic EMT-level emergency care rendered be different if you could. Consider any abdominal pain or cramp to be serious in the child patient. Intermittent cramps may be just as serious a problem as having steady cramps or pain. Fever, vomiting, blood in the stools, and "lumps" in the abdomen all indicate that the problem could be very serious. The child may be dehydrated. In severe cases, the signs of shock may be present. Treat the child as you would an adult with acute abdomen (see p. 408). Remember, you will have to provide much more emotional support. Transport the child to a medical facility as soon as possible. If the parents cannot decide if they want their child to be transported, lead them away from the child and explain why it is important for the child to be seen by a physician.

Diarrhea and Vomiting

Diarrhea and vomiting are commonly associated with childhood illnesses. Both can cause dehydration that worsen the child's condition and may lead to life-threatening shock. Any pediatric patient with diarrhea or vomiting should be transported and seen by a physician. Do not give the child anything by mouth, even if he appears to have dry skin and mucous membranes. To do so may induce vomiting. Providing needed fluids for the patient (rehydration) will be done at the medical facility, usually by intravenous techniques.

When transporting the patient, be prepared to provide oral suctioning. Save all vomitus and rectal discharge.

Poisonings

Children are often the victims of accidental poisoning, often resulting from the ingestion of household products or medications. The procedures described in Chapter 14 apply to infant, child, and adult (a patient under age 10 receives only one tablespoon of syrup of ipecac, if allowed). There are some special types of poisonings not often associated with adult patients, however. These special cases include:

- Aspirin Poisoning—Look for hyperventilation, vomiting, and sweating. The patient's skin may feel hot. In severe cases, you may note seizures, coma, or shock.
- Acetaminophen Poisoning—Many medications have this compound, including Tylenol, Comtrex, Bancap, Excedrin P.M., and Datril. The child may be restless (early) or drowsy. Nausea, vomiting, and heavy perspiration may occur. The loss of consciousness is possible.
- Lead Poisoning—This usually comes from ingesting pieces of lead-based paints. Look for nausea with abdominal pain and vomiting. Muscle cramps, headache, muscle weakness, and irritability are often present.
- Iron Poisoning—Iron compounds such as ferrous sulfate are found in some vitamin tablets and liquids. As little as one gram of ferrous sulfate can be lethal to a child. Within 30 minutes to several hours, the child will show nausea and vomiting, often accompanied by bloody diarrhea. Typically the child will develop shock; however, this may be delayed for up to 24 hours as the child at first appears to be getting better.
- Petroleum Product Poisoning—The patient

will usually be vomiting, with coughing or choking taking place. In most cases, you will smell the distinctive odor of a petroleum distillate (e.g., gasoline, kerosene, heating fuel). Aspiration pneumonia is a serious problem for victims of petroleum poisoning.

REMEMBER: Care for poisonings as directed by your local poison control center and on-line medical command.

Sudden Infant Death Syndrome

In the United States, **sudden infant death syndrome** (SIDS) occurs to between 6,500 and 7,500 apparently healthy babies each year. These babies were receiving proper care and frequently pass physical examinations within days of their sudden death. The problem may possibly be related to nerve cell development in the brain or the tissue chemistry of the respiratory system or the heart. Some relationships have been drawn to family history of SIDS and respiratory problems, but there is still no accepted reason given for why these babies die.

The cause of death in SIDS can usually be related to respiratory failure. When asleep, the typical SIDS patient will show periods of cardiac slowdown and temporary cessation of breathing known as *sleep apnea* (ap-NE-ah). Exhaustion, respiratory disease, and overheating have been demonstrated as causing increased episodes. During sleep, the SIDS baby will have episodes of apnea. Eventually, the infant will stop breathing and will not start again on its own. Unless reached in time, the episode can be fatal.

As an EMT, you are to provide basic cardiac life support measures for the possible SIDS patient. Be certain that the parents receive emotional support and that they believe all that is possible is being done for the child at the scene and in transport.

Parents who lose a child to SIDS often suffer intense guilt feelings from the moment they find the child. If a parent expresses such guilt, remind them that SIDS occurs to apparently healthy babies who are receiving the best of parental care. In cases of SIDS, do not be embarrassed to express your sorrow for their loss, but do so only after a *physician* has officially informed them of the child's death.

REMEMBER: Speaking with a suspicious tone or asking inappropriate questions may only increase the parents' sorrow or guilt.

Table 15–2. **HOW TO DISTINGUISH BETWEEN SIDS AND CHILD ABUSE AND NEGLECT***

Sudden Infant Death Syndrome	*Child Abuse and Neglect*
Incidence: Deaths: 6,500 to 7,500/year Highest: 2 to 4 months of age When: Winter months	*Incidence*: Deaths: 1,000 to 4,000/year Deaths in Infants: 300/year When: No seasonal difference
Physical Appearance: • Exhibits no external signs of injury. • Exhibits "natural" appearance of dead baby: —Lividity—settling of blood; frothy drainage from nose/mouth —Small marks, e.g., diaper rash looks more severe —Cooling/rigor mortis: takes place quickly in infants (about 3 hours) • Appears to be well-developed baby, though may be small for age. • Other siblings appear normal and healthy.	*Physical Appearance*: • Distinguishable and visible signs of injury. —Broken bone(s) —Bruises —Burns —Cuts —Head trauma, e.g., black eye —Scars —Welts —Wounds • May be obviously wasted away (malnutrition). • Other siblings may show patterns of injuries commonly seen in child abuse and neglect.
May Initially Suspect SIDS • All of the above characteristics PLUS • Parents say that infant was well and healthy when put to sleep (last time seen alive).	*May Initially Suspect Child Abuse/Neglect* • All of the above characteristics PLUS • Parents' story does not "sound right" or cannot account for all injuries on infant.

NOTE: The determination of whether the child is or is not a SIDS victim is the responsibility of the medical examiner or medical coroner. **It is NOT the responsibility of the Emergency Medical Technician.**

* *Support Systems Manual*, National SIDS Foundation, 1989, pp. i–xii.

Infant death and child abuse are emotionally hard on EMTs. After providing basic life support, transporting the child, and doing all you can for the parents, take care of yourself. Talk with other EMTs. If your squad or service has a counselor, see this person for advice. You may think that you can handle the sorrow by yourself, but experienced EMTs know better. Unless you resolve the impact of an infant death, the problems created will compound with others caused by the stress of being an EMT and could lead to "burn out."

SUMMARY

An infant is anyone under 1 year of age. Traditionally, a child is anyone from 1 to 8 years of age; however, this does not mean that all factors applying to the care of adults can be used for individuals from 8 to 18.

Remember that you are a professional. Learn to control your emotions at the scene so that you can provide prompt and efficient care. You will need to provide emotional support to the patient, parents, and bystanders in cases of pediatric emergencies.

When conducting a primary survey, establish responsiveness by gently shaking or tapping the infant or child. Take care in establishing an adequate airway. When needed, deliver rescue breathing and interposed ventilations by the mouth-to-mask, mouth-to-mouth, and nose technique for infants and small children. The mouth-to-mask or mouth-to-mouth method may be used for larger children. Abdominal thrusts can be used to clear the airway of a child. Once the child is unconscious, use the combined procedures of abdominal thrusts, visualized removal of foreign objects, and reattempts to ventilate. For the infant, use four back blows and four chest thrusts. Once the infant is unconscious, attempt to clear the airway by providing two breaths, four back blows, four chest thrusts (as you would in CPR), finger sweeps (only when you can see the object and you use your little finger for probing), and reattempt to ventilate.

Rescue breathing is provided to the infant at the rate of one breath every 3 seconds. For the child patient, the rate is one breath every 4 seconds.

Establish an infant's pulse by feeling for the brachial pulse. Use the carotid pulse for children. For infants in cardiac arrest, compress the sternum along the midline, one finger-width below an imaginary line drawn directly between the nipples. Use the tips of two or three fingers to compress ½ to 1 inch. Provide at least 100 compressions per minute with 1 interposed ventilation every 5 compressions.

For the child in cardiac arrest, compress the sternum along the midline, directly between the nipples. Use the tips of two or three fingers for the very small young child and the heel of one hand for older children. Compress the sternum 1 to 1½ inches. Provide 80 to 100 compressions per minute with 1 interposed ventilation every 5 compressions.

An infant is considered to be in shock if he has lost 25 ml or more of blood or his systolic blood pressure falls below 70 mmHg. A child is considered to be in shock if he has lost 500 ml or more blood, or if his systolic blood pressure falls below 50 mmHg (preschooler), 60 mmHg (to age 12), or 70 mmHg (teenager).

Take your time with the interview when the patient is a child. Talk to the parents, but also direct questions to the child. Show the child, the parents, and the bystanders that you are a concerned professional. Tell the child what you are going to do before you do it. Do not lie to the child. Tell him when he may experience pain. Apply the correct values for vital signs to infants and children (see Table 15–1). Do not use adult vital sign figures for infants and children.

When conducting a physical examination of a conscious infant or young child patient, use the toe-to-head approach. The older child is assessed by the head-to-toe approach. Take special care to look for head injuries, signs of skull fracture, cervical spine injuries, unusual breathing sounds, abdominal tenderness, and rectal bleeding. Always conduct a neurologic assessment. You may have to treat the infant as if he were an unconscious patient and depend on response to painful stimuli.

In cases of head injury, note drowsiness, speech problems, vomiting, headache, unequal pupils, seeing double, clear or bloody fluids in the nose or ears, convulsions, and a stiff or sore neck (within days of the injury). Be certain that the parents are aware of what to look for if they do not allow you to transport the child. Obtain a signed release form.

Treat a bike fork compression injury as you would a fractured ankle. Immobilize with a pillow splint and transport.

Always be on the alert for possible child abuse. Look for indications of injuries and behavior that may lead you to suspect physical or sexual abuse. Report all suspicions to the emergency department staff. Do a complete survey so that you will detect all obvious injuries and indications of past abuse. Remember to maintain patient and family confidentiality.

Do not underestimate the significance of fever, seizures, respiratory problems, diarrhea, vomiting, and abdominal pain in infants and children.

Croup usually occurs to young children, often

following a cold or other respiratory infection. The patient will have a "seal bark" cough and respiratory distress. Oxygen (humidified) and transport are the major elements of care. Epiglottitis *must* always be considered to be a life-threatening emergency. The child will have a sudden onset of high fever and pain on swallowing (usually he will drool). The typical patient will assume a tripod position. Handle the patient gently, provide oxygen (humidified), and transport immediately. DO NOT PLACE ANYTHING IN THE CHILD'S MOUTH. Constantly monitor the child and be prepared for total airway obstruction and respiratory arrest.

Remember that many children are accidental poisoning victims. Be on special alert for aspirin, acetaminophen, lead, iron, and petroleum product poisonings. Follow the instructions of your local poison control center and on-line medical command.

Sudden infant death syndrome (SIDS) victims must receive resuscitative measures. The parents will need strong emotional support. If they express feelings of guilt, tell them that SIDS occurs to thousands of apparently healthy babies each year. Even with the very best of care, these babies die. Do not be embarrassed to express your own sorrow.

NOTE: Nearly 10% of the average EMS System's patients are children. If you lack experience in dealing with children, you may be able to improve your communication skills and methods for handling children by doing volunteer clinical work at your local hospital's pediatric ward. You also may arrange to take an ambulance to your local schools to show the children. Not only will you improve your skills in dealing with children, you also will be able to show the children that the EMT is their friend.

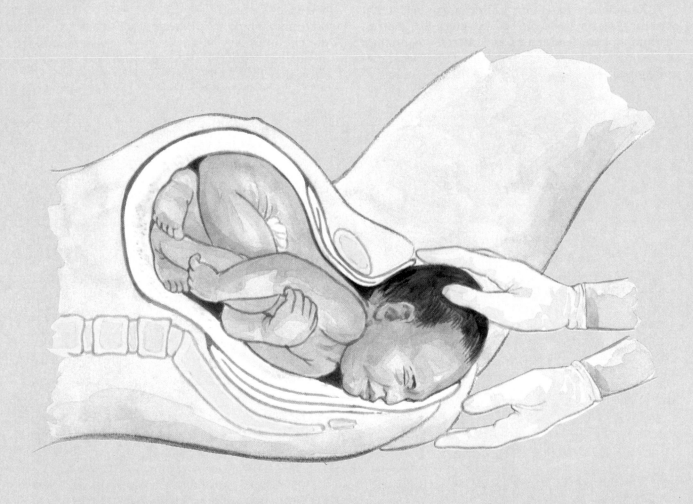

CHAPTER 16

Childbirth

OBJECTIVES As an EMT, you should be able to:

1. Name the components of the sterile emergency obstetric pack and describe the uses for each item. (p. 437)
2. Name and locate the anatomical structures of pregnancy. (pp. 437–438)
3. List and describe the three stages of labor. (p. 438)
4. Describe how to evaluate the mother before delivery. (pp. 439–440)
5. Describe how to prepare the mother, the delivery scene, and personnel prior to delivery. (pp 440–441)
6. Describe, step by step, what the EMT should do during each of the three stages of labor. (pp. 439, pp. 441–442, and p. 447)
7. Describe the care given to both mother and infant after delivery, including airway and umbilical cord care. (p. 442, and pp. 444–448)
8. List the possible complications of delivery and state what the EMT should do in each situation. (pp. 449–456)
9. Describe the courses of action taken by the EMT in cases of multiple births, premature births, abortions (miscarriages), and stillbirths. (pp. 455–456)
10. List those emergencies involving birth that require immediate transport. pp. 449–450 and pp. 454–455)
11. Describe what the EMT can do to comfort parents during normal and abnormal deliveries. (pp. 440–442, p. 448, pp. 450–451, and p. 455)

SKILLS As an EMT, you should be able to:

1. Evaluate a woman in labor and assist her in the delivery of her child.
2. Provide postdelivery care for the newborn, including proper airway and umbilical cord care.
3. Provide resuscitative measures for newborns in respiratory and cardiac arrest.
4. Assist in delivery of the placenta.
5. Provide postdelivery care for the mother,

including emotional support, and provide care of the afterbirth.

6. Provide emergency care and needed basic cardiac life support procedures for abnormal deliveries, including breech and premature birth.

7. Properly provide oxygen for the newborn when required.

8. Record all vital information needed for the live birth or fetal death certificate.

TERMS you may be using for the first time:

Abortion – spontaneous (miscarriage) or induced termination of pregnancy.

Afterbirth – the placenta, membranes of the amniotic sac, part of the umbilical cord, and some tissues from the lining of the uterus that are delivered after the birth of the baby.

Amniotic (am-ne-OT-ic) **Sac** – the "bag of waters" that surrounds the developing fetus.

Breech Presentation – when the baby appears buttocks or both legs first during birth.

Cephalic (se-FAL-ik) **Presentation** – when the baby appears head first during birth. This is the normal presentation.

Cervix (SUR-viks) – the neck of the uterus that enters the birth canal.

Crowning – when part of the baby is visible through the vaginal opening.

Eclampsia (e-KLAMP-se-ah) – a severe complication of pregnancy that produces convulsions and coma.

Ectopic (ek-TOP-ik) **Pregnancy** – when implantation is not in the body of the uterus, occurring instead in the oviduct (fallopian tube), cervix, or abdominopelvic cavity.

Fetus (FE-tus) – the baby as it develops in the womb.

Labor – the three stages of delivery that begin with the contractions of the uterus and end with the expulsion of the placenta.

Perineum (per-i-NE-um) – the surface area between the vulva and anus.

Placenta (plah-SEN-tah) – the organ of pregnancy where exchange of oxygen, foods, and wastes occurs between mother and fetus.

Pre-eclapmsia (pre-e-KLAMP-se-ah) – a complication of pregnancy that can lead to convulsions and coma.

Premature Infant – any newborn weighing less than 5.5 pounds or being born before the 37th week of pregnancy.

Umbilical (um-BIL-i-cal) **Cord** – the fetal structure containing the blood vessels that travel to and from the placenta.

Uterus (U-ter-us) – the womb where the fetus develops.

Vagina (vah-JI-nah) – the birth canal.

Vulva (VUL-vah) – the female external genitalia.

CHILDBIRTH

The Role of the EMT

Participating in the delivery of a baby is usually a wonderful and exciting event for the EMT. In most cases, you will be dealing with a natural event, not an emergency.

Seldom is childbirth outside of a medical facility an emergency, except perhaps to an untrained attendant! Many people in our society presently believe that birth is meant to occur in a hospital delivery room. Although it is true that hospital care of mother and newborn does reduce the chance of problems and can correct most immediate complications, keep in mind that the vast majority of babies ever born on this planet were delivered away from any type of medical facility. This holds true today, for the majority of the world's women do not have access to modern medical facilities for the purpose of giving birth.

Birth is a natural process. The anatomy of the human female and the anatomy of the baby allow for the process to occur with few immediate problems. Nonetheless, EMTs need to know the procedures that can help mother and baby before, during, and after delivery, as well as the techniques that can be employed when complications arise.

REMEMBER: EMTs do not deliver babies . . . mothers do! Your primary role will be one of *helping* the mother as she delivers her child.

Equipment and Supplies

Assisting the mother and providing care is much easier if a few basic items are kept as part of the ambulance supplies. You will need a sterile obstetric kit that contains the items required for preparation of the mother, delivery, and initial care of the newborn. This kit should include:

- Several pairs of sterile surgical gloves
- 5 towels or sheets for draping the mother
- 1 dozen 4 x 4 gauze pads (sponges)
- 1 small rubber-bulb syringe
- 3 cord clamps or hemostats
- Umbilical cord tape
- 1 pair of surgical scissors
- 1 baby blanket
- Several individually wrapped sanitary napkins

In addition, you will find use for a stainless steel basin, two large plastic bags, and disposable masks, paper gowns, caps, and eye protection.

Occasionally, EMTs assist in the delivery of a baby without using a sterile delivery pack. Remember that most babies have been born without such packs. A few simple supplies are used to assist the mother:

- Clean sheets and towels to drape the mother and wrap the newborn

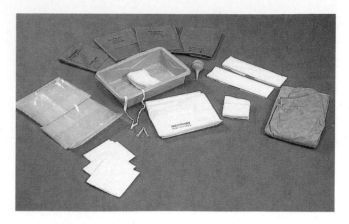

FIGURE 16–1. Contents of a disposable obstetric kit.

- Heavy flat twine or new shoelaces to tie the cord (*do not* use thread, wire, or light string since these may cut through the cord)
- A towel or plastic bag to wrap the placenta after its delivery
- Clean, unused rubber gloves. If none are available, carefully wash your hands, if at all possible. The lack of gloves will mean possible exposure to infectious diseases.

Anatomy of Pregnancy and Delivery

The developing baby is called a **fetus** (FE-tus). During pregnancy, the fetus grows in its mother's **uterus** (U-ter-us), a muscular organ often called the womb (Figure 16–2). When the mother is in labor, the muscles of the uterus contract at ever-shortening inter-

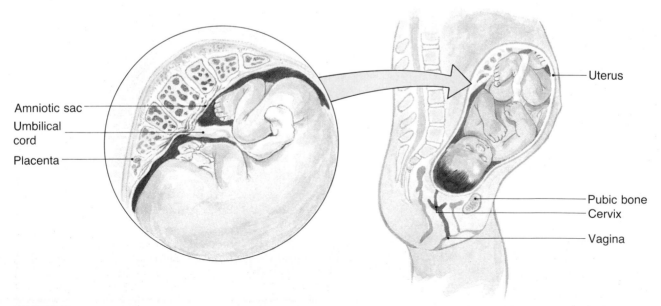

Amniotic sac
Umbilical cord
Placenta

Uterus

Pubic bone
Cervix

Vagina

FIGURE 16–2. The structures of pregnancy.

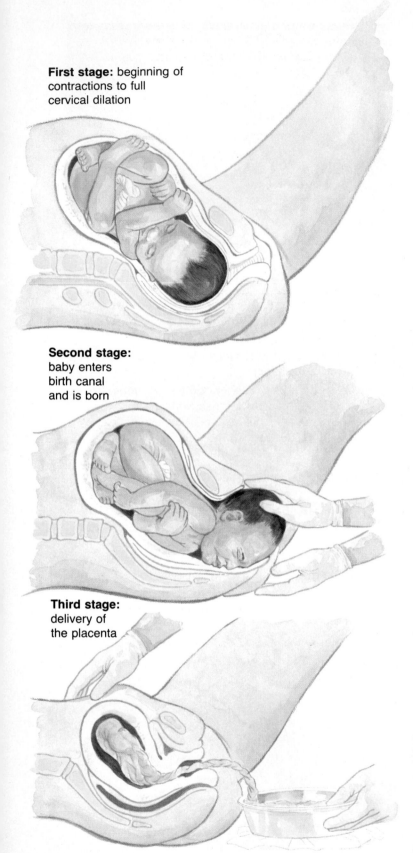

First stage: beginning of contractions to full cervical dilation

Second stage: baby enters birth canal and is born

Third stage: delivery of the placenta

FIGURE 16–3. The three stages of labor.

vals and push the baby through the neck of the uterus known as the **cervix** (SUR-viks). The cervix must dilate some 4 inches during labor to allow the baby's head to pass into the **vagina** (vah-JI-nah) or birth canal so that delivery can take place.

More than just the fetus develops within the uterus during pregnancy. Attached to the wall of the uterus is a special organ called the **placenta** (plah-SEN-tah). Composed of both maternal and fetal tissues, the placenta serves as an exchange area between mother and fetus. Oxygen and foods from the mother's bloodstream are carried across the placenta to the fetus. Carbon dioxide and certain other wastes cross from fetal circulation to maternal circulation. Since the placenta is an *organ of pregnancy,* it is expelled after the baby is born.

The mother's blood does *not* flow through the body of the fetus. The fetus has its own circulatory system. Blood from the fetus must be sent through the placenta and returned back into its body. This is done by way of the blood vessels contained in the **umbilical** (um-BIL-i-kal) **cord.** The umbilical cord is fully expelled with the birth of the baby and the delivery of the placenta.

While developing in the uterus, the fetus is enclosed and protected within a thin, membranous "bag of waters" known as the **amniotic** (am-ne-OT-ik) **sac.** This sac contains one–two quarts of liquid called amniotic fluid, which allows the fetus to float during development. In the vast majority of cases, the amniotic sac breaks during labor and the fluid gushes from the birth canal. This is a normal condition of childbirth.

Crowning occurs when the **"presenting"** part of the baby first bulges from the vaginal opening. The presenting part of the baby usually is the head. The normal head-first birth is called a **cephalic** (se-FAL-ik) **delivery.** If the buttocks or both feet of the baby deliver first, the birth is called a **breech birth.**

The Stages of Labor

There are three stages of labor (Figure 16–3):

1. *First stage*—starts with regular contractions and ends when the cervix is fully dilated.
2. *Second stage*—the time from when the baby enters the birth canal until it is born.
3. *Third stage*—begins when the baby is born until the afterbirth (placenta, umbilical cord, and some tissues from the amniotic sac and the lining of the uterus) is delivered.

The contractions of the uterus that occur during the first stage of labor move the baby downward and *dilate* the cervix. The cycle of contractions starts far apart and becomes shorter as birth approaches. Typically, these contractions range from every 30 minutes down to 3 minutes apart, or less. Labor pains may accompany the contractions.

As the fetus moves and the cervix dilates, the amniotic sac usually breaks. The full dilation of the cervix signals the end of the first stage of labor. Most women giving birth for the first time will remain in this first stage for an average of 16 hours. However, some women may remain in this stage for no more than 4 hours.

There may be a watery, bloody discharge (not bleeding) of mucus associated with the first stage of labor. Part of this initial discharge will be from a mucous plug that was in the cervix. This is usually mixed with blood and is called the "bloody show." It is not to be wiped away. Watery, bloody fluids discharging from the vagina are typical for all three stages of labor.

The second stage of labor begins after the full dilation of the cervix. During this time, contractions become increasingly more frequent. Labor pains may become more severe. In the second stage of labor, the cramping and abdominal pains associated with the first stage of labor still may be present, but most women report a major new discomfort, that of feeling they have to move their bowels. This is caused as the baby's body moves and places pressure on the rectum. The moment of birth is nearing and the EMT will have to decide whether to transport or to keep the mother where she is and prepare to assist with delivery.

Labor Pains

The contractions of the uterus produce normal labor pains. Most women report the start of labor pains as an ache in the lower back. As labor progresses, the pain becomes most noticeable in the lower abdomen, with the intensity of pain increasing. The pains come at regular intervals, lasting from 30 seconds to one minute. When the uterus starts to contract, the pain begins. As the muscles relax, there is relief from the pain. Labor pains may start, stop for awhile, then start up again.

As an EMT, you must time the following characteristics of labor pains:

- *Contraction time*—the time from the beginning of contraction to when the uterus relaxes.
- *Interval*—the time from the start of one contraction to the beginning of the next (start to start).

Some women experience *false labor*, complete with pain, as early as four weeks prior to true labor. The pain is caused by changes in the uterus as it adjusts in size and shape. False labor pains are usually different from true labor pains. In most cases, they are confined to the lower abdomen, with no back involvement and do not show the regular interval pattern of true labor pains. Some women in false labor will have false labor pains that begin in the lower back.

The Normal Delivery

Evaluating the Mother

A simple series of questions, an examination for crowning, and determination of vital signs will allow you to make the decision for transport. However, do not let the "urgency" of this decision upset the mother. Your patient needs emotional support at this time. Your calm, professional actions will help her feel more at ease and assure her that the required care will be provided for both her and the unborn child.

Begin to evaluate the mother:

1. Ask her name and age.
2. Ask if this is her *first* pregnancy. The average time of labor for a woman having her first baby usually lasts about 16 to 17 hours. The time in labor is considerably shorter for each subsequent birth.
3. Ask her how long she has been having labor pains, how often she is having pains, and if her "bag of waters" has broken. At this point, with a woman having her first delivery, you may think that you can make a decision about transport. You should continue with the evaluation procedure. Also, you should begin to time the frequency and length of the contractions.
4. Ask her if she is straining or if she feels as though she needs to move her bowels. If she says yes, this usually means that the baby has moved into the birth canal and is pressing the vaginal wall against the rectum. Birth will probably occur very soon. The mother may tell you that she can feel the baby trying to move out through her vaginal opening. In such cases, birth is probably very near.
5. Examine the mother for **crowning.** This is a visual inspection to see if there is bulging at the vaginal opening or if the presenting

part of the baby is visible. Crowning means birth is imminent.

6. Feel for uterine contractions. You may have to delay this procedure until the patient tells you she is having labor pains. Tell her what you are going to do, then, place the palm of your gloved hand on her abdomen, above the navel. This can be done over the top of the patient's clothing. You should be able to feel her uterus and its contraction. All contractions should be timed. The uterus and the tissues between this organ and the skin will feel more rigid as the delivery of the baby nears.

7. If you do not have a partner taking vital signs, do so yourself at this time. Alert the medical facility staff if the mother's vital signs are abnormal.

Examining for crowning may be very embarrassing to the mother, the father, and any required bystanders. For this reason, it is very important that you fully explain what you are doing and why. Be certain that you protect the mother from the stares of bystanders. In a polite, but firm, manner, ask everyone who does not belong at the scene to leave. Carefully help the patient remove enough clothing to allow you an unobstructed view of the vulva (VUL-vah), or external genitalia.

REMEMBER: A professional appearance coupled with a professional approach to a problem instills confidence in patients and bystanders alike.

If this is the woman's first delivery, she is not straining, and there is no crowning, there is little reason why she cannot be transported to a medical facility for delivery. On the other hand, if this is not her first delivery, and she is straining, crying out, and complaining about having to go to the bath-

room, birth will probably occur too soon for transport. If the mother is having labor pains from contractions about 2 minutes apart, birth is very near. Crowning certainly means that it is too late to transport the mother.

You may find a patient who is afraid of transport because she believes that birth will occur along the way. Assure her that you believe there is enough time before delivery. Let her know that you are trained to assist with the delivery and that the ambulance is well equipped to handle her needs and care for the newborn should she deliver en route.

If your evaluation of the patient leads you to believe that birth is too near at hand for transport, prepare the mother for delivery. Remember, as part of the preparation, the patient will need emotional support.

REMEMBER: Do not allow the mother to go to the bathroom, even though she says that she has to move her bowels. Birth is probably only a few minutes away. Do not allow the mother to hold her legs together or use any other "folkway" method to attempt to delay the delivery.

Supine Hypotensive Syndrome

Near term, the weight of the uterus, coupled with the infant's weight, placenta, and amniotic fluid, approximates 20–24 pounds. Should the mother be in a supine position, this heavy mass will tend to compress the inferior vena cava reducing venous return to the heart causing dizziness (vertigo).

To counteract or avoid the possible drop in blood pressure, all third trimester patients should be transported on their left side (left lateral recumbent position). A pillow or rolled blanket should be placed behind the back to maintain proper positioning. A severe drop in blood pressure should alert the EMT to the possibility of internal hemorrhage.

Preparing the Expectant Mother

When your evaluation leads you to believe birth is imminent, you must immediately prepare the mother for delivery. To do so, you should:

1. Control the scene so that the mother will have privacy (her coach may remain). If you are not in a private room and transfer to the ambulance is not practical (crowning is present), ask bystanders to leave.

2. Place the mother on a bed, sturdy table, or the ambulance stretcher. You will need about two feet of work space below the woman's legs to place and initially care for the newborn. Space is limited on the ambulance

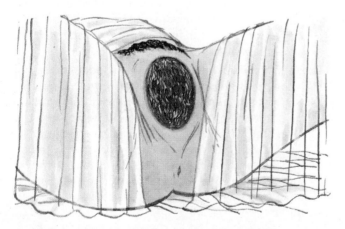

FIGURE 16–4. Crowning of the infant's head occurs in the second stage of labor.

stretcher, but having the patient positioned there may speed transport if complications arise.

NOTE: *Do not* delay positioning the patient. If time permits, and the mother is to be placed on a table or other hard surface, lay down a folded blanket, towels, or even newspapers with a sheet over them to make a cushion. If delivery is to be on a bed and time permits, firm up the mattress with plywood, table leaves, or other such rigid materials that can be placed between the mattress and the springs. Such firmness will tend to keep blood and other fluids from pooling in the work area. A rubber sheet, plastic bag, or newspapers placed under the sheet will help prevent the mattress from becoming soaked. *Do not* leave the patient to find these materials.

3. Remove any of the patient's clothing or underclothing that obstructs your view of the vaginal opening. Put on sterile gloves from the obstetric kit. Use sterile sheets or sterile towels to cover the mother as shown in Figure 16–5. Clean sheets, clean cloths, towels, or material such as tablecloths can be used if you do not have an obstetric kit.

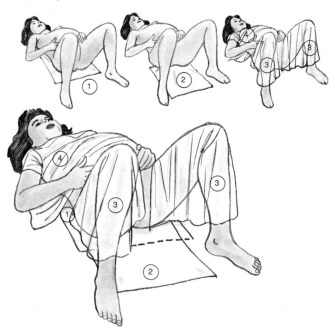

PLACEMENT OF SHEETS OR TOWELS
① One under the buttocks
② One under the vaginal opening
③ One on each thigh
④ One on the abdomen so that it drapes each thigh

FIGURE 16–5. Preparing the mother for delivery.

4. Have the mother lie down on her back with her thighs spread, her knees flexed, and her feet flat. Use one or two pillows to elevate her head and shoulders. A folded blanket should be used to lift her buttocks approximately 2 inches above the supporting surface. This hip elevation is desired to make the delivery easier for the mother and the EMT.

5. Position your partner, the father, or someone the mother agrees to have assist you at the mother's head, opposite from the side where you will be working (work on the mother's right if you are right-handed, or on her left if you are left-handed). This person should stay alert to help turn the mother's head should she vomit. As well, this person should provide emotional support to the mother, soothing and encouraging her.

6. Position the obstetric pack on a table or chair located on the same side as where you will be working. All items must be within easy reach.

7. If time allows, put on any protective items such as a mask or gown.

NOTE: If delivery is to take place in an automobile, position the mother flat on the seat. Arrange her legs so that she has one foot resting on the seat and the other foot resting on the floor.

Delivering the Baby

Position yourself to the mother's side in such a way that you have a constant view of the vaginal opening. Be prepared for the baby to come at any moment. See if there is crowning, that is, if part of the baby's head becomes visible with each contraction. *Do not* assume that birth will be delayed if the baby is not visible or if the area of the baby seen is "less than the size of a fifty-cent piece."

Be prepared for the patient to experience discomfort. Delivering a child may be a natural process, but it may be accompanied by pain. Your patient may also have intense feelings of nausea. If this is her first child, she may be very frightened. All these factors may cause your patient to be uncooperative at times. You must remember that the patient is in pain and she probably feels ill. She will need emotional support.

During delivery, talk to the mother. Encourage her to relax between contractions. Continue to time each contraction from the beginning of one contraction to the beginning of the next contraction. Encourage her not to strain unless she feels she must. Remind her that her feeling of a pending bowel movement is usually just pressure caused by the baby moving into her birth canal. Encourage her to breathe deeply through her mouth. She may feel better if she pants, although she should be discouraged from breathing rapidly and deeply enough to bring on hyperventilation. If her "bag of waters" breaks, remind her that this is normal.

NOTE: Until there are signs of complications, consider the delivery to be normal if there is a cephalic presentation.

The steps for assisting the mother with a normal delivery are:

1. Continue to keep someone at the mother's head in case she vomits. If no one is on hand to help, be alert for vomiting.

2. Position your gloved hands at the mother's vaginal opening when the baby's head starts to appear. *Do not* touch her skin.

3. Place one hand below the baby's head as it is delivered. Spread your fingers evenly around the baby's head (see Scan 16–1), remembering that its skull contains "soft spots" or **fontanelles.** Support the baby's head, but avoid pressure to these soft areas of the skull. Use your other hand to help cradle the baby's head. This slight pressure may help prevent an explosive delivery. **DO NOT PULL ON THE BABY!**

4. If the umbilical cord is wrapped around the baby's neck, *gently* loosen the cord. Even though the umbilical cord is very tough, if you are too rough with the cord, it may tear. Try to place two fingers under the cord at the back of the baby's neck. Bring the cord forward, over the baby's upper shoulder and head. If you cannot loosen and reposition the cord, the baby cannot be delivered. Immediately clamp the cord in two places using the clamps provided in the obstetric kit. Be very careful not to injury the baby. With extreme care, cut the cord between the two clamps. Gently unwrap the ends of the cord from around the baby's neck.

5. If the amniotic sac has not broken by the time the baby's head is delivered, use your finger to puncture the membrane. Pull the membranes away from the baby's mouth and nose.

6. Most babies are born face down and then rotate to the right or left. Support the baby's head so that it does not touch the mother's anal area. When the entire head of the baby is visible, continue to support the head with one hand and reach for the rubber bulb syringe. Compress the syringe BEFORE placing it in the baby's mouth. Carefully insert the tip of the syringe about 1 to 1½ inches into the baby's mouth and release the bulb to allow fluids to be drawn into the syringe. Control the release with your fingers. Withdraw the tip and discharge the syringe's contents onto a towel. Repeat this procedure two or three times in the baby's mouth and once or twice in each nostril. The tip of the syringe should not be inserted more than ½ inch into the baby's nostril.

7. The upper shoulder (usually with some delay) will deliver next, followed quickly by the lower shoulder. You must support the baby throughout this entire process. Gently guide the baby's head downward, to assist the mother in delivering the baby's upper shoulder. If the lower shoulder is slow to deliver, assist the mother by gently guiding the baby's head upward.

8. Support the baby throughout the entire birth process. Once the feet are delivered, lay the baby on its side with its head slightly lower than its body. This is done to allow blood, fluids, and mucus to drain from the mouth and nose. Keep the baby at the same level as the mother until the umbilical cord is cut.

9. Note the exact time of birth.

CAUTION: Babies being born are slippery! Make certain that you offer proper support. Some deliveries are explosive. *Do not* squeeze the baby, but do provide adequate support. You can prevent an explosive delivery by using one hand to maintain slight pressure on the baby's head.

Assessing the Newborn

The *vigor* of an infant should be assessed at 1 and 5 minutes after it is born. If you arrive after the birth, it is still your responsibility to make the assessments based on your first observations and those made 5 minutes later. Care for the infant and the mother should not be delayed. The assessment is meant to take place while these other activities are being performed.

Your system may call for a general or a specific evaluation protocol. A general evaluation usually calls for noting ease of respiration, crying, movement, and skin color. A newborn should be breathing easily, crying (vigorous crying is a good sign), moving its extremities (the more active, the better), and show blue coloration at the hands and feet only. Five minutes later, these signs should still be apparent, with

SCAN 16—1 NORMAL DELIVERY

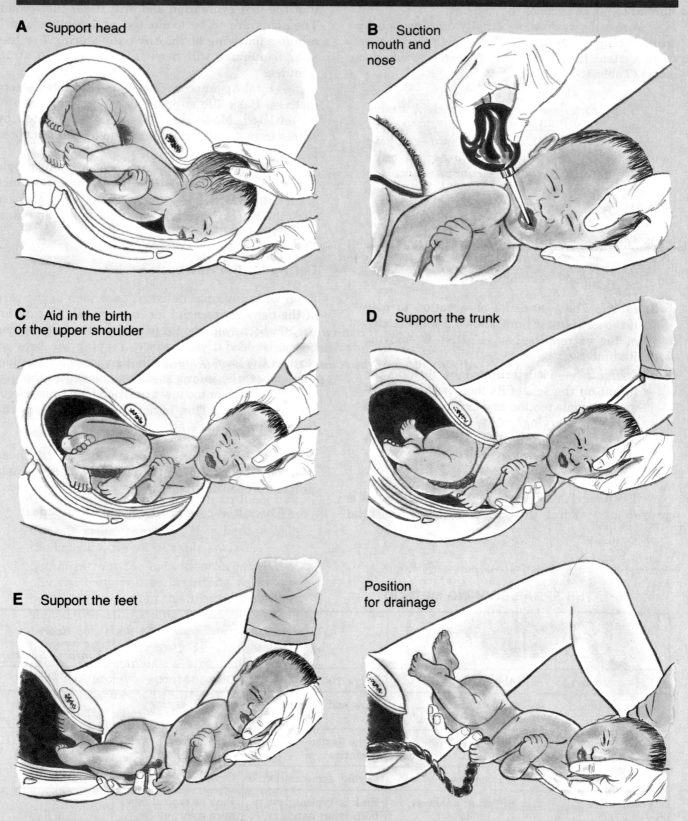

A   Support head

B   Suction mouth and nose

C   Aid in the birth of the upper shoulder

D   Support the trunk

E   Support the feet

Position for drainage

NOTE: Assist the mother by supporting the baby throughout the entire birth process.

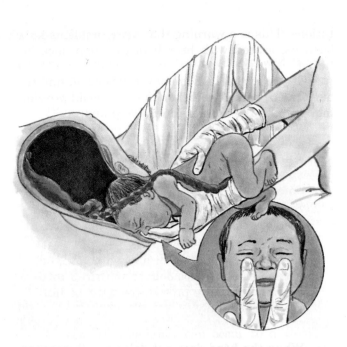

FIGURE 16–17. Procedures in a breech birth.

airway and transport mother and child as a unit. Administer oxygen to the mother. Take extreme care to maintain the airway being provided for the infant. You may be able to keep the mother on her back if she is delivering (follow local guidelines).

REMEMBER: *Do not* attempt to deliver the baby by pulling on its legs.

Prolapsed Umbilical Cord

A prolapsed umbilical cord is a TRUE EMERGENCY, usually seen early in labor. During delivery, the umbilical cord presents first. The cord is squeezed between the vaginal canal walls and the head of the baby. The cord is pinched, and oxygen supply to the baby may be totally interrupted. Such an emergency requires IMMEDIATE TRANSPORT to a medical facility, keeping the mother in an exaggerated shock position with a pillow or blanket under her hips. Be certain to provide her with a high concentration of oxygen to increase the concentration carried over to the infant. Check the cord for pulses and wrap the exposed cord, using a sterile towel from the obstetric kit. The cord must be kept warm or spasms may occur and interrupt circulation. The best results are obtained if this towel is kept moist with *sterile saline* and wrapped again with a dry towel to prevent evaporative heat loss.

It will be necessary for you to insert several fingers of a gloved hand into the mother's vagina so that you can gently push up on the baby's head to keep pressure off of the cord. You will be pushing

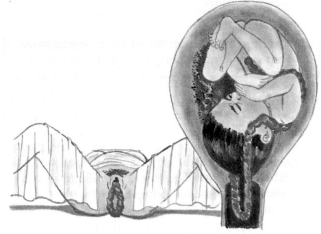

- Elevate hips, administer oxygen and keep warm
- Keep baby's head away from cord
- Do not attempt to push cord back
- Wrap cord in sterile moist towel
- Transport mother to hospital, continuing pressure on baby's head

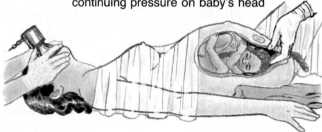

FIGURE 16–18. Prolapsed umbilical cord.

up through the cervix. This may be the only chance that the baby has for survival, so continue to push up on the baby until you are relieved by a physician. You may feel the cord pulsating when pressure is released.

Limb Presentation

If, on evaluation of the mother, you find an upper or lower limb presenting, transport the mother immediately to a medical facility. Keep her in a left lateral recumbant position with her feet slightly elevated or the delivery position (follow local guidelines). This also applies if there is a compound presentation of an arm and a leg or a shoulder and an arm. Administer a high concentration of oxygen to the mother.

There is often a prolapsed cord with the compound presentation. Follow the same procedures as you would for any delivery involving a prolapsed cord. Remember, you have to keep pushing up on the baby until relieved by a physician. The baby must be kept off of the cord if it is to survive.

On rare occasions, a baby will have shoulders too large to fit through the pelvic bones (symphysis pubis) and the hollow of the sacrum. The head will deliver, but the shoulders become wedged. Suction the baby's mouth and nose and carefully transport without delay. Provide oxygen to the mother.

REMEMBER: For a limb presentation, do not try to pull on the limb or replace the limb into the vagina. *Do not* place your gloved hand into the vagina, unless there is a prolapsed cord as well.

Multiple Birth

Multiple birth, usually in the form of twins, is not considered to be a complication, provided that the deliveries are normal. Twins are generally delivered in the same manner as a single delivery, one birth following the other. If the mother is under a physician's care, she will probably be aware that she is carrying twins. Without this information, you should consider a multiple birth to be a possibility if the mother's abdomen appears unusually large before delivery, or it remains very large after delivery of the baby. If the birth is multiple, labor contractions will continue and the second baby will be delivered shortly after the first. Usually, this is within minutes of the first birth. The placenta or placentas are delivered normally.

When assisting in the delivery of twins, clamp or tie the cord of the first baby to prevent bleeding from the second baby via the cord. Assist the mother with the delivery of the second baby, then provide care for the babies, umbilical cords, placentas, and the mother as you would in a single baby delivery. The babies will probably be smaller than in a single birth, so special care should be taken to keep them warm during transport. When delivering twins, identify the infants as to order of birth (1 and 2 or A and B).

Premature Birth

By definition, a **premature baby** is one that weighs less than 5½ pounds at birth, or one that is born

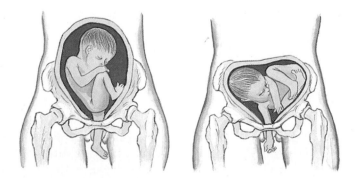

FIGURE 16–19. Limb presentation.

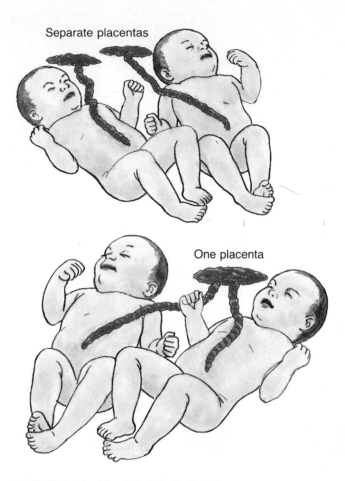

FIGURE 16–20. Multiple births.

before the 37th week or prior to the ninth month of pregnancy. Since you will probably not be able to weigh the baby, you will have to make a determination based on the mother's information and the baby's appearance. By comparison with a normal full-term baby, the head of a premature infant is much larger in proportion to the small, thin, red body.

Premature babies need special care from the moment of birth. The smaller the baby, the more important is the initial care. You should take the following steps when providing care for the premature infant:

1. Keep the baby warm. Once breathing, the baby should be wrapped snugly in a warm blanket. Additional protection can be provided by an outer wrap of plastic (keep away from the face) or aluminum foil. Premature babies lack fat deposits that would normally keep them warm. Some EMS systems in cold regions are using a plastic wrap or bag for the infant, covered by a blanket. This helps maintain warmth and allows for easier visual inspection of the clamped cord to check

for bleeding. A cap of stockinette can be placed on the baby's head to help reduce heat loss.

2. **Keep the airway clear.** Continue to suction fluids from the nose and mouth using a rubber bulb syringe. Keep checking to see if additional suctioning is required.

3. **Watch the umbilical cord for bleeding.** Examine the cut end of the cord carefully. If there is any sign of bleeding, even the slightest, apply another clamp or tie closer to the baby's body.

4. **Provide oxygen.** Deliver the oxygen into the top of an aluminum foil tent placed over the baby's head. *Do not* blow a stream of oxygen directly on the baby's face. If available, use a humidified source of oxygen. Remember, this procedure keeps the oxygen concentration below the harmful level for the time of transport.

5. **Avoid contamination.** The premature infant is susceptible to infection. Keep it away from other people. Do not breathe on its face. When available, disposable paper gowns, caps, and masks should be worn.

6. **Transport the infant in a warm ambulance.** The desired temperature is between 90°F and 100°F. Use the ambulance heater to warm the patient compartment prior to transport. In the summer months, the air conditioning should be turned off and all compartment windows should be closed or adjusted to keep the desired temperature.

7. **Call ahead and alert the medical facility.**

When a premature infant carrier is available, make certain that you are completely familiar with its use. Some require you to fill hot water bottles that are covered and placed in the carrier. The infant is to be wrapped in a blanket and aluminum foil or plastic wrap and a blanket. The carrier must be properly secured in the ambulance prior to transport.

In some areas, a mobile intensive care unit may be able to respond and transport the baby.

The Stillborn Infant

As noted earlier, some babies die up to several hours before birth. These babies are not to receive resuscitation. Any other babies who are born in pulmonary or cardiac arrest are to receive basic cardiac life support measures. When death appears to be imminent, you should prepare to provide life support.

Nothing is quite so sad as a baby born dead or one that dies shortly after birth. It is a tragic

- Keep warm by wrapping in blanket and then in aluminum foil
- Clear mouth and nose of fluid and mucus

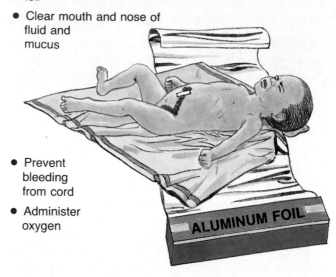

- Prevent bleeding from cord
- Administer oxygen

FIGURE 16–21. Premature infants need special care.

moment for both the parents and the emergency care personnel. Your thoughtfulness may provide the distraught parents with spiritual comfort. Christian parents may ask you to baptize the baby if death appears likely. This is acceptable practice for emergency personnel. Regardless of your own religious belief, you should comply with the parents' request. Ask the parents if they know the exact words of baptism for their denomination. Say exactly what they tell you. If they are not sure, simply sprinkle drops of water on the baby's head and say: "I baptize thee in the name of the Father, and of the Son, and of the Holy Spirit." In some cases, the parents may request that you modify the above by saying, ". . . and of the Holy Ghost."

Needless to say, resuscitative efforts should be continued during and after the baptism and continued until transfer at the hospital.

You must keep accurate records of the time of stillbirth and the care rendered for completion of the fetal death certificate. It is a good idea to note if the baby was baptized by EMS personnel.

SUMMARY

The fetus developing in the uterus is surrounded by the amniotic sac. While developing, the fetus receives nourishment and oxygen through the placenta. It is connected to the placenta by way of the umbilical cord.

The first stage of labor starts with contractions and ends with the full dilation of the cervix. The second stage of labor ends with birth. The third stage ends with the delivery of the placenta.

Evaluate the mother to see if she is about to deliver. Consider if this is her first baby, how far apart the contractions are, if she feels pressure or feels as if she may have a bowel movement, if her "bag of waters" has broken, or if she feels the baby moving into her vagina.

If you believe that birth will occur shortly, provide the mother with as much privacy as possible, position her on her back, with the buttocks elevated, her knees bent, feet flat, and legs spread apart. Remove any clothing obstructing your view of the vaginal opening. See if any part of the baby is visible or visible on contractions. This is crowning. If the head appears first, this is a cephalic presentation.

Assist the mother as she delivers her baby. Carefully support the head of the infant as it is born. Provide support for its entire body and head as birth proceeds.

If you notice the umbilical cord around a baby's neck, gently loosen the cord with your fingers. When the cord will not loosen, you will have to clamp it in two locations and cut between the clamps.

If the amniotic sac does not break, puncture it and pull it away from the baby's mouth and nose.

Remember to record the exact time of birth and to assess the newborn at 1 and 5 minutes after it is born.

In caring for the newborn, clear the baby's airway and make certain that the baby is breathing. If it is not breathing, gently but rigorously rub its back. Should this fail to produce spontaneous respirations, you will have to "encourage" the child to breathe by snapping your index finger on the soles of its feet. (Never lift and spank the baby.) For non-breathing babies with a brachial pulse, provide mouth-to-mask or mouth-to-mouth and nose resuscitation. If there is no pulse, provide CPR. If CPR is necessary, you will have to clamp and cut the cord.

If the environment is cold, you may have to partially wrap the newborn before cutting the cord. Do not tie, clamp, or cut a cord until the baby is breathing on its own, unless you have to provide CPR for the infant.

Always wrap the newborn in a blanket to keep it warm.

Assist the mother as she delivers the placenta and save all tissues for transport. Help control vaginal bleeding with clean pads over her vaginal opening and massage her abdomen over the site of the uterus. Remove all wet towels and sheets. Wipe clean the mother's face and hands.

REMEMBER: Throughout the entire birth process, provide emotional support to the mother.

Be ready for complications during a delivery. When the buttocks or both legs appear first, this is a breech presentation. Provide an airway with your fingers. Maintain this airway until the baby is born or until you hand the mother over to trained professionals at a medical facility. Transport mothers with prebirth bleeding, prolapsed umbilical cords, or limb presentations to a medical facility as soon as possible. If there is a prolapsed cord, you will have to insert several fingers into the vagina to push the baby off the cord.

Administer a high concentration of oxygen to all women having complications with birth.

If there is severe bleeding before delivery, place a pad over the vaginal opening, treat for shock, administer a high concentration of oxygen, and transport as soon as possible.

Expect a multiple birth if contractions continue after a baby is born. Tie or clamp the umbilical cord of the first child before the next one delivers.

Keep all premature babies warm, maintain a clear airway, monitor the cord for bleeding, provide oxygen to a tent over the baby's head, and protect from contamination.

In cases of miscarriage and abortion, be certain to provide emotional support to the mother. Place a pad over her vaginal opening if there is bleeding. Save all blood-soaked pads and any passed tissues. Care for shock and provide a high concentration of oxygen.

In cases of stillborns, remain professional and provide emotional support to the mother, father, and other family members. Unless there is evidence that the baby died several hours before birth, provide basic cardiac life support for all babies who are in cardiac arrest.

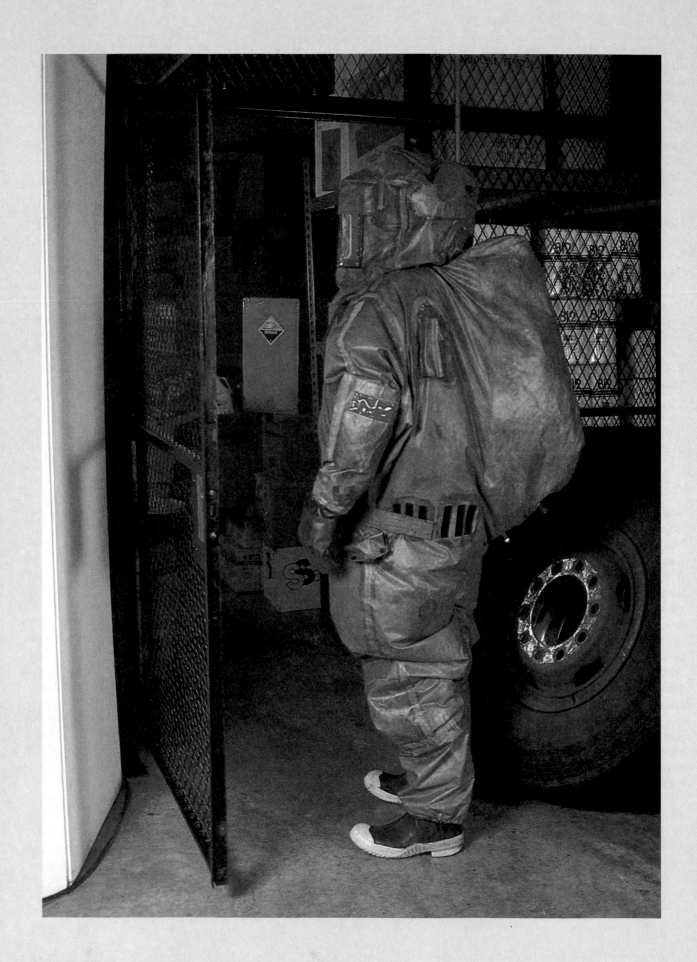

CHAPTER 17

Burns and Hazardous Materials

As an EMT, you should be able to:

1. Define *first-*, *second-*, and *third-degree burns*. (p. 461)
2. State the factors used in determining the severity of burns. (p. 462)
3. Define *Rule of Nines* and fill out a body chart for both adult and child patients. (pp. 462–463)
4. List the factors used to distinguish among critical, moderate, and minor burns. (p. 463)
5. Describe proper care for thermal, chemical, and electrical burns. (pp. 464–468 and p. 470)
6. Describe the proper care for thermal and chemical burns to the eyes. (pp. 467–468)
7. Describe the emergency care provided for smoke inhalation victims. (pp. 468–469)
8. Describe basic care procedures for the victim of an electrical accident. (p. 470)
9. Describe the EMT's role in hazardous materials accidents. (pp. 470–473)
10. Describe the care procedures for radiation accidents. (pp. 475–476)

SKILLS **As an EMT, you should be able to:**

1. Assess a patient's burns as first-, second-, or third-degree.
2. Use the Rule of Nines to determine the severity of a burn.
3. Provide care for thermal, chemical, electrical, and radiation burns.
4. Provide care for patients suffering from smoke inhalation.
5. Provide care for special emergencies, including electrical, hazardous materials, and radiation accidents according to your EMS system guidelines.

TERMS **you may be using for the first time:**

Alkali – a substance that is basic, as opposed to being neutral or acid.

Dynamic Pressure – energy released as an airborne shock wave.

First-degree Burn – a burn involving only the epidermis.

Ionizing Radiation – the product of atomic decay, including alpha particles, beta particles, and gamma rays.

Overpressure – an increase in pressure above normal atmospheric pressure limits.

Second-degree Burn – a burn involving the epidermis and the dermis but not penetrating through the dermis.

Third-degree Burn – a full-thickness burn with damage extending through the dermis.

ENVIRONMENTAL FACTORS

Nearly any element or combination of elements in our daily lives can cause injury. From a practical point of view, environmental emergencies are those related to:

- Fire
- Excessive heat
- Excessive cold
- Water and ice
- Electricity
- Hazardous chemicals
- Radiation

Often, it is the combination of two or more of the above that causes serious injury and complicates emergency care efforts. Excessive heat can cause shifts in the regulatory mechanisms of the body, leading to a true emergency. This can be combined with the burns received from fires. Water is not only a danger in terms of drowning; its temperature may bring about injury due to excessive cold. Electricity not only will burn the skin, but it will also change vital chemical activities within the body.

The skin is the first line of defense against the environment. For this reason, many environmental injuries involve the skin. The eyes sustain injuries usually avoided by other body organs. Thus the eyes also are involved in many environmental emergencies. The airway opens the respiratory system to the outside, making the lining of the airway susceptible to damage from many environmental factors. Respiratory injury can extend from the nasal membranes to the alveoli of the lungs.

Body organs and their chemical activities can be altered because of environmental factors. Radiation can affect the cells deep within the body. Electricity can disrupt nerve, muscle, and heart actions. Many hazardous materials can destroy or alter the cells that make up the body's tissues. Sometimes this action is rapid and dramatic; at other times it is slow and subtle.

As an EMT, you must be prepared to provide care for a variety of environmental emergencies. Keep in mind that such emergencies can occur anywhere, at any time.

EMS System Responsibilities

EMTs assess and provide care for patients having received injuries due to environmental factors. However, EMTs are not usually trained to combat all of the environmental sources of injury or to control all the various types of scenes involving environmental factors. Keep this in mind and remember that your safety must be the first consideration.

Typically, EMTs are trained to control the fire scene but not to fight fires. They are capable of handling certain electrical emergencies but are limited in rescue procedures. Water rescue, hazardous materials rescue, and radiation accident rescue all require specialized training. Even when other branches of emergency and rescue services attend victims, special training is required to guarantee the safety of the emergency care provider in such hazardous accidents.

REMEMBER: Do only what you have been trained to do. "Heroic" efforts can place you and fellow rescuers in danger and may even delay proper care for the patient.

Burns

You must be able to classify, evaluate, and care for burn injuries.

For most cases involving burns, the first thought is of injury to the skin. Since the skin is the part of the body constantly in direct contact with the environment, such an assumption is partly valid, but burns can do much more than injure the skin.

Injuries due to burns often involve structures below the skin, including muscles, bones, nerves, and blood vessels. The eyes can be injured beyond repair when burned. Respiratory system structures can be damaged producing airway obstruction due to tissue swelling, respiratory failure, and respiratory arrest. In addition to the physical damage caused by burns, patients also may suffer emotional and psychological problems that begin at the emergency scene and may last a lifetime.

When caring for the burn patient, do not limit your thinking only to the damage caused by the burn. A medical emergency or an accident may have led to the situation in which the patient received his burns. The patient may have had a heart attack while smoking a cigarette. The unattended cigarette may have caused the fire that produced the patient's burns; however, the heart problem should not go undetected. Someone trying to escape a fire may fall and suffer serious spinal damage and fractures. These problems also should be detected. The patient assessment should not be overlooked in order to go immediately to burn care procedures.

Classifying Burns

Burns can be classified according to the agent causing the burn. The source of the burn also can be used to make the classification more specific. For example, the source of the burn can be heat. This can be reported as "thermal burns from contact with a radiator." You should report the *agent* causing the burn and, when practical, the *source* of the agent. The agent of burn can be:

- Thermal—including flame, radiation or excessive heat from fire, steam, hot liquids, and hot objects
- Chemicals—including various acids, bases, and caustics
- Electricity—including AC current, DC current, and lightning
- Light—typically involving the eyes, with burns caused by intense light sources or ultraviolet light (includes sunlight)
- Radiation—usually from nuclear sources. Ultraviolet light also can be considered to be a source of radiation burn.

Never assume the source of the burn. What may appear to be a thermal burn could be from radiation. You may find minor thermal burns on the patient's face and forget to consider light burns to the eyes. Always gather information from your observa-tions of the scene, bystanders' reports, and the patient interview.

Burns involving the skin can be classified as partial-thickness and full-thickness burns. **Partial-thickness burns** can involve the epidermis, or the epidermis and upper dermis, but they do not include burns that pass through the dermis to damage underlying tissues (see Chapter 8). A **full-thickness burn** will pass through epidermis and dermis, causing injury to the subcutaneous layers. Both partial- and full-thickness burns are described using an evaluation system employing the term *degree*, with burns involving the skin classified as first-, second-, or third-degree. The least serious burn is the first-degree burn.

- *First-degree Burn*—a superficial injury that involves only the epidermis. It is characterized by reddening of the skin and perhaps some swelling. The patient will usually complain about pain at the site. The burn will heal of its own accord, without scarring. Since the skin is not burned through, this type of burn is evaluated as a *mild-partial-thickness burn*.
- *Second-degree Burn*—The first layer of skin is burned through and the second layer is damaged, but the burn does not pass through to underlying tissues. There will be deep intense pain, intense reddening, blisters, and a mottled (spotted) appearance to the skin. Burns of this type cause swelling and blistering for 48 hours after the injury as plasma and tissue fluids are released and rise to the top layer of skin. A second-degree burn is called a *partial-thickness burn*. Intense pain will always accompany this type of burn. When treated with reasonable care, second-degree burns will heal themselves, producing very little scarring.
- *Third-degree Burn*—This is a *full-thickness burn*, with all the layers of the skin damaged. Some third-degree burns are difficult to tell from second-degree burns; however, there are usually areas charred black or areas that are dry and white. The patient may complain of severe pain, or if enough nerves have been damaged, he may not feel any pain at all (except at the periphery of the burn where adjoining second-degree burns may be causing pain). This type of burn may require skin grafting. As third-degree burns heal, dense scars form.

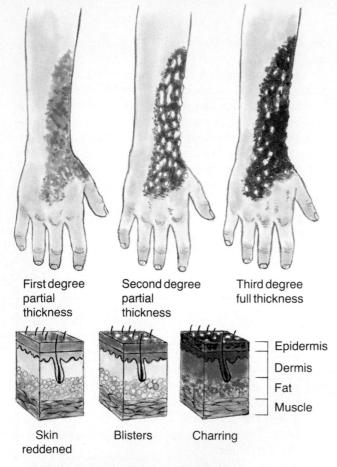

First degree
partial
thickness

Second degree
partial
thickness

Third degree
full thickness

Epidermis

Dermis

Fat

Muscle

Skin
reddened

Blisters

Charring

FIGURE 17–1. Severity of burns.

Determining the Severity of Burns

When determining the severity of a burn, consider the following factors:

- Source of the burn
- Body regions burned
- Degree of burn
- Extent of burn area
- Age of the patient
- Other patient illnesses and injuries

The source of the burn can be significant in terms of patient assessment. A minor burn caused by nuclear radiation is of more concern than one caused by thermal sources. Chemical burns are of special concern since the chemical may remain on the skin and continue to burn for hours, or even days, eventually entering the bloodstream. This is sometimes the case with certain alkaline chemicals.

Any burn to the face is of special concern, since it may involve injury to the airway or injury to the eyes. The hands and feet also are areas of special concern because scarring may cause loss of movement of fingers or toes. Special care is required to reduce aggravation to these injury sites by patient movement and to prevent the damaged tissues from

sticking to one another prior to transfer at the hospital. When the groin, buttocks, or medial thighs are burned, the chances for bacterial contamination present unusual problems that can be far more serious than the initial damage to the tissues.

Circumferential burns are burns that encircle the body or a body part. These burns can be very serious. When they occur to an extremity, there may be an interruption of circulation to the tissues distal to the burn site. The burn healing process can be very complicated with circumferential burns. This is particularly true when the burns occur to joints, the chest, and the abdomen where scarring encircles the part and tends to limit normal functions.

The degree of the burn is important. In second- and third-degree burns, the outer layer of the skin is penetrated. This can lead to contamination of exposed tissues and the invasion of the circulatory system by harmful chemicals and microorganisms.

It is important that you be able to estimate roughly the extent of the burn area. The amount of skin surface involved can be calculated quickly by using the **"Rule of Nines."** Each of the following areas represents 9% of the body surface: the head and neck, each upper limb, the chest, the abdomen, the upper back, the lower back and buttocks, the front of each lower limb, and the back of each lower limb. These make up 99% of the body's surface. The remaining 1% is assigned to the genital region.

These figures apply only to adults. The system for infants and children is shown in Figure 17–2. At the emergency scene, it is more practical to consider the infant's head and neck as 18%; each upper limb, 9%; the chest and abdomen, 18%; the entire back, 18%; each lower limb, 14%; and the genital region, 1%. True, this adds up to 101%, but it is only used to give a rough determination. Note how the head of the infant receives an 18% value. The head of an infant or child is much larger in relationship to the rest of the body than the head of the adult.

Age is a major factor in burn cases. Infants, children under age 5, and adults over age 60 have the most severe body reactions to burns and different healing patterns than other age groups. Burn intensity and body area involvement that would be classified as minor to moderate for a young adult may be fatal for the infant or the aged.

The infant and young child have a surface area that is much greater in proportion to the total body size when compared with the older child and adult. This factor means that a burn will produce a greater body fluid loss for the patient under age 5. In late adulthood, the body's ability to cope with injury is reduced by aging tissues and failing body systems.

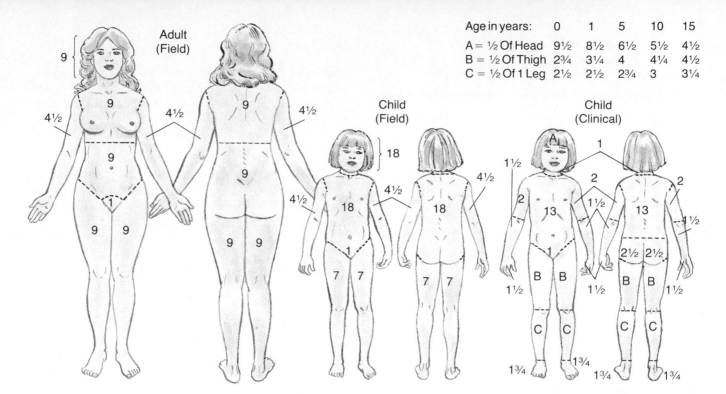

Age in years:	0	1	5	10	15
A = ½ Of Head	9½	8½	6½	5½	4½
B = ½ Of Thigh	2¾	3¼	4	4¼	4½
C = ½ Of 1 Leg	2½	2½	2¾	3	3¼

FIGURE 17–2. The Rule of Nines.

The ability of tissues to heal from any injury is lessened and the time of healing is increased.

NOTE: An adult's reactions to the burn and the complications associated with burn injury healing increase significantly after age 35.

Obviously, patients with respiratory illnesses will be placed in greater jeopardy when exposed to heated air or chemical vapors. Likewise, the stress of an environmental emergency leading to a burn will undoubtedly be of concern for patients with heart disease. Patients with respiratory ailments, heart disease, or diabetes will react more severely to burn damage. What may be a minor burn for a healthy adult could be of major significance to these types of patients.

Injuries other than burns may compromise the individual's health. When the stress of a burn is added, the seriousness of the emergency may lead to shock or some other life-threatening problem. All burns are to be treated as more serious if accompanied by other injuries. If you discover that the patient is hypotensive, always assume that he has other serious injuries. Attempt to determine the patient's problem through standard assessment techniques.

Classifying the Severity of Burns

Burns must be classified as to severity to determine the order of care, type of care, and order of transport and to supply the emergency department with as much information as possible before they receive the patient. In some cases, the severity of the burn

may determine if the patient is to be taken directly to a hospital with special burn care facilities.

Once the factors affecting severity have been noted, the following classification can be used:

Critical Burns

- All burns complicated by injuries of the respiratory tract, other soft tissue injuries, and injuries of the bones
- Second- or third-degree burns involving the face, hands, feet, groin, or major joints
- Third-degree burns involving more than 10% of the body surface
- Second-degree burns involving more than 30% of the body surface
- First-degree burns involving more than 75% of the body surface

Moderate Burns

- Third-degree burns that involve less than 10% of the body surface, excluding face, hands, feet, groin, or major joints
- Second-degree burns that involve 15% to 30% of the body surface
- First-degree burns that involve 20% to 75% of the body surface

Minor Burns

> - Third-degree burns involving less than 2% of the body surface, excluding face, hands, feet, groin, or major joints.
> - Second-degree burns that involve less than 15% of the body surface
> - First-degree burns that involve less than 20% of the body surface

Emergency Care for Burns

Many injuries and medical emergencies receive care before burns. Usually, if a burn patient without respiratory involvement is given a high priority, it is because of the development of shock. Airway obstruction, severe breathing difficulties, respiratory arrest, cardiac arrest, severe bleeding, shock, spinal injuries, severe head injuries, open chest wounds, and open abdominal wounds take priority over burns. This holds true for the individual patient with any of these emergencies as well as burns or when deciding the order of treatment and transport at the multiple-patient scene.

Certain *medical* problems are cared for before burns. These include heart attack, stroke, heat stroke, poisoning, and abnormal childbirth. Again, this applies to both the single-patient and the multiple-patient scene.

Burns involving the respiratory tract are considered *high-priority emergencies*. This is the only burn that most EMS Systems rate as highly as the injuries and medical problems listed previously. Immediate transport is called for if the patient has burns that can be classified as being critical. Since age can be a factor, immediate transport is usually recommended for any child or elderly patient with deep or extensive second- or third-degree burns. Likewise, a patient with known chronic respiratory disease, heart disease, past history of stroke, or diabetes will usually be considered for immediate transport.

If more than one patient is injured, transport is generally done in the order of estimated severity, but some consideration is given to the benefits of awaiting care. Patients with respiratory tract injury, or complications involving respiration or heart action, are typically given first transport. Some systems next transport those patients with severe burns covering 60% to 80% of the body surface. They justify waiting on patients with severe burns over 80% or more of the body on the grounds that death is likely and the other patients have a higher chance of survival if transported as soon as possible. Pain is also a consideration for order of transport. Remember that third-degree burn patients with the most serious burns will often have no pain due to the damage of nerve endings. It may seem cruel to let a second-degree burn patient in pain wait, but if the third-degree burn patient has more serious injuries, he is to be transported first.

NOTE: The order of patient care and transport varies according to locality. The above is only one example. Follow your local guidelines. More will be discussed about the triage of patients in Chapter 20.

REMEMBER: If in doubt when evaluating a burn, overclassify. Should you be uncertain as to whether a burn is first-degree or second-degree, consider the burn to be second-degree. If you are uncertain as to whether a burn is second-degree or third-degree, consider it third-degree. The actual severity of some burns may not be known for several hours.

Treating Thermal Burns

WARNING: *Do not* attempt to rescue persons trapped by fire unless you are trained to do so and have the equipment and personnel required. The simple act of opening a door might cost you your life. In some fires, opening a door or window may greatly intensify the fire or even cause an explosion.

As an EMT, you will have to care for thermal burns caused by scalding liquids, steam, contact with hot objects, flames, and flaming liquids and gases. On rare occasions, you may be called to care for sunburn which can be severe when involving infants and young children. These patients may also have other heat-related injuries.

EMTs must manage burns correctly until the patient can be transferred to the care of the staff of a medical facility. *Never* apply ointments, sprays, or butter to the burn site. To do so would delay treatment. *Do not* apply ice to any burn.

The basic care for thermal burns is set forth in the Scan 17–1. Local protocols may vary somewhat depending on the procedures used at the local burn center or medical facility. For example, some EMS Systems state that all third-degree burns are to be wrapped with dry sterile dressing or a burn sheet. Some burn centers recommend moist dressings for partial-thickness burns to 9% or less of the body and dry dressings for more severe cases. This is now being adopted by most EMS Systems.

Table 17–1 is an example of a protocol for the field management of burn patients.

Treating Chemical Burns

WARNING: Some scenes where chemical burns have taken place can be very hazardous. Always evaluate the scene. There may be large pools of dangerous chemicals around the patient. Acids could

Table 17–1. MARYLAND PROTOCOL FOR FIELD MANAGEMENT OF BURN PATIENTS*

1. Eliminate source of burn
   a. Flame—Wet, smother, or remove smoldering clothing.
   b. Tar—Cool area until burning has stopped. Do not remove tar.
   c. Electrical—Remove from electrical source with nonconductive material.
   d. Chemical—Immediately wash area with copious amounts of water (for at least 10 to 20 minutes *prior* to transport). (Call engine company if necessary.)
2. Assess patient
   a. Airway (respiratory injury)—Look for singed nasal hairs, facial burns, soot in mouth, etc. (closed-space accident).
   b. Perform routine primary survey (be alert for associated trauma). Treat trauma as if burn did not exist. The use of PASG is appropriate when indicated for associated injuries.
   c. Obtain history (mechanism of injury and circumstances of injury).
   d. Determine depth and percent of body area burned ("rule of nines"—"rule of palm").

NOTE: If transfer to the Burn Center is desired, or if there is a question concerning treatment, contact Burn Center via EMS communications.

   e. Indications for transfer to Burn Center:
      (1) Second- and third-degree burns:
         (a) Greater than 10% in patients under 10 or over 50 years old.
         (b) Greater than 20% in other age groups.
         (c) Burns of the face, hands, feet, or perineum.
      (2) Electrical burns.
      (3) Chemical burns.
3. Management
   a. Remove all jewelry and clothing necessary to evaluate burn.
   b. Wrap the patient in a clean, *dry* sheet.

NOTE: As an exception to the above, if the burn area is small (less than 9%), moist dressings for patient comfort are optional.

   d. After irrigation of chemical burns, cover with dry sheet.
   e. After initial cooling of tar, cover with dry dressings.
   f. For an inhalation injury, administer 100% oxygen per mask or nasal cannula.
4. Transport
   a. Maintain warm environment and continuously monitor vital signs.
   b. Utilize a helicopter if patient is more than 30 minutes from the Burn Center by ground.
   c. If patient has sustained an electrical injury, place patient on cardiac monitor and obtain consultation.
   SPECIAL WARNINGS
   1. Do not give patient with greater than 20% body surface area burns any fluid by mouth.
   2. Do not give any medication intramuscularly, subcutaneously, or by mouth without consultation unless a cardiac emergency exists.
   3. Do not place ice on *any* burn.

* *The Maryland Way, EMT-A Skills Manual.* Maryland Institute for Emergency Medical Services System, Baltimore, Maryland.

be spurting from containers. Toxic fumes may be present. If the scene will place you in danger, *do not* attempt a rescue unless you have been trained for such a situation and have the needed equipment and personnel at the scene.

Chemical burns require *immediate* care. It is hoped that people at the scene will begin this care before you arrive. At many industrial sites, workers and First Responders are trained to provide initial care for accidents involving the chemicals in use. Most major industries have emergency deluge-type safety showers to wash dangerous chemicals from the body. This will not always be the case. Be prepared for situations in which nothing has been done and there is no running water near the scene.

Immediate action is called for with chemical burns. The primary procedure of care is to WASH AWAY the chemical by using flowing water (one exception is dry lime. Brush it away. (DO NOT WASH.) Simply wetting the burn site is not enough. Continuous flooding of the affected area is required, using a copious, but gentle flow of water. Avoid hard sprays that may damage badly burned tissues. Continue to wash the area for several minutes, removing contaminated clothing, shoes, socks, and jewelry from the patient AS YOU APPLY THE WASH.

WARNING: Protect yourself during the washing process. Wear rubber or latex gloves (if none are available, use the gloves from an obstetric kit) and control the wash to avoid splashing.

Once you have washed the burned areas, apply a sterile dressing or burn sheet, treat for shock, and transport the patient. When possible, find out the

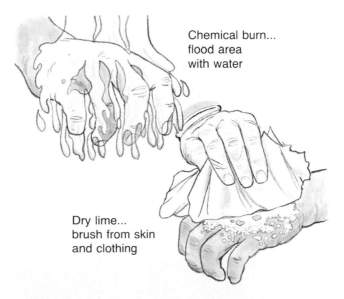

Chemical burn... flood area with water

Dry lime... brush from skin and clothing

FIGURE 17–3. Emergency care for chemical burns.

SCAN 17–1 CARE FOR THERMAL BURNS

1   STOP THE BURNING PROCESS!!

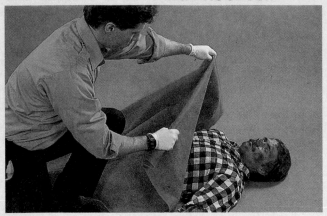

Flame—wet down, smother, or remove clothing.

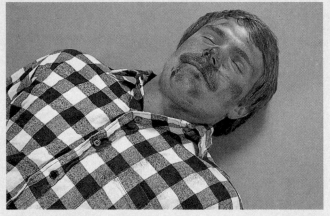

Semisolid (grease, tar, wax)—cool with water . . . do **not** remove substance

2

Ensure an
open airway

Assess breathing
• Look
• Listen
• Feel

3

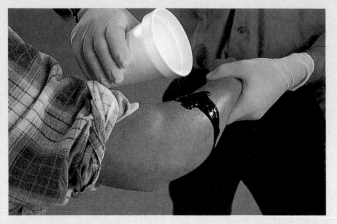

Look for airway injury: soot deposits, burnt nasal hair, and facial burns.

4

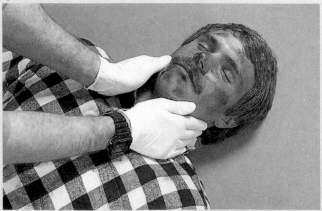

Complete the patient assessment.

5

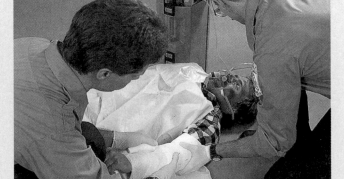

Treat for shock. Provide a high concentration of oxygen. Treat more serious injuries.

6

Evaluate Burns — Degree
  — Rule of Nines
  — Severity

Remove clothing, if necessary.

Decide if special transport is needed.

Type of Burn	Tissue Burned			Color Changes	Pain	Blisters
	Outer Layer of Skin	2nd Layer of Skin	Tissue Below Skin			
1st Degree	Yes	No	No	Red	Yes	No
2nd Degree	Yes	Yes	No	Deep Red	Yes	Yes
3rd Degree	Yes	Yes	Yes	Charred Black or White	Yes/No	Yes/No

7

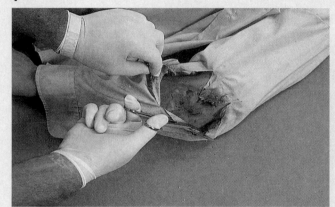

Do not clear debris. Remove clothing and jewelry.

8

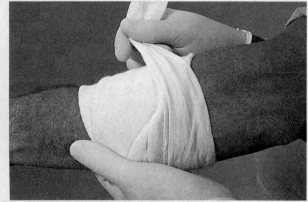

Wrap with dressing: • Less than 9%—moisten
• 9% plus—dry

9A

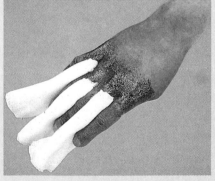

If hands or toes are burned—separate digits with sterile gauze pads. Moisten pads with sterile water. Apply loose dressings.
• Hand should be placed in position of function

9B

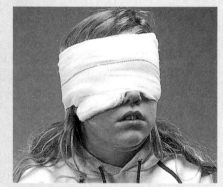

Burns to the eyes—Do not open eyelids if burned. Be certain burn is thermal, not chemical. Apply moist sterile gauze pads to both eyes.

FOLLOW LOCAL BURN CENTER PROTOCOL, AND TRANSPORT ALL BURN PATIENTS AS SOON AS POSSIBLE.

exact chemical or mixture of chemicals involved in the accident. Be on the alert for delayed reactions that may cause renewed pain or interfere with the patient's ability to breathe.

Should the patient complain of increased burning or irritation, wash the burned areas again with flowing water for several minutes. Avoid removing dressings once they are in place.

Many of the chemicals used in industrial processes are mixed acids. Their combined action can be immediate and severe. The pain produced from the initial chemical burn may mask any pain being caused by renewed burning due to small concentrations left on the skin. When the chemical is a strong acid (e.g., hydrochloric acid or sulfuric acid), a combination of acids, or an unknown, play it safe and continue washing even after the patient claims he is no longer experiencing pain.

There are some special situations:

- If dry lime is the burn agent, *do not* wash the burn site with water. To do so will create a corrosive liquid. Brush the dry lime from the patient's skin, hair, and clothing. Make certain that you do not contaminate the eyes or airway. Use water *only* after the lime has been brushed from the body, contaminated clothing and jewelry have been removed, and the process of washing can be done quickly and continuously with running water.
- Carbolic acid (phenol) does not mix with water. When available, use *alcohol* for the initial wash of unbroken skin, followed by a long steady wash with water. (Follow local protocols.)
- Concentrated sulfuric acid and water produce heat when water is added to the acid, but it is still preferable to wash rather than leave contaminant on the skin. An initial wash with mild soapy water can be used if the burns are not severe when you begin to provide care.
- Hydrofluoric acid is used for etching glass and in many other manufacturing processes. Since burns may be delayed, treat all patients who may have come into contact with the chemical. First apply a bicarbonate of soda solution and then flood with water. If burning sensations are severe on your arrival, immediately begin the water wash. *Do not* delay care and transport to find neutralizing agents. (Follow local protocols.)

Anytime a patient is exposed to a caustic chemical and may have inhaled the vapors, provide a high concentration of oxygen (humidified, if available) and

transport as soon as possible. This is very important when the chemical is an acid that is known to vaporize at standard environmental temperatures (e.g., hydrochloric acid or sulfuric acid).

Chemical Burns to the Eyes   A corrosive chemical can burn the globe of a person's eye before he can react and close the eyelid. Even with the lid shut, chemicals can seep through onto the globe. To care for chemical burns to the eye, you should:

1. IMMEDIATELY flood the eyes with water. Often, the burn will involve areas of the face as well as the eye. When this is the case, you will have to flood the entire area. Avoid washing chemicals back into the eye or into an unaffected eye.
2. Keep running water from a faucet, low pressure hose, bucket, cup, bottle, rubber bulb syringe, IV setup, or other such source flowing into the burned eye.* The flow should be from the medial (nasal) corner of the eye to the lateral corner. Since the patient's natural reaction will be to keep the eyes tightly shut, you may have to hold the eyelids open.
3. Start transport and continue washing the eye for 20 minutes or until arrival at the medical facility.
4. After washing the eye, cover both eyes with moistened pads.
5. Wash the patient's eyes for 5 more minutes if he begins to complain about renewed burning sensations or irritation.

WARNING: *Do not* use neutralizers such as vinegar or baking soda in a patient's eyes.

Smoke Inhalation

Smoke inhalation is a serious problem associated with the scenes of thermal and chemical burns. The smoke from any fire source contains many poisonous substances. Modern building materials and furnishings often contain plastics and other synthetics that release toxic fumes when they burn or are overheated. It is possible for the substances found in smoke to burn the skin, irritate the eyes, injure the airway, cause respiratory arrest, and, in some cases, cause cardiac arrest.

As an EMT, you will most likely see irritation of the eyes and injury of the airway associated with smoke. Irritations to the skin and eyes may be treated by simple flooding with water. Your first priority will be the patient's airway. The patient

---

* Some eye bath stations may run dirty water at first due to the age of the piping. Run water until clear.

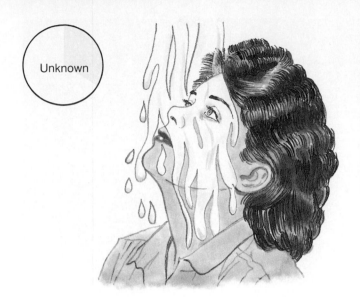

FIGURE 17–4. Care of chemical burns to the eyes.

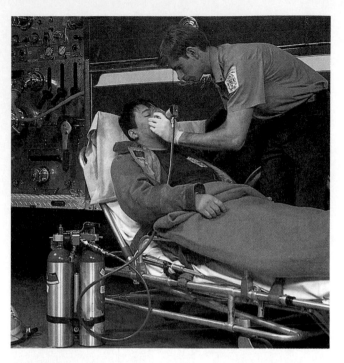

FIGURE 17–5. Care for smoke inhalation.

usually will have difficulty breathing, often accompanied by coughing. Note if his breath has a "smoky" smell or the odor of chemicals involved at the scene. Look for black (carbon) residue in the patient's mouth and nose, and be on the alert for this residue in any sputum coughed up by the patient.

In cases of smoke or toxic gas inhalation, you should:

1. Move the patient to a safe area.
2. Do a primary survey and supply life support measures as needed.
3. Administer oxygen in a high concentration and continue this throughout transport. Use a humidified source if available. A nonrebreather mask is recommended.
4. Care for possible spinal injuries and any other injury or illness requiring care at the scene.
5. Provide care for shock. Most conscious patients arc able to breathe more easily when kept in a semi-seated position.
6. Stay alert for behavioral changes. Some patients may try to jump up or push you aside as they recover from the effects of the smoke. Most patients become very restless. A few become violent.
7. Transport as soon as possible, providing a high concentration of oxygen and monitoring the patient's vital signs.

NOTE: The body's reaction to toxic gases and foreign matter in the airway can often be delayed. Convince all smoke inhalation patients that they *must* be seen by a physician.

Injuries Due to Electricity

WARNING: The scenes of injuries due to electricity are often very hazardous. If the source of electricity is still active, *do not* attempt a rescue unless you have been trained to do so and have the necessary equipment and personnel.

Electric current, including lightning, can cause severe damage to the body. The skin is burned where the energy enters the body and where it flows into a ground. Along the path of this flow, tissues are damaged due to heat. Significant chemical changes take place in the nerves, heart, and muscles, and the body processes are disrupted or completely shut down. The victim of an electrical accident may have any or all of the following symptoms and signs:

- Burns where the energy enters and exits the body
- Disrupted nerve pathways displayed as paralysis
- Muscle tenderness, with or without muscular twitching
- Respiratory difficulties or arrest (the tongue may swell and obstruct the airway)
- Irregular heartbeat or cardiac arrest
- Elevated blood pressure or low blood pressure with the symptoms and signs of shock
- Restlessness or irritability if conscious, or loss of consciousness
- Visual difficulties

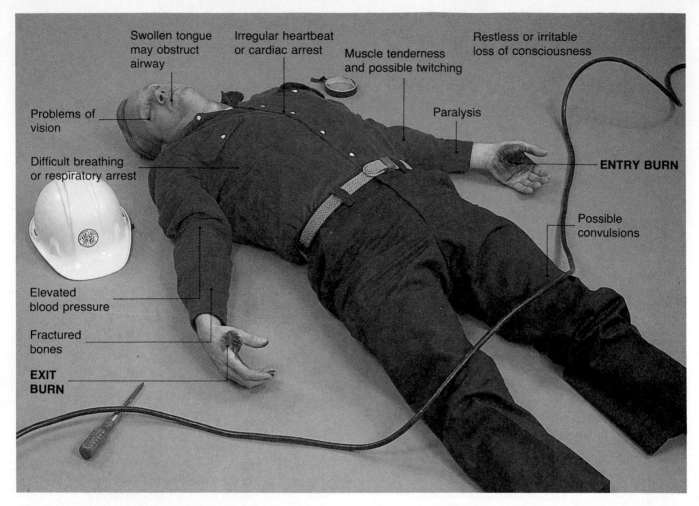

FIGURE 17–6. Injuries due to electrical shock.

Labels in figure:
Swollen tongue may obstruct airway
Irregular heartbeat or cardiac arrest
Muscle tenderness and possible twitching
Restless or irritable loss of consciousness
Problems of vision
Paralysis
Difficult breathing or respiratory arrest
ENTRY BURN
Possible convulsions
Elevated blood pressure
Fractured bones
EXIT BURN

- Fractured bones and dislocations from severe muscle contractions or from falling. This can include the spinal column.
- Seizures (severe cases)

As with all patients, establishing and maintaining an open airway will be your primary responsibility, followed by assurance of circulation. As you provide care, remember to look for the signs of spinal injury, dislocations, and fractures.

Patients who are victims of electrical accidents may require care for electrical burns. To care for such burns, you should:

1. Make certain that you and the patient are in a SAFE ZONE.
2. Provide airway care (remembering that electrical shock may cause severe swelling along the airway).
3. Provide basic cardiac life support as required.
4. Care for spinal injuries, head injuries, and severe fractures.
5. Evaluate the burn, looking for at least two external burn sites: contact with the energy source and contact with a ground.
6. Cool the burn areas and smoldering clothing the same as you would for a flame burn.
7. Apply dry sterile dressings to the burn sites.
8. Care for shock and administer oxygen.
9. Transport as soon as possible. Some problems have a slow onset. If there are burns, there also may be more serious hidden problems. In any case of electrical shock, problems with the heart may develop.

REMEMBER: The major problem caused by electrical shock is usually not the burn. Respiratory and cardiac arrest are real possibilities. Be prepared to provide basic cardiac life support measures.

Hazardous Materials

WARNING: *Do not* attempt a rescue when an accident involves hazardous materials unless you have been trained to do so, have the needed equipment, and have the personnel necessary to ensure a safe scene. Many excellent courses are offered in hazardous materials. As an EMT, you would do well to take a hazardous materials course as part of your continuing education. You should follow the guidelines set by the DOT and the Superfund Amendments and Reauthorization Act (SARA).

Table 17–2. EXAMPLES OF HAZARDOUS MATERIALS

Material	Possible Hazard
Benzene (benzol)	Toxic vapors; can be absorbed through the skin; destroys bone marrow.
Benzoyl peroxide	Fire and explosion.
Carbon tetrachloride	Damages internal organs.
Cyclohexane	Explosive—eye and throat irritant.
Diethyl ether	Flammable; can be explosive; irritant to eyes and respiratory tract; can cause drowsiness or unconsciousness.
Ethyl acetate	Irritates eyes and respiratory tract.
Ethylene dichloride	Strong irritant.
Heptane	Respiratory irritant.
Hydrochloric acid	Respiratory irritant; exposure to high concentration of vapors can produce pulmonary edema; can damage skin and eyes.
Hydrofluoric acid	Vapors can cause pulmonary edema and severe eye burns; vapors and liquid can burn skin; vapors can be lethal. There may be delayed reactions.
Hydrogen cyanide	Highly flammable—very toxic through inhalation or absorption.
Methyl isobutyl ketone (hexose)	Irritates eyes and mucous membranes.
Methylene chloride	Damages eyes.
Nitric acid	Produces a toxic gas (nitrogen dioxide); skin irritant; can cause self-ignition of cellulose products (e.g., sawdust).
Organochloride (Chlordane, DDT, Dieldrin, Lindane, Methoxychlor)	Irritates eyes and skin; fumes and smoke are toxic.
Perchloroethylene	Toxic if inhaled or swallowed.
Silicon tetrachloride	Water-reactive to form toxic hydrogen chloride fumes.
Tetrahydrofuram (THF)	Damages eyes and mucous membranes.
Toluol (toluene)	Toxic vapors; can cause organ damage.
Vinyl chloride	Flammable and explosive; listed as a carcinogen.

One of the undesirable aspects of our modern world is the growing number of hazardous materials. They are needed for the industrial manufacturing of essential and beneficial products. Hazardous materials also can be the waste products of manufacturing. Even though safety procedures have been established and followed for the most part, accidents involving hazardous materials do occur. They take place at factories, along railroads, and on local, state, and federal highways.

You must understand that as an EMT, you will be highly skilled in emergency care. However, without specialized training, you are still a layperson when it comes to hazardous materials. Special training is required to understand hazardous materials, to work at the scene of accidents involving these materials, and to render the scene safe. You cannot judge the state of a container or the probability of explosion without the benefit of specialized training. *Do not* believe that you can use safety equipment unless you have been trained in the care, field testing, and actual use of the equipment. With hazardous material accidents, you may be able to do nothing more than stay a safe distance away from the scene and wait for expert help to arrive.

Should you arrive first at the scene of a hazardous materials accident and you are trained to do so, ESTABLISH A SAFE ZONE. Keep unauthorized people out of this zone and try to convince them to leave the immediate area. Stay upwind from the site and avoid being downhill in case there are flowing liquids or gases that are burning or otherwise unsafe. Make sure that you do not set up your position in a low-lying area in case fumes are escaping and hanging close to the ground. Likewise, avoid placing yourself higher than the accident scene so that you will not be in the path of escaping gases or heated air. Be alert to the fact that a sewer system can rapidly spread the hazardous materials over a large area.

CALL FOR THE HELP THAT YOU WILL NEED. The support services required at the scene of a hazardous materials accident may include fire services, special rescue personnel, local or state hazardous materials experts, and law enforcement personnel for crowd control. If the accident has taken place at an industrial site or along a railway, the company experts in hazardous materials need to be notified. Much of this can be done by a single call to your dispatcher.

Local backup support will want to know certain facts, including:

- Type of hazardous material—gas, liquid chemical, cooled chemical, dry chemical, radioactive liquid, radioactive gases, or solid radioactive materials

- Specific name of the material, or its identification number
- How much material is at the scene
- Current state of the material—escaping as a gas, leaking as a liquid, being blown into the air, in flames, or apparently still contained
- How long you estimate that the scene has been dangerous (when did the incident begin?)
- Other hazardous materials near the scene
- Estimated number of possible patients in the danger zone

You do have sources of information. Vehicle drivers, plant and railroad personnel, and perhaps even bystanders may be able to tell you the name of the hazardous material. In many cases, there will be a colored placard (Figure 17–7) on the vehicle, tank, or railroad car. This placard will have a four-digit identification number. Older placards are usually orange and have an identification number preceded by the letters UN or UA. Your dispatcher may have access to the name of the material through this identification number. There also may be an invoice, shipping manifest (trains), or bill of lading (trucks) that can confirm the identity of the substance.

WARNING: *Do not* approach the scene to obtain this information. If it is safe to do so, placard information may be obtainable by observation with binoculars.

The Chemical Transportation Emergency Center (CHEMTREC) has been established in Washington, D.C. by the Chemical Manufacturers Association. They can provide your dispatcher or you with information about the hazardous material. They have a 24-hour, toll-free telephone number for the continental United States: 800–424–9300. In the Washington, D.C. area, the number is 202–483–7616. CHEMTREC will accept collect calls. When you call, keep the line open so that changes in the scene can be reported to CHEMTREC and the center can confirm that they have contacted the shipper or manufacturer. CHEMTREC will be able to direct you as to your initial course of action. If there is no identification number and no one knows what is being carried, you may have no other choice than to wait for experts to arrive at the scene.

WARNING: Recent studies by the Office of Technology Assessment have shown that some states report 25% to 50% of the identification placards have been found to be incorrect. These same studies indicate that many shipping documents also are inaccurate or incomplete. Do only what you have been trained to do, following the directions of hazardous materials experts.

Initial actions at the scene can be directed according to information sent to you by your dispatcher, hazardous materials expert, or CHEMTREC. Often, this initial action is based on the procedures presented in *Hazardous Materials, The Emergency Response Handbook* (DOT P 5800.2), published by the United States Department of Transportation. When you call your dispatcher or CHEMTREC:

1. Give your name and call back number.
2. Explain the nature and location of the problem.
3. Report the identification number if there is a safe way for you to obtain this information.
4. When possible, supply the name of the shipper or manufacturer.
5. Describe the type of container.
6. Report if the container is on railcar, truck, open storage, or housed storage.
7. Give the carrier's name and the name of the consignee.
8. Report local conditions, including the weather.
9. Keep the line of communication open at all times.

During the entire process, you are to keep in a safe area. *Do not* walk in any spilled materials. *Do not* think that the scene is safe simply because

FIGURE 17–7. Hazardous material placards.

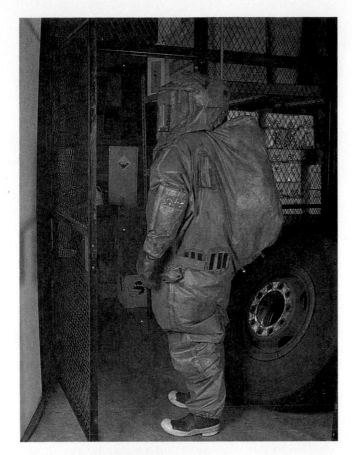

FIGURE 17–8. Special equipment is required at a hazardous material accident.

the substance does not have any apparent color or odor. Do what you can to keep people away from the scene.

As soon as possible, decide who will take charge of the scene. If this has not been decided in planning sessions prior to the incident, you or another professional at the scene should become the incident commander (IC) until experts arrive to take over responsibility at the scene.

Providing Emergency Care

After a safety zone is created, you may do the following, if trained to do so:

1. Put on 100% full-body protective clothing and a self-contained breathing apparatus (you must know how to check out and properly wear such equipment) (Figure 17–8).
2. Isolate the accident area and keep the safe zone clear of unauthorized and unprotected personnel.
3. Evaluate the scene in terms of possible fire or explosion (this takes special training).

4. Move any patients as soon as possible. If the scene offers no immediate danger (expert judgment is required to determine this), begin life support measures within the danger zone.
5. Provide basic life support. For pulmonary resuscitation and CPR, use oxygen with a demand valve or a bag-valve-mask and oxygen reservoir so that you do not have to take off your own protective gear.
6. Administer oxygen to any patient having difficulty breathing.
7. IMMEDIATELY flush with water the skin, clothing, and eyes of anyone coming into contact with the hazardous material. Continue the wash for no less than 20 minutes.
8. Remove clothing, shoes, and jewelry from all patients and personnel. Flush the person's skin with water. Remove your protective gear as recommended by local guidelines.
9. Transport the patient(s) as soon as possible, providing care for shock, administering oxygen, and taking all steps necessary to maintain normal body temperature.

NOTE: After reading this section, you may well ask, "What can I do other than wait for experts to arrive?" Some materials will allow you to act. This is why you need to provide your dispatcher with all the information available. There are materials that will require experts to respond before you can gain access and provide care. Remember, you are an EMT, not an expert in hazardous materials.

Radiation Accidents

WARNING: An EMT is not expected to be an expert in radiation accidents. Do *only* what you have been trained to do. Every state has a procedure for emergency services to follow when radioactive substances are involved in an accident. All emergency care personnel must learn and understand these procedures, especially if duties are performed in heavily traveled transportation corridors.

Radiation is a general term that applies to the transmission of energy. This can include nuclear energy, ultraviolet light, visible light, heat, sound, and x-rays. When we speak of radiation accidents, we are referring to **ionizing radiation.** This radiation is from an atomic source and is used to generate electricity, provide isotopes for medicine and industry, and make nuclear weapons. Whenever atomic materials are made or used, there is a certain amount of waste material and contaminated material produced. The sources of radiation seen in accidents include not only radioactive materials in use but also radioactive waste materials.

In most cases of radiation accidents, industrial experts will be promptly available to provide you with instructions for your safety and the care of the patient. Away from the industrial site, local rescue experts or state and federal officials may direct your activities. When in doubt, call your dispatcher to secure directions, or obtain assistance by calling the nearest Federal Radiological Emergency Response coordinating office, Disaster and Emergency Services, or Civil Defense.

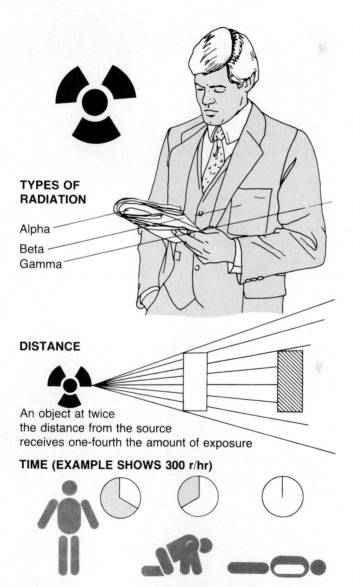

TYPES OF RADIATION

Alpha

Beta

Gamma

DISTANCE

An object at twice the distance from the source receives one-fourth the amount of exposure

TIME (EXAMPLE SHOWS 300 r/hr)

FIGURE 17–9. Factors determining radiation received.

Types of Radiation

The three major types of ionizing radiation include **alpha particles**, **beta particles**, and **gamma rays**. Neutron radiation also exists, but this is rarely encountered, being primarily found in association with nuclear reactor fuels. Neutrons can penetrate deep within the tissues and cause serious tissue damage and death.

Alpha particles do little damage since they can be absorbed (stopped) by a layer of clothing, a few inches of air, paper, or the outer layer of skin. This is a low-energy source of radiation. Beta particles are higher in energy level and cannot be stopped by clothing (including turnout gear). The danger of exposure to alpha and beta radiation cannot be taken lightly. Irradiated dust particles and smoke can be inhaled into the lungs, particles can contaminate open wounds, and irradiated foodstuffs can be ingested. Once inside the body, they continue to cause cell damage until they are removed or until they decay.

Gamma rays and x-rays can be considered the same thing. Gamma radiation is extremely dangerous, carrying high levels of energy able to penetrate thick shielding. The rays easily pass through clothing and the entire body, inflicting extensive cell damage.

Since ionizing radiation cannot be seen, felt, or heard, some sort of detection instrument is needed to measure the radiation given off by a radiation source. The most commonly used device is the Geiger counter. The rate of radiation is measured in *roentgens* (RENT-gens, also REN-chens) *per hour* (R/hr) or *milliroentgens per hour* (mR/hr) (1,000 mR = 1 R).

Effects of Radiation on the Body

Simply stated, ionizing radiation causes changes in the body cells. Depending on the dosage received, the changes can be in cell division, cell structure, and cell chemical activities. If enough radiation is absorbed, leukemia and other cancers may result. At a certain dosage level, death is a certainty.

Determining exposure, absorption, and damage done by radiation requires highly specialized training. Look at the problem in a practical manner. If you are working for one hour in an area where the Geiger counter reading is 100 R/hr, you will probably tolerate the dose with no ill effects. Should your exposure be 200 R/hr, you may become ill. Increase this to 300 R/hr and you will become very ill. At 400 R/hr, you will probably die in a short time.

How much radiation a person receives depends on the source of radiation, the length of time exposed, the distance from the source, and the shielding between the person and the source. The amount of radiation at the patient's initial location may be 300 R/hr. If you are only exposed for 20 minutes, this is the same radiation equivalent as working one hour at a 100 R/hr scene. The amount of radiation may drop off quickly as the patient is decontaminated and as you move the patient away from his initial position. If you wear protective gear, the amount of radiation absorbed will be considerably less than the Geiger counter reading.

Keep in mind that if care requires 60 minutes at a scene of 300 R/hr, three EMTs can take turns providing the care, provided that they are under the direction of a radiation expert. Each EMT will be exposed for only 20 minutes, so the exposure per person does not exceed the equivalent of working for 1 hour at 100 R/hr.

Types of Radiation Accidents

As an EMT, you may respond to two types of radiation accidents: clean and dirty.

In the **clean accident,** the patient is exposed to radiation but is not contaminated by the radioactive substance, particles of radioactive dust, or radioactive liquids, gases, or smoke. If the patient has not been contaminated or is properly decontaminated before you arrive, there is little danger to you, provided that the source of radiation is no longer exposed at the scene. The body itself does not become radioactive.

The **dirty accident,** often associated with fire at the scene of a radiation accident, exposes the patient to radiation and contaminates him with radioactive particles or liquids. The scene may be highly contaminated, even though the primary source of radiation is shielded when you arrive. If you are the first to arrive, you may have to wait for technical assistance unless you have radiation detection instruments and know how to use them. Otherwise, what you consider to be a clean accident may be a dirty one.

Rescue and Care Procedures

Your duties at the scene should include:

1. Protecting yourself from exposure.
2. Noting any hazard labels that indicate there may be a radiation hazard.
3. Alerting your dispatcher so you can obtain expert assistance.
4. Carrying out those rescue procedures you are trained to do when appropriate equipment is at the scene.

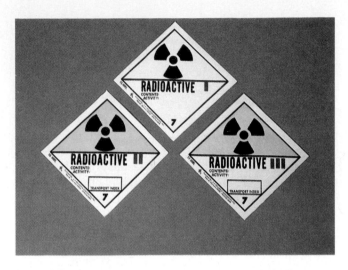

FIGURE 17–10.   Radiation hazard labels.

5. Providing emergency care for the decontaminated patient.
6. Helping prevent the spread of radiation through the control of contaminated articles.

When arriving at the scene, look for RADIATION HAZARD LABELS (Figure 17–10). These labels have a purple "propeller" on a yellow background. Notify your dispatcher immediately to inform the proper authorities and to send technical assistance to the scene. If your dispatcher tells you to leave the scene, or if a radiation expert tells you to leave, do so promptly and safely. Otherwise, park upwind, as far from the scene as practical, behind any shielding of considerable mass. Thick metal or concrete walls, earth banks, and even heavy vehicles and construction equipment offer some additional shielding.

You will have to wait for technical assistance unless you are trained to measure the radiation level and have the proper protective clothing and breathing equipment to allow a rescue. If you are trained to rescue the patient, remember to approach from upwind, avoiding when possible any dust clouds or smoke. If radiation levels are high, extricate the patient as quickly as possible, even when this means no survey, no immediate basic life support, and no splinting "where he lies." The rule is to *"get in and out quickly."*

Before care can be given, the patient must be decontaminated. Move the patient to the edge of the ACCIDENT ZONE (this is determined by local standards). Quickly remove the patient's clothing, shoes, and jewelry. If possible, place these articles in a plastic bag and place the bag in a metal container that has a tightly fitting lid. After removing the patient's clothing, remove your own protective garments and breathing apparatus. Bag these articles and place them in the container and close the lid. Some breathing apparatus may be too large to fit in this container. If this is the case, leave the apparatus next to the container. Make certain that someone guards this container so that it can be removed properly.

Care can now be rendered, provided the level of radiation on the patient's skin does not exceed locally set limitations. Place yourself and the patient in a shielded area.

There are four types of radiation accident patients that may require your care:

1. *Clean/patient received an external dose of radiation.* The patient is no danger to the EMT.
2. *Dirty/patient received an internal dose of radiation.* After external cleansing there is no danger to the EMT. Should rescue breathing be required before decontamination, use oxygen and a demand valve or a bag-valve-mask unit with oxygen reservoir.
3. *Dirty/patient externally contaminated.* There is danger to the EMT. Avoid contact until patient decontamination is possible. Unless radiation levels are high, basic life support and care for life-threatening problems is possible. Use oxygen with a demand valve or a bag-valve-mask unit for rescue breathing.
4. *Dirty/external surface contamination and wounds.* Take care not to contaminate yourself during care. Use oxygen with a demand valve or a bag-valve-mask unit if rescue breathing is required. The wounds should be cleaned separately from the adjacent skin. Dress the wounds.

Anytime that a patient is suspected of having received internal contamination, save all vomitus and body wastes for transport. Keep them in a sealed, properly labeled metal container. Swab the anterior portions of the patient's nostrils, and place the swabs in a sealed metal container. Label the container. Take nothing from the scene unless directed to do so by the radiation officer in charge.

Transport and Decontamination

Before you can transport the patient, he should be washed. Ask for a safe area to do this that will be guarded in case of contaminated water runoff. Before transport, cover the ambulance stretcher mattress with a blanket. Wrap the patient in the blanket and fashion a head covering from a towel. Only the patient's face should show when he is ready for transport. Transport the patient to the medical facility in accordance with your local radiation accident plan. You should radio ahead to alert the staff to the situation and to give your estimated time of arrival.

Decontamination or disposal of the equipment and clothing left at the scene will be done by those in charge of the radiation accident. Your ambulance, clothing, and supplies will be decontaminated by radiation experts. This is one reason why keeping an accurate ambulance equipment and supply inventory is so important. The experts must know what you used at the scene. You may be asked to help in the process, but you do not have the training to ensure a proper job.

This leaves the most important decontamination procedure—your own personal decontamination. Shower (do not bathe) with copious quantities of water, carefully washing your entire body. Pay particular attention to your hair, orifices, and parts of the body that usually rub together (e.g., medial arm and lateral chest). Allow the shower to run for some time after you complete washing to flush contaminants deep into the sanitary system. Have yourself checked by radiation experts and a physician.

NOTE: There is always some degree of risk when providing care at the radiation accident scene and when trying to provide care for the contaminated patient. Be *certain* to follow all local guidelines to the letter.

Explosions

Fire and hazardous materials often lead to explosions. An *explosion* is defined as the rapid release of energy. The magnitude of an explosion depends on several factors, including the type of explosive agent, the space in which the agent is detonated, and the degree of confinement of the explosion.

The damage done is a result of the shock wave that is generated during the release of energy. As the wave extends outward in all directions, two types of pressure are generated. **Overpressure** is the pressure increase above the normal atmospheric pressure. Overpressure surrounds an object as the shock wave hits it and tends to crush the object inward. **Dynamic pressure** may be compared to a strong wind, striking each object in its path as the shock wave moves outward. Objects are pushed over or torn apart, and debris is picked up and propelled outward.

Injury is usually related to the distance from the point of detonation. The closer the victim, the more injuries. Typical injuries can include ruptured ear drums, ruptured internal organs, internal bleeding, contusions of the lungs (due to rapid pressure changes), burns, lacerations, impaled objects, fractures, and crush injuries.

Explosions often produce superheated air that can cause severe respiratory system damage and thermal burns. When providing care at the scene of an explosion, be alert for these problems.

Basic life support is the first priority of care. A complete patient assessment is the only way you can detect most major injuries. There may be a delay in the appearance of some serious injuries while transporting. Always assume that there are internal injuries.

SUMMARY

Burns can be caused by heat (thermal), chemicals, electricity, light, and radiation.

As an EMT, you must be able to classify burns in terms of first-, second-, and third-degree. See Scan 17–1 for the factors involved in this classification.

Care for all burns, keeping in mind that burns are more serious for children, the elderly, injured patients, and those with a chronic illness. Always remember to monitor vital signs, since the respiratory system and also the circulatory system may be involved.

Any burn to the hands, feet, groin, or face is to be considered as a serious burn (exception: simple sunburn). If a whole area of the body is involved, such as the chest, you are to consider this to be a serious burn. Second- and third-degree burns that involve a major joint also must be considered to be serious. Learn to use the Rule of Nines in evaluating burns. Consider critical:

- Any burn that is complicated by injuries to the respiratory tract, soft tissues, and bones
- Second- or third-degree burns to the face, groin, hands, feet, or major joint
- Third-degree burns that involve more than 10% body surface
- Second-degree burns that involve more than 30% body surface
- First-degree burns that involve more than 75% body surface

When in doubt, OVERCLASSIFY . . . consider a questionable first-degree burn to be second degree and a questionable second-degree burn to be third degree.

Care for minor burns with cold water and a sterile or clean dressing. Do not soak major burns in cold water. Wrap the affected areas in sterile or clean dressings. Treat for shock and transport.

If the patient's eyes or eyelids are burned, cover the eyelids with sterile or clean pads. Moisten with sterile water. Use sterile or clean pads to separate burned fingers and toes before dressing.

The care for chemical burns involves flooding with water. Do not use water if the cause of the burn is dry lime. Instead, BRUSH AWAY the chemical from the patient's skin and clothing. After washing or brushing, apply dressings, treat for shock, and transport.

When the eyes are involved in cases of chemical burns, take immediate action and flood with water. Use running water for 20 minutes in cases of unknown agents, acid burns, and alkali burns. Many localities use a rule of 20 minutes or until transfer at the medical facility.

In the care for patients with electrical burns, your primary concern should be with breathing and pulse. For the actual care of the burn, remember to look for at least two external burn sites. One will be where the electricity entered the patient's body and the other will be the site where the electricity exited. Apply sterile or clean dressings, provide care for shock, and transport.

Smoke contains many poisonous substances. Move the patient to a safe atmosphere and aid in breathing by administering oxygen. Have the patient seen by a physician.

Hazardous materials should be handled by experts. Learn to look for hazardous materials placards. Provide care only when safe to do so. If trained to do so, establish a safe zone and call for the help that you will need. When you can provide care, direct your attentions to basic life support and decontamination of the patient.

Radiation accidents require expert assistance. Learn to look for radiation hazard labels. Alert your dispatcher and request the help that you will need. Park in a shielded area, wear protective clothing, and use a protective breathing apparatus. *Get in and out quickly.* Remove the patient's clothing and your contaminated gear. Provide care and decontaminate the patient. Make certain that you shower to decontaminate yourself.

Explosions can cause serious multiple injuries. Basic life support is the priority in care. A complete patient assessment is essential to provide proper care.

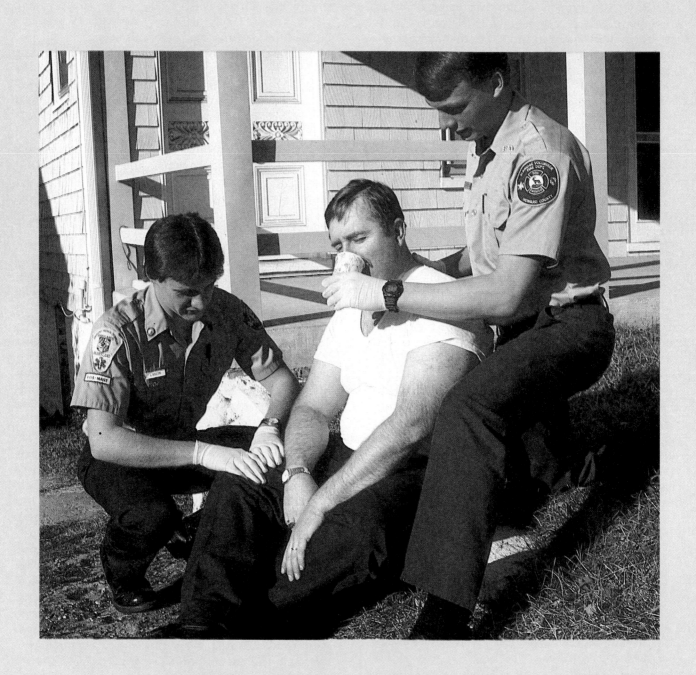

CHAPTER 18

Environmental Emergencies

SECTION ONE:
Heat- and Cold-Related Emergencies

OBJECTIVES   As an EMT, you should be able to:

1. Use symptoms and signs to distinguish between heat cramps, heat exhaustion, and heat stroke. (p. 482)
2. List the steps in caring for heat cramps, heat exhaustion, and heat stroke. (p. 482)
3. State how to distinguish among incipient, superficial, and deep frostbite. (pp. 483–484)
4. Describe emergency care for incipient,

superficial, and deep frostbite. (pp. 485–486)
5. State the symptoms and signs of hypothermia. (pp. 485–487)
6. Distinguish between mild and severe hypothermia. (pp. 485–487)
7. Describe the care procedures for mild and severe hypothermia. (pp. 486–487)

SKILLS   As an EMT, you should be able to:

1. Detect, classify, and care for heat cramps, heat exhaustion, and heat stroke.
2. Detect an emergency due to cold exposure.
3. Recognize problems due to cold exposure in terms of:
   • Mild hypothermia

   • Severe hypothermia
   • Incipient frostbite (frostnip)
   • Superficial frostbite (frostbite)
   • Deep frostbite (freezing)
4. Provide care for patients with emergencies due to exposure to cold.

TERMS   you may be using for the first time:

Deep Frostbite – freezing of body tissue.
Heat Cramps – a condition brought about by loss

of body fluids and salts due to profuse perspiration. The patient complains of muscle cramps.

Heat Exhaustion – heat prostration. A form of shock caused by the loss of fluids and salts.

Heat Stroke – commonly called "sun stroke." A life-threatening emergency that occurs when the body's temperature-regulating mechanisms fail during exposure to heat. The patient stops sweating in response to the high temperatures around him, which stops needed heat loss through evaporation.

Hyperthermia (HI-per-THURM-i-ah) – having an increase in body temperature above normal.

Hypothermia (HI-po-THURM-i-ah) – a generalized cooling that may reduce the body temperature to a point at which the body can no longer generate enough heat to support life.

Incipient Frostbite – frostnip; very mild localized changes to the skin caused by exposure to cold. This is the first stage of frostbite.

Superficial Frostbite – commonly called "frostbite," in which exposure to cold damages the skin and subcutaneous layers.

EMERGENCIES DUE TO EXCESSIVE HEAT

The body's chemical activities take place in a limited temperature range. They cannot occur with the efficiency needed for life if the body temperature is too high or too low. Heat is generated as a result of the constant chemical processes within the body. A certain amount of this heat is required to maintain normal body temperature. Any heat that is not needed for temperature maintenance must be lost from the body or **hyperthermia** (HI-per-THURM-i-ah), an abnormally high body temperature, will be created. If allowed to go unchecked, this will lead to death.

Heat is lost by the body through the lungs or the skin.

   a. Lungs
   • *Respiration*—The air we exhale is warm. As the body overheats, respirations become more rapid as the body tries to rid itself of excess heat.

   b. Skin
   • *Radiation*—Process of heat being lost into the atmosphere in the form of rays.
   • *Evaporative Heat Loss*—Perspiration is given off from glands in the dermis of the skin. As this perspiration evaporates, the skin is cooled and heat is lost in the process.
   • *Conduction*—Heat is lost directly to the surrounding medium—air or water.

Consider what can happen to the body when it is placed in a hot environment. Air being inhaled is warm, possibly warmer than the air being exhaled. The skin may actually absorb more heat than it radi-

ates. If high humidity is added, the evaporation of perspiration slows. To make things even more difficult, consider all this in an environment that lacks circulating air or a breeze that would speed up radiation and evaporative heat loss. What exists now is the environment often associated with emergencies due to excessive heat, or *hyperthermia*. This is why a "heat wave" greatly increases EMS responses for heat-related emergencies.

Since evaporative heat loss is reduced in a humid environment, *moist heat* can produce dramatic body changes in a short time. However, moist heat usually tires individuals very quickly, frequently stopping them from overexerting and harming themselves. Yet some people continue to push, running the risk of placing their bodies in a state of emergency.

Dry heat often deceives individuals. They continue to work or remain exposed to excess heat far beyond the point that their bodies can tolerate. This is the reason why you may see problems caused by dry heat exposure that are worse than those seen in moist heat exposure.

The same rules of care apply to heat-related emergencies as to any emergency. You will still have to perform patient surveys and interviews. *Do not overlook other possible problems.* Collapse due to heat exposure may result in a fall that can fracture bones. A history of high blood pressure, heart disease, or lung problems may have quickened the effects of heat exposure. What may appear to be a problem related to heat exposure could be a heart attack. Age, diseases, and existing injuries all must be considered when evaluating the patient. Always consider the problem to be greater if the patient is a child, elderly, or injured or has a chronic disease.

Common Heat Emergencies

There are three common emergencies brought about by exposure to excessive heat:

1. HEAT CRAMPS—brought about by long exposure to heat. The emergency scene temperature does not have to be much greater than what would be considered to be a "normal" environmental temperature. The individual perspires heavily, often drinking large quantities of water. As the sweating continues, salts are lost by the body, bringing on painful muscle cramps. Researchers are trying to determine if the loss of water alone is enough to have the patient develop heat cramps. Many medical authorities still believe that it is a combination of water and salt loss that brings on the condition.

2. HEAT EXHAUSTION—the typical heat exhaustion patient is a healthy individual who has been exposed to excessive heat while working or exercising. This is a form of shock brought about by fluid and salt loss. This problem is often seen with firefighters, construction workers, dock workers, and those employed in poorly ventilated warehouses. Heat exhaustion is more of a problem during the summer and reaches a peak during prolonged heat waves. This condition may develop into heat stroke and requires large volumes of fluid replacement to manage.

3. HEAT STROKE—this is a TRUE EMERGENCY, brought about when a person's temperature-regulating mechanisms fail and his body cannot rid itself of excess heat. The problem is compounded when the patient fails to sweat in response to fluid and salt loss due to heat. Athletes, laborers, and others who exercise or work in hot environments are common victims. The elderly who live in poorly ventilated apartments without air conditioning and children left in cars with the windows rolled up are common victims of heat stroke.

   More cases of heat stroke are reported on hot, humid days. However, many cases occur from exposure to dry heat. Even though heat stroke is commonly called "sun stroke," it can be caused by excessive heat other than from the sun. ALL cases of heat stroke are serious and the patient must be rapidly cooled and transported. Ice should be carried in the EMS unit during times of high environmental temperatures.

The symptoms and signs of heat cramps, heat exhaustion, and heat stroke are compared in Scan 18–1. Care procedures also are listed. Some factors require special consideration:

- Fluids—Patients with heat cramps or heat exhaustion are to be given water or commercial electrolyte fluids. Most local protocols require water or half-strength electrolyte solution be provided for heat exhaustion patients. You are to follow the procedures ordered by your EMS System's medical board.
- Cooling—Rapid cooling for heat stroke is recommended. Place cool compresses or ice packs on the wrist, ankle, or to the head, neck, axilla, and groin. For school-age children, cooling is started using tepid (lukewarm) water. This water can then be replaced with cooler water at the recommendation of the emergency department physician.
- Transport—Transport as soon as possible if:

1. There are the symptoms and signs of heat stroke.
2. There are the symptoms and signs of heat exhaustion.
3. The patient's condition worsens.
4. The patient does not respond to care.
5. You believe that the patient will return to the same environment and activity. A patient with heat cramps could become a patient with heat exhaustion or heat stroke on your next run.
6. You believe that the patient may have other medical problems.

Beware of what you are told by some patients. They may not believe heat-related emergencies are serious. Many simply want to return to work or do not wish to miss time from work. Interview the patient, take vital signs, and do the appropriate survey. Make certain that the patient has stable vital signs within normal limits. If you have any doubts, tell the patient why he should be transported and seek his permission. You may have to spend a little time with some patients to gain their confidence.

Condition	Muscle Cramps	Breathing	Pulse	Weakness	Skin	Perspiration	Loss of Consciousness
Heat cramps	Yes	Varies	Varies	Yes	Moist-warm No change	Heavy	Seldom
Heat exhaustion	No	Rapid Shallow	Weak	Yes	Cold Clammy	Heavy	Sometimes
Heat-stroke	No	Deep, then shallow	Full Rapid	Yes	Dry-hot	Little or none	Often

1 HEAT CRAMPS

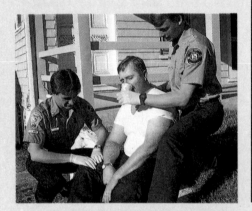

SYMPTOMS AND SIGNS:
Severe muscle cramps (usually in the legs and abdomen), exhaustion, sometimes dizziness or periods of faintness.

EMERGENCY CARE PROCEDURES:
• Move patient to a nearby cool place
• Give patient salted water to drink or half-strength commercial electrolyte fluids
• Massage the "cramped" muscle to help ease the patient's discomfort, massaging with pressure will be more effective than light rubbing actions. (Optional in some EMS systems).
• Apply moist towels to the patient's forehead and over cramped muscles for added relief
• If cramps persist, or if more serious signs and symptoms develop, ready the patient and transport

2 HEAT EXHAUSTION

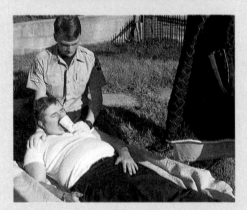

SYMPTOMS AND SIGNS:
Rapid and shallow breathing, weak pulse, cold and clammy skin, heavy perspiration, total body weakness, and dizziness that sometimes leads to unconsciousness.

EMERGENCY CARE PROCEDURES:
• Move the patient to a nearby cool place.
• Keep the patient at rest.
• Remove enough clothing to cool the patient without chilling him (watch for shivering)
• Fan the patient's skin.
• Give the patient salted water or half-strength commercial electrolyte fluids. Do not try to administer fluids to an unconscious patient.
• Treat for shock, but do not cover to the point of overheating the patient.
• Provide oxygen if needed
• If unconscious, fails to recover rapidly, has other injuries, or has a history of medical problems, transport as soon as possible.

3 HEATSTROKE

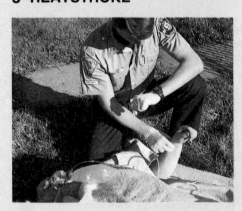

SYMPTOMS AND SIGNS:
Deep breaths, then shallow breathing; rapid strong pulse, then rapid, weak pulse; dry, hot skin; dilated pupils; loss of consciousness (possible coma); seizures or muscular twitching may be seen.

EMERGENCY CARE PROCEDURES:
• Cool the patient—in any manner—rapidly, move the patient out of the sun or away from the heat source. Remove patient's clothing and wrap him in wet towels and sheets. Pour cool water over these wrappings. Body heat must be lowered rapidly or brain cells will die!
• Treat for shock and administer a high concentration of oxygen.
• If cold packs or ice bags are available, wrap them and place one bag or pack under each of the patients armpits, one behind each knee, one in the groin, one on each wrist and ankle, and one on each side of the patient's neck.
• Transport as soon as possible.
• Should transport be delayed, find a tub or container—immerse patient up to the face in cooled water. Constantly monitor to prevent drowning.
• Monitor vital signs throughout process.

EMERGENCIES DUE TO EXCESSIVE COLD

As noted in the section on heat-related emergencies, the human body generates heat, trying to keep a temperature of 98.6°F (37°C). This involves a balance of the heat being generated, the heat lost, and the heat absorbed from the environment. If the environment is too cold, body heat can be lost faster than it can be generated. The body attempts to adjust by reducing respirations, perspiration, and circulation to the skin. Muscular activity will increase in the form of shivering to generate more heat. The rate at which foods that serve as fuel are burned within the body increases to produce more heat. At a certain point, enough heat will not be available to all parts of the body, leading to damage of exposed tissues, a general reduction of body functions, or the cessation of a vital body function. An EMT's actions can prevent long rehabilitation due to cold-related injuries, can keep body parts from becoming nonfunctional, and may even save the patient's life.

Cold-related emergencies can be the result of local cooling or general cooling. **Local cooling** injuries are those affecting particular parts of the body. They are grouped under the heading of **frostbite. General cooling** affects the entire body. This problem is known as **hypothermia** (HI-po-THURM-i-ah).

The body can lose heat by **conduction.** This is a direct transfer of heat from the warm body into the cold environment. Heat also can be lost by **convection** as cool air passes over the body surface and carries away body heat. If a person's body or protective clothing becomes wet, **water chill** becomes a problem. Water conducts heat away from the body 240 times faster than still air. The effects of a cold environment also can be made worse by **wind chill.** The more wind, the more heat loss by the body. Wind increases the effects of cold temperatures. For example, if it is 10°F outside and there is a 20 mph wind, the amount of heat lost by the body is the same as if it were −25°F.

When evaluating the effects of cold temperatures on a patient, you must consider temperature, wind chill, water chill, exposed areas of the body, clothing, length of exposure, health of the patient, existing injuries, age, and how active the patient was during the exposure. Patients with injuries or chronic illnesses will show the effects of cold much sooner than healthy persons. Those under the influence of alcohol or other substances tend to be affected more rapidly and more severely than the average person. The elderly will be more quickly affected.

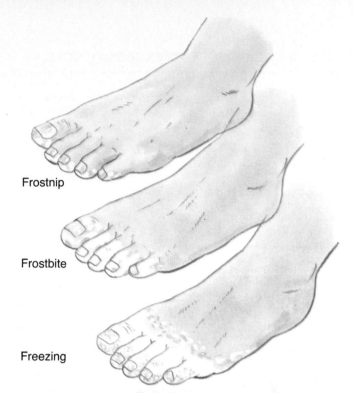

Frostnip

Frostbite

Freezing

FIGURE 18–1. **The three degrees of frostbite.**

The unconscious patient lying on the cold ground will tend to have greater cold-related problems than one who is conscious and able to walk about.

Local Cooling

Local cooling is **frostbite.** Most commonly affected are the ears, nose, hands, and feet. When a part of the body is exposed to intensely cold air or liquid, blood flow to that particular part is limited by the constriction of blood vessels. When this happens, tissues do not receive enough warmth to prevent freezing. Ice crystals can form in the skin. In the most severe cases, *gangrene* (localized tissue death) can set in and ultimately lead to the loss of the body part.

There are three degrees of frostbite:

- FROSTNIP—this is incipient (the first stage of) frostbite, brought about by direct contact with a cold object or exposure of a body part to cold air. Wind chill and water chill also can be major factors. This condition is not serious. Tissue damage is minor and the response to care is good. The tip of the nose, the tips of the ears, the upper cheeks, and the fingers (all areas generally exposed) are most susceptible to frostnip.
- SUPERFICIAL FROSTBITE—commonly called "frostbite." The skin and subcutaneous layers become involved. If frostnip goes untreated, it becomes superficial frostbite.

Table 18–1. EXPOSURE TO EXCESSIVE COLD

Condition	Skin Surface	Tissue under Skin	Skin Color
Frostnip	Soft	Soft	Initially red, then white
Frostbite	Hard	Soft	White and waxy
Freezing	Hard	Hard	Blotchy, white to yellow-gray to blue-gray

- FREEZING—this is deep frostbite in which the skin, the subcutaneous layers, and the deeper structures of the body are affected. Muscles, bones, deep blood vessels, and organ membranes can become frozen.

As an EMT, you will need to know the symptoms, signs, and care procedures for all three degrees of frostbite (Table 18–1). Notice how the symptoms and signs of frostbite are progressive. First, the exposed skin reddens, or in dark-skinned individuals, the skin color lightens and approaches a blanched (reduced color or whitened) condition. Then, as exposure continues, the skin takes on a gray or white, blotchy appearance. Exposed skin surfaces become numb, due to reduced circulation. If the freezing process is allowed to continue, all sensation is lost and the skin becomes dead white.

Frostnip/Incipient Frostbite

The symptoms and signs of frostnip include:

- Slow onset—Frostnip usually takes some time to develop.
- Patient unawareness—Most people with frostnip are not aware of the problem until someone indicates that there is something unusual about their skin color. The frostnip site is usually numb.
- Skin color changes—The area of the skin affected will at first redden, then it blanches (becomes white). Once blanching begins, the color change can take place very quickly.
- The affected area will feel numb to the patient.

Emergency care for frostnip is simple . . . warm the affected area. Usually, the patient can apply warmth from his own bare hands, blow warm air on the site, or, if the fingers are involved, hold them in the armpits. During recovery from frostnip, the patient may complain about "tingling" or burning sensations, which is normal. If the condition does not respond to this simple care, begin to treat for frostbite.

Superficial and Deep Frostbite

The symptoms and signs of superficial frostbite are:

- The affected area of the skin appears white and waxy.
- The affected area will feel frozen, but only on the surface. The tissue below the surface *must* still be soft and have its normal "bounce." Do not squeeze or "poke" the tissue. The condition of the deeper tissues can be determined by gently feeling the affected area. Do the assessment as if the affected area had a fractured bone.

The symptoms and signs of freezing include:

- The skin will turn mottled or blotchy. The color will turn to white, then grayish yellow, and finally a grayish blue.
- The tissues feel frozen to the touch, without the underlying resilience characteristic of superficial frostbite.

Initial care for superficial frostbite and for deep frostbite is the same:

- When the patient can be transported to a medical facility without delay, protect the frostbitten area by covering the site of injury and handling the affected part as gently as possible.

When practical, transport should be as soon as possible, but if transport must be delayed, get the patient indoors and keep him warm. Do not allow the patient to smoke. Smoking causes blood vessels to constrict, decreasing circulation in the damaged tissues. Likewise, discourage the consumption of alcoholic beverages. Rewarm the frozen part as to local protocol, or request orders from the emergency department physician. To rewarm the affected part, you will need a container to heat water and a second container to immerse the entire site of injury *without* the limb touching the sides or bottom of this container. If you cannot find a suitable container, fashion one from a plastic bag supported by a cardboard box or wooden crate (Fig. 18–2). Proceed as follows:

1. Heat some water to a temperature between 100° and 105°F. You should be able to put your finger into the water without experiencing discomfort.

2. Fill the container with the water and prepare the injured part by removing any clothing, jewelry, bands, or straps.

3. Fully immerse the injured part. *Do not* allow the frostbitten area to touch the sides or bottom of the container. *Do not* place any pressure on the affected part. When the water cools below 100°F, remove the limb and add more warm water. The patient may complain of some pain as the affected area rewarms or he may experience some period of intense pain. The presence of pain is usually a good indicator of successful rewarming.

4. If you complete rewarming of the part (it no longer feels frozen and is turning red or blue), gently dry the affected area and apply a sterile dressing. Place pads of dressing material between fingers and toes before dressing hands and feet. Next, cover the site with blankets or whatever is available to keep the affected area warm. *Do not* allow these coverings to come in direct contact with the injured area or to put pressure on the site. Best results can be obtained if you first build some sort of framework on which the coverings can rest.

5. Keep the patient at rest. *Do not* allow the patient to walk if a lower extremity has been frostbitten or frozen.

6. Make certain that you keep the entire patient as warm as possible without overheating. Cover the head with a towel or small blanket to reduce heat loss. Leave the patient's face exposed.

7. Continue to monitor the patient.

8. Assist circulation by rhythmically and carefully raising and lowering the affected limb. (Follow local guidelines.)

9. Transport as soon as possible with the affected limb slightly elevated. Keep the entire patient warm.

NOTE: Never listen to bystanders' myths and folktales about the care of frostbite. *Never* rub a frostbitten or frozen area. *Never* rub snow on a frostbitten or frozen area. There are ice crystals at the capillary level. Rubbing the injury site may cause these crystals to seriously damage the already injured tissues.

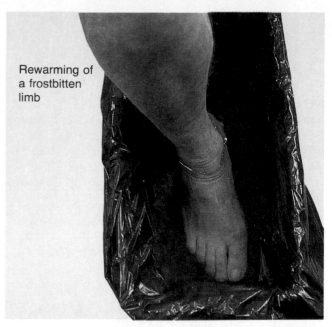

Rewarming of a frostbitten limb

FIGURE 18–2. Rewarming the frozen part.

Do not thaw a frozen limb if there is any chance it will be refrozen.

General Cooling/Hypothermia

The general cooling of the human body is known as **systemic hypothermia.** Exposure to cold reduces body heat. With time, the body is unable to maintain its proper core (internal) temperature. If allowed to continue, hypothermia leads to death. Be aware that hypothermia can develop in temperatures *above* freezing.

Hypothermia is often a serious problem for the aged. During the winter months, many older citizens attempt to live in rooms that are kept too cool. Failing body systems, chronic illnesses, poor diets, and a lack of exercise combine with this cold environment to bring about hypothermia.

The symptoms and signs of hypothermia include:

- Shivering (early stages when body core temperature is above 90°F)
- Feelings of numbness
- Drowsiness and unwillingness to do even the simplest of activities. A decreased level of consciousness may be observed.
- Slow breathing and pulse rates (seen in cases of prolonged hypothermia)
- Failing eyesight (seen in cases of prolonged hypothermia)
- Coordination difficulties (the patient may stagger)

- Unconsciousness, usually the patient has a "glassy stare" (seen in extreme cases)
- Freezing of body parts (seen in the most extreme cases). Action must be taken immediately, since the patient may be near death.

NOTE: Rewarming a patient with mild hypothermia in the field is allowed by some EMS Systems but not all. This can prove to be a *dangerous* process if the patient's condition is more serious than believed. If you are allowed to rewarm a patient with mild hypothermia, do not delay transport. Rewarm the patient while en route.

The care of *mild hypothermia* requires you to:

1. Do patient surveys and interviews to determine the extent of the problem.
2. Keep the patient dry. Remove any wet cloth-

Table 18–2. STAGES OF SYSTEMIC HYPOTHERMIA

Body Temperature (core), °F	°C	Symptoms
99–96	37–35.5	Intense, uncontrollable shivering.
95–91	35.5–32.7	Violent shivering persists. If victim is conscious, he has difficulty speaking.
90–86	32–30	Shivering decreases, is replaced by strong muscular rigidity. Muscle coordination is affected. Erratic or jerky movements are produced. Thinking is less clear. General comprehension is dulled. There may be total amnesia. The victim is generally still able to maintain the appearance of psychological contact with his surroundings.
85–81	29.4–27.2	Victim becomes irrational, loses contact with his environment, and drifts into a stuporous state. Muscular rigidity continues. Pulse and respirations are slow and patient may develop cardiac arrhythmias.
80–78	26.6–18.5	Victim becomes unconscious. He does not respond to the spoken word. Most reflexes cease to function. Heartbeat becomes erratic.
Below 78	25.5	Cardiac and respiratory centers of the brain fail. Ventricular fibrillation occurs; probably edema and hemorrhage in the lungs; death.

ing and replace the articles with dry items, or wrap the patient in dry blankets.

3. Use heat to raise the patient's core body temperature. This should be done during transport, but if transport is delayed, move the patient to a warm environment if at all possible. Gently apply heat to the patient's body in the form of heat packs, hot water bottles, electric heating pads, hot air, radiated heat, and your own body heat and that of bystanders. DO NOT WARM THE PATIENT TOO QUICKLY. Rapid warming will circulate peripherally stagnated cold blood and rapidly cool the vital central areas of the body, possibly causing serious heart problems (ventricular fibrillation.)

The process used to rewarm the patient should be CORE REWARMING. This means that you must avoid rewarming the limbs. Heat should be applied to the trunk of the body, armpits, and groin. If the limbs are warmed first, blood will collect in the extremities due to vasodilation and cause a fatal form of hypovolemic shock. If you rewarm the trunk and leave the lower extremities exposed, you can control the rewarming process and help prevent most of the problems associated with the procedure.

If transport must be delayed, a warm bath is very helpful, but you must keep the patient alert enough so that he does not drown. *Constant* monitoring is necessary for unconscious patients. Again, do not warm the patient too quickly.

4. Keep the patient at rest. *Do not* allow the patient to walk. Such activity may set off severe heart problems, including ventricular fibrillation. Since the patient's blood is coldest in the extremities, exercise could quickly circulate this blood to lower the core temperature.
5. Provide care for shock and provide oxygen. *Do not* use oxygen from a cold cylinder unless there is no other choice. If a cold cylinder must be used, realize that the temperature delivered to the patient will be warmer than what is found in the cylinder. Cold cylinder oxygen will warm once it leaves the cylinder and expands in the regulator.
6. If the patient is alert, *slowly* give him warm liquids. When warm fluids are given quickly, circulation patterns change sending blood away from the core to the skin and extremities.
7. Except in the mildest of cases (shivering),

transport the patient, with the head lower than the feet. Continue to provide oxygen and monitor vital signs.

8. *Never* allow a patient to remain in, or return to, a cold environment. Hypothermia will probably recur.

NOTE: You will not be providing very much help to patients suffering from general cooling if you simply wrap them in blankets. Their bodies can no longer generate enough heat to make such care useful. Provide external heat sources, but rewarm the patient slowly. Handle the patient with great care, the same as you would if there were unstabilized cervical spine injuries.

DO NOT TRY TO REWARM THE PATIENT WITH SEVERE HYPOTHERMIA. Even if you rewarm the patient slowly, you may cause the patient to develop lethal ventricular fibrillation. For the patient with *severe hypothermia*, you should:

1. Handle the patient as gently as possible. Rough handling may cause ventricular fibrillation.
2. Place the patient in a head-down position. Make certain that he has an open airway.
3. Provide a high concentration of oxygen that has been passed through a warm water humidifier. If need be, the oxygen that has been kept warm in the passenger compartment can be used. If there is no other choice, oxygen from a cold cylinder may be used.
4. Wrap the patient in blankets. If available, use insulating blankets.
5. Transport IMMEDIATELY.

In extreme cases of hypothermia, you will find the patient unconscious, with no discernable vital signs (take one minute to assess the carotid pulse). The patient will feel very cold to your touch (the core temperature of the body may be below 80°F), but it is possible that the patient is still alive!* Begin CPR immediately! The patient may not reach biological death for over 30 minutes. The staff at the emergency department will not pronounce a patient biologically dead until after he is rewarmed as resuscitative measures are being applied. This means that you cannot assume that a severe hypothermia patient is dead on the basis of body temperature and lack of vital signs.

* The lowest temperature recorded for an accidental hypothermia patient who survived is 64.4°F.

Other Cold-Related Injuries

Chilblains

Chilblains are lesions that occur from repeated prolonged exposures of bare skin to temperatures of 60°F or lower. The lesions are in the form of red, swollen areas that the patient reports as hot, tender, and itchy. Chilblains are chronic; that is, they linger. There is no emergency care procedure for chilblains other than to protect the injured area and try to prevent recurrence. Keep in mind that the role of the EMT does not include diagnosis. Therefore, you should recommend that the patient be transported to a physician to receive the appropriate treatment and to make certain that chilblains is the problem.

Trench Foot

Sometimes called immersion foot, trench foot is a condition that develops when the lower extremities remain in cool water for a prolonged period. The affected part of the limb becomes swollen and appears waxy and mottled. It feels cold to the touch and to the patient. The patient may complain of numbness.

To provide care, remove wet shoes and stockings. Do not open any blisters that may have developed. Gently rewarm the extremity, and wrap it lightly with sterile dressing. The extremity may become red and hot. Dress the affected limb, placing strips of dressing between the toes. Keep the limb slightly elevated. Severe disability can occur with trench foot. Make certain that you transport the patient to a medical facility.

Protecting the Accident Victim from Cold

The injured patient is more susceptible to the effects of cold. As an EMT, you should begin to protect the accident victim before extrication and throughout care and transport. The major course of action is to prevent additional body heat loss. Although it may be neither practical nor possible to replace wet clothing, you can at least create a barrier to the cold with blankets, a salvage cover, an aluminized blanket, a survival blanket, or even articles of clothing. A plastic trash bag can serve as protection from wind and water, and it will help prevent heat loss. Keep in mind that the greatest area of heat loss may be the head. Provide some sort of head covering for the patient.

When the patient's injuries allow, place a blanket between his body and the cold ground. If the patient will remain in the trapped wreckage for a period of time, plug holes in the wreckage with blankets or salvage covers. If available, use a 500-watt incandescent lamp to generate heat within the wreckage.

When administering oxygen to patients exposed to cold, keep the cylinder inside the warm ambulance when possible.

SUMMARY

Exposure to excessive heat can bring about heat cramps, heat exhaustion, or heat stroke. Heat cramps are seldom a serious problem. Some cases of heat exhaustion can turn serious. All cases of heat stroke are serious. HEAT STROKE IS A TRUE EMERGENCY. See Scan 18–1 for the symptoms and signs of all three conditions. You must be able to tell one condition from the others.

Care for heat cramps includes cooling the patient, giving water or half-strength commercial electrolyte fluids (check local protocol), and massaging cramped muscles. In cases of heat exhaustion, you must cool the patient, give water or half-strength commercial electrolyte fluids (check local protocol), administer oxygen if needed, and treat for shock.

Heat stroke requires you to cool the patient as rapidly as possible. Do not delay transport . . .

cool the patient while en route. Use ice bags, cold packs or soaked sheets, and additional cool water. Remember, TRANSPORT IMMEDIATELY. This is a TRUE EMERGENCY.

Exposure to cold can cause incipient frostbite (frostnip), superficial frostbite (frostbite), or deep frostbite (freezing). The signs for each of these conditions are given in Table 18–1.

Often, the patient can use his own body heat to warm frostnipped areas of the body. Frostbite requires gentle handling of the affected part, keeping the patient warm, dressing the site, and transporting to a medical facility. If transport is delayed, the affected area will have to be rewarmed by immersing it in warm water (100° to 105°F). Keep the water warm, but still comfortable to your touch. The same basic care also applies to freezing.

Excessive cold can bring about hypothermia. Shivering, feelings of numbness, and drowsiness are most frequently noted in hypothermia. Care for mild hypothermia involves using external heat sources to raise the patient's body temperature slowly (follow local protocol). Hypothermia can be very serious. If the patient becomes unconscious, has problems with breathing, has a slowed pulse rate, has frozen body parts, or is in cardiac arrest, provide needed basic life support, wrap him in an insulated blanket, and transport as soon as possible. *Do not* try to rewarm the patient with severe hypothermia.

SECTION TWO
Water- and Ice-Related Accidents

OBJECTIVES   As an EMT, you should be able to:

1. List the common types of injuries associated with swimming and diving accidents. (p. 491)
2. List, in correct order, the methods to use when attempting to reach a patient in the water. (pp. 491–492)
3. State the basic order of care procedures for patients who are near-drowning victims. (p. 492)
4. Describe the techniques of resuscitation applied to the near-drowning victim. (pp. 492–493)
5. Describe, step by step, how to turn a patient

in the water and place him on a long spine board. (p. 494)
6. State the basic care procedures for diving accident victims with possible neck or spinal injury. (pp. 493 and 495)
7. Describe two special types of problems faced when dealing with patients who have had scuba diving accidents and tell what should be done for each type of problem. (pp. 495–496)
8. Describe basic ice rescue procedures. (pp. 496–497)

SKILLS   As an EMT, you should be able to:

1. Evaluate a patient who is the victim of a swimming or diving accident.
2. Solve the basic problems faced in reaching the patient in water- and ice-related accidents.
3. Apply resuscitation skills and other basic life

support measures to the near-drowning patient and to the diving accident victim.
4. Work as a member of a team to turn a patient in the water and to place him on a long spine board.

TERMS you may be using for the first time:

Air Embolism – gas bubbles in the bloodstream.

Asphyxia (as-FIK-si-ah) – to suffocate from lack of air.

Decompression Sickness – the "bends"; nitrogen is trapped in the body's tissues, possibly finding its way into the bloodstream.

Laryngospasm (lah-RING-go-spaz'm) – spasms of the larynx set off when water passes the epiglottis.

Mammalian Diving Reflex – a reaction that occurs when the face is submerged in cold water. Breathing is inhibited, the heart rate slows, and major blood flow is sent to the brain, heart, and lungs.

ACCIDENTS INVOLVING THE WATER

WARNING: *Do not* attempt a water rescue unless you have been trained to do so and are a very good swimmer. Except for shallow pools and open, shallow waters with uniform bottoms, the problems faced in water rescue are too great and too dangerous for the poor swimmer and untrained person to attempt. If this bothers you—having to stand by not being able to help—then take a course in water safety and rescue. Otherwise, if you attempt a rescue, you will probably become a victim yourself rather than the person who rescues and provides care.

Drowning and Near-Drowning

Drowning is immediately brought to mind when one hears of water-related accidents. This is a valid association, since drowning must be the number one consideration in terms of water-related accidents. Even if the first problem faced by a person in the water may be an injury or a medical emergency, the danger of drowning becomes the first concern.

The process of drowning begins as a person struggles to keep afloat in the water. He gulps in large breaths of air as he thrashes about. When he can no longer keep afloat and starts to submerge, he tries to take and hold one more deep breath. As he does, water may enter the airway. There is a series of coughing and swallowing actions, and the victim involuntarily inhales and swallows water. As water flows past the epiglottis, it triggers a reflex spasm of the larynx. This **laryngospasm** (lah-RING-go-spazm) seals the airway so effectively that no more than a small amount of water ever reaches the lungs. Unconsciousness soon results from hypoxia.

About 10% of the people who drown die from true asphyxia, or simply suffocation from the lack of air. In the remaining victims, the person attempts a final respiratory effort and draws water into the lungs, or the laryngospasms subside with the onset of unconsciousness and water freely enters the lungs. What happens next depends on whether the victim is in fresh water or salt water.

In fresh-water drowning, the water washes away a chemical found on the inner surface of the alveoli (surfactant). This chemical is needed to maintain the elasticity of the lungs. As it is washed away, the alveoli collapse and air exchange is no longer possible (see atelectasis, pp. 174–175). Ventricular fibrillation (or some other lethal heart arrhythmia) occurs. This heart action is lethal and is probably the cause of death in many fresh-water drownings.

In salt-water drownings, water is taken from the bloodstream and moved into the lungs, causing pulmonary edema to develop. As much as one-fourth of the total blood volume may be lost as fluids move into the lungs. Hypoxia becomes a major problem. Death is often the result of the hypovolemic shock that occurs with circulatory collapse.

The initial care procedures will be the same, regardless of the type of water causing the accident. Transport of the near-drowning patient should not be delayed. As an EMT, you should start using the term *near-drowning*. Obviously, if the patient is breathing, coughing up water, he has not drowned but nearly drowned. This is only part of what we mean as near-drowning. If a victim has "drowned" in layperson's terms, he is not necessarily biologically dead. Resuscitative measures may be able to keep the patient biologically alive long enough for more advanced life support measures to be used to save the patient's life. Only when sufficient time has passed to render resuscitation useless is the victim truly drowned.

The phrase *"sufficient time"* has a different meaning today when applied to clinically dead patients. The concept of 4 to 6 minutes is no longer valid for some cases of cold-water near-drowning

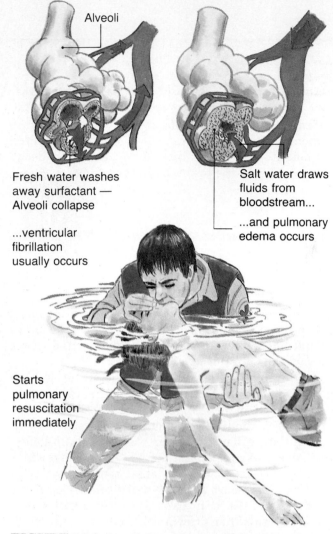

Alveoli

Fresh water washes away surfactant — Alveoli collapse

...ventricular fibrillation usually occurs

Starts pulmonary resuscitation immediately

Salt water draws fluids from bloodstream...

...and pulmonary edema occurs

FIGURE 18.2–1. **Salt water and fresh water have different effects on the body. The initial care procedures are the same. Begin pulmonary resuscitation as soon as possible.**

and hypothermia. We now know that patients in cold water can be resuscitated after 30 minutes or more in cardiac arrest. Once the water temperature falls below 70°F, biological death may be delayed. The colder the water, the better are the patient's chances for survival, unless hypothermia produces lethal complications. More will be said about this later in the chapter.

Water-Related Injuries

Many different types of injuries occur on, in, or near the water. Boating, waterskiing, diving board, and scuba diving accidents can produce fractured bones, bleeding, soft tissue injuries, and airway obstruction. Automobiles may come to rest in the water, with the passengers receiving the same types of injuries normally associated with motor vehicle accidents.

However, this type of accident is made more complex by the presence of the water, and, in some cases the additional cold.

A medical emergency may take place while someone is in the water or on a boat. Knowing how the accident occurred may give clues to help detect medical emergencies. As with all patients, the patient survey and interview may be critical in deciding the procedures followed when providing care.

An EMT must consider how accidents occur. Learn to associate the problems of drowning to scenes other than the pool and the beach. Remember, bathtub drownings do happen. Only a few inches of water are needed for the adult to drown. Even less is required for an infant.

As an EMT, remember to look for the following when your patient is the victim of a water-related accident:

- Airway obstruction—This may be from water in the lungs, foreign matter in the airway, or swollen airway tissues (common if the neck is injured in a dive). Spasms along the airway may be present in cases of near-drowning.
- Cardiac arrest—Often related to respiratory arrest or occurring before the near-drowning.
- Signs of heart attack—Through overexertion, the patient may have greater problems than obvious near-drowning. Some untrained rescuers are fooled into thinking that chest pains are due to muscle cramps produced during swimming.
- Injuries to the head and neck—These are expected to be found in boating, waterskiing, and diving accidents, but they are also very common in swimming accidents.
- Internal injuries—While doing the patient survey, stay on the alert for fractured bones, soft tissue injuries, and internal bleeding (which may be missed during the first stages of care).
- Hypothermia—The water does not have to be very cold and the length of stay in the water does not have to be very long for hypothermia to occur (in some cases of near-drowning, the patient may have a better chance for survival in cold water).
- Substance abuse—Alcohol and mind-altering drug abuse are closely associated with adolescent and adult drownings. Elevated blood alcohol levels have been found in over 30% of drowning victims. The screening for drug abuse has not been as extensive as that done for alcohol, but research indicates that

mind-altering drugs are a contributory factor in many cases in certain areas of the country.

Emergency Care for Water-Related Accidents

Reaching the Patient

Unless you are a very good swimmer and trained in water rescue, *do not* go into the water to save someone. Such training is available from the American Red Cross and the YMCA in the form of water safety and rescue courses.

The basic order of procedures for a water rescue is to REACH AND PULL, THROW, TOW, and, as a last resort, GO into the water.

When the patient is responsive and close to shore or poolside, begin the rescue by holding out an object for him to grab; then **PULL** him from the water. When doing this, your position must be secure to avoid being pulled into the water. Of all the items that could be used for such a rescue, line (rope) is considered the best choice. If no line is available, use a branch, fishing rod, oar, stick, or other such object. Remember that a towel, blanket, or even an article of your own clothing can work quite well. In cases in which there is no object near at hand or conditions are such that you may have only one opportunity to grab the person (e.g., strong currents), position yourself flat on your stomach and extend your hand or leg to the patient (not recommended for the nonswimmer). Again, make certain that you are working from a secure position.

Should the person be alert, but too far away for you to reach and pull from the water, **THROW** an object that will float (Figure 18.2–2). A personal flotation device (PFD or lifejacket), or ring buoy (life preserver) is best, if available. The primary course of action is to throw anything that will float and to

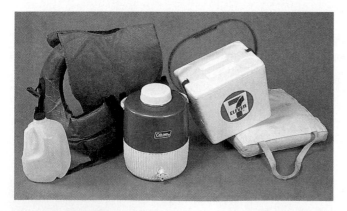

FIGURE 18.2–2. Throw the patient any object that will float.

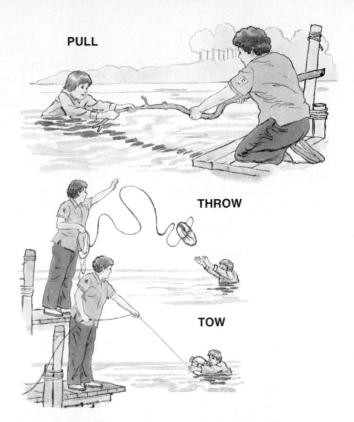

FIGURE 18.2–3. If you can, REACH AND PULL the patient from the water. If this fails, THROW him anything that will float and try to TOW him from the water.

do so as soon as possible. Buoyant objects that may be at the typical water-related accident scene include foam cushions, plastic jugs, logs, plastic picnic containers, surf boards, flat boards, large beach balls, and plastic toys. Two empty, capped, plastic milk jugs can keep an adult afloat for hours. Inflatable splints can be used if there is nothing at the scene that will float.

Once the conscious patient has a flotation device or floating object to hold onto, try to find a way to **TOW** him to shore (Figure 18.2–3). From a safe position, throw the patient a line or another flotation device attached to a line. If you are a good swimmer and you know how to judge the water, wade out to no deeper than your waist should you find it necessary to cut down the distance for throwing the line. You must be wearing a personal flotation device and have a safety line that is secured on shore.

In cases in which the near-drowning victim is too far from shore to allow for throwing and towing, or the patient is unresponsive, you may be able to **GO** by boat to the patient. *Do not* attempt this if you cannot swim. Even if you are a good swimmer, wearing a personal flotation device while in the boat is REQUIRED. In cases in which the patient is conscious, tell him to grab an oar or the stern (rear end) of the boat. You must exercise great care when helping the patient into the boat. This is even more tricky when in a canoe. Should the canoe tip over, stay with the canoe and hold onto its bottom and side. Most canoes will stay afloat.

If you take a boat to the patient and find that he is unresponsive, you can conduct a quick primary survey from your position in the boat and look for obvious signs of neck or spinal injury before trying to pull him from the water. Of course, this is a judgment call. Should conditions be such that you may lose the chance to grab the patient, then these emergency care procedures must be delayed until after you have the patient safely in the boat.

When reaching and pulling, throwing, and towing fail and a boat is not at the scene, you can **GO** into the water and swim to the patient. YOU MUST BE A GOOD SWIMMER, trained in water rescue and lifesaving.

Care for the Patient

You may have to provide care for patients who are out of the water when you arrive, in the water when you arrive but rescued by others, or in the water when you initiate care. When needed, begin PULMONARY RESUSCITATION without delay. CPR will not be effective if the patient is still in the water.

Do not be surprised to find resistance to the ventilations you attempt to provide to the near-drowning patient. You will probably have to apply more force than you would for other patients. Be sure that no foreign objects are in the patient's airway (obstruction may be due to laryngospasms). Remember, you must provide air to the patient's lungs as soon as possible.

A patient with water in the lungs usually will have water in the stomach. If there is enough water in the stomach, there will be added resistance to your efforts to provide pulmonary resuscitation or the interposed ventilations of CPR. Since the patient may have spasms along the airway, or swollen tissues in the larynx or trachea, you may find that some of the air you provide will go into the patient's stomach. Remember, the same problem will occur if you do not properly open the airway or you are too forceful in providing ventilations. Current American Heart Association guidelines do not call for you to attempt to relieve water or air from the patient's stomach. Doing so could drive materials from the stomach into the patient's airway.

Humans have something in common with many other mammals: a process called the **mammalian diving reflex.** When a person dives into cold water, the body reacts to the submersion of the face. Breathing is inhibited, the heart rate slows (bradycardia), and a series of complex functions begin that shut off major blood flow to most parts of the body except the heart, lungs, and brain. Whatever oxygen remains in the blood supply is made available to the brain. The colder the water, the more oxygen we tend to divert to the brain. Therefore, for this reason, do not think that a near-drowning victim should not receive resuscitative care if he has not been breathing for 10 minutes or more. Many such patients have been resuscitated. Recent studies have shown that some fresh-water near-drowning patients have been resuscitated, without brain damage, after 30 minutes or more without breathing. The colder the water, the better the patient's chances. Infants and young children have the best chance for survival.

The Patient Rescued by Others

In all cases of water-related accidents, assume that the unconscious patient has neck and spinal injuries. When the patient is rescued by others while you wait, or is out of the water when you arrive, you should:

1. DO A PRIMARY SURVEY, protecting the spine as much as possible.
2. Provide pulmonary resuscitation, if needed, as soon as possible. Do not forget to check for airway obstruction. Protect yourself! Use a pocket face mask with one-way valve or bag-valve-mask unit.
3. Provide CPR, if needed, as you would for any patient in cardiac arrest.
4. If the patient has an open airway, adequate breathing, and a pulse, look for and control all profuse bleeding. Since the patient's heart rate may have slowed down, take a pulse for 60 seconds in all cold water rescue situations.
5. When resuscitative measures are needed, begin them immediately and continue throughout transport. Initial and periodic suctioning may be needed. The near-drowning patient receiving pulmonary resuscitation or CPR should be transported as soon as possible. For all other patients . . .
6. Cover the patient to conserve body heat and complete a SECONDARY SURVEY. Uncover only those areas of the patient's body involved with the stage of the survey. Care for any problems or injuries detected during the survey, in the order of their priority.
7. Provide care for shock, administer a high concentration of oxygen, and transport the patient as soon as possible. Stay on the alert

for fluids in the mouth that will require suctioning. When transport is delayed and you believe that the patient can be moved to a warmer place, do so without aggravating any existing injuries. *Do not* allow the near-drowning patient to walk.

Information from the scene and while en route supplied to dispatch or the medical center is critical in cases of near-drowning. The staff needs to know if this is a fresh- or salt-water drowning and if it took place in cold or warm water. They also need to know if the drowning is related to a diving accident. You may be asked to transport the patient to a special facility or to a center having a hyperbaric chamber when decompression therapy is needed.

The Patient with Possible Spinal Injuries

Injuries to the cervical spine are seen with many water-related accidents. Most often, these injuries are received during a dive or when the patient is struck by a boat, skier, or ski. Even though cervical spine injuries are the most common of the spinal injuries seen in water-related accidents, there can be injury anywhere along the spine.

When a patient is unconscious, you may not be able to detect spinal injuries. In water-related accidents, you are to **ASSUME** that the unconscious patient has neck and spinal injuries. Should the patient have head injuries, also assume that there are neck and spinal injuries. Keep in mind that a patient found in respiratory arrest or cardiac arrest will need resuscitation started before you can immobilize the neck and spine. Also, realize that you will not be able to carry out a complete survey for spinal injuries while the patient is in the water. Take care to avoid aggravating spinal injuries, but do not delay basic life support. Do not delay removing the patient from the water if the scene presents an immediate danger. When possible, keep the patient's neck rigid in a straight line with the body's midline. Use the *jaw-thrust* for pulmonary resuscitation.

If the patient with possible spinal injuries is still in the water and you are a good swimmer, able to aid in the rescue, secure the patient to a long spine board before removing him from the water. Steps for this procedure are shown on Scan 18.2–1. This type of rescue requires *special training* in the use of the spine board while in the water. This rigid device can "pop up" very easily from below the water surface. Make certain that you know how to control the board and how to work in the water.

Pulmonary resuscitation can begin while the patient is in the water. CPR requires that the patient be out of the water, in a boat, or on land. There is some debate over the value of beginning CPR in the water when the patient is on a long spine board. There is no evidence to prove that this will be effective, and the procedure will probably slow down the rescue and increase the risk to the rescuers.

NOTE: Be realistic when dealing with near-drowning patients. Many of these patients cannot be resuscitated and will have already drowned. Even when you provide the best of care, some patients will die. However, you must try to resuscitate the patient. There is no way that you will be able to decide if the patient can or cannot be resuscitated. Do your best, to the level of your training. Successful resuscitation is possible!

Diving Accidents

Diving Board Accidents

Water-related accidents often involve injuries that occur when individuals attempt dives or enter the water from diving boards. In the majority of these accidents, the patient is a teenager. Basically the same types of injuries are seen in dives taken from diving boards, poolsides, docks, boats, and the shore. The injury may be due to the diver striking the board or some object on or under the water. If an improper dive is made, injury may result from impact with the water.

Most diving accidents involve the head and neck, but you will also find injuries to the spine, hands, feet, and ribs occurring in many cases. Any part of the body can be injured because of the odd position that the diver may be in when he strikes the water or an object. This means that you must perform *both* the primary and secondary surveys on all diving accident patients unless you are providing life support measures. Do not overlook the fact that a medical emergency may have led to the diving accident.

Care for diving accident patients is the same as for any accident patient, if they are out of the water. Care provided in the water and in removing the patient from the water is the same as for any patient who may have neck and spine injuries. Remember, assume that any unconscious or unresponsive patient has neck and spinal injuries. There can be delayed reactions with patients having spinal injuries. Compression along the spine may cause a patient with no apparent injuries to suddenly exhibit indications of nerve impairment. Often this begins as a numbness or tingling sensation in the legs.

SCAN 18.2–1 WATER RESCUE—POSSIBLE SPINAL INJURY

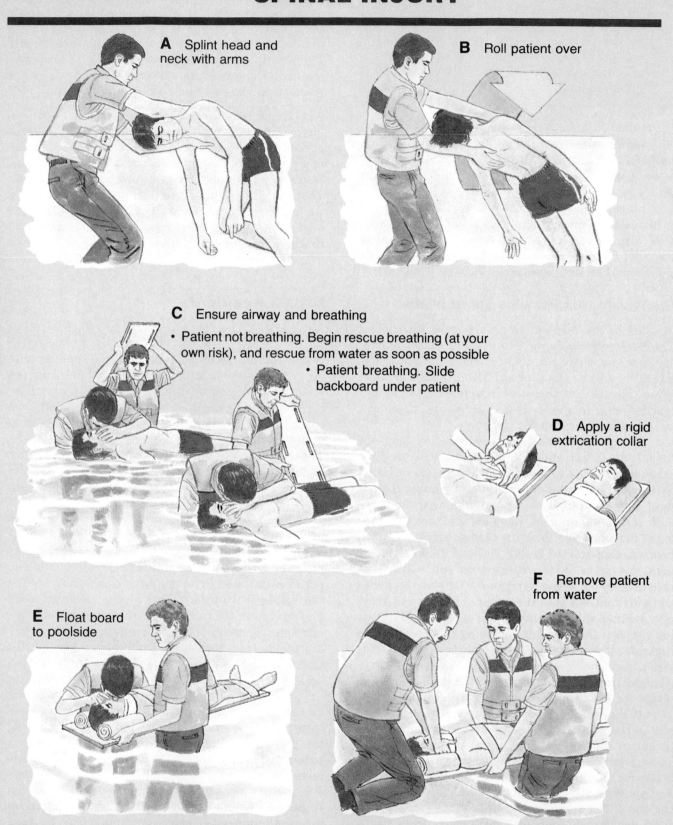

A Splint head and neck with arms

B Roll patient over

C Ensure airway and breathing

• Patient not breathing. Begin rescue breathing (at your own risk), and rescue from water as soon as possible

• Patient breathing. Slide backboard under patient

D Apply a rigid extrication collar

E Float board to poolside

F Remove patient from water

NOTE: The use of gloves and protective breathing masks or units is not practical for patients receiving in-water care.

Scuba Diving Accidents

NOTE: The National Diving Accident Network (DAN) was formed to assist rescuers with the care for underwater diving accident patients. The staff, available on a 24-hour basis, can be reached by phoning (919) 684–8111. Collect calls will be accepted for actual emergencies. DAN can give you or your dispatcher information on assessment and care and how to transfer the patient to a hyperbaric trauma care center.

Scuba (self-contained underwater breathing apparatus) diving accidents have increased with the popularity of the sport, especially since many untrained and inexperienced persons are attempting dives. Today, there are more than 2 million people who scuba dive for sport or as part of their industrial or military job. Added to this are a large number who decide to "try it one time," without the benefits of lessons or supervision. Well-trained divers seldom have problems. Those with inadequate training place themselves at great risk.

Scuba diving accidents include all types of body injuries and near-drownings. In many cases, the scuba diving accident was brought about by medical problems that existed prior to the dive. There are two special problems seen in scuba diving accidents. They are air emboli in the diver's blood and the "bends."

Air embolism is the result of gases leaving a damaged lung and entering the bloodstream. Severe damage to the lungs may lead to a spontaneous pneumothorax. Air emboli (gas bubbles in the blood) are most often associated with divers who hold their breath because of inadequate training, an equipment failure, underwater emergency, or when trying to conserve air during a dive. However, a diver may develop an air embolism in very shallow water (as little as 4 feet). The onset is rapid, with many of the symptoms and signs of a cerebrovascular accident. Expect to find any or all of the following:

- Personality changes
- The senses become distorted, often giving the impression that the patient is intoxicated on alcohol. Blurred vision is common.
- Chest pains
- Numbness and tingling sensations in the extremities
- Generalized or specific weakness—possible paralysis
- Frothy blood in mouth or nose
- Convulsions
- Rapid lapse into unconsciousness

- Sounds may be heard in the chest indicating gases are trapped outside the lungs, in the thoracic cavity.
- Respiratory arrest
- Cardiac arrest

An automobile accident victim trapped below water may take gulps of air from air bubbles held inside the vehicle. When freed, the patient may develop air emboli the same as the scuba diver.

The "bends" are really part of what is called **decompression sickness,** usually caused when the diver comes up too quickly from a deep, prolonged dive. The quick ascent causes nitrogen gas to be trapped in the body tissues. It is common for this trapped nitrogen to find its way into the patient's bloodstream. The onset of "bends" in scuba divers takes from 1 to 48 hours to appear, with about 90% of the cases occurring within 3 hours of the dive. Because of this delay, carefully consider all information gathered from the patient interview and reports from the patient's family and friends. This information may provide the only clues that will allow you to relate the patient's problems to a scuba dive.

Another way of detecting decompression sickness can be gained during the interview stage of patient assessment. Divers increase the risk of decompression sickness if they fly within 12 hours of a dive.

The symptoms and signs of decompression sickness include:

- Fatigue
- Deep pain to the muscles and joints (the "bends")
- Itchy blotches on the skin (mottling)
- Numbness or paralysis
- Choking
- Coughing
- Labored breathing
- Behavior similar to intoxication (e.g., staggering)
- Chest pains
- Collapse leading to unconsciousness
- Skin rashes that keep changing in appearance (in some cases)

NOTE: The well-trained scuba diver wears a preplanned dive chart. The chart may provide you with useful information concerning the nature and duration of the dive. This chart must be transported with the patient.

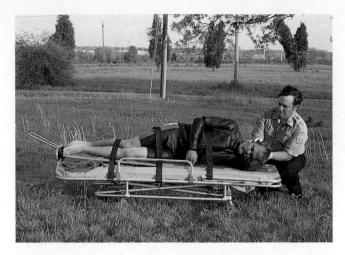

FIGURE 18.2–4. Positioning the patient after a scuba diving accident.

Do not try to diagnose if the patient's problem is air embolism or decompression sickness. Rapidly transport *all* patients with possible air emboli, decompression sickness, or possible pneumothorax. Alert dispatch or the medical center for specific directions concerning where to take the patient. You may be sent directly to a hyperbaric trauma center.

Be certain to maintain an open airway. Administer the highest possible concentration of oxygen by non-rebreathing mask. Manage shock, keeping the patient warm. Positioning of the patient is critical, to avoid damage to the brain by gas bubbles in the blood (Figure 18.2–4). As noted under the care for neck vein wounds (see p. 345), proper positioning will help trap gas bubbles in the right atrium. Place the patient on the left side in a head-down position (this should *not* be tried if there are any signs of neck or spinal injuries). Make certain that the patient's head is placed downward by slanting the entire body (about 15 degrees) rather than simply lifting the legs. Continue to monitor the patient. You may have to reposition the patient to ensure an open airway.

ACCIDENTS INVOLVING ICE

Every winter the deaths of numerous persons who fall through ice while skating or attempting to cross an ice-covered body of water are reported. Often, the ice-related accident scene becomes a multiple-rescue problem as individuals try to reach the victim and also fall through the ice.

There are several ways in which you can reach a patient who has fallen through ice:

- Flotation devices can be thrown to the victim.
- A rope in which a loop has been formed can be tossed to the victim. He can put the loop around his body so that he can be pulled onto the ice and away from the danger area.
- A spine board can be used to spread the rescuer's weight over a larger area to allow crawling out on the ice to reach the patient (this is very risky).
- A small, flat-bottomed aluminum boat is probably the best device for an ice rescue. It can be pushed stern first by other rescuers and pulled to safety by a rope secured to the bow (front end). The primary rescuer will remain dry and safe should the ice break. The patient can be pulled from the water or allowed to grasp the side of the boat.
- A ladder is an effective tool often used in ice rescue. It can be laid flat and pushed to the victim, then pulled back by an attached rope. The ladder also can serve as a surface on which a rescuer can spread out his weight if he must go on the ice to reach the victim. The ladder should have a line that can be secured by a rescuer in a safe position. Any one on the ladder should have a safety line.

When attempting to rescue the victim, remember that he may not be able to do much to help in the process. The effects of the cold water may slow his mental and physical capabilities in a matter of minutes.

You should *never* enter the water through a hole in the ice in order to find the victim. Whenever possible, *do not* work alone when trying to perform an ice rescue. If you must work alone, do not walk out onto the ice, but throw a rope, or push a ladder to the victim (Figure 18.2–5). *Never* go onto ice that is rapidly breaking. *Your best course of action will be to work with others, from a safe ice surface or the shore.* When there is no other choice, you and

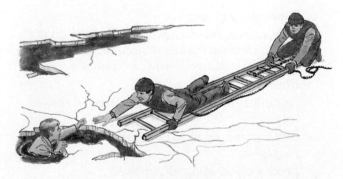

FIGURE 18.2–5. The safest way to perform an ice rescue is to work with others.

your fellow rescuers can elect to form a human chain to reach the victim. However, this is not the safest method to employ, even when all the rescuers are wearing PFDs and using safety lines.

Expect to find injuries to most patients who have fallen through the ice. Fractures to bones of the lower extremities are common. Hypothermia may be a problem. Remember that blanket wraps are of little help to patients with mild hypothermia. They require the slow application of an external source of heat. Transport *all* patients who have fallen through ice. The patient with severe hypothermia should not be rewarmed in the field.

There may be injuries that are difficult to detect and problems due to the cold that may be delayed. Keep ice-related accident patients as warm as possible without overheating. Treat for shock and transport as soon as possible.

SUMMARY

WARNING: DO NOT ATTEMPT A WATER OR ICE RESCUE UNLESS YOU CAN SWIM. DO NOT GO INTO THE WATER UNLESS YOU ARE A GOOD SWIMMER AND HAVE BEEN TRAINED IN WATER RESCUE.

Near-drowning is the number one problem faced in all water-related and ice-related accidents. However, injuries of all types do occur and medical problems may have caused the accident.

Often associated with water and ice accidents are airway obstruction, cardiac arrest, heart attacks, head and neck injuries, internal injuries, and hypothermia.

If the victim is in the water, try to REACH and PULL him out, THROW him something that will float, TOW him from the water, or take a boat to GO out to him. If you go by boat to reach the person in the water, you should be a good swimmer, wearing a personal flotation device. If you are trained to do so, GO in the water and swim to the patient.

Consider any unconscious patient to have neck and spinal injuries. Care for any patient already out of the water as required by your primary and secondary surveys and your interviews. Take special care to protect possible neck and spinal injuries.

When providing mouth-to-mouth resuscitation, use the jaw-thrust method to protect possible neck and spinal injuries.

If you are a good swimmer and have been trained in water rescue, you may be able to start pulmonary resuscitation while the patient is in the water. Remember, mouth-to-mouth resuscitation places the rescuer at risk. Starting CPR while the patient is in the water will probably be ineffective. If you are alone and must row a cardiac arrest victim to shore, delay CPR and reach shore as quickly as possible in order to provide uninterrupted, effective CPR.

Many patients in cardiac arrest can be resuscitated even after 10 minutes in arrest. If the water is cold enough, they may survive more than 30 minutes before reaching biological death.

When patients in water are found unconscious, work to apply an extrication collar and to place the patient on a spine board for floating and lifting from the water. Begin pulmonary resuscitation as soon as possible. Effective CPR is very difficult to perform while the patient is still in the water.

Whenever possible try to support the patient's back and keep the neck rigid and in line with the midline of the body.

All patients in water- or ice-related accidents should be managed for shock, kept as warm as possible without overheating, and given oxygen if needed. *Do not* allow the near-drowning victim to walk.

Dispatch or the medical facility will need to know if the accident was in fresh or salt water and if it was a cold- or warm-water accident. Obtain directions for transport. You may have to take the patient to a special facility.

Diving accidents usually produce head, neck, and spinal injuries. The hands, feet, and ribs also are frequently injured.

Scuba diving accidents may involve air embolism, decompression sickness, or pneumothorax. In cases of possible gas bubbles in the blood, look for unusual behavior, distorted senses, convulsions, sudden loss of consciousness, and signs of air being trapped in the chest cavity. For decompression sickness, expect a delayed reaction, difficult breathing, coughing, choking, chest pains, and changes in the appearance of the skin (blotches or changing rashes). Deep pains in the muscles and joints (the "bends") are typical symptoms in decompression sickness.

In cases of scuba diving accidents, if the possibility of air emboli exists, or if the patient is having the "bends," place the patient on the left side, with the body slanted to keep the head in a slight downward position. Provide the highest concentration of oxygen possible, provide care for shock, and keep the patient warm. Find out if the patient is to be taken to a special care facility.

If you must perform an ice rescue, you should be trained to do so and have the personnel and the equipment you will need. Try to throw a line or extend a pole to the victim. With the help of others, you may be able to reach the victim by crawling along a ladder.

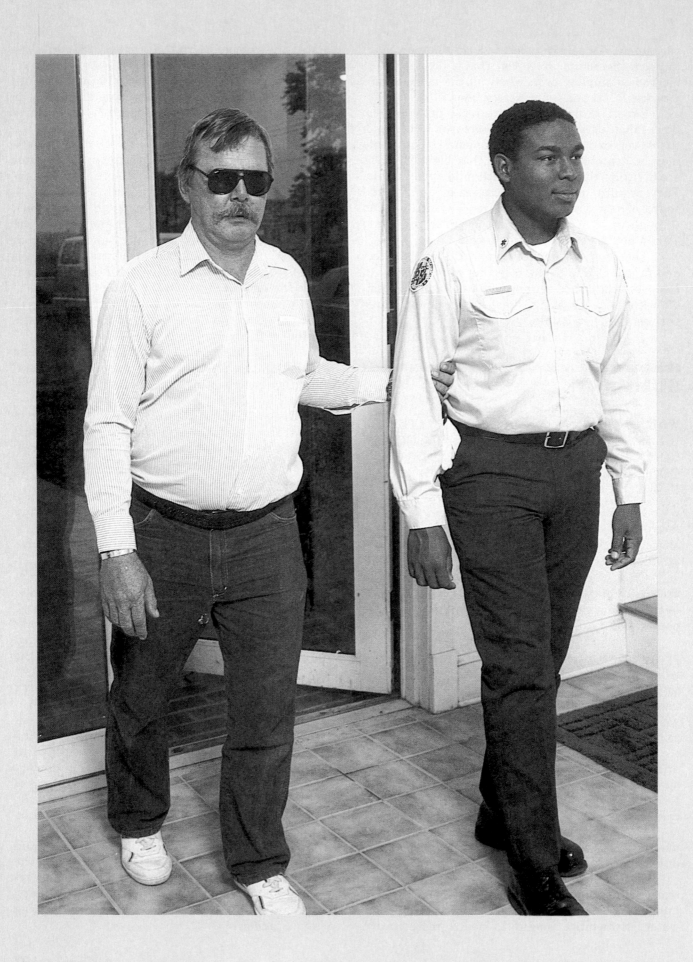

CHAPTER 19

Special Patients and Behavioral Problems

OBJECTIVES   As an EMT, you should be able to:

1. Define *special patient* in terms that apply to emergency care. (p. 500)

2. Define *personal interaction*. (p. 501)

3. Define *crisis* from a patient's point of view. (p. 501)

4. List FIVE things an EMT should do when trying to initiate crisis management procedures. (p. 501)

5. State the questions the EMT should ask himself in order to control emotional involvement. (p. 502)

6. List the general principles of communication. (pp. 502–503)

7. Describe the modifications in the approach to care that are made when dealing with elderly patients. (p. 503)

8. State how the EMT can establish communication with a deaf patient. (p. 503)

9. Describe how an EMT should modify care procedures when the patient is blind. (p. 504)

10. Describe what the EMT can do to establish communication with a non-English-speaking patient. (pp. 504–505)

11. Describe how the EMT should treat a disabled patient. (p. 505)

12. Describe how the EMT should establish communication with the developmentally disabled, mentally retarded, or confused patient. (p. 505)

13. Define *stress reaction, psychiatric emergency,* and *emotional emergency.* (p. 505 and p. 508)

14. State the special problems faced by the patient's family and the EMT in cases of sudden death. (p. 507)

15. State the special problems faced by the patient, his family, and the EMT in cases of terminal illness. (pp. 507–508)

16. List the indications of *EMT stress syndrome* (post-traumatic stress disorder). (p. 511)

17. List some ways the EMT can relieve stress. (pp. 511–512)

18. Make a list of the terms you can use to describe what you consider to be unusual behavior. (p. 508)

19. Describe how personal interaction relates to caring for patients in emotional emergencies. (p. 508)

20. List at least five injuries or medical problems that may produce behaviors similar to those

usually seen in a psychiatric emergency. (p. 509)

21. Describe the actions to be taken by the EMT if the patient is aggressive. (p. 509)
22. Describe the actions to be taken by the EMT when caring for a patient who may attempt suicide. (p. 510)
23. State the role of the EMT at the crime scene in relation to patient care and the chain of evidence. (p. 510)
24. Describe what special factors must be considered when providing care for the victim of assault, spouse abuse, and attempted murder. (p. 511)
25. Describe what special factors must be considered when providing care for the rape victim. (p. 511)

SKILLS As an EMT, you should be able to:

1. Use personal interaction with patients experiencing a crisis or having an emotional emergency.
2. Initiate crisis management when appropriate.
3. Conduct an efficient interview with elderly patients.
4. Establish effective communication with deaf patients.
5. Provide care and comfort for the blind patient.
6. Establish communication with the non-English-speaking patient.
7. Establish communications with the mentally retarded, developmentally disabled, or confused patient.
8. Determine if a patient is possibly having an emotional emergency.
9. Provide proper care for the aggressive patient and the patient about to attempt suicide, when your own safety is ensured.
10. Provide care at the controlled crime scene, helping to preserve the chain of evidence.
11. Provide care for rape victims that considers their emotional needs, privacy, comfort, and dignity.
12. Apply stress reduction techniques to prevent *EMT stress syndrome* (post-traumatic stress disorder).

TERMS you may be using for the first time:

Crisis – any event seen as a crucial moment or turning point in the patient's life.

Emotional Emergency – a situation in which a patient behaves in a manner that is not considered usual (typical) for the occasion. The patient's behavior is often not considered to be socially acceptable. The patient's emotions are strongly evident, interferring with his thoughts and behavior.

Personal Interaction – acting in a calm, professional manner to talk with the patient and listen to what he is saying so that emotional support can be provided and accepted.

THE MANAGEMENT OF SPECIAL PATIENTS

Every patient cared for by an EMS System is considered to be special. A patient is a *unique individual*, with his own specific problems and his own ways of attempting to deal with those problems. In emergency care, "*special patients*" are those who require care procedures that are modifications of what is usually done for most patients or care procedures that are specifically designed to deal with a particu-lar problem. Some of these patients have already been discussed. Caring for a child requires the EMT to modify interview and physical examination procedures. The same is often the case if you are dealing with a drug abuse or alcohol abuse patient. Care procedures change once a patient is thought to have a neck or spinal injury. This trauma patient becomes special, requiring the EMT to use procedures of evaluation and care specifically designed for the problem of spinal injury.

Most special patients require you to apply special communications skills and to provide emotional support. How you speak to a patient, what you say, how you express concern, how you listen, and how you indicate that you are listening are very important in special patient emergency care. Collectively, this is **personal interaction,** a skill that takes time to develop and is dependent on experience with many different types of patients.

The process of personal interaction is of great importance when dealing with children, the elderly, deaf patients, blind patients, drug and alcohol abuse patients, patients with emotional emergencies, victims of crime and sexual abuse, and patients who have been injured by friends or members of their own families. Each of these patients may believe that the emergency they are experiencing is a crisis and they are unable to control any aspect of the situation. Efficient personal interaction may be the key to providing effective total patient care.

The Concept of Crisis

When you are called to the scene of an accident or an illness, you consider the situation to be an emergency. To the patient, the situation may be a **crisis,** a crucial moment, or a turning point in his life. Bystanders may consider the emergency to be a crisis because they believe that what is happening is beyond their control and their ability to help.

Whenever a crisis exists, whether it is real or imagined, it must be managed. As an EMT, you will find yourself having to initiate the first steps in crisis management, working with the patient, his family, and friends to begin to deal with the crisis. Your professional attitude, your skills at personal interaction, and the emergency care you provide will help the patient begin to deal with the crisis.

Simply put, a person in a crisis is upset. Emotional stress is a part of every person's response to injury and illness. For the conscious and alert patient, this emotional stress can be a significant factor, steadily deteriorating the patient's physical and mental stability. If you provide emotional support, you can lessen the emotional stress. By doing so, you not only help the patient begin to cope with a problem but you also improve his mental and physical well-being. This could keep an emotional emergency from growing worse, or it may be the primary reason why a trauma patient relaxes and avoids developing serious shock.

Any emergency may require you to practice the skills of crisis management, so remember:

1. Look and act like a *professional* provider of emergency care.
2. Act in a *calm professional* manner. Be careful not to react to what may be meaningless insults or to overreact to what the patient may do or say. Remember, the patient in need of your care is not at his best.
3. Talk *with* the patient and *listen* to what he is saying. Let him know that you are there to help. This tells the patient you are concerned, he is important, and you recognize that he truly has a problem.
4. Avoid improper conversation. You should never offer a simple solution to the patient's problem or tell him that everything is going to be fine. You should avoid comparing yourself with the patient or telling the patient your own problems. You should not confront the patient and tell him that he is wrong or he is not making sense.
5. *Do* something for the patient. The idea that "actions speak louder than words" is very true in emergency care. Asking if the patient is in pain, controlling minor bleeding, or dressing a minor wound helps a patient deal with the emergency, even if he sees it as a crisis.

Be realistic in caring for patients. You do not have the time to sit down with the patient and go through every phase of crisis intervention, step by step. The sooner you can calmly transport the patient to a medical facility, the sooner he will receive medical care and crisis management help from trained and experienced professionals. Your role with the patient is not a problem-solving role but one of providing some emotional support and taking the patient to where the patient care team can assess his needs and problems. Never think for a moment that because you are good at working with people or good at solving your own problems you can assess patients' abilities to handle crises and determine what they must do to solve problems.

Even though the time you have with a patient is limited, the emotional support you can provide is of great importance. Let the patient know that you are concerned and that you care. To the best of your abilities and training, answer questions asked by the patient. Do not lie to the patient, but try to be positive about his situation.

It is important for the patient to believe that you are concerned about him because he is a person, not just an emergency care problem for you to solve.

Make certain that you use his name. When possible, do not just talk to the patient but have a conversation with him. Avoid spending most of the time talking with your partner. Some EMTs develop the habit of stopping conversation with the patient after the initial interview. They provide physical care, reserving conversation for other members of the EMS System. Emotional support cannot be provided unless you develop personal interaction with the patient.

Anyone wishing to become an EMT should be cautioned about becoming emotionally involved with what is happening at the emergency scene. This was discussed earlier in regard to illness and injury, but it also can be a major problem when dealing with patients who are under severe emotional distress. Unless you remain professional, you can become emotionally involved to the point where you cannot provide prompt and efficient care. Your approach to emotional involvement may also harm your emotional stability. Trying to deny that you are emotionally affected could lead to serious problems. Too many EMTs needlessly experience "burn out" in the profession because of this. More will be said about this later when we consider stress reactions.

When you arrive at the scene of injury, illness, or emotional crisis, make certain that you know why you are there and what you can do. Ask yourself, "Why am I here?" Odds are you were not at the scene when the problem occurred or began but rather that you were called to the scene. "Why was I called to the scene?" The call was made because someone was in need of emergency care. "What does the patient need?" The patient may need many things, ranging from love and understanding to a solution for a family problem. However, the patient also needs professional-level emergency care. "What am I trained to do as a professional?" You are trained to provide emergency care, including emotional support. Once people recognize that there is a problem and they start to do something, crisis management begins.

There may be one more question you find yourself asking. That question is, "Did I make a difference?" Almost certainly you did. The reaction of the patient may not have been what you had hoped for and there may not have been any "miracle" turnaround in terms of emotional stress, but you probably helped the patient at the scene and during transport. Your help was not only in terms of illnesses and injuries but also in his efforts to cope with emotional stress. The very fact that you transported the patient to a facility where he could gain access to total patient care must be considered a major helping factor. In addition to this, the emotional support that you provided before transfer at the medical facility probably helped the patient deal with the emergency and made him more receptive to the support offered by other members of the patient care team.

Problems with Communication

Difficulties in talking with people can be part of any patient–EMT interaction. However, EMTs report that they have experienced special problems when interviewing children, older patients, deaf patients, blind patients, patients who speak a foreign language, and patients who are mentally retarded, developmentally disabled, or confused. Interviewing children was covered in Chapter 15.

Communication is simply the act of having your thoughts, needs, and desires understood by another person. This is a two-way process, requiring a sender and a receiver, with the receiver responding back to the sender. The form of communication can be verbal (oral or written), nonverbal (using body language: eye contact, gestures, posture, touching, physical proximity), or a combination of both. As an EMT, you must strive to establish effective communications by:

- *Ensuring contact*—Never assume that you have established communications. Identify yourself, ask if you can help, and give the patient a chance to respond. You cannot develop a rapport with a patient unless you are sure, verbally or nonverbally, that he is listening and understands what you are trying to express.

- *Being direct*—Let the patient know that you are taking responsibility for his care. Explain what you are doing and what you are looking for. Answer his questions honestly. Do not play down the fact that injury or medical problems exist. Do not give the false hope that nothing is wrong or that everything is OK or will be OK.

- *Communicating at the proper level*—Make certain that you are using terms that are understood by the patient. ("Are you having trouble breathing?" is more meaningful than "Do you have dyspnea?") Ask questions so that the patient may participate in his own care and you can assess his understanding of the situation and what you are trying to do.

- *Using nonverbal communication skills*—Keep eye contact with the patient. Realize that some people may feel threatened by this eye contact and adjust such contact to suit the patient. Smile when appropriate. Stay relaxed enough so that the patient believes you have confidence in yourself and you have an interest in him and his problem. Allow the patient to be comfortable with you and your desire to help. Until then, give the patient his "space." Some people cannot tolerate the close physical proximity of another person until they have established some form of comfortable communication.

The Geriatric Patient

Never stereotype patients. Too often, we have a preconceived notion of how someone will act, think, and react. In many cases, a determining factor of how we believe someone will behave is based on age. As in any age group, late adulthood is made up of individuals of all types and personalities. A person is the total of all his experiences. Someone in late adulthood probably has experienced more than someone in early or middle adulthood. This means that you will find more variations with older patients. Realize that you will probably find that older patients approach things differently than you do.

You should provide care for the older patient as you would for any adult. Make certain that you properly identify yourself as an Emergency Medical Technician, trained to help. Although you may think that all "old people are alike," the older patient may think that all young people are alike . . . too inexperienced to help. Ask the patient to tell you his name and use it frequently, never resorting to "old timer," "pops," "grandma," or other such phrases. REMEMBER, you are talking with an adult, one who has faced other emergencies in life.

As people age, diminished hearing becomes a problem. A hearing problem may prove to be the reason why an older patient is unresponsive to your questions. Stay alert for the possibility of this problem, but do not assume that an older person cannot hear what you are saying. Avoid shouting whenever possible. Maintain eye contact, speaking directly to the patient. Begin by speaking in your normal voice. When in doubt, ask if he can hear you. If need be, speak directly into his ear.

Words become more important to people as they grow older. People in late adulthood spend more time thinking about what you say and what they are going to say in response. Younger people detect that the conversation is going more slowly than it does with members of their own age group. Consequently, the younger person assumes that the older individual is thinking more slowly or that something must go wrong with the mental processes as a person ages. This slowness in conversation has been shown to have nothing to do with the mind's slowing down. Older people, through experience, know that words can have many different meanings during a conversation and even more meanings after a conversation is over. They simply spend more time in conversation because experience has taught them to place a *high value* on what is said. Do not rush the conversation.

You will find that many older people are out of practice in the art of face-to-face communication. In today's society, it is easy for an older person to become isolated, with little opportunity for conversation. This will change the patient's speech patterns. You may find an older patient changing topics or seeming to drift slowly away from the topic of your question. In some cases, this may be due to changes in the circulation to the brain (arteriosclerosis—hardening of the arteries). However, more often than not, this is simply because the older patient is out of practice in the art of conversation.

As an EMT, you must remember that the older patient is an adult who has gone through other emergencies in his life. *Older people know what works for them.* After you are certain that there are no life-threatening problems, allow the older patient to have some control of the pace of the survey and interview.

If the patient's spouse or close friend is at the scene, think of yourself as having more than one patient. You may be caring for a husband while his wife of 30 years watches in total fear, believing that death will take him away. Provide emotional support to *both* individuals. Be watchful of partners and friends, for the stress of the situation could set off a heart attack, convulsion, respiratory problem, or some other medical emergency.

The Deaf Patient

It is unfortunate, but most of us have little experience in communicating with the deaf and almost no skills to help us talk to them. This is true even though there are several million totally deaf people in our country, and many more who have some serious degree of hearing loss.

Seldom will you find a deaf person embarrassed about being deaf. Usually, it is the person with normal hearing who has this problem during a conversation with the deaf person. Even experienced EMTs find themselves embarrassed when trying to interview a deaf patient. The embarrassment usually comes from being asked to do something new or to do something one cannot do well. However, sometimes the uneasy feelings are due to guilt, as if the EMT had done something to cause the person's deafness. The deaf individual does not blame you for his deafness.

Remember that any patient might not be able to hear you. He may be able to speak clearly but still not be able to hear. In most cases, a deaf person will tell you that he is deaf or point to his ear and shake his head to indicate, "No, I cannot hear." Some patients may try to speak to you in sign, using their hands and fingers to make communicating gestures. When in doubt, write out, "Are you deaf?" on a card or piece of paper.

Once you are aware of the patient's deafness, see if the patient can read lips. Either write this out or ask him, "Can you read lips?" When speaking to the lip-reading deaf patient, make certain that your face is in bright light (use a flashlight if you have to) and speak slowly, but without distorting how you would normally form words. When you ask a question, point to your mouth to alert the person to the fact that he will have to read your lips. Never turn away from the deaf person while you speak.

Many deaf people cannot read lips or find the process to be very difficult in an emergency. Your best methods of communication will be through writing and using gestures. If you point to an area on your body and make a face as if you are in pain and point back to the individual, he will usually understand your question. If you are examining the patient, point to your own body before you attempt to do something to his body.

Throughout the entire care of a deaf patient, try to remain face to face and keep direct physical contact (touching). Hold his hand, keeping one of your hands free to gesture or to gain his attention by a gentle tap on the shoulder. Point out the arrival of additional help or other events that may have gone unnoticed.

Some deaf persons can speak clearly, some can speak in a voice that may take a little practice to understand, and others may not be able to speak at all. If the patient cannot speak, use written communication. Should the deaf patient be able to speak, listen very carefully to what he is saying. If you cannot understand something that has been said, do not pretend to understand. This could be a serious mistake in gaining information and patient confidence. Always indicate that you do not understand by shaking your head in an obvious "no" gesture.

The Blind Patient

Blind people are seldom embarrassed by their blindness. Again, it is the inexperienced person trying to communicate with the blind who usually becomes embarrassed. Think for a moment. Why should it be difficult to converse with a blind person? After all, he can hear what you are saying and he is usually very aware of the world around him. Many EMTs claim that the survey and interview of blind patients are really not much different from those of sighted patients. If you remember to tell the blind patient what you are going to do before you do it, if you keep voice and touch contact throughout the period of care, and if you keep the blind person informed of what is happening around him (e.g., the source of strange noises, the arrival of additional help), you will find little extra difficulty in caring for the blind patient.

Try to remember three things when dealing with the blind:

• *Do not* shout or speak loudly. Being blind does not mean the person cannot hear.
• *Do not* change the words you would normally use in speaking to a patient. People often become upset if they use the words "see" or "look" when they are with a blind person. Blind people also use these words. Your blind patients will know that you are not trying to embarrass them.
• Keep in contact through speech or touch.

Should you have to move a blind patient who can walk on his own, lead him while he holds onto your arm. The best placement for this patient would be standing slightly behind you, off to your side. Alert the blind patient of steps and other hazards. Never push the blind patient, always lead him (Figure 19–1).

The Non-English-Speaking Patient

Establishing patient confidence and carrying out a useful patient assessment can be extremely difficult if your patient does not speak English. If a bystander can be of help, use him to help you communicate with the patient. If no such help is on hand, point to yourself and say your name. Let the patient see your patch or badge. Try to find out your patient's name. Usually, if you point to yourself and say your name and then point to the patient, he will understand and respond with his name. Point to the part of a patient's body you need to touch or examine. Use gestures to indicate there may be pain or to ask if there is pain. Throughout the entire process, speak to the patient. He may understand more English than is at first apparent.

If you are an EMT whose service area includes communities of non-English-speaking individuals, learn a few simple phrases to help you gain patient confidence and provide emergency care. In many cases, those persons who live in the community would welcome the opportunity to help you and other EMTs learn their language as it applies to the emergency

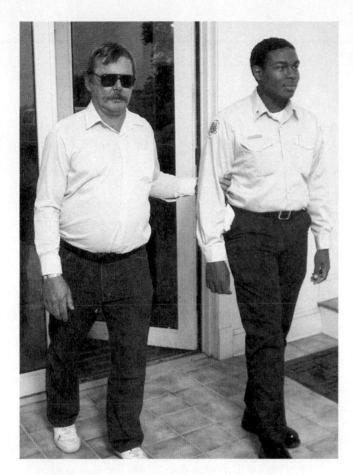

FIGURE 19–1. A blind person is led, not pushed.

situation. Table 19–1 is a guide to allow you to work with others in developing the needed foreign language skills for your area. Additional help may be sought from the American Red Cross, which has a multilanguage book for the EMT.

The Disabled Patient

The typical disabled patient will have an orthopedic or neurologic disability. This type of patient can present special problems in physical assessment since it is difficult to determine injury to a body part that does not function properly or will not respond to neurologic tests. When caring for the physically disabled trauma patient, you will have to *assume* injury, provide care accordingly, and transport so a physician can make the proper determination of the patient's problem.

In regard to communication, very little is different for interacting with the physically handicapped. Do not avoid questioning the patient about his handicap. Use the terms *handicap* and *disability*. Never use the terms *cripple*, *crippled*, or *lame*.

Let the physically handicapped patient do what he can for himself. If something is appropriate for the nonhandicapped patient to do, then it is appropriate for the handicapped patient who can do the task.

Not all handicaps involve body movement and functions. Some patients are handicapped by mental retardation or developmental disabilities. There will be times when this is easy to detect. At other times you may not be able to tell if these disabilities may be the cause of the patient's behavior or if you are dealing with a "normal" patient who is somehow confused. When dealing with a patient who is confused or may be mentally retarded or developmentally disabled, you should:

1. Begin by speaking to the patient as you would to any patient in his age group.
2. Ask questions and evaluate the patient's response. This will help you determine:
   - Patient understanding
   - If you are using terms at the appropriate level
   - If you need to reexplain anything that you have told the patient
3. Listen carefully to the patient, reassessing his level of understanding.
4. Slow the pace of the conversation. This type of patient often gives delayed responses to questions and actions.

Behavioral Problems

In an emergency, most patients will behave in a manner considered to be "normal" for the situation. However, using the term *normal* forces you to imply that certain medical and philosophical judgments have been made. It is more appropriate to say that the patient is behaving in a "typical" manner, or behaving "as expected." This provides you with a very broad method of initially assessing patients. Based on your training and experience, you will be able to classify patients, simply stating that they are either "behaving as expected" or "behaving in an unusual manner."

At the scene of accident or illness, you may have to provide care for:

- Stress reactions
- Emotional emergencies
- Psychiatric emergencies

Stress Reactions

An emergency is a stressful situation. You should expect that most distressed patients will display cer-

Table 19–1.

English	French	German	Spanish	Italian
Hello	Bonjour	Guten Tag	¡Hola!	Pronto
My name is	Je m'appelle	Ich heisse	Mi nombre es (Me llamo)	Mi chiamo
I am an emergency technician	Je suis infirmier de salle d'urgence	Ich bin Medizin-Techniker für Notfälle	Yo soy un enfermero (una enfermera)	Sono un tecnico del pronto soccorso
I am here to help you	Je suis ici pour vous aider	Ich bin hier um Ihnen zu helfen	Estoy aquí para ayudarle	Sono quí per aiutarLa
Do you understand?	Comprenez-vous?	Verstehen Sie?	¿Me comprende?	Comprende?
I do not understand	Je ne comprends pas	Nein, ich verstehe Sie nicht	¡No comprendo!	No, non capisco
What is your name?	Comment vous appelez-vous?	Wie heissen Sie?	¿Cuál es su nombre? (¿Cómo se llama usted?)	Come si chiama (Lei)?
Mr.	Monsieur	Herr	Señor	Signore
Mrs.	Madame	Frau	Señora	Signora
Miss	Mademoiselle	Fräulein	Señorita	Signorina
Are you sick?	Etes-vous malade?	Sind Sie krank?	¿Está usted enfermo? (enferma)	È malato(a)?
Are you injured?	Etes-vous blessé?	Sind Sie verletzt?	¿Está usted herido? (herida)	È ferito(a)?
Are you a diabetic?	Etes-vous diabétique?	Sind Sie zuckerkrank?	¿Es usted diabético? (diabética)	È diabetico(a)?
Yes/No	Oui/Non	Ja/Nein	Si/No	Si/No
Do you have a doctor?	Avez-vous un docteur?	Haben Sie einen Hausarzt?	¿Tiene usted un doctor?	Ha un medico di famiglia?
Who is your doctor?	Qui est votre docteur?	Wer ist Ihr Arzt?	¿Quién es su doctor?	Chi è il Suo dottore?
Where do you live?	Où habitez-vous?	Wo wohnen Sie?	¿Dónde vive usted?	Dove abita (Lei)?

Translation by Denise Guback, Translator, University of Illinois-Champaign.

tain emotions such as fear, grief, and anger. These are typical **stress reactions** at the accident scene and common reactions to serious illness.

The emergency patient initially displays a mixture of emotions. As you begin to take control of the situation and start to treat him as an individual, his reactions to stress tend to change. In the vast majority of cases, *personal interaction* will inspire confidence in your ability to help. The patient will begin to calm down and may even begin to feel that he can cope with the emergency.

The inexperienced EMT may rush the patient interview, becoming too concerned with the physical assessment. True, it is critical that an EMT detect and attempt to correct life-threatening problems, but these aspects of care must be accomplished in a calm professional manner.

As you begin an interview, be prepared to spend some time with the patient. Let him know that you are there to help. If you rush through conversations, the patient may think he has lost control of the situa-

tion. He also may believe that you are concerned about the problem, not him as an individual.

Whenever you care for a distressed emergency patient who is acting in a manner you would expect:

1. Act in a calm manner, giving the patient time to gain control of his emotions.
2. Quietly and carefully evaluate the situation.
3. Keep your own emotions under control.
4. Honestly explain things to the patient.
5. Let the patient know that you are listening to what he is saying.
6. Stay alert for sudden changes in behavior.

Basically, you are applying *crisis management* techniques to help the patient deal with stress. If the patient does not begin to interact with you, or

English	French	German	Spanish	Italian
What is your telephone number?	Quel est votre numéro de téléphone?	Was ist Ihre Telefonnummer?	¿Cuál es el número de su teléfono?	Qual 'è il Suo numero di telefono?
Do you have a priest? (Rabbi? Minister?)	Avez-vous un prêtre? (un rabbin, un pasteur?)	Haben Sie einen Priester? (Rabiner, Pastor)	¿Conoce usted un sacerdote? (Rabbi, pastor)	Conosce un sacerdote? (rabbino, ministro?)
I need to examine you for injuries	J'ai besoin de voir vos blessures	Ich muss Ihre Verletzungen untersuchen	Tengo que examinarle para ver si tiene heridas	Devo esaminarLa per eventuali ferite.
Is that all right?	D'accord?	Sind Sie damit einverstanden?	¿Está de acuerdo?	Va bene?
I am going to measure your blood pressure	Je vais prendre votre tension artérielle	Ich nehme Ihren Blutdruck	Le voy a tomar la presión arterial	Devo misurarLe la pressione del sangue
I need to adjust your clothing	J'ai besoin d'ajuster vos vêtements	Ich muss Ihre Kleider lockern	Necesito quitarle (sacarle) parte de la ropa	Devo sbottonarLe il vestito
I am going to touch the injury site. It may cause pain. Do you understand?	Je vais toucher l'endroit de vos blessures. Cela peut faire mal. Comprenez vous?	Ich werde Ihre Wunde anfassen. Es wird Ihnen vielleicht weh tun. Verstehen Sie?	Le voy a tocar la parte herida y tal vez le cause dolor. ¿Me comprende?	Ora devo toccare la ferita. Potrebbe sentire dolore. Comprende?
Does this hurt?	Cela fait mal?	Tut es weh?	¿Le duele ésto?	Fa male?
Can you move your foot? (leg, hand)	Pouvez-vous remuer le pied? (la jambe, la main?)	Können Sie Ihren Fuss bewegen? (Ihr Bein, Ihre Hand)	¿Puede usted mover el pie? (la mano)	Può muovere il piede? (la gamba, la mano?)
Can you feel that?	Pouvez-vous sentir cela?	Fühlen Sie das?	¿Siente usted cuando le toco?	Sente dove La tocco?
I have finished the examination. Can I go ahead with emergency care procedures?	J'ai terminé mon examen. Puis-je continuer avec les premiers soins d'urgence?	Ich habe die Untersuchung durchgeführt. Kann ich jetzt mit der Erstversorgung beginnen?	He terminado de examinarle. ¿Puedo comenzar con los tratamientos de emergencia?	Ho finito la visita. Posso cominciare con le procedure d'emergenza?
Don't move!	Ne bougez pas!	Bleiben Sie still!	¡No se mueva!	Non ti muovere!

if he does not calm down, then you must assume that he is having a problem of a more serious nature than an expected stress reaction.

Sudden Death   Any emergency involving patient death produces a great amount of stress for the patient's family, bystanders, and the EMTs. Death without warning due to trauma or medical causes can produce intense reactions from the patient's family. Be prepared to deal with any or all of the following:

- Grief
- Denial
- Guilt
- Anger and hostility
- Crying, sometimes completely uncontrollably
- Hysteria
- Physical illness, including nausea, vomiting, and fainting.

There may be little you can do for the family and bystanders since you will probably be initiating basic life support. Tell the family what you must do. Keep them informed of the care being provided. Do not offer false hope.

Watch for indications that the stress of the situation is affecting you or your partner (use the "buddy system"). Indications of immediate stress reactions include physical illness, feelings of helplessness, anger, guilt, or frustration, avoidance of the fact of death, using "gallows" humor, or taking a cold (hyperclinical) approach to the emergency.

Terminal Disease   The process of dying can produce more stress on a family than the loved one's death. The patient and the family may display one of the following responses to the dying process:

- Denial—the person is not going to die
- Bargaining—if God lets the person live, or if someone will cure the patient, something

will be done in return (e.g., "If you let me live, I will dedicate my life to help feed the starving people of the world.")

- Anger
- Depression
- Acceptance

Usually the early reaction to the news of terminal illness is denial, with acceptance being the last stage. It is not unusual for the family to lag behind the patient in response to the dying process by at least one stage.

When providing care for the terminally ill, ask the patient how long he has known that he is dying. Find out if he is prepared for death or if he wishes to speak to someone about death and dying. The emergency department staff should be informed of the request so that a referral can be made. The family should be asked the same questions. Do not isolate the family from the patient. Should death occur while the patient is under your care, and there is a "living will" request not to resuscitate, provide or withhold basic life support according to local protocol (see Chapter 1, p. 21).

Emotional Emergencies

We use the term **emotional emergency** to indicate situations in which the patient is not acting as expected, displaying his emotions to a point where they interfere with his thoughts and behavior. However, he is responding to people around him and is not showing any indications of being dangerous to himself or to others. He may be extremely frightened compared with most patients in a similar situation. Perhaps he is unable to calm his excited state after an accident. At first, you may assume that the patient's behavior is a typical stress reaction to the emergency. However, the patient does not calm down during the interview and the beginning of care procedures. You must reconsider the stress of the emergency and try to establish some level of *personal interaction*. Once this is tried and the patient's behavior is still a concern, you may conclude that his behavior appears to be unusual.

Each patient is a unique individual. His behavior may be related to an undetected illness or injury, or he may simply need more time to cope with the emergency and respond to your efforts. What you observe could be part of a mental illness, but you cannot draw such a conclusion. At this point in assessment, all you can say is that you believe the patient is acting in an unusual manner and seems to be experiencing some kind of emotional emergency.

The emotional emergency may be an independent problem, or it may be the result of an accident, injury, illness, or disaster. As an independent event, the display of emotions may be due to a psychiatric problem. Before you jump to the conclusion that the patient has a "psychological" problem or that the patient is "abnormal," consider your role as an EMT. A simple observation and some knowledge of terminology is not enough for you to reach any immediate conclusions. You must be able to rule out stress reactions, physical injury, and illness.

As an EMT, use terms such as *excited*, *fearful*, *confused*, *overactive*, *unpredictable*, *agitated*, *aggressive*, and *detached*. Avoid terms such as *mentally ill*, *psychotic*, *phobic*, *paranoid*, *manic*, *neurotic*, and *schizophrenic*. Also avoid going to the other extreme by using terms such as *crazy*, *nuts*, *wacko*, *loony*, and other nonprofessional words often associated with mental illness and emotional problems.

Often, the patient characterized as having an emotional emergency simply needs more time to cope with the stress of an emergency. *Personal interaction* is your main course of action for a patient with an emotional emergency. Usually for this type of patient, you will have to spend more time talking with him and listening than would be necessary for most patients undergoing a stress reaction. The patient may improve if he thinks that he has more control over the situation. Give him time to answer your questions. When appropriate, let him decide which arm will be used for the blood pressure determination and how he would like to be positioned for transport.

Psychiatric Emergencies

As an EMT, you cannot make a medical diagnosis. Therefore, you cannot declare a patient to be mentally ill, or state that he is having a psychiatric emergency. Once you believe that apparent illness, injury, stress reaction, and emotional emergency are not the sources of a behavioral problem, then, in basic EMT-level emergency care, you can *assume* that a patient may be having a psychiatric emergency if he:

- Tries to hurt himself
- Tries to hurt others
- Withdraws, no longer responding to people or to his environment
- Continues to express rage and hostility
- Continues to act depressed, sometimes crying and expressing feelings of worthlessness
- Apparently wishes to take no actions to help himself or to allow himself to be helped

This can only be an assumption, since you cannot detect all possible illness and injury in the field.

Also, the patient may not be responding to your attempts at personal interaction at the scene, but he may respond very well to your efforts or those of another professional once he arrives at the medical facility.

If you arrive at the scene to find a patient displaying violent behavior, you cannot rule out illness or injury as the cause; however, you should immediately assume that this is a possible psychiatric emergency and not a stress reaction.

The assessment and care of the patient having a possible psychiatric emergency requires you to stay calm and to act in a strictly professional manner. Carefully observe the patient; listen to what he is saying. Detect whatever symptoms and signs are evident, making certain that throughout the entire process of care that you can eliminate the possibilities of head injury, stroke, insulin shock, drug reactions, high fever, and other such medical emergencies.

Talk to the patient and let him talk to you. Make certain that he knows that you hear what he is saying. *Do not* threaten the patient or argue with him. Try to provide reassurance by telling him that you are there to help. Speak in a calm, direct manner, keeping eye contact whenever possible. Again, this is the method of *personal interaction*, your first line of action in trying to care for a patient having a possible psychiatric emergency. *Do not* leave the patient alone. Unless life-threatening illness or injury requires you to act differently, spend additional time talking with the patient. You are the first professional to begin both the physical and mental health care of the patient. The more *reassurance* you can provide for the patient, the easier it will be for the emergency department staff to continue with his care.

Aggressive Behavior

Aggressive or disruptive behavior may be caused by trauma to the brain and nervous system, metabolic disorders, stress, alcohol, drugs, or psychological disorders. Sometimes you will know that you will be dealing with an aggressive patient from the information you receive from dispatch. Other times the scene may provide quick clues (e.g., drugs, unclean conditions, broken furniture). Neighbors, family members, or bystanders may tell you that the patient is dangerous or that he is angry. The patient's stance or how he has positioned himself in the room may give you an early warning of possible violence. On rare occasions, you may start with an apparently calm patient who quickly turns aggressive.

When a patient acts as if he may hurt himself or others, your first concern must be YOUR OWN SAFETY.* In such cases, alert the police. *Do not* isolate yourself from your partner or other sources of help. MAKE CERTAIN THAT YOU HAVE AN ESCAPE ROUTE. Should a patient become violent, retreat and wait for police assistance. *Do not* put yourself in danger by taking any action that may be considered threatening by the patient. To do so may bring about hostile behavior directed against you or others.

Always be on the watch for weapons or indications that the patient wishes to use physical force. Stay in a safe area until the police can control the scene.

DO NOT TRY TO RESTRAIN A PATIENT UNLESS IT IS LEGAL FOR YOU TO DO SO. In most localities, an EMT cannot legally restrain a patient, move him against his will, or force him to accept emergency care. You cannot restrain a patient even when his family asks you to do so. The restraint and forcible moving of patients is within the jurisdiction of law enforcement officers. Once the patient is under control, the police can order you to transport the patient to the appropriate medical facility or, in some states, the order can come from a physician. In some jurisdictions, a physician can order a patient to be restrained; however, the physician is not empowered to order you to do this if taking such actions may place you in danger.

REMEMBER: Each EMS System has its own standard operating procedures for dealing with aggressive patients and patients who may hurt themselves or others. Always follow your local guidelines.

DO NOT TRY TO RESTRAIN A PATIENT UNLESS THERE IS SUFFICIENT PERSONNEL TO DO THE JOB. You must be able to ensure your safety and the safety of the patient.

If you help the police or a physician restrain a patient, make certain that the restraints are *humane* restraints. Handcuffs and plastic "throwaway" criminal restraints should not be used because of the soft tissue damage they can inflict. Initially, the police may have to use such restraints; however, these types of restraints can be replaced with leather cuffs and belts (these are not authorized for use in all states). An ambulance should carry leather cuffs, a waist-size belt, and at least three short belts. Soft restraints for the wrists and ankles can be made from gauze roller bandage.

Do not remove police restraints until you and the police are certain that the gauze or leather restraints will hold the patient. Once soft restraints are placed on a patient, *do not* remove them, even

---

* **WARNING:** Some patients may act adversely to your uniform, believing you to be a law enforcement officer.

if the patient appears to be acting rationally. The patient may display the same aggressive behavior after the restraints are removed. The removal of restraints is the responsibility of the emergency facility staff and the police.

NOTE: Never secure a patient to a stretcher in a position that will not allow the patient to be turned in case of vomiting. The patient must be secured so that his wrists and ankles remain secured but his body can be turned.

Attempted Suicide

Each year in this country, some 20,000 people commit suicide. Many more suffer both physical and emotional injuries in suicide attempts. Anyone may become suicidal if emotional distress is severe, regardless of age, sex, race, ethnic origin, or economic and social status.

People attempt suicide for many reasons, including the death of a loved one, financial problems, a terminated love affair, poor health, loss of esteem, divorce, fears of failure, and alcohol and drug abuse. They attempt to end their lives by any of a variety of methods. Most often, they try to do so with sedatives and hypnotic drugs. Less common are those individuals who attempt to die by hanging, jumping from high places, ingesting poisons, inhaling gas, wrist-cutting, self-mutilation, or stabbing or shooting themselves.

Providing Care for Attempted Suicide Whenever you find yourself having to care for a patient who has attempted suicide or is about to attempt suicide, your first concern is your *own* safety. Make certain that the scene is safe and the patient does not have a weapon. *Unless you are a trained law enforcement officer following standard operating procedures, you have no business dealing with someone who has a weapon.* Should you see that a patient has a weapon, withdraw carefully, if you can. Do not frighten him with any sudden moves. Do not threaten him in any way. Above all, do not try to be a hero and attempt to seize the weapon.

If you cannot withdraw to safety, your best course of action is to try to talk to the individual and keep him engaged in conversation until additional help arrives. Again, do not do anything foolhardy that will result in your getting hurt.

For all cases of attempted suicide, make certain that the police are alerted. If your own safety is secure, establish visual and verbal contact with the patient as soon as possible. Talk with the patient in a calm, professional manner, making certain that the patient knows you are listening to what he is saying. Make no threats and offer no indication of using force.

Do not argue with the patient or criticize him. Do not point out that he is not making sense or that he contradicts something he said earlier in the conversation. Never joke about the patient's situation. Ask if you can help. If he seems in doubt, tell him that you wish to help him. Ask if he is hurt or in pain. Stay calm and keep face-to-face contact whenever possible. Keeping the patient in a conversation is probably the only way you can get him to relax and grant you his confidence.

Do not leave the patient alone. Unless there is a physical emergency that must be cared for, sit down and spend some time with the patient. Talk with him, but do not try to direct all the conversation. It is likely that the patient has a need to tell you his story. You should provide reassurance, but be certain to avoid pity. As you gain the patient's confidence, tell him that you wish to help and explain what questions he must answer and what must be done as part of the physical assessment. Let the patient know that you think it would be best if he went with you to the hospital. Tell him how you need his cooperation and help. If the patient indicates increasing fear or aggression, do not push the issues of the examination or transport. Instead, try to reestablish the conversation and give the patient more time before you tell him again that going to the hospital is a good idea.

Victims of Crime

As in all aspects of emergency care, your first concern must be your own safety. If you arrive at the scene and a crime is in progress or the criminal is still active at the scene, *do not* attempt to provide care. Wait until the police arrive and they tell you that the scene is safe.

Your first priority at the controlled crime scene is to provide emergency care. While doing so, you must try to preserve the *chain of evidence* that will go from the crime scene to the courtroom. Touch only what you need to touch. Move only what must be moved to protect the patient and to provide proper care. Do not use the telephone unless the police tell you that you may do so. Unless you have police permission, move the patient only if he is in danger or if he must be moved to provide proper care (e.g., to a hard surface for CPR).

When approaching a crime victim, clearly identify yourself by name and state that you are an Emergency Medical Technician arriving to help. This may prove to be very important if you are the first person to see the victim since the crime. The patient may be very frightened and disoriented. He could think that you are the criminal still at the scene or returning to the scene.

Do not burden the patient with questions about the crime. Keep to your duties involving the care of the patient, remembering that one of the most important things you can do when caring for the victim of a crime is to provide emotional support and reassurance. Be prepared for the patient to show outrage or disbelief. The patient may withdraw, become depressed, or display rage or hysteria. Severe reactions often are noted in cases of assault and attempted murder.

In cases in which you are called to the scene of a domestic dispute, wait for police assistance. Domestic disputes are dangerous calls because the people involved often act unpredictably. The call to have you respond was probably placed because someone has been beaten or injured by some act of violence. If the violent person is still on the scene, he may turn his aggression toward you. Sometimes, it is the victim of the aggressive act who will attack you because you are an outsider interfering with a family matter.

If the crime is rape, do not wash the patient nor allow the patient to wash. Ask the patient not to change clothing, use the bathroom, or take any liquids or food. To do so may destroy evidence. Obviously, you may not physically prevent anyone from doing these things, but you can explain why such activities may break the chain of evidence. The patient will probably cooperate and follow your requests. *Emotional support* is a must in cases of rape. The privacy, comfort, and *dignity* of the patient must be considered from the beginning of care. The degree of future emotional problems faced by the rape victim may well depend on how the patient is initially treated by the professionals who respond to help.

REMEMBER: As an EMT, you may have a legal duty to report any situation in which injury is a possible result of crime or was received in the commission of a crime. In most localities, you should not leave the crime scene until the police give you permission to do so.

EMT STRESS SYNDROME

Caring for patients suffering from stress reactions and other behavioral emergencies can cause you to suffer delayed reactions to stress (post-traumatic stress disorder). This is commonly know as *EMT*

stress syndrome. It is much the same as any stress syndrome, except it is associated with the stress generated at accidents, medical emergencies, disasters (see Chapter 20), incidents involving death, crime scenes, and emotional and psychiatric emergencies. This syndrome can lead to "burn out."

Some of the indications of stress syndrome include:

- Irritability
- Feeling unappreciated
- Fatigue
- Inability to concentrate
- Lack of enthusiasm, perhaps wanting to quit
- Insomnia or nightmares
- Loss of appetite and/or interest in sexual activities
- Decrease in social activities
- Alcohol or drug abuse
- Avoidance of change and new ideas
- Physiologic reactions, such as nausea, symptoms and signs of ulcers, colitis, frequent headaches, and muscle aches

The ways to prevent, reduce, or stop the development of stress syndrome include:

- Peer support—Talk with other EMTs about situations that bother you.
- Family and friend support—Let them know the "what, how, and why" of any incident that was stressful.
- Be willing to show and accept your emotional reactions.
- Seek professional counseling—If your EMS System does not offer this service, see your family doctor. Since stress syndrome is a part of every level of health care, odds are that your physician will know how to help you or refer you to someone for help.
- Assess the reasons why you became an EMT and why you have continued to be one. Is being an EMT still what you want? Before deciding to leave the service, talk with a professional counselor about other solutions.
- Take some time off—Take a vacation from being an EMT. A little change in schedule or environment may help you sort out your problems and give you a better perspective of your role as an EMT.

- Use continuing education to reestablish your confidence.
- Keep things in perspective—Not everything about being an EMT is serious. Keep a sense of humor. Do not become hyperclinical.

Your family and friends can be of significant help if they understand what you do and the stress it can cause. Do not expect a great deal of help if you have let being an EMT lead to family problems (e.g., feelings of being ignored or prioritized, no family activities). The members of your family and your friends can be of help if you plan time to share with them and make certain that you do not reprioritize them for the sake of your career or your interest in emergency medical service. Let them share in what you do by inviting them to your station or squad (show off new equipment and procedures). Have them participate in social activities that are part of being an EMT. Tell them what you do and why you believe it is important to both you and the community. Help them receive training in first aid, basic life support, or first responder–level care or to become EMTs if they so desire.

Stress syndrome is best prevented by sharing your experiences with family and friends and with other health care providers who understand what you do.

SUMMARY

Special patients are those who require modified approaches to care and special procedures designed to consider a specific problem. Often, the EMT will find that these patients require an extra effort in terms of communication and emotional support.

What is an emergency to you may be a crisis for the patient. The patient sees the event as a crucial moment or a turning point in his life. For such situations, crisis management must be initiated by the EMT.

Your main method to employ in crisis management is personal interaction. You have to act in a calm, professional manner, talking with the patient and listening to what he says. As you provide emotional support, you must do something for the patient. Providing even the simplest of care measures is useful in helping to manage the crisis.

The stress of helping others in a crisis can affect your own emotional stability. Remember that you have been trained to provide professional-level emer-

gency care. The patient may need many things, one of which is your professional help. Keep in mind that you do make a difference.

Problems with communication can occur when providing emergency care. When dealing with elderly patients, remember that patients in late adulthood have faced other emergencies. The elderly patient may set a pace of the interview and examination different from yours. The older patient knows what works, so allow him some control. During the entire process of care, it is important to remember that words have more meaning and value to the older patient. Never assume that an older patient cannot hear you or think clearly. Keep in mind that you will have to provide emotional support for the patient, family, and friends.

Always make certain that a patient is able to hear you. If the patient is deaf, establish this fact and then find out if the patient can read lips or if you will have to use writing and gestures for communication. Try to maintain face-to-face contact with the deaf person.

When dealing with blind patients, do not raise your voice. Talk as you would to any patient, and keep both verbal and physical contact with the patient throughout all stages of care.

Some of your patients may not speak English. Use the help of bystanders whenever you can. If there is a large community of non-English-speaking people in your locality, learn some of the basic words and phrases needed to help you provide emergency care.

Most patients will exhibit stress reactions during an emergency. They tend to calm down as you interact with them and begin care. Emotional emergencies are those in which the patients have an emotional reaction to a situation that you do not consider to be usual. In many cases, such patients simply need longer to cope with the emergency than do most patients. Any patients who act as if they wish to hurt themselves or others are having a psychiatric emergency. This classification also applies to patients who continue to express withdrawal, rage, hostility, depression, or an unwillingness to take any action.

Personal interaction is your best approach as you provide care. Make certain that the problem is not due to an injury or medical emergency. You must eliminate the possibilities of head injury, stroke, insulin shock, drug reactions, high fever, and other problems.

In cases involving psychiatric emergencies, maintain a professional manner and talk calmly with the patient. Do not leave the patient alone. Indicate that you are listening to what he says and let him tell his story. If the patient is violent, wait for police assistance. Never try to provide care for a patient who has a weapon. Do not try to illegally restrain or transport the patient.

Provide care for the victims of crime only when the crime scene is controlled and you are certain of your own personal safety. Preserve the chain of evidence whenever possible. Touch only what you need to touch, and move the patient only when care or safety requires him to be moved.

Emotional support is a must in cases of rape. The privacy, comfort, and dignity of the patient must be carefully considered from the beginning of care. Explain to the patient why she should not change clothing, wash, go to the bathroom, or take any liquids or food.

As an EMT, you may have a legal duty to report any situations in which injury may be due to crime or may have been received during the commission of a crime.

In all special care situations, your safety comes first.

Learn to recognize the indications of EMT stress syndrome. Interact with your peers, family, friends, and professional counselors to prevent this syndrome or to stop it before it can lead to burn out and other problems.

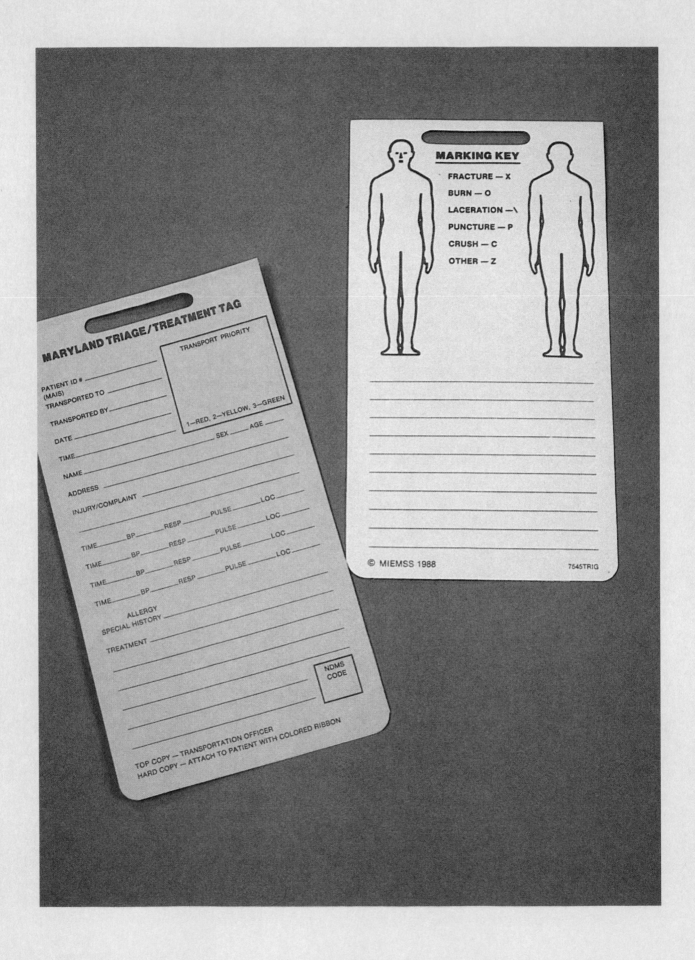

Triage and Disaster Management

WARNING: The procedures of patient assessment may bring you into contact with patient blood or body fluids. Be certain to wear protective latex gloves, and follow all local guidelines established to prevent the spread of disease.

OBJECTIVES   As an EMT, you should be able to:

1. Define *triage* and classify various illnesses and injuries as to priority. (pp. 516–517)
2. State when triage is needed. (p. 516)
3. List and describe the FOUR major steps of an initial triage plan to be performed by the first rescuers to arrive at a multiple casualty incident. (pp. 518–519)
4. Relate given signs to specific illnesses and injuries. (pp. 519–520)

5. Define *disaster* and *disaster plan*. (p. 520)
6. List and define the SEVEN periods (stages) of a disaster. (pp. 521–522)
7. Describe the impact of a disaster on EMS personnel and what can be done to reduce this impact. (p. 523)
8. Describe a model disaster scene operation. (pp. 523–525)

SKILLS   As an EMT, you should be able to:

1. Initiate and conduct triage for a multiple patient emergency.
2. Apply assessment skills to triage.

3. Provide triage, emergency care, and transport as defined by your locality's disaster plans.

TERMS   you may be using for the first time:

Disaster – any emergency involving illness and injury that taxes the resources of an EMS system.
Disaster Plan – a plan worked out in advance that describes how the various services will respond and

what they will do in cases of specific types of disasters in their locality.
Triage – a process used to sort patients in terms of priority for care and transport, based on the severity of illness and injury.

Gurgling: airway obstruction, lung disease, lung damage due to excessive heat

Coughing blood: chest wound, rib fracture, internal injury

- Blood Pressure (vital sign)

  High: chronic hypertension, head injury, severe pain, drug withdrawal

  Low: chronic hypotension, shock, internal bleeding, chest injury, drug abuse

- Skin temperature (vital sign)

  Cool, moist: shock, bleeding, heat loss, heat exhaustion

  Cool, dry: exposure to cold

  Cool, clammy: shock, heart attack

  Hot, dry: heat stroke, high fever

  Hot, moist: fever, infectious disease

- Skin color

  Red: high blood pressure, heat stroke, diabetic coma, minor burn

  Cherry red: carbon monoxide poisoning (rare, limited to late stages)

  White, pale, ashen: shock, heart attack, excessive bleeding, heat exhaustion, fright, insulin overdose, or insulin shock

  Blue: heart failure, airway obstruction, lung disease, certain poisonings

- Pupils

  Dilated, unresponsive to light: cardiac arrest, unconsciousness, shock, bleeding, heat stroke, use of certain types of drugs (LSD, uppers)

  Constricted: damage to the central nervous system, use of certain types of drugs (heroin, morphine, codeine)

  Unequal: stroke, head injury

  Lackluster: shock, coma

- State of consciousness

  Confusion: fright, anxiety, illness, minor head injury, alcohol or drug abuse, mental illness, shock, epilepsy, hypoxia

  Stupor: moderate to severe head injury, alcohol or drug abuse, stroke

  Brief unconsciousness: minor head injury, fainting, epilepsy

  Coma: stroke, anaphylactic shock, severe head injury, poisoning, drug or alcohol abuse, diabetic coma, heat stroke

- Paralysis or loss of sensation

  One side of body: stroke, head injury

  Upper limbs: spinal injury in neck

  Lower limbs: spinal injury along back

  Upper and lower limbs: spinal injury in neck and possibly along back

  No pain, obvious injury: spinal cord or brain damage, shock, hysteria, drug or alcohol abuse

Disasters

Fires, floods, hurricanes, earthquakes, and tornadoes come to mind when one thinks of a disaster. So, too, do airplane crashes, train wrecks, or any accidents in which many people are injured. To the EMS system, a **disaster** is any occurrence involving or having the potential to cause many injuries. To be a true disaster, the event must tax the resources of the local EMS system and rescue support systems.

To provide prompt and efficient care during a disaster, the personnel involved must be trained for such an event and have practiced the techniques and procedures to be used during the disaster. In addition, a **disaster plan** should be developed for each possible disaster that may occur within a community. A disaster plan worked out in advance will allow for all agencies, personnel, and support services to work together to meet the needs of the patients and the community. (See Figure 20–3.) When a disaster occurs, the EMS system personnel must know each aspect of disaster management:

- Who is in authority for the overall plan
- Who controls each aspect of the management of the particular disaster
- How is transportation and communication set up and regulated
- What needs to be done
- Where specific procedures should be done
- Who is needed to do a particular job or procedure
- What are the support services, where are they located, and how can they be reached
- Who are additional sources of help

The Phases of a Disaster— How People React

Any disaster can be divided into phases based on the way individuals and the community respond to it. The phases of a disaster are called periods. They can *vary* according to the type of disaster; however, most include the following:

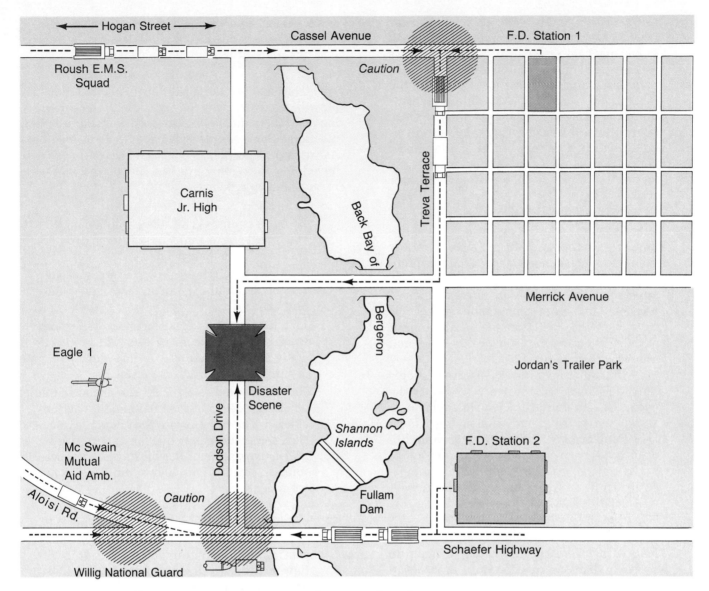

FIGURE 20–3. **Disaster management requires preplanning, involving all appropriate agencies.**

1. WARNING PERIOD—Some disasters give warning of their approach. When the onset of a disaster is sudden, as in earthquakes and airplane crashes, people may respond better to the sudden emergency than they do when warned in advance, even though their initial response after the disaster impacts may be more severe. Apparently, some individuals are not able to cope with the anxiety and apprehension that intensifies as a known disaster approaches. For these people, the warning phase is followed by a period of ALARM, not a period of action. During this phase, you may have to interact with "helpless" people, giving them specific tasks to do for their own safety and emotional stability.

2. THREAT PERIOD—This is a critical decision-making time for many individuals. They have to ask if the threat is real, and if so, when will the disaster materialize. A person may find himself thinking: "Will I be killed or hurt?" "Will my family be killed or hurt?" "Will I lose everything?" "Can I escape in time?" These and a host of other questions precipitate decisions that are important to survival. Making such decisions can bring about an emotional crisis for some people, particularly for those individuals who find day-to-day decision making to be difficult.

3. IMPACT PERIOD—When the disaster strikes, people may, at first, be stunned. Then they begin to realize its magnitude as as they see injury, death, and destruction. Some people panic, but this is rare. On the other hand, some wander aimlessly about, unable to cope with the problem or even to follow the directions of others. A few individuals begin to step forward after the impact period to assume leadership, and it is these few that the others follow after a disaster strikes.

4. INVENTORY PERIOD—During this phase of a disaster, people try to assess what has happened to them, producing a great variety of emotional responses. Depending on a number of factors, survivors may exhibit fear, anger, sorrow, depression, anxiety, apprehension, and other emotions. Most people start their recovery after feeling the impact of their inventory, but some carry emotional scars for their entire lives.

   Immediately after a disaster, people tend to feel isolated and overwhelmed by the event. Observers have noted that some men stand and stare, some women hug themselves and display a rocking motion, and children have been seen to display regressive behavior (e.g., an eight-year-old may temporarily act like a five-year-old). Many individuals try to engage themselves in some sort of purposeful activity.

5. RESCUE PERIOD—Once people begin to help with the rescue and start to clean up property damage, their feelings of isolation and being overwhelmed may begin to fade. During this post-disaster phase, the survivors help each other to cope. Emotional "shock" is still a problem, but in some people apathy and withdrawal are noted. Most of these individuals *begin* to overcome their problems once they join others in helping to rescue victims, provide comfort to others, and to reestablish shelter and other needs.

6. REMEDY PERIOD—The morale of survivors usually picks up during this period as they work together with rescue personnel to get the community back on its feet. A spirit of cooperation often prevails. The period of remedy is often the longest postdisaster phase, as reconstruction takes place.

7. RESTORATION PERIOD—In this final phase, the individuals of a community *regain the stability* that they enjoyed prior to the disaster. How long it takes for a community to reach *equilibrium* depends on the nature of the disaster, the degree of destruction, and the amount of help available.

Throughout the disaster, keep in mind that people will change the way they react, with some improving and others displaying progressively more severe reactions. Some people will have *delayed reactions*. As you assess people, realize that reassessment will have to be an ongoing process. As you interact with victims during a disaster:

- Be professional—This does not mean that you have to be formal, but stay alert to detect their problems and needs.
- Talk with victims—Always acknowledge their individual existence, fears, questions, and needs.
- Listen to victims—Reassurance often comes from having someone listen. This is especially true for victims who are near panic, argumentative, or overly active.
- Provide needed care—Both the physical and emotional needs of the victims must be considered. The more severe the emotional reaction, the greater the need for understanding and conversation. You will have to reassess injuries, medical problems, and emotional reactions.
- Provide food and drink—When possible, provide warm food and drink for all victims who do not have injuries or medical problems that contraindicate anything by mouth. This will have a calming effect, provide reassurance, and help you in your efforts to assume a leadership role.
- Design tasks for the victims—Be certain to give the active and overly active something to do. If you do not, these people may set out on their own and disorganize the disaster plan. Try to have those who are injury free but act helpless or dazed help others with simple tasks. If you do not, these patients may suffer severe withdrawal or depression that will require constant monitoring.
- Keep victims together—Until the scene is organized and communications are well established, keep the victims in groups. Use tasks, food and drink, and reason to keep people together. Explain that if everyone stays put, it will be easier to reunite families and loved ones. Do not let anyone believe that he is alone or a stranger during a disaster.

The Impact on EMS Personnel

During a disaster, emergency care personnel have to cope with their own fears and their worries about the safety of their families, friends, and property. Added to this emotional stress are the effects of seeing destruction, providing care for the injured and sick, and having to deal with the dead victims of the disaster. Throughout the entire emergency operation, emergency personnel often have to keep their emotions in check, trying to cope with the stress they are experiencing. Include the factors of exhaustion and exposure to environmental elements and you have the potential for severe emotional crises.

The problem of emotional disturbance in rescue workers was never given much thought in the past. Today, it is considered a real threat to mental health, enough so that crisis intervention teams who work with rescuers' problems are now part of most disaster planning. Three things are now done to help reduce stress on emergency personnel:

1. EMS personnel are given work schedules for the disaster operation. These schedules contain regular rest periods.
2. Rescue efforts are organized so that someone in authority can constantly watch rescuers for signs of emotional distress and physical fatigue. If a supervisor sees that one of the workers may be having emotional problems or is physically exhausted, he can require the worker to take a longer than usual rest period. Following the rest period, the worker can be assigned to a less stressful task.
3. Rescuers are encouraged to eat and sleep whenever they can and to engage in conversations with other workers. The talking helps, but individuals should avoid using "gallows humor" as an attempt to find a safety valve for dealing with stress. What seems to be harmless jokes about the disaster, fellow workers, and superiors may upset some workers at the time. Many rescuers report that this type of humor continues to bother them long after the disaster is over.

Remember that you can never fully predict how you will act in a disaster. If you are mentally prepared for what will happen in a disaster, and for what you will be doing during disaster operations, the chance that you will become an emotional casualty is reduced. Realize that you will do a more effective job as a provider of emergency care if you:

- Attend crisis intervention training programs.
- Participate as both rescuer and victim in disaster training programs.
- Know the forms of disaster most likely to strike your community.
- Know how your community's resources will be mobilized at the time of the disaster, and know what help is immediately available.
- Understand that there are limits to what a rescuer or an EMS system can do in a disaster.

Disaster Scene Operations

Each locality has its own standard operating procedures for disaster operations and multiple-casualty incidents. The following is a general *example* of the operations at a disaster scene (Fig. 20–4).

1. The first arriving ambulance is the command post, which should be stationed in a safe area. The EMTs on board then begin immediate triage of the injured, and the EMTs become the initial triage officers. It is important that this first arriving unit *does not* transport regardless of what has taken place. The ambulance is the command post with communications to hospitals, dispatchers, and all other emergency service units that will be arriving and in need of instruction. Supplies from this unit are to be used in the initial care of the injured. This unit will be replaced as other fire and rescue personnel set up a field command post.
2. Communications are established with hospitals, medical facilities, dispatchers, and other emergency services units. This requires a multichannel radio transmitter. Separate units for each channel in use may be needed for simultaneous communications.
3. The EMTs on the first ambulance to arrive automatically become triage officers. They continue this duty until a qualified triage officer arrives, for example, a physician from a nearby major medical facility. If a triage team arrives with this person, the EMTs can begin patient care; otherwise, they should continue to assist with triage.
4. Hazard control must begin as soon as possible. There must be close coordination between rescue personnel, EMTs, firefighters, and law-enforcement officers. If the scene is not safe, triage and patient care will have to be delayed.

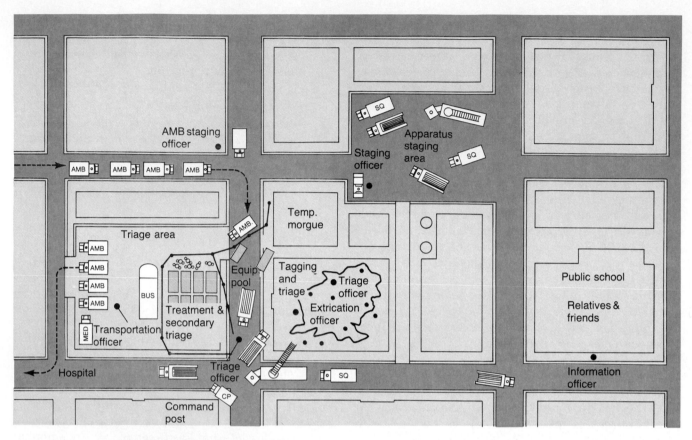

FIGURE 20–4. The disaster scene.

5. Extrication may be difficult or delayed. Those doing the extrication must work closely with the EMTs so that triage and care can begin as soon as possible and so that patients are not injured during disentanglement operations.

6. When possible, patients are removed from wreckage according to the severity of their injuries, but this is not always practical.

7. A triage point or points should be set up in a safe area. At least one of these triage points should be in the immediate area of the command post. Triage areas are to be located so that all patients are funneled through triage before they are taken to ambulances for transport.

8. A staging area is set up for incoming ambulances. These ambulances are not to go to the triage areas. This will reduce congestion and allow for quicker transport.

9. All ambulance drivers should stay with their vehicles. EMTs should report to the triage officer. When reporting, the EMTs should carry portable equipment with them, including trauma kits, spine boards, splints, folding stretchers, and other removable supplies and equipment.

10. The ambulance supplies and equipment should be placed in a supply pool near the treatment area. A rescue worker must be placed in charge of this equipment. When possible, ambulances can be directed to this equipment pool prior to reporting to their staging point.

11. Incoming EMTs should be assigned to patient care activities.

12. Volunteers can and should be used to help free EMTs, rescuers, firefighters, and police from tasks that take them away from their main duties.

13. A second triage area should be set up to determine the order of transport for treated patients. This area must be placed so that all patients go from initial triage and care through the transport triage. The patient must be brought through this second triage before ambulances are called from the staging area. This is also often called the *field hospital*.

14. Patients should be packaged for transport

and ambulances should be called, as needed, from the staging area.

15. The command post or central communications should determine the hospital to which a particular ambulance should go. When a hospital reaches its capacity, the command post can be notified.

16. Patients should be transported with an EMT providing care.

17. As ambulances discharge their patients at a medical facility, they need to call the dispatcher or command post to see if they should return to the scene. On returning to the scene, they should report directly to the staging area and let the command post know that they have arrived.

18. A special area should be set up to receive relatives and friends of the disaster victims. Someone must be placed in charge of this area and must make certain that only reliable information is passed on to those waiting to hear about friends and relatives. Emergency care should be available at the information center in case a friend or relative has a medical emergency.

19. Since dead victims will not be removed from the scene until all the injured patients have been transported, a temporary morgue should be established out of sight. Someone must stand guard to prevent unauthorized persons from disturbing the bodies.

SUMMARY

Triage is a method of sorting patients into categories for receiving care and transport. The sorting is done based on the severity of patients' illnesses and injuries.

Highest priority (immediate) includes respiratory arrest, airway obstruction and severe breathing difficulties, cardiac arrest (witnessed), life-threatening bleeding, severe head injuries (patient unconscious), open chest and abdominal wounds, severe shock, burns involving the respiratory tract, severe medical problems (including heart attack and stroke), unconsciousness, fractured cervical vertebrae (stabilize), joint fractures with no distal pulse, fractured femurs, and open eye wounds.

Secondary priority includes severe burns, injuries to the spine other than cervical, moderate bleeding, conscious patients with head injuries, multiple fractures, back injuries, stable drug overdose, and normal childbirth.

Low priority (delayed) includes minor bleeding, minor fractures and soft tissue injuries, moderate and minor burns, and obvious mortal wounds.

Most systems have a fourth category, obvious death.

A modified rapid triage such as the START plan can be used for multiple casualty incidents. Patients can be quickly assessed based on their ability to move, adequate respirations, adequate perfusion, and possible brain injury. Patients can be classified as *immediate*, *delayed*, and *dead*. Basic airway maintenance and the control of serious bleeding can be started during the triage process.

Patient assessment is very important during triage. Vital signs and other key signs are used. Pulse, respiration, blood pressure, skin temperature, skin color, pupils, state of consciousness, paralysis, and loss of sensation are used in making assessments.

A disaster is any emergency that taxes the resources of the EMS system. To be an effective EMT, you must be familiar with your local disaster plans. These plans indicate who is in authority, who controls and carries out certain duties, how communications and transportation will be done, what specifically must be done, what procedures are to be used, and what are the support services and other sources of help.

People react to a disaster in many different ways. Often, specific behavior can be associated with the period of the disaster. As an EMT you may have to give people directions and tasks for their own safety and emotional stability and help the survivors by assuming a leadership role. Remember that your own emotional health can be affected. Take needed rest periods and set aside time to talk with fellow rescue workers.

The disaster scene will need a command post, multichannel radio communications, triage points and areas for care, transport triage points, a staging area for ambulances, an equipment pool, an area to receive friends and relatives of the victims, and a protected area to be used as a temporary morgue.

REMEMBER: A disaster taxes the resources of the EMS system. Disaster management depends on all personnel performing the right task at the right time. If you are in the first ambulance to arrive, your actions during the first few minutes of operation may well influence the outcome of the disaster.

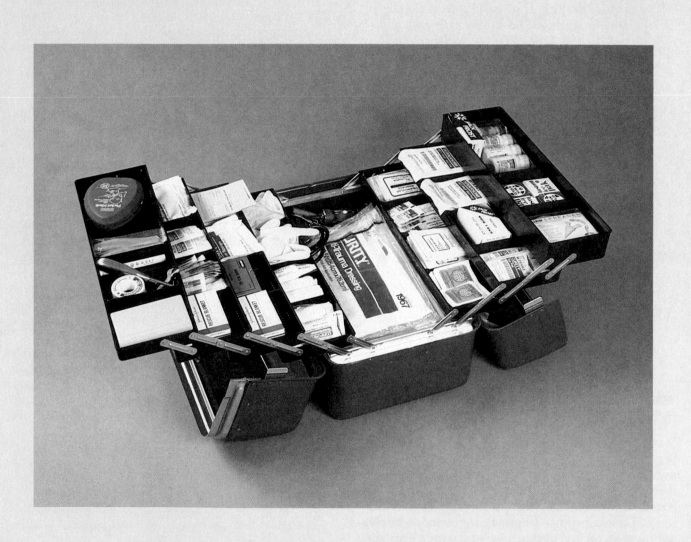

Preparing for the Ambulance Run

OBJECTIVES As an EMT, you should be able to:

1. List and give uses for the items that should be included in each of the following categories of supplies and equipment:
   - Basic supplies (p. 528)
   - Equipment for the transfer of patients (pp. 528–529)
   - Equipment for airway maintenance, ventilation, and resuscitation (p. 529)
   - Oxygen therapy equipment (p. 529)
   - Suction equipment (pp. 529–530)
   - Equipment for cardiac compression (p. 530)
   - Supplies and equipment for the immobilization of fractures (p. 530)

   - Supplies for wound care (pp. 530–531)
   - Supplies and equipment for the treatment of shock (p. 531)
   - Supplies for childbirth (p. 531)
   - Equipment for the treatment of newborns (p. 531)
   - Supplies for the treatment of acute poisoning (p. 531)
2. List the steps that should be included in a pre-shift ambulance inspection. (pp. 532–535)

SKILLS As an EMT, you should be able to:

1. Identify supply and equipment items carried on an ambulance.
2. Use the items carried on the ambulance during patient care activities.

3. Conduct a preshift ambulance inspection.

THE AMBULANCE

It is doubtful that anyone really knows when a wheeled conveyance was first used to move a sick or injured person from one place to another. "Body wagons" were used throughout medieval times, especially when thousands fell victim to a plague. As you can imagine, those conveyances were used to transport the dead, not the living.

During the Napoleonic Wars hand-drawn and horse-drawn carts were given the designation "ambulance" and used for the singular purpose of transporting wounded soldiers. Military leaders decided that it would be better to transport wounded soldiers to safe places behind front lines rather than risk the lives of physicians in the midst of the fighting.

Ambulances evolved from horse-drawn wagons to motor vehicles in 1906, and motorized ambulances were extensively used on the battlefields of France and Flanders during World War I.

From the conclusion of World War I until the late 1960s, hearses were traditionally used as ambulances because they were the only vehicles in which a person could be transported lying down. It is likely that ambulances would still be built on long wheel base passenger car chassis if it were not for a report made in 1966 on the state of pre-hospital emergency care. In *Accidental Death and Disability: The Neglected Disease of Modern Society* the need for ambulances better suited to the purpose of transporting sick and injured persons to medical facilities was detailed. The personnel of public and private agencies were inspired to establish and refine design criteria, and from their efforts have come guidelines for the manufacture of modern ambulances.

Ambulance Supplies and Equipment

Even though it is especially designed and constructed, an ambulance is only another truck if it does not have the proper equipment for patient care and transportation.

Following are lists of supplies and equipment that should be carried in an ambulance so that EMTs can provide the correct care for a variety of illness and injury situations. The lists are based on recommendations of the American College of Surgeons and the U.S. Department of Transportation.

Basic Supplies

The ambulance should be provided with linens and blankets that serve not only to protect patients and keep them warm but also to reduce the possibility of contamination (when used in sufficient numbers).

There should be:

- Two pillows
- Four pillow cases
- Four sheets
- Two spare sheets
- Four blankets (the number may vary according to local climatic conditions)

Certain items should be carried to assist in the care of a patient's personal needs.

- Six disposable emesis bags
- Two boxes of tissues
- A bedpan
- A urinal
- Four towels
- A package of disposable drinking cups
- Unbreakable containers of drinking water

Other basic supplies include:

- One package of wet wipes
- Four liters of irrigation fluid
- Four soft restraining devices (upper and lower extremities)
- One package of plastic garbage bags for waste or severed parts
- Latex disposable gloves
- Disinfectant cleaner

The following items should be carried for patient-monitoring activities:

- An adult sphygmomanometer kit with separate cuffs for average-sized and obese persons
- A pediatric sphygmomanometer kit with separate cuffs for children and infants
- A dual-head stethoscope
- Disposable skin temperature indicating devices

Equipment for the Transfer of Sick and Injured Persons

Three carrying devices should be included.

1. The *wheeled ambulance stretcher* is designed so that a sick or injured person can be trans-

ported in the prone, supine, or recumbent position. Also called a cot or gurney, the wheeled stretcher should have a number of features. It should be adjustable in height. It should be adjustable so that a patient can be transported in a number of positions: with the foot end elevated, with the head end elevated, sitting, and semi-sitting. It should have detachable supports for intravenous fluid containers. Restraining devices should be provided so that a patient can be prevented from falling off the stretcher or sliding past the foot end or head end.

2. A *folding ambulance stretcher* should be carried so that a second patient can be transported in the ambulance in a prone, supine, or lateral position. Some ambulances have stretchers that can be carried flat or folded into a stair chair; thus the stretcher serves two purposes.

3. A *folding stair chair* should be carried for times when a sick or injured person must be moved down stairs or through hallways too narrow for conventional wheeled or portable ambulance stretchers.

An excellent device for picking up seriously injured persons with a minimum of body movement is the *scoop-style stretcher* (orthopedic stretcher). The components of one model scoop stretcher can be formed into an upper body immobilization device.

When the ambulance personnel are responsible for removing sick or injured persons from locations where the usual patient-carrying devices cannot be used, a *basket stretcher* should be either carried on the ambulance or kept in quarters in a place where it will be immediately available.

Equipment for Airway Maintenance, Ventilation, and Resuscitation

A number of devices should be carried for maintaining an open airway.

- Oropharyngeal airways in sizes suitable for adults, children, and infants
- Soft rubber nasopharyngeal airways in sizes 14 through 30
- An esophageal obturator airway or an esophageal gastric tube airway, if approved for use by protocol or the unit's medical advisor

The following devices should be carried for artificial ventilation efforts:

- Two manually operated, self-filling, bag-valve-mask units (one adult and one pediatric). The units should be capable of delivering 100% oxygen to a patient by the addition of a reservoir. Masks of various sizes should be carried, and the masks should be designed to ensure a tight face seal. The masks should be clear so that an attending EMT can see vomitus and the clouding caused by exhalations during ventilation efforts.
- A pocket face mask with one-way valve should be available for times when oronasal ventilation is necessary but direct contact with the patient is either impossible or undesirable. The mask should have an oxygen inlet.
- A commercially available jaw block should be carried so that the mouth of a convulsing person can be kept open.

Oxygen Therapy Equipment

It is recommended that an ambulance be provided with two oxygen supply systems (one fixed and one portable) so that oxygen can be supplied to two patients, both at the scene of an emergency and during transportation to a medical facility.

The fixed oxygen delivery system is provided to supply oxygen to a patient within the ambulance. A typical installation consists of a minimum 3,000-liter reservoir, a two-stage regulator, and the necessary yokes, reducing valve, non-gravity-type flowmeter, and humidifier. The oxygen delivery tubes, transparent masks, and controls should all be situated within easy reach of an EMT working at a patient's head. The system should be capable of delivering at least 10 liters of oxygen per minute, and the system must be adaptable to the bag-valve-mask units carried on the ambulance.

The portable oxygen delivery system should have a capacity of at least 300 liters. It, too, must have the necessary hardware and masks of all sizes. The system should be capable of delivering at least 10 liters of oxygen per minute, and there should be a spare 300-liter cylinder. Many ambulances are equipped with portable units that can be used for resuscitation and suctioning as well as oxygen delivery.

Suction Equipment

An ambulance should be provided with both a fixed suction system and a portable suction device.

The fixed suction system should be sufficient to provide an air flow of over 30 liters per minute at the end of the delivery tube. A vacuum of at least 300 mm Hg should be reached within 4 seconds after the suction tube is clamped. The suction should be controllable. The installed system should have a large-diameter, nonkinking tube fitted with a rigid tip. There should be a spare nonbreakable suction bottle, and a container of water for rinsing the suction tubes. There should be an assortment of sterile catheters. As with the oxygen delivery system, the suction tube and controls should be located within easy reach of an EMT working at a patient's head.

The portable suction unit can be one of the many models powered by motor, hand or foot action, oxygen, vacuum, or compressed air. A portable unit should be fitted with a nonkinking tube that has a rigid tip.

Equipment for Assisting with External Chest Compression

A CPR board can be obtained from an emergency care equipment supplier. When in position under a patient, a CPR board positions the patient's head in a constant open airway position and provides the rigid back support that is necessary for external chest compressions to be effective.

In the event that a CPR board is not available, the short spine board that is generally carried on an ambulance for the immobilization of neck and back injuries can provide rigid support during CPR efforts.

Supplies and Equipment for the Immobilization of Fractures

A well-equipped ambulance carries a variety of devices that can be used to immobilize skeletal injuries:

- A rigid, hinged, half-ring lower extremity traction splint with limb support straps, a padded ankle hitch, and a traction strap with a buckle
- Any of a variety of commercially available traction devices for the immobilization of fractured femurs
- A number of padded board splints for the immobilization of upper and lower extremities. Recommended are two 3 × 54-inch splints, two 3 × 36-inch splints, and two 3 × 15-inch splints.

Other devices that might be carried for the immobilization of injured extremities are:

- Air-inflatable splints, vacuum splints, wire ladder splints, cardboard splints, canvas lace-up splints, soft rubberized splints with aluminum stays and Velcro fasteners, padded aluminum roll-up splints (for extremi-

ties), and splints that are inflated with cryogenic gas (**WARNING**: Improper use may lead to frostbite!)
- A number of tongue depressors to use to immobilize fractured fingers
- Triangular bandages for use with splints, spine boards, and for making slings and swathes
- Several rolls of soft roller bandage for securing the various splints
- Chemical cold packs for use on fractured extremities
- A long spine board for full-body immobilization. The long spine board can also be used for patient transfer activities.
- One 6-foot, 1-inch spliced rope sling for pulling a patient onto the long spineboard from under vehicles, off the floor of a vehicle, or any area where the patient could not be lifted safely
- Rigid cervical and extrication collars in a variety of sizes
- A vest-type immobilizing device for persons who have possible spinal injuries
- Six 9-foot by 2-inch web straps with aircraft-style buckles for securing patients to carrying devices
- A suitable device, such as a head immobilizer or rolled blanket, for stabilizing the head of a person who has a known or suspected cervical spine injury

The number and types of immobilizing devices carried on an ambulance are mostly decided by local policy on the recommendation of the unit's medical advisor.

Supplies for Wound Care

A variety of dressing and bandaging materials should be carried on an ambulance.

- Sterile gauze pads (2 × 2 inches and 4 × 4 inches)
- Sterile universal dressings (often called multitrauma dressings) approximately 10 × 36 inches when unfolded
- Soft self-adhering roller bandages in 4- and 6-inch widths × 5 yards
- Sterile, nonporous, nonadherent occlusive dressings for the sealing of sucking chest wounds and eviscerations

- Aluminum foil (sterilized in separate package) for use as occlusive dressing and also to maintain body heat of newborn infants
- Sterile burn sheets or prepackaged burn kit
- Adhesive strip bandages for minor wound care (1 × ¾ inch and 1 × ½ inch), individually packaged (Band-Aids)
- Adhesive tape (1- and 3-inch rolls)
- Large safety pins for the securing of bandages, slings and swathes
- Bandage scissors
- Latex disposable gloves

Supplies and Equipment for the Treatment of Shock

In the past, the treatment for shock was usually limited to the elevation of a person's feet and the conservation of body heat. Today, many EMTs are qualified to provide more definitive anti-shock measures; consequently, ambulances are equipped with the following:

- Pneumatic counterpressure devices (also called anti-shock trousers, MAST garments), sized for adults and children
- Aluminum blankets (survival blankets) for maintaining body heat

Supplies for Childbirth

A sterile childbirth kit should be carried. In some areas, ambulances carry kits provided by local medical facilities. In other areas, ambulances are provided with commercially available disposable obstetric kits. Whatever the source, an obstetric kit should contain the following items:

- A pair of surgical scissors
- Four umbilical cord clamps or umbilical tape
- A rubber bulb syringe (3 oz.)
- Twelve 4 × 4 inch gauze pads
- Four pairs of latex gloves
- Five towels
- A baby blanket (receiving blanket)
- Sanitary napkins
- Two large plastic bags

In addition to the latex gloves included in the obstetric kit, an ambulance should be provided with items that can be worn by EMTs to minimize contamination of the mother and baby during and after childbirth, including:

- Two surgical gowns
- Two surgical caps
- Two surgical masks

Equipment for the Transfer of Newborns

It is not necessary to carry an incubator on every ambulance; however, each ambulance squad should be able to acquire an incubator from a local medical facility or neonatal ambulance without delay. If an incubator is not available, supplies and equipment should be stored in quarters and available for immediate use when it is necessary to care for a newborn. Included in the inventory should be:

- A small portable crib or a bassinet
- Three hot water bottles
- A quilted pad
- A baby blanket
- A room thermometer
- A rubber suction tube with trap
- Two umbilical clamps (umbilical tape may be required)
- A rubber suction bulb
- A rubber funnel with tube
- A portable oxygen cylinder with delivery hardware
- A bottle of 70% alcohol

Supplies for the Treatment of Acute Poisoning

A number of poison control kits are available from emergency care equipment suppliers. Whether purchased intact or hand-made, a poison control kit should include these items:

- Syrup of ipecac (if allowed in your system)
- Activated charcoal (if allowed in your system)
- Drinking water that can be used to dilute poisons and assist with the administration of charcoal
- Paper cups and other equipment for oral administration
- Equipment for irrigating a person's eyes with sterile water
- Constriction bands for snakebites

Special Equipment for Qualified EMTs, Paramedics, and Physicians

Depending on state laws and local protocols, some ambulances are provided with locked kits of supplies and equipment that can be used by paramedics or physicians, especially in rural areas. Among the kits that might be carried are:

- IV fluid infusion kits
- Tracheal intubation kit
- Pleural decompression kit
- Drug injection kit
- Tracheostomy or cricothyrotomy kit
- Portable cardiac monitor and defibrillator
- Venous cutdown kit
- Minor surgical repair kit
- EMT holster

The supplies and equipment listed above are for emergency care efforts. Ambulances should also be provided with personal protective gear for the EMTs, equipment for warning, signaling and lighting, hazard control devices, and tools for gaining access and disentanglement. Since these items are rescue related, they are listed and described in Chapter 27.

When you have an opportunity, compare the items listed in this chapter with the inventory of your ambulance. Learn where each item is stored so that you can reach it quickly in any emergency situation. Learn what every item is for and when it should be used. If the item is a mechanical device, learn not only what it is for and when it should be used but also how it works and how it should be maintained.

Organizing Supplies and Equipment for Immediate Use

The items on the preceding lists can be stored in compartments throughout the ambulance, but when emergency care items are stored in *kits*, they are immediately accessible. There is no need to go from compartment to compartment gathering up armloads of supplies and equipment. There are a variety of kits available from equipment vendors; however, you can make your own kits by fitting out readily available plastic or metal boxes and soft-sided bags.

A jump kit is the most useful of all the kits that might be carried on an ambulance (see Figs. 21–1 and 21–2). It should contain all the supplies and equipment that may be needed to initiate primary life-saving measures, such as airways, a pocket mask with one-way valve or bag-valve-mask unit, bulky dressings, and soft roller bandages. Airways, pocket masks and ventilation adjunct devices, bag-valve-mask units, and suction catheters can be carried in an airway maintenance and ventilation equipment kit. A wound care kit might include a variety of bandages and dressings, occlusive materials, tape, bandage shears and related materials. Other supplies and equipment can be carried in an obstetric kit, a shock kit, a rescue kit of hand tools, and so on.

Ensuring that the Ambulance Is Ready for Service

The most modern well-equipped ambulance is not worth the room it takes up in a garage if it is not ready to respond at the time of an emergency. A state of readiness results from a planned preventive maintenance program that includes periodic servicing. Oil should be changed regularly, tires should be rotated, the vehicle should be lubricated, and so on. These are important steps, to be sure; but the one step that can ensure that an ambulance is continually ready for service is the pre-shift inspection.

Let us say that you and your partner have just reported for duty. As soon as it is practical, speak with the crew members going off duty. Learn whether they experienced any problems with either the ambulance or the equipment during their shift. Check the run reports to see what supplies and equipment were used during the preceding shift. Make notes to inspect the equipment and to see that any expendable items used have been replaced. Then make a thorough bumper-to-bumper inspection of the ambulance. Use a checklist if one is provided by your service.

- *Inspect the body of the vehicle.* Look for damage that could interfere with safe operation. A crumpled fender, for example, may prevent the front wheels from turning the maximum distance.
- *Inspect the wheels and tires.* Remember that ambulance tires take a beating when they meet curbs, stones, and potholes. At accident scenes they may contact shards of glass and sharp pieces of metal and other debris. Check for damaged wheels and damaged sidewalls. Look for signs of abnormal wear. Check the tread depth. Use a pressure gauge to ensure that all tires are properly inflated. Be sure to include the spare wheel in your inspection, and don't forget to inspect the inside walls of all tires.
- *Inspect windows and mirrors.* Look for broken glass and loose or missing parts. See that mirrors are clean and properly adjusted for maximum visibility.
- *Check the operation of the doors.* Ensure that every door will open and close properly and that all latches and locks are operational.
- *Inspect the components of the cooling system.* (**WARNING:** Allow the engine to cool before removing any pressure caps.) Check the level of the coolant. Inspect the cooling system hoses for leaks and cracks.

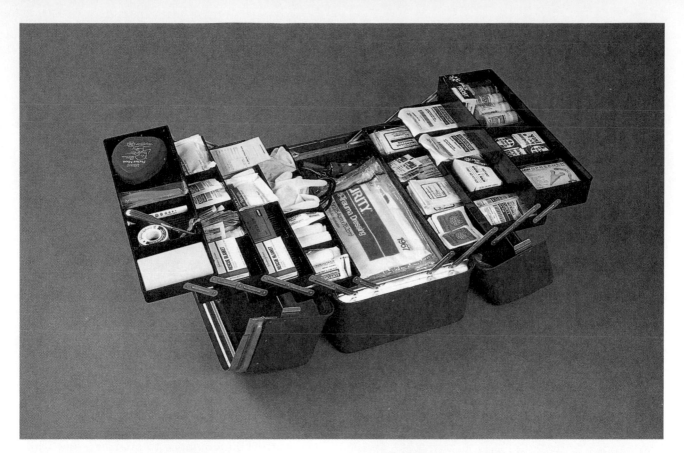

FIGURE 21–1.   A specially prepared trauma or jump kit with equipment to initiate primary life-saving measures.

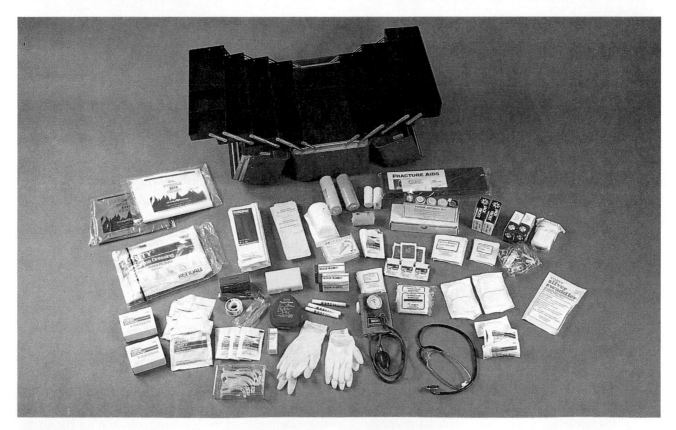

FIGURE 21–2.   Supplies in the primary life-saving trauma or jump kit.

- *Check the level of the other vehicle fluids,* including the engine oil and the brake, power steering and transmission fluids. Do not forget to check the level of the windshield washer fluid.
- *Check the battery.* If the battery has removable fill caps, check the level of the electrolyte. If the battery is the sealed type, determine its condition by checking the indicator port. Inspect the battery cable connections for tightness and signs of corrosion.
- *Inspect the interior surfaces and upholstery for damage.* See that interior surfaces are clean.
- *Check the windows for operation.* See that the interior surface of each window is clean.
- *Test the horn.*
- *Test the siren for the full range of operation.*
- *Check the seat belts.* Examine each belt to see that it is not damaged. Pull each belt from its storage spool to ensure that the retractor mechanisms work. Buckle each belt to ensure that the latches work properly.
- *Adjust the seat for comfort and optimum steering wheel and pedal operation.*
- *Observe the dash-mounted indicator lights.* See that each is working.
- *Check the fuel level.* An ambulance should be refueled after each run, however short. How much fuel was used on a run is less relevant than how much fuel may be needed for the next response.

The next steps require you to start the engine. Pull the ambulance from quarters if engine exhaust fumes will be a problem. Set the emergency brake and put the transmission in "park." Have your partner chock the wheels. Then:

- *Check the dash-mounted indicators again.* See if any light remains on to indicate a possible problem with oil pressure, engine temperature, or the vehicle's electrical system.
- *Check dash-mounted gauges for proper operation.*
- *Depress the brake pedal.* Note whether pedal travel seems correct or excessive.
- *Test the parking brake.* Move the transmission lever to a drive position. Replace the lever to the "park" position as soon as you are sure that the parking brake is holding.
- *Turn the steering wheel from side to side.* Note whether the movement is smooth or jerky.
- *Check the operation of the windshield wipers and washers.* The glass should be wiped clean each time the blade moves.
- *Turn on the vehicle's warning lights.* Have your partner walk around the ambulance and check each flashing and revolving light for operation. Turn off the warning lights.
- *Turn on the other vehicle lights.* Have your partner walk around the ambulance again, this time checking the headlights (high and low beams), turn signals, four-way flashers, brake lights, backup lights, side and rear scene illumination lights, and ICC marker lights.
- *Check the operation of the heating and air-conditioning equipment.* While you check the operation of the equipment in the driver's compartment, have your partner check the equipment in the patient's compartment.
- *Operate the communications equipment.* Test portable as well as the fixed radios and any radio-telephone communication equipment.

Return the ambulance to quarters, and while you are backing, have your partner note whether the backup alarm is operating (if the ambulance is so equipped).

Shut off the engine and complete your inspection by checking the patient space and equipment compartments:

- *Check the interior of the patient compartment.* Look for damage to the interior surfaces and upholstery. Be certain that any needed decontamination has been completed and that the compartment is clean.
- *See that the emergency care supplies and equipment and the rescue equipment listed on the inventory are in the ambulance and ready for use.*

This last check should be more than merely a quick glance into storage cabinets and compartments. It should be an item-by-item inspection of everything carried on the ambulance, with findings recorded on a printed checklist.

Not only should items be identified during the ambulance inspection, they should also be checked for completeness, condition, and operation. The pressure of oxygen cylinders should be checked. Air splints should be inflated and examined for leaks. Suction and ventilation equipment should be tested for proper operation. Rescue tools should be examined for rust and dirt that may prevent them from working properly. Battery-powered devices should be operated to ensure that the batteries have a proper charge, and so on.

When you are finished with your inspection of the ambulance and its equipment, complete the inspection report. Correct any deficiencies, replace missing items, and if you can, repair nonworking items. Make your supervisor aware of any deficiencies that cannot be immediately corrected.

Finally, clean the unit if necessary. Maintaining the ambulance's appearance enhances your organization's image in the public's eye. If you take pride in your work as an EMT, show it by taking pride in the appearance of your ambulance as well.

When you are physically and mentally prepared to respond, when the ambulance is fully maintained and ready for a run, and when supplies and equipment are available for virtually any sort of emergency, then you can truly say that your unit is ready for service.

SUMMARY

A variety of supplies and equipment should be carried on an ambulance so that EMTs can cope with virtually every illness and injury situation.

Basic supplies and equipment should include items that an EMT can use to protect the patient and keep him warm, care for a patient's personal needs, and measure vital signs.

Equipment for patient transfer should include devices that EMTs can use to lift and carry sick or injured persons to the ambulance in a prone, supine, recumbent, or sitting position.

Equipment for airway maintenance, ventilation, and resuscitation should include airways and artificial ventilation devices, fixed and portable oxygen delivery systems, fixed and portable suction systems, and either a CPR board or a spine board that can be placed under a patient during CPR efforts.

Supplies and equipment for immobilizing fractures should include traction devices for lower extremities, padded board splints for both upper and lower extremities, other rigid and soft splints, long and short spine boards, web straps, triangular bandages and soft roller bandages, and head immobilization devices.

Supplies and equipment for wound care should include a variety of dressing and bandaging materials, occlusive dressings, tape, bandage shears, and safety pins.

Supplies and equipment for the treatment of shock should include pneumatic countershock devices and aluminum survival blankets.

Supplies and equipment for childbirth should include a sterile obstetric kit and sterile garments for the EMTs.

If an incubator is not available, there should be a store of supplies and equipment ready for times when a newborn must be transported to a distant medical facility.

Supplies for the treatment of poisoning should include syrup of ipecac, activated charcoal, drinking water, and items for oral administration. Constriction bands for the care of snakebites should be carried.

Special advanced life support equipment should be carried when the ambulance will be staffed by a qualified EMT, paramedic or physician.

A thorough inspection of an ambulance and its supplies and equipment should be made by EMTs at the beginning of each shift to ensure that the unit is ready for service.

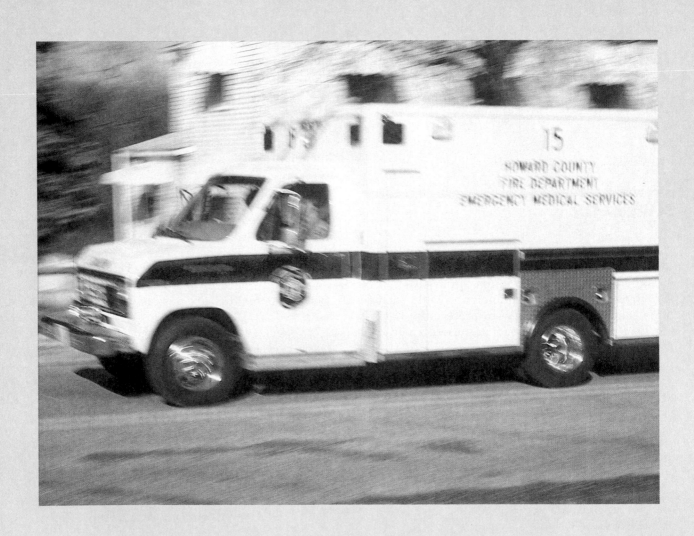

Responding to the Call for Help

OBJECTIVES   As an EMT, you should be able to:

1. List at least FOUR advantages of the universal number concept of emergency reporting. (p. 539)

2. Diagram in the manner of Figure 22–1 the pathways that citizen calls for emergency assistance take in the local jurisdiction. (p. 539)

3. List SIX questions that an EMS dispatcher should ask a caller who is requesting an ambulance for a sick or injured person. (p. 540)

4. List 14 questions that an EMS dispatcher might ask a caller who is reporting a motor vehicle accident. (pp. 540–541)

5. List at least SIX times when a person should not drive an ambulance. (p. 542)

6. List at least SIX privileges usually granted by state statutes to the operators of emergency vehicles. (pp. 542–543)

7. Describe an effect that a continuously sounded siren may have on other motorists and on patients. (p. 543)

8. List at least THREE suggestions as to the proper use of sirens. (p. 543)

9. Explain what special driving skills or actions an ambulance driver should take for each of the following situations:

- When roads are wet with rain (p. 544)
- When the ambulance must be driven through standing water (p. 544)
- When roads are covered with ice or snow (pp. 544–545)
- When visibility is poor (p. 545)
- When there is an object on the road (p. 546)
- When there is an animal on the road (p. 546)
- When there are persons on the road (p. 546)
- When a tire blows out (p. 547)
- When there is a loss or reduction of steering ability (p. 547)
- When brakes fail (pp. 547–548)
- When there is a loss of accelerator control (p. 548)

10. List at least EIGHT steps that an ambulance driver might take to promote a safe response at night. (pp. 546–547)

11. Explain how an ambulance driver might avoid each of these accidents:
- An accident with the vehicle ahead (p. 549)
- An accident with the vehicle behind (p. 550)
- An accident with an approaching vehicle (p. 551)

- An accident at an intersection (pp. 551–552)
- An accident with a vehicle being passed (p. 552)
- An accident with a passing vehicle (p. 552)

12. Explain how an ambulance driver can avoid backing accidents. (p. 552)
13. Explain how each of the following factors can affect an ambulance response:
    - Day of the week (p. 553)
    - Time of day (p. 553)
    - Weather (p. 553)
    - Detours (p. 553)
    - Railroads (p. 553)
    - Bridges and tunnels (p. 553–554)
    - Schools (p. 554)
14. List the observations that the attending EMT may make and the actions he might take during a response to a motor vehicle accident:
    - As the ambulance leaves quarters (p. 554)
    - During the response (p. 554)
    - As the ambulance approaches the scene (p. 554)
    - When the ambulance is within sight of the accident scene (p. 555)
    - As the approach continues (p. 555)
15. Define *danger zone* as it applies to a motor vehicle accident activity. (p. 555)
16. Define the limits of the danger zone for each of the following situations:
    - When there are no apparent hazards (p. 555)
    - When fuel has been spilled (p. 557)
    - When an accident vehicle is on fire (p. 557)
    - When wires are down (p. 557)
    - When a hazardous commodity is involved (p. 557)
17. Describe the manner in which an ambulance should be parked:
    - On a call to assist a sick or injured person (p. 557)
    - At the scene of a motor vehicle accident (p. 557)

TERMS you may be using for the first time:

Braking Distance – the number of feet a vehicle travels from the start of braking action until it comes to a full stop.

Central Dispatch – one dispatch headquarters that receives all emergency calls and relays information to the needed services (fire department, rescue squad, police department, etc.).

Danger Zone – the area at the emergency scene in which rescue personnel, patients, and bystanders may be exposed to hazards such as fire, dangerous chemicals, explosion, downed electrical wires, or radiation.

Hydroplaning – during wet driving conditions, a film of water develops between the tires and the road surface, causing the tires to ride on the water rather than the road surface.

Reaction Distance – the number of feet a vehicle travels from the time a driver decides to stop until his foot applies pressure to the brake pedal.

Stopping Distance – the number of feet a vehicle travels from the moment a driver decides to stop until the vehicle actually stops. It is the total of reaction distance and braking distance.

Universal Number Calling – one-number calling, where the number 911 is used to gain access to central dispatch.

RECEIVING THE CALL FOR HELP

Initiating Emergency Service Responses

Figures 22–1a and b show that there are several ways in which a citizen can call for emergency service assistance.

In many areas of the country, a person needs only to dial 911 to access a community's ambulance service, fire department, rescue squad, police depart-

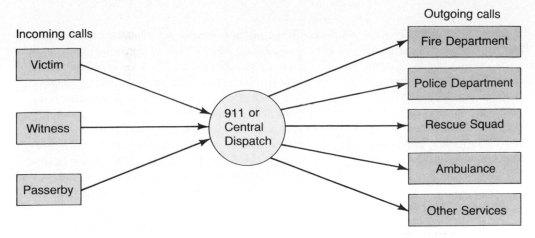

FIGURE 22–1a. Routings of a citizen's call for help. When all requests for assistance follow a direct route from caller through central dispatch (universal one-number concept) to the proper agency, an efficient flow of information helps ensure the proper prompt response.

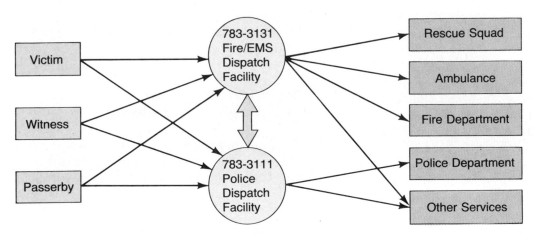

FIGURE 22–1b. Routings of a citizen's call for help. Many communities are served by separate dispatching facilities. Direct telephone and radio links between the centers help reduce the problems caused by misdirected calls.

ment, or other emergency service. A trained dispatcher records information from callers, decides which service is needed, and alerts that service.

There are distinct advantages to the universal number concept:

- Citizens do not have to look for emergency service numbers in a telephone directory, if a telephone directory is available, that is. Today few public telephone installations have directories.
- With one-number calling, there is no need for a citizen to decide which emergency service to call if he is unfamiliar with the area.
- There is no chance that calls for help placed through a telephone company operator will be misdirected.
- The delays that often result when one service

is called when another service is needed are eliminated, as when a person calls the police department when he needs an ambulance.

- One-number emergency telephone centers are usually manned by dispatchers who are specially trained to elicit information from distraught and excited callers.

In other parts of the country two dispatch centers are provided, one for the police and the other for the fire, rescue, and ambulance services. Even though a caller may dial the police department when he needs an ambulance, the possibility of a delay in response is minimized because of cross-communication capabilities.

In still other areas of the country a request for emergency medical service may follow a roundabout route from caller to ambulance headquarters.

A family member or neighbor, a witness to an accident, or even the sick or injured person himself may reach a small dispatch center (which, in fact, may be someone's home or business), the ambulance garage, the local fire department, or the police department, depending on which of the many available numbers the caller dials. Valuable time is lost when calls for help are routed in this manner, especially if calls have to be shuffled between agencies.

Obtaining Routine Information

It is essential that the dispatcher obtain as much information as he or she can. Everything that is learned about the situation will be (or should be) truly important to the crew that responds to the call for help.

The dispatcher should ask these questions when answering a call for help:

1. *Do you have an emergency?* Ask this question as soon as you have identified your organization and yourself. It will tell you that you will be handling an emergency. It will also cause the caller to get his thoughts in order and may even help to calm or slow him down.
2. *What is the exact location of the sick or injured person (or emergency)?* Here you must elicit as much information as possible. You must ask for the house or building number, and if the building is an apartment house, the apartment number. Ascertain the street name with the direction designator (e.g., north, east): when you alert the ambulance crew you should provide them with the nearest cross street as well as the location of the emergency. Finally, learn the name of the development or subdivision.
3. *What is the nature of the emergency?* This is an important question, especially if you have protocols to follow with regard to the type of emergency. If you learn that the caller is reporting a vehicle accident, for example, you may wish to ask questions that you would not ask a person requesting an ambulance for a sick person. You may even have different forms to fill in for different types of calls.
4. *Can you tell me the (sick or injured) person's name and age?* With this question you should be able to learn both the person's name and sex. If you are unable to determine sex from the first name, ask whether the sick or injured person is male or female.

5. *What is your name and what number are you calling from?* This is an important question. If the person refuses to give his name and number, you will have reason to suspect the validity of the call and follow whatever protocol has been established for possible false calls. Moreover, you will be able to learn the location of the number from the telephone company if the ambulance crew is unable to locate the sick or injured person at the given address or if the call proves to be false.
6. *Will you be at that number if I need more information?* Being able to contact the caller again is important if there is any question about the location given for the sick or injured person. Such may be the case when several streets within a community have the same name or when you fail to learn whether the building is on North Main Street or South Main Street.

Obtaining Information about a Vehicle Accident

The procedure for obtaining information about a motor vehicle accident may vary slightly. In this case you should attempt to learn everything you can about the accident with questions such as:

1. *What is the exact location of the accident?* If the accident has occurred in a built-up area, you should be able to learn a street address or the names of the nearest two streets that intersect. But if the accident has occurred in a rural area you may have a problem learning the exact location, especially when the caller is not familiar with the area. The person reporting the accident may say something like, "There has been an accident about three miles north of town." You must try to pinpoint that "three miles north of town" by asking questions about the nearest crossroad or the name of a nearby store, if there is one, or what landmarks are visible from the caller's point of view (e.g., mileposts, water towers, large silos, or radio antennas). If the caller cannot provide concrete information you must determine the number of the telephone he is using. The telephone company should be able to provide the location of the phone.
2. *What number are you calling from?*
3. *What is your name?*

4. *How many and what kind of vehicles are involved?* Many kinds of vehicles are involved in traffic accidents, and certain vehicles may require special attention from responding emergency service units. Determine, if possible, how many accident vehicles are passenger cars, buses, or trucks. If you learn that a truck is involved, try to determine what type the truck is—for example, a box cargo truck, a tank truck, or a dump truck. Valid descriptions of accident vehicles help emergency service personnel plan their response and first-on-the-scene activities.

5. *How many persons do you think are injured?* A fact important to a response plan is information about injuries. When you as a dispatcher learn that some people have been injured in an accident, you may assume that "some" means two or three and send a single ambulance. If you learn from the initial caller that five people have been injured, then you may deem it necessary or prudent to send two or three ambulances at the same time. Time, and perhaps lives, will be saved by your knowing precisely the number of people injured in a vehicle accident.

6. *Do the accident victims appear trapped?* Knowing that persons are trapped and knowing what the rescue capabilities of the ambulance are will help you to formulate a decision whether to send a rescue unit on the initial response.

Next, attempt to learn something about the scene. Ask the caller these questions about traffic conditions on the scene:

- *Is traffic moving?*
- *How many lanes are open?*
- *How far is traffic backed up?*

If you can inform responding units that all lanes of a particular road leading to the accident scene are blocked, drivers can select alternate response routes.

Then attempt to learn whether hazards have been produced by the accident by asking these questions:

- *Are any of the vehicles on fire?*
- *Are any of the vehicles leaking fuel?*
- *Are any electrical wires down?*
- *Do any of the vehicles appear unstable? Is any vehicle on its side or top?*

- *Does a truck appear to be carrying a hazardous cargo?*

It takes a little time to gather this information, but what you learn from a caller will enable you to alert the proper services, and what information you pass on will enable ambulance, fire, rescue, and other emergency service personnel to plan effective responses.

Transmitting Information to the Ambulance Squad

This is how you might dispatch an ambulance to the location of an injured person:

> Ambulance Company 11—An emergency call for a 34-year-old male who has fallen. Respond to the Acme Paper Company Warehouse located at 123 Madison Street. The cross street is Maple.

Repeat the message to minimize any question as to its content, and give the time.

The person receiving the message at the ambulance quarters should identify his station, note the information on a form provided for that purpose, and confirm the message.

DRIVING THE AMBULANCE

Neither this nor any other textbook can fully prepare you for the task of driving an ambulance; books can only offer suggestions. Nor can you become a good ambulance driver through experience alone.

If you aspire to drive an ambulance, make every effort to attend a formal emergency vehicle driver training program that has both classroom and in-vehicle road sessions. In the classroom you will learn how a vehicle operates, how it behaves on different types of roads, the proper use of audible and visual warning devices, laws regarding the operation of emergency vehicles, and so on.

On the driving range, you will learn, among other things, how to make a safe response, how to change lanes quickly and safely, how to recover from skids, and how to back the vehicle.

If you do not have an opportunity to attend a formal driver training course, attend the defensive driving course that is offered by local safety councils and law enforcement agencies. You will at least learn how to prevent accidents by staying alert for problems caused by other motorists, changing road conditions, and hazards. Then spend time behind the wheel driving under the guidance of a good ambulance driver—one who practices defensive driving, cares for safety, and has a clean driving record.

To be a good ambulance driver, you should:

- *Be physically fit.* You should not have any impairment that prevents you from turning the steering wheel, operating the gear shift, or depressing the floor pedals. Nor should you have any medical condition that might disable you while driving, such as a heart condition or uncontrolled diabetes or epilepsy.

- *Be mentally fit, with your emotions under control.* Some emergency service personnel undergo personality changes when they drive an emergency vehicle, or when they are put in charge of an emergency situation. If you fit in this category, do not drive an ambulance.

- *Be able to perform under stress.*

- *Have a positive attitude about your ability as a driver,* but do not think that you are the best in the world.

- *Be tolerant of other drivers.* Always keep in mind that people react differently when they see an emergency vehicle. Accept and tolerate the bad habits of other drivers without flying into a rage. Appreciate the need for cooperation, and cooperate yourself.

To be a safe ambulance driver:

- *Do not drive without corrective lenses if you have defective vision.* If you need them to drive your car, you need them to drive the ambulance!

- *Do not drive while you are taking medications that can cause drowsiness.* These medications include such items as over-the-counter cold remedies.

- *Do not take "pep-pills."* They cause temporary euphoria and interfere with concentration.

- *Do not drive if you are taking pain killers or tranquilizers.* They can dull your senses, cause inattention, and induce sleep.

- *Do not drive if you have been drinking.* Alcohol dulls reflexes and impedes judgment.

- *Do not drive if you are preoccupied with personal problems.* You will not be able to concentrate on the driving task if you are constantly thinking about bills, family problems, or job problems.

Understanding the Law

Every state has statutes that regulate the operation of emergency vehicles. Although the wording of the statutes may vary, the intent of the laws remains essentially the same. Emergency vehicle operators are generally granted certain privileges with regard to speed, parking, passage through traffic signals, and direction of travel. However, the laws also clearly state that if an emergency vehicle operator does not drive with regard for the safety of others, he must be prepared to pay the consequences for his actions.

Following are some points usually included in laws that regulate the operation of ambulances:

- An ambulance driver must have a valid driver's license and must have completed a formal emergency vehicle and defensive driver training program.

- Privileges granted under the law to the operators of ambulances apply when the vehicle is responding to an emergency or is involved in the emergency transport of a sick or injured person. When the ambulance is not on an emergency call, the laws that apply to the operation of non-emergency vehicles also apply to the ambulance.

- Even though certain privileges are granted during an emergency, an ambulance driver is not relieved from the duty to operate the vehicle with regard to the safety of all persons. The privileges granted do not provide immunity to the driver in cases of reckless driving or disregard for the safety of others.

- Privileges granted during emergency situations apply only if the driver is using warning devices in the manner prescribed by law.

Most statutes allow ambulance drivers to:

- Park the vehicle anywhere so long as it does not damage personal property or endanger lives.

- Leave the ambulance standing in the middle of a street or intersection.

- Proceed past red stop signals, flashing red stop signals, and stop signs. Some states require that emergency vehicle operators come to a full stop, then proceed with caution. Other states require only that a driver slow down and proceed with caution.

- Exceed the posted speed limit as long as life and property are not endangered. In most jurisdictions, this is limited to 5 to 10 mph over the posted limit.

- Pass other vehicles in designated no-passing zones after promptly signaling, ensuring that the way is clear, and taking precautions to avoid endangering life and property.
- With proper caution and signals, disregard regulations that govern direction of travel and turning in specific directions.

Again, these are just some of the privileges granted to ambulance drivers. Do not assume that they are granted in your state. Obtain a copy of the motor vehicle rules and regulations and study them carefully before you start to drive the ambulance.

Using the Warning Devices

Ambulance drivers, like the drivers of other emergency vehicles, become so obsessed with the idea that sirens and flashing lights will clear the roads that they may often overlook hazards and take chances. Audible and visual warning devices do serve a purpose; however, safe emergency vehicle operation can be achieved only when the proper use of warning devices is coupled with sound emergency and defensive driving practices.

Using the Siren

Although the siren is the most commonly used audible warning device, it is also the most misused. Consider the effects that sirens have on other motorists, patients in ambulances, and ambulance drivers themselves:

- Motorists are less inclined to give way to ambulances when sirens are continually sounded. Many operators feel that the right-of-way privileges granted to ambulances by law are being abused when sirens are sounded.
- The continuous sound of a siren may cause a sick or injured person to suffer increased fear and anxiety, and his condition may actually worsen as stress builds.
- Ambulance drivers themselves are affected by the continuous sound of a siren. Tests have shown that inexperienced ambulance drivers tend to increase their driving speeds from 10 to 15 miles per hour while continually sounding the siren. In some reported cases, drivers using a siren were unable to negotiate curves that they could pass through easily when not sounding the siren.

Many states have statutes that regulate the use of audible warning signals, and where there are no such statutes, ambulance organizations usually create their own regulations. If your organization does not, you may find some of the following suggestions helpful when you think it is necessary to use the siren during an ambulance run:

- Use the siren sparingly, and only when you must. The more you use the siren, the greater the chance that other motorists will be indifferent to its sound.
- Never assume that all motorists will hear your signal. Buildings, trees, and dense shrubbery may effectively block siren sounds. Improved soundproofing keeps outside noises from entering vehicles, and if the radio or tape system is on, the likelihood that an outside sound will be heard is further diminished.
- Always assume that some motorists will hear your siren but that they will choose to ignore it.
- Be prepared for the erratic maneuvers of other drivers. Some drivers panic when they hear a siren.
- Do not pull up close to a vehicle and then sound your siren. Such action may cause the driver to jam on his brakes so quickly that you will be unable to stop. Use the horn when you are close to a vehicle ahead.
- Never use the siren indiscriminately, and never use it to scare someone.

NOTE: Some states require the use of the siren at all times when the ambulance is responding in the emergency mode.

Using the Horn

All ambulances must be equipped with a horn. Experienced drivers find that in many cases the judicious use of the horn clears traffic as quickly as using the siren. The guidelines for using a siren apply to the use of an ambulance's horn as well.

Using Visual Warning Devices

There is general agreement among ambulance operators that all visual warning devices should be in operation when an ambulance is responding to emergency calls and whenever a patient is in the ambulance.

There is disagreement, however, as to whether warning lights should be on when the ambulance is responding to a nonemergency call or when the unit is returning to quarters. Some operators believe that if warning lights are used at all times, motorists will become so accustomed to flashing and revolving lights that they will disregard the signals altogether.

Unless the policy of your organization dictates otherwise, consider using the headlights to supplement warning lights when you think that the ambulance needs greater visibility during daylight hours. Headlights can often be seen at a far greater distance than colored flashing and revolving lights, which blend in with illuminated signs, traffic signals, and the taillights of other vehicles.

Do not use four-way flashers when the vehicle is moving to gain visibility for your ambulance, however. In most states this practice is illegal; moreover, it may interfere with the operation of turn signals.

REMEMBER: Audible and visual warning signals merely ask the drivers of other vehicles to give way to an emergency vehicle. They do not demand that drivers give way, and they certainly cannot physically clear the road.

Special Driving Techniques for Inclement Weather

Rain, sleet, and snow all make driving dangerous. Seeing is difficult, and so is stopping. In a panic-stop situation, a vehicle will travel twice as far on rain-slicked pavement as it will on dry pavement once the brakes are applied. On an ice-covered road, expect to travel five times as far as you would when making a quick stop on a dry road.

Driving in Rain

- Keep in mind that roads are most slippery just after it starts to rain.
- Avoid sudden acceleration, sudden braking, and sudden turns of the steering wheel.
- Wipe your mirrors from time to time to enhance rear vision.
- Reduce the likelihood of hydroplaning by having good tires and driving at reduced speeds during wet weather. Hydroplaning is a dangerous condition that often occurs when a vehicle with worn tires is operated over 35 mph on a wet road. The tires ride on a film of water instead of the road surface, and steering becomes virtually impossible. If you do start to hydroplane while driving on a wet road:
  - Do not jam on the brakes; you will only go into a skid.

- Do not turn the steering wheel from side to side in an attempt to "bite through" the film of water.
- Hold the wheel steady and decelerate slowly until you regain control.

Driving Through Standing Water

You may have to drive the ambulance through large pools of water when a road is flooded and roadside drainage is poor.

The best way to avoid the problems that often result when a vehicle is driven through deep standing water is to avoid the water altogether. If this is not possible, drive slowly to prevent water from splashing into the engine compartment and short circuiting the vehicle's ignition system. When clear of the pool of water, dry the brake linings by lightly tapping the brake pedal several times. Continue to tap the pedal until there is no tendency for the vehicle to pull to one side, an indication of wet brake linings.

Driving During Winter Storms

Prepare for poor winter driving conditions before you have to go on a call.

- Ensure that the ambulance engine is operating properly. This reduces the chance that you will break down during a storm. Keep the battery charged.
- Ensure that the heater and defroster are working.
- Equip all four wheels of the ambulance with studded tires if they are legal in your state. Carry chains if studded tires are not legal.
- Carry a shovel and sand in the ambulance.
- Carry booster cables and two tow chains.

If you must drive for considerable distances during winter storms, consider carrying a storm kit that includes additional blankets or sleeping bags, matches and candles for light, high-calorie nonperishable foods (such as those available from camping supply stores).

When it turns cold:

- Keep an eye on the temperature. Wet ice and freezing rain occur at temperatures between 28° and 40°F.
- Avoid sudden movements of the steering wheel and sudden braking. Either action can cause the vehicle to skid.
- Drive slowly on slippery roads.
- When it is necessary to bring the ambulance

to a stop, do not jam on the brakes; you will lose your ability to steer the vehicle.

- Pump the brakes. You will retain the rolling friction that must exist between the road and wheels in order for a vehicle to turn or stop within a desired distance.
- If the ambulance begins to skid, steer in the direction needed to regain control (see Figure 22–2).

Keep in mind these points about slippery roads:

- Perfectly dry roads can be as slippery as those covered with ice and snow. Gravel roads, for example, are notoriously slippery when traveled at high speeds, as are dirt roads.
- When the temperature drops to below freezing, elevated roads and bridges ice before other roadways.

Driving When Visibility is Poor

Fog, rain, and snow contribute to highway disasters. Massive chain-reaction pileups often result when drivers cannot see far enough ahead to stop their vehicles before hitting something. Accidents also result when poor visibility causes drivers to pass stop signals at intersections and to enter unfamiliar curves at too high a speed.

Slow and careful driving is always in order during inclement weather. However, there may be a time when visibility is reduced all of a sudden, as when entering a patch of fog or when rainfall suddenly becomes heavy. In such cases:

- Turn on your headlights (low beams) during daylight hours—not so you can see better, but so you can be better seen!
- Use ambulance's wipers to improve visibility.
- Watch carefully for slow-moving or stopped vehicles ahead.
- Do not attempt to pass slow-moving vehicles when visibility is poor. To do so may force them off the road.
- Slow down when you have to, but not quickly! Make sure that following drivers know that you are slowing by tapping your brake pedal several times.
- If visibility is so poor that you cannot proceed with at least a degree of safety, pull off the road into a safe place. Turn on the ambulance's four-way flashers. Remain there until conditions improve.

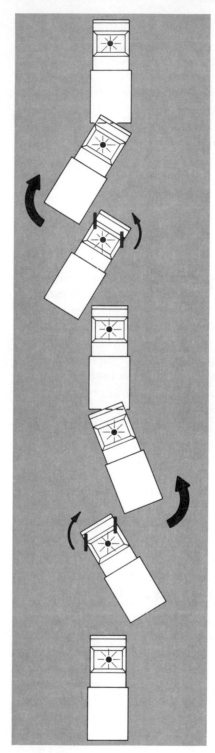

1. The vehicle is going straight.

2. The back end of the vehicle skids around to the left (the vehicle is still moving forward at an angle).

3. You'd steer left, in the direction you want the vehicle to go relative to the way it's facing.

4. The vehicle is back on course.

5. The back end fishtails to the right.

6. To control fishtailing in the opposite direction, you'd countersteer right to help you get back on course.

7. Steering control is re-established

FIGURE 22–2. Steering in a skid is intended to keep front wheels pointed in the direction you want to travel. (From B. J. Childs and D. J. Ptacnik, _Emergency Ambulance Driving._ Brady Communications Company, Englewood Cliffs, N.J., 1985.)

Sharing the Road

Seldom do you drive anywhere without seeing something on the road, whether it is debris from a truck, pieces of blown tire, an animal, a cyclist, or a person walking. Here are some suggestions that you might find helpful when you have to share the road with something or someone.

When There is an Object on the Road

If you travel at a safe speed and maintain the proper distance between the ambulance and the vehicle ahead, you can significantly reduce the danger of striking an object lying on the roadway. If you see an object on the road and you cannot stop before reaching it:

- Do not attempt to straddle the object unless you are absolutely sure that you can do so safely; the object may be taller than it appears. If it contacts the undercarriage of the ambulance, the object may damage the steering mechanism and/or the drive shaft, and it may even puncture the gas tank.
- Do not steer to the left; you may enter the lane of opposing traffic.
- Decelerate and steer to the right. If you can pass the object safely, do so. Be careful driving onto the shoulder of the road, however. If the shoulder is soft or depressed, you may lose control of the vehicle.
- If it appears that the object will pose a problem for other motorists, advise your dispatcher of the situation by radio and ask him to notify the appropriate agency.

When There is an Animal on the Road

Animals in the roadway are commonly seen. In urban areas, dogs and cats are usually the problem. Larger animals such as deer and horses may be seen in rural areas. It may seem cruel, but you may have to hit smaller animals. If you jam on the brakes, you may lose control of the ambulance. If you try to steer around the animal, you may hit another moving vehicle, a parked vehicle, or even a person along the side of the road. When transporting a patient, keep in mind that he may not be able to tolerate the additional stress brought about by a sudden stop or a rapid swerve of the ambulance.

Whenever you see an animal that may wander onto the road surface, slow down! Tap the horn several times. Application of the siren may frighten the animal, causing it to jump into the path of the ambulance. BE ON THE ALERT FOR CHILDREN

RUNNING AFTER THE ANIMAL. If you can steer the ambulance around the animal without risk to life or property, steer in the opposite direction to which the animal is running.

Large animals such as horses, deer, and cattle should be avoided by combined steering and braking actions. Collision with a large animal may produce as much damage as striking another motor vehicle. Remember to steer in the opposite direction of a running animal. If you see a horse and rider, slow down. While still at a distance, tap the horn to alert the rider. Do NOT use the siren. If the horse and rider are on a bridge or overpass, proceed with caution at a slow speed.

When There are People on the Road

As you respond to emergency calls, always keep in mind that people are attracted to siren-sounding emergency vehicles, and it is not unusual for adults and children alike to run into the road.

Drive at a slow speed in residential areas. You will probably have to travel slower than the posted speed limit to avoid children who may run out into the street to see the ambulance. The best way to prevent a terrible accident is to stay alert and drive slowly when you see that someone is likely to run onto the road.

Driving at Night

Dawn and dusk are the most dangerous times to drive for many reasons:

- Less light is available, thus vision is restricted.
- Drivers are often fatigued, less alert, less able to react quickly, and more likely to make mistakes.
- There are drivers especially older persons, who do not see well at night. Some persons have problems associated with reduced light; some are temporarily blinded by headlights.
- Many drivers have problems with contrast and depth perception at night.
- There are more motorists under the influence of alcohol and drugs at night.

Before you have to drive an ambulance at night:

- Make certain that the headlights, taillights, turn signals, and clearance lights are all working. Check the dash lights so you will be able to read the instruments. Keep the dash lights dim, especially if they reflect on the windshield.

- Make certain that the windshield, side windows, and rearview mirrors are clean.
- Drive more slowly than you would during the day.
- Drive defensively. Assume that other drivers will make mistakes. Give them more room on the road and more time to make decisions.
- Do not stare into the headlights of other vehicles.
- Do not continually focus your eyes on an object. Keep them moving.
- Dim your lights within 500 feet of an approaching vehicle and when you are within 300 feet of a vehicle ahead of you.
- Never use high beams when entering a curve.
- Refrain from flicking your high beams on and off to ask an approaching motorist to dim his lights. Even a short burst of a bright light can temporarily blind some drivers.

Coping with Mechanical Problems

No matter how well you maintain your ambulance, some mechanical malfunction can happen when you least expect it. Be prepared for a variety of problems.

Tire Blowout

When tires are periodically and properly inspected, blowouts are rare occurrences. Nonetheless they do happen. If you are driving an ambulance and a tire suddenly deflates:

- Hold the steering wheel firmly while you brake slowly to prevent wheel lock-up.
- Pull completely off the road before coming to a stop. If you have stopped in a lane of traffic, turn on your warning lights and initiate traffic control measures.
- Notify your dispatcher of the situation.

Loss or Reduction of Steering Ability

The complete loss of the ability to steer a vehicle is rare and results from some mechanical problem such as the parting of a tie rod end or the separation of the universal joint at the steering box.

If you are driving and you suddenly lose the ability to steer the ambulance:

1. Bring the vehicle to a complete stop as quickly as you can.
2. Turn on your warning lights and initiate traffic control measures.
3. Notify your dispatcher of the situation.

If you are traveling at high speed when you lose the ability to steer your vehicle, be prepared for a skid or even a rollover. Since there are no mechanisms to hold the front wheels in a straight line, a bump in the road, a pothole, or even a high crown could cause the wheels to change direction and put the vehicle into an uncontrollable turn.

A more common problem is the reduction in steering ability that results when fluid in the power steering unit is lost, when the power steering pump belt slips or breaks, or when a hydraulic line fails.

If you are driving and suddenly discover that steering becomes difficult, steer to the shoulder or the side of the road and stop. Steering may be difficult because there is no power assist; however you should be able to maintain full control of the vehicle. Shut off the motor and turn on your warning lights. Look under the hood to see if you can discover the problem.

If it appears that a broken fan belt or loose hydraulic line will not interfere with any moving parts, restart the motor and continue to your destination at a slower speed. Again, steering will be difficult but not impossible, and you will have to turn corners at a very low speed so you do not drift from your lane.

If you cannot continue on your way, park in a safe place if you can. If not, turn on your warning lights and initiate traffic control measures.

Brake Failure

The loss of braking ability is probably the most severe problem for an ambulance driver. Brake failure is a dangerous situation in itself; however the danger is compounded by the fact that the loss of brakes is seldom discovered until it is time to slow or stop the vehicle.

If while driving an ambulance with an automatic transmission you suddenly discover that the brakes have failed:

1. Turn on your warning lights and audible signal with the hope that drivers ahead will pull out of your way.
2. Do not jam on the parking brake. You may cause the rear wheels to lock.
3. Pump the brake pedal vigorously. You may be able to develop enough pressure in the brake system to stop the vehicle.

If this fails:

- Shift to the lowest gear. The engine will slow the vehicle somewhat.
- Continue on as far as you can while the vehicle slows.

When the vehicle has slowed considerably, or before you get so close to another vehicle or object that a collision will be inevitable, or before you must turn a corner at a dangerously high speed:

- Gently apply the parking brake. Since parking brakes are cable operated, you will not experience the smooth slowing action of service brakes. You will be braking two wheels instead of four, and if the cable to one brake is tighter than the cable to the other brake, there will be the tendency for the vehicle to pull to one side. Counter this pull with the steering wheel.

When the vehicle has slowed to the speed where you can do so safely:

- Steer the vehicle to the side or shoulder of the road and bring it to a stop.

If you are driving a vehicle equipped with a manual transmission and you discover that you have no brakes:

- Do not attempt to shift to a lower gear unless you are skilled in double-clutching and downshifting, especially if you are traveling downhill. With the transmission in neutral your vehicle will become a runaway and you will have little hope of stopping it with the parking brake.
- Pump the brake pedal vigorously. You may be able to develop enough pressure in the brake system to stop the vehicle.
- If pumping the brake fails, allow the engine to slow the vehicle for as long as you can before risking collision.
- Gently apply the parking brake.
- When the vehicle has slowed sufficiently, steer to the side or shoulder of the road and bring the vehicle to a stop.
- Notify your dispatcher of the situation and request assistance. Do not under any circumstances attempt to move the vehicle once you have stopped.
- If you are stopped in a traffic lane, leave your flashing and revolving lights on and set out flares or other devices to warn approaching motorists.

NOTE: Ambulance drivers must be trained in emergency braking procedures. You would do well to practice the technique just described at different speeds in a large, level parking lot (under the supervision of a qualified driving instructor). Thus you will be able to determine exactly how your vehicle will behave when you must use the parking brake to stop.

Loss of Accelerator Control

Mechanical malfunctions in a vehicle's acceleration system cause a variety of problems. A disconnected ball joint will cause the engine to slow to its idle speed. A broken carburetor linkage will cause the engine to run at full speed. In either case, movement of the accelerator pedal will have no effect whatsoever.

If while driving you suddenly lose speed that cannot be regained by depressing the accelerator pedal, shift into neutral and steer to the side or shoulder of the road. If you must continue on for a short distance to reach a safe place, re-engage the transmission. You will be able to creep along at least at idle speed.

If the engine suddenly speeds for no reason:

- Shift into neutral.
- Steer to the side or shoulder of the road.
- Shut off the ignition to prevent a runaway engine.
- Notify your dispatcher of the situation.

If you are required to stop in a traffic lane, turn on your warning lights and initiate traffic control measures.

The Effect of Speed on an Ambulance Run

Several times thus far you have been admonished to drive slowly, as when visibility is poor and when the road surface is slippery.

At this point you may be inclined to say something like, "How will I ever get a seriously ill or injured person to a hospital if I poke along?"

We are not suggesting that you "poke along." We are suggesting that you drive with these facts in mind:

- The use of excessive speed increases the probability of an accident.
- Speed reduces the chance of avoiding a hazardous situation because of the increase in stopping distance.

Stopping distance is the number of feet that a vehicle travels from the instant that the driver decides to stop until the moment that the vehicle actually stops. It is dependent on several factors, including the speed and condition of the vehicle, road conditions, and the alertness of the driver.

Stopping distance is the total of *reaction distance* and *braking distance*. **Reaction distance** is the number of feet the vehicle travels from the moment that the driver decides to stop until his foot applies pressure to the brake pedal. **Braking distance** is the number of feet that the vehicle travels from the start of the braking action until the vehicle comes to a complete stop. Table 22–1 shows the stopping distances for various vehicles.

Now, what effect does speed have on an ambulance run? Consider a five-mile trip to a hospital from where a sick or injured person was picked up.

Assuming that you will not have to stop or slow down, at 60 miles per hour you will be able to cover the five miles in 5 minutes. At 50 miles per hour it will take 6 minutes to reach the hospital.

At 60 miles per hour the ambulance will travel

TABLE 22–1. The Stopping Distances of Standard Passenger Cars and Trucks on Dry, Clean, and Level Pavement

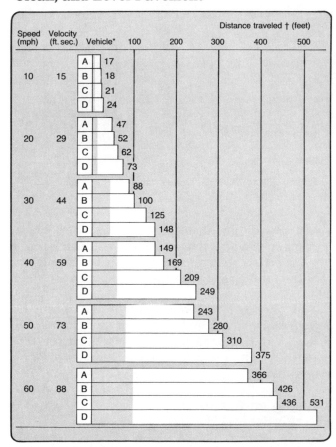

* (A) Standard passenger cars, (B) Light 2-axle trucks, (C) Heavy 2-axle trucks and buses, (D) 3-axle trucks and combinations.

† ☐ Driver reaction distance—based on a reaction time of ¾-second, a typical reaction for most drivers under most conditions.

☐ Vehicle stopping distance—based on provisions for the Uniform Vehicle Code for 20 mph.

more than 425 feet before the driver can bring the vehicle to a complete stop once he perceives a dangerous situation. But at 50 miles per hour the driver will be able to stop the ambulance in less than 300 feet. The one minute gained in response time is not worth the risk of accident brought about by the 25% increase in stopping distance.

Drive Defensively

Ambulances, like all other vehicles, can become involved in a variety of accidents. An ambulance may strike a tree, a utility pole, or perhaps a parked car if the driver tries to turn a corner at too high a speed. Or, an ambulance may roll over or plunge down an embankment when the right-side wheels drop from the roadway onto a depressed shoulder. Seldom do accidents like these occur without producing injuries to the occupants. However, most fatalities and injuries, and the greatest amount of property damage, occur when an ambulance is involved in a collision with another vehicle.

There are seven common ways in which an ambulance can be involved in a collision with another vehicle: (1) with a vehicle ahead; (2) with a vehicle behind; (3) with an approaching vehicle; (4) with a vehicle at an intersection; (5) with a vehicle being passed; (6) with a vehicle that is passing; and (7) with a vehicle or object while backing up (see Figure 22–3).

Some tips for avoiding such accidents follow.

Avoiding an Accident with the Vehicle Ahead

Drivers of other vehicles react to the approach of an ambulance from behind in several ways. One operator may pull his vehicle to the right as he is supposed to do, while another operator may drive his vehicle sharply to the left. Still another operator may jam on his brakes and stop in the middle of the roadway! To avoid hitting a vehicle ahead of you:

- Stay alert for signs of what the driver ahead is planning to do. A flashing turn signal usually indicates a driver's intent to turn, and lighted brake lamps usually indicate that a driver is either slowing or stopping his vehicle. Movement into another lane may tell of a driver's intent to get out of your way. However, do not be lulled into a false sense of security by such signals and movements. Drivers sometimes do just the opposite of what they have signaled.
- Carefully watch the driver who has not signaled or initiated any movement at all. He may not have heard or seen your approach,

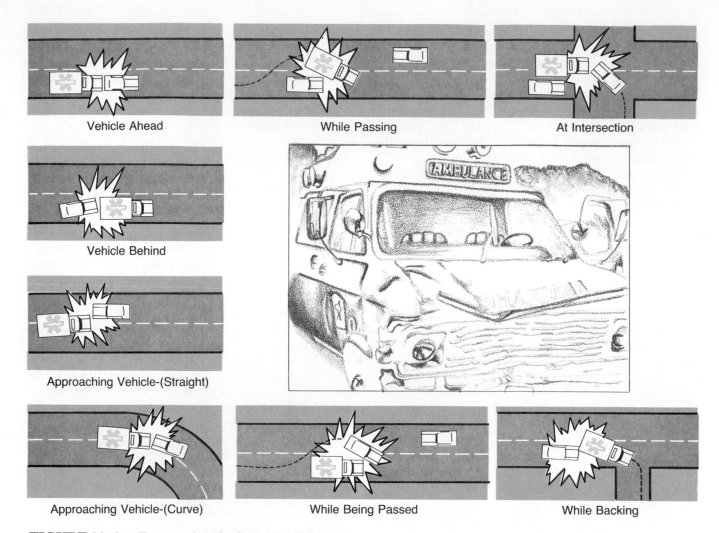

Vehicle Ahead

While Passing

At Intersection

Vehicle Behind

Approaching Vehicle-(Straight)

Approaching Vehicle-(Curve)

While Being Passed

While Backing

FIGURE 22–3.   Types of ambulance accidents.

and he may suddenly jam on his brakes when he looks into his rearview mirror and sees that you are right behind him.

- Do not concentrate solely on the vehicle immediately in front of you. Instead, watch the line of vehicles for some distance ahead.
- Stay a safe distance from the vehicle ahead. Some ambulance drivers have a tendency to drive dangerously close behind other vehicles. If a car or truck ahead stops suddenly, a rear-end collision is almost inevitable. Maintaining one vehicle length for every 10 miles per hour of speed between your ambulance and the vehicle ahead gives you room to maneuver if the other driver decides to brake suddenly.
- Decelerate as soon as you perceive a dangerous situation. Remember that a good driver keeps a foot poised over the brake pedal whenever he senses a potentially dangerous situation. When it is necessary to brake sud-

denly, do not jam on the brakes. Instead, pump them so that the wheels do not lock, an action that contributes to skidding and the total loss of steering capability.

If you think that you cannot brake in time to avoid a collision, attempt to steer around the vehicle ahead. A well-trained and experienced driver can change lanes in a relatively short distance, even in a heavy truck.

Avoiding an Accident with the Vehicle Behind

A motorist who tailgates is asking for trouble. One who tailgates an ambulance is inviting disaster! Why a driver will tailgate an ambulance is a matter for conjecture. Some drivers probably just want to see where the ambulance is going. Other motorists undoubtedly follow ambulance and other emergency vehicles closely just so they can move quicker through traffic. However, the reasons for tailgating are not as important as what can be done about this dangerous practice.

When you are operating an ambulance that is not on an emergency call, there are a number of steps that you can take to discourage or prevent tailgating.

- Slow down and pull to the right. Thus you encourage the tailgater to pass you.
- Slow down and increase the distance between your ambulance and the vehicle directly ahead. Then if the driver ahead brakes suddenly, you will not have to, nor will the tailgater.
- If these tactics fail to discourage or prevent tailgating, you can always pull over, stop, and let the tailgater go around you.

When you are responding to an emergency situation and a vehicle behind you is tailgating, reduce the danger of collision in this manner:

- Maintain a safe distance between the ambulance and the vehicle ahead.
- Use directional and hand signals to make the driver behind fully aware of your intentions at all times. When you must stop, brake smoothly.

Avoiding an Accident with an Approaching Vehicle

An accident with an approaching vehicle is most deadly, even at low speeds. When two vehicles hit squarely head on, inertia causes occupants to continue to move forward even though the vehicle has stopped. An unrestrained driver is thrust forcefully against the steering wheel, and an unrestrained passenger is sometimes propelled completely through the windshield opening. Even when head-on collisions occur slightly off center, the results can be disastrous.

Head-on collisions often occur on straight roads when a driver steers into an oncoming traffic lane in an effort to pass slow-moving vehicles. If you find that you are caught in traffic on a straight roadway:

- Slow down and stay in the correct lane.
- Sound a warning signal.
- Pass when the drivers ahead of you have had the chance to pull their vehicles to the right.

Centrifugal force contributes to head-on collisions on curves. When the roadway curves to the right, there is a tendency for a vehicle to drift to the left and enter the lane of oncoming traffic. On a left-hand curve, you face the possibility of an oncoming vehicle moving into your lane. Drift is more pronounced at high speeds, and unless drifting is corrected, a head-on crash is almost certain. To avoid an accident with a vehicle on a curved roadway:

- Slow down as you enter the curve. If the road curves to the right, keep the ambulance close to the right edge of the roadway. When the road curves to the left, stay in the middle of the lane.
- Do not brake on a curve. If your speed is sufficient, braking may cause a dangerous skid.
- Steer around the curve and apply power as you approach the straightaway.

Avoiding an Accident at an Intersection

One third of all motor vehicle accidents occur at intersections. By following some simple suggestions you can reduce the possibility of such a collision.

- Know where you must turn. This will eliminate the need for a sudden stop or a sudden swerve that can contribute to an accident. Remember that complete familiarity with the response district and the routes to every area within the district is the responsibility of every ambulance driver.
- Be alert for unmarked intersections. Motorists ahead may suddenly change lanes as they approach those intersections. Watch for drivers to pull suddenly into intersections from side streets and driveways.

When approaching a controlled intersection:

- Try to time your arrival so that you can enter the intersection with the signal in your favor.
- Slow down at the intersection.
- Signal your intention to turn.
- Look in both directions, first to the left, then to the right, and then to the left again.
- When it is safe to turn, go!

Be especially watchful for other emergency vehicles that may reach an intersection at the same time you do. When an intersection is controlled by a traffic signal, the emergency vehicle that has the green light in its favor generally proceeds through the intersection first. At intersections without traffic signals, a vehicle usually yields to the one on the right.

WARNING: When stopping at an intersection before making a left turn, keep your wheels in a straight line until you are ready to move. Then, if you are hit from behind, the ambulance will be pushed in a relatively straight line instead of being forced into the lane of oncoming traffic.

Avoiding an Accident with a Vehicle Being Passed

There are few instances when an ambulance does not have to pass vehicles traveling in the same direction. Follow some simple guidelines to ensure your safety and the safety of persons in your care.

- Check oncoming traffic before starting to pass. Bear in mind that if your ambulance and an approaching vehicle are both traveling at 55 mph, the distance between vehicles is closing at slightly less than 2 miles a minute!
- Check the traffic ahead moving in the same direction as the ambulance. Although it may appear to be safe to pass one or more vehicles, it may not be safe to reenter the lane if traffic is congested. Your sudden swerve to the right may cause a driver behind to stop short, with the result being a chain of rear-end collisions. Or, you may force another vehicle off the road.
- Make other motorists aware of your intention to pass by operating both the directional signal and horn or other audible warning device.
- When it is safe to do so, move into the adjacent lane.
- Signal, and then reenter the line of traffic.

Avoiding an Accident with a Passing Vehicle

An accident with a passing vehicle usually occurs when an ambulance is on a nonemergency run or when it is returning to quarters.

As a thoughtful and considerate ambulance driver, you should help other motorists pass your vehicle just as you expect them to help you pass. When a motorist behind you signals his intent to pass your ambulance:

- Pull to the right as far as you can safely and allow the following driver to pass.
- Slow down so the driver has plenty of room to safely reenter the traffic lane.

Avoiding an Accident While Backing

Unfortunately, many ambulances are damaged in accidents that occur when they are being backed, as into a driveway, against a loading dock, or even into quarters.

To avoid a backing accident:

- Have your partner or another person guide you as you back. Watch for his signals.
- If there is no one to guide you, use the side mirrors as you back the ambulance. Backing by mirrors is a little tricky at first, but once you have mastered the technique, backing will be easy.
- Do not under any circumstance lean out of the ambulance and look backward while you operate in reverse.

Escorts and Multiple-Vehicle Responses

When the police provide an escort for an ambulance, you may think that the chances of having an accident are greatly reduced. In some cases, this may be true; however, the same dangers exist while under escort and new ones may be created. Too often, the inexperienced ambulance driver follows the escort vehicle too closely and is unable to stop should the lead vehicle(s) have to make an emergency stop. The inexperienced driver may assume that other drivers know that his vehicle is following the escort. Many times, other drivers will pull out in front of the ambulance just after the escort vehicle passes their position. Because of the dangers involved with escorts, most EMS Systems recommend no escorts unless the driver is not familiar with the location of the patient (or hospital) and must be given assistance from the police.

New dangers exist in cases of multiple vehicle responses. These dangers can be the same ones that are generated by escorted responses, especially when the responding vehicles travel in the same direction, close together.

In multiple-vehicle responses, a great danger exists when two vehicles approach the same intersection at the same time. Not only may they fail to yield for each other; other drivers may yield for the first vehicle but not the second. Obviously, great care must be exercised at intersections during multiple vehicle responses.

NOTE: Be certain to follow your local protocols for the use of warning lights and sirens during escorts and multiple-vehicle responses. If everyone approaching the scene does not follow the proper protocols, the confusion generated may cause the vehicle drivers and other motorists to make serious errors in judgment.

Factors that Affect Response

Movies and television programs often depict ambulance runs as effortless responses over straight, traffic-free roadways in good weather during daylight hours. How easy the operation of an ambulance would be if this were always the case! In reality, an ambulance response can be affected by a number of factors (see Figure 22–4).

Day of the Week

This has a direct bearing on the flow of traffic within a given area. Weekdays are the days of heaviest traffic flow because people are commuting to and from work. On Saturday, commuter traffic generally diminishes, but traffic increases around urban and suburban shopping centers. Sunday traffic is generally minimal, although superhighways and interstate roads may be crowded in the late afternoon and evening.

Time of Day

There was a time not too long ago when traffic patterns were quite predictable. During morning rush hours vehicles moved persons from suburbs to cities, and in the evening the traffic pattern was reversed. Emergency vehicle operators were reasonably sure that if they opposed the flow of traffic their progress

would be relatively unimpeded. Likewise they knew that travel in the same direction as traffic would be difficult.

Today the situation is much different. Downtown areas are still major employment centers, but so, too, are suburban shopping malls, office complexes, and industrial parks. Accordingly, traffic over major arteries tends to be heavy to and from suburban and urban areas during normal commuter hours. Ambulance operators can expect blocked intersections, packed roads, and crawling vehicles regardless of the direction in which they must travel.

Weather

Adverse weather conditions seriously affect ambulance responses. Rain and fog reduce driving speeds and thus increase response times. Icy roads increase response times even more, and a heavy snowfall can temporarily prevent any response at all!

Detours

The movement of vehicles can be seriously impeded by road construction and maintenance activities. Detours and lane restrictions may last only a few hours or they may be in force for months and even years.

A detour often affects the operation of emergency vehicles less than the closing of one or more lanes of a multilane highway. An ambulance can continue to travel over a detour, but when several lanes of a highway are merged into one, there is often no way for an ambulance to move around slow-moving or stopped vehicles or to pull off the road in favor of an alternate route. Thus there is no escaping the traffic jam. Neither siren-sounding nor light flashing can move vehicles out of the way when there is no place for them to go.

Railroads

Although many road grade crossings have been replaced with overpasses, there are still more than a quarter-million in the United States. Thus there are still many opportunities for traffic to be blocked by long, slow-moving freight trains. The problem is not limited to small towns; whole sections of cities can be completely isolated by trains several times a day. Obviously an ambulance or other emergency vehicle cannot pass a grade crossing until a train clears it.

Bridges and Tunnels

Bridges are erected to allow the flow of vehicles over natural and man-made dividers, and tunnels are dug so that traffic can flow under such dividers. However, traffic over bridges and through tunnels slows

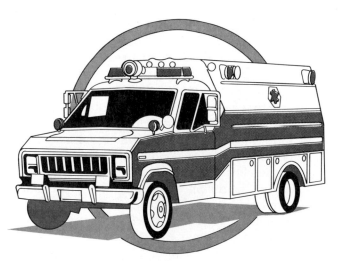

1. Day of the week
2. Time of the day
3. Weather
4. Detours
5. Railroads
6. Bridges and Tunnels
7. Schools
8. Alternate Routes

FIGURE 22–4. Factors that affect response.

during rush hours, and when an accident occurs on a bridge or in a tunnel, the flow of vehicles, including emergency vehicles, may stop altogether, even for an extended period.

Schools

Schools contribute to traffic slowdowns. The reduced speed limits in force during school hours slow the flow of vehicles. Crossing guards also disrupt the flow of traffic, and it is a natural reaction of drivers to slow down when an area is congested with children.

School buses also slow traffic. When a bus makes frequent stops along a two-lane road, traffic can back up behind the bus for a considerable distance. Vehicles on the road cannot resume normal speed until the bus turns off or allows the traffic to pass.

REMEMBER: Emergency vehicles attract children, who often venture out into the street to see them. The driver of every emergency vehicle should slow down when approaching a school or playground.

When it appears that an ambulance will be delayed in reaching a sick or injured person because of these or other factors, the driver should consider taking an alternate route or requesting the response of another ambulance.

Selecting an Alternate Route

Knowing that a variety of changing conditions *can* affect an ambulance response is not enough. You must have a plan for times when changing conditions *do* affect response.

Obtain detailed maps of your service area. On the maps, indicate usually troublesome traffic spots such as schools, bridges, tunnels, railroad grade crossings, and heavily congested areas. Also indicate temporary problems such as road and building construction sites. Mark in both long- and short-term detours.

Using another color, indicate alternate routes to areas normally served by bridges and tunnels. Mark alternate routes to industrial areas that may be partially isolated by long trains. Indicate snow routes, and so on.

Hang one map in quarters and place another map in the ambulance. Then when you must travel past a problem area in response to an urgent call for help you will be able to select an alternate route that will get you to your destination quickly and safely.

RESPONDING TO THE SCENE OF A VEHICLE ACCIDENT

Let us say that your ambulance has just been dispatched to the scene of a motor vehicle accident. Your partner is driving. If he is a good driver, one who concentrates fully on the driving task, he will spend every minute of the trip employing the special skills that are required for the safe response of an ambulance.

But what will you do during the response? Here are some suggestions:

- Confirm the location of the accident with your dispatcher.
- Ask whether there are any further details. While you were preparing to leave quarters, the dispatcher may have been able to elicit additional important bits of information from the initial and subsequent callers.
- Listen for other units on the radio. Knowing that other units are responding will cause you to be watchful for them as you travel to the scene.
- Listen for status reports. Messages from first-arriving units often provide facts about the nature and severity of accidents, facts that will help you to formulate a plan of action even before you arrive on the scene.
- Picture in your mind the location of rescue equipment on the unit. The few seconds that you can save in acquiring rescue tools may mean the difference between life and death.
- As you near intersections, look and listen for other emergency service units approaching from side streets. Remember that other units may be responding along with yours, or they may be responding to a different call. Remember also that in urban settings, sounds bouncing off of buildings can blend siren noises in such a way that you will not be able to determine the direction of an approaching emergency vehicle.
- Look for signs of an accident-related power outage—signs that will suggest that wires are down at the accident scene. During daylight hours, look into the windows of stores and office buildings that would normally be lighted at the time. At night, suspect a power interruption when you see that dwellings and businesses are dark when you would expect them to be illuminated.

- Observe traffic flow. If there is no opposing traffic, suspect a blockade at the accident scene. Remember that all lanes of the road may be blocked for some distance from the crash site.
- Look for smoke in the direction of the accident scene—a sign that fire has resulted from the accident. If you see smoke, note the color; it will be a clue as to what is burning. Black smoke results from burning petroleum products and foamed plastics. Burning hay and vegetable products produce white smoke. White or gray smoke results when wood, paper, and cloth products burn.
- When you are within sight of the accident scene, look at the involved vehicles. If you see that a truck has been damaged, look for fumes or vapor clouds. If you see anything suspicious, stop the ambulance immediately. If you have binoculars on the ambulance, scan the vehicle for hazardous material warning placards. If you see such placards, notify your dispatcher and request advice, or consult the on-board reference book. If you elect to continue on, go directly to a safe place.
- Look for accident victims on or near the road. A person may have been thrown from a vehicle as it careened out of control, or an injured person may have walked away from the wreckage and collapsed on or near the roadway.
- Look for smoke that you may not have seen at a distance—indication of a developing fire.
- Look for broken utility poles and downed wires. At night, direct the beam of a spotlight or handlight on poles and wire spans as you approach the scene. Keep in mind that wires may be down several hundred feet from the crash vehicles.
- Be alert for persons walking along the side of the road toward the accident scene. "Rubberneckers" (excited children in particular) are often oblivious to vehicles approaching from behind. Be especially watchful at night. You may not be able to see persons dressed in dark clothing until they are well within the stopping distance of your vehicle.
- Watch for the signals of police officers and other emergency service personnel. They may have information about hazards or the location of injured persons.
- Sniff for odors as you approach the scene. The odor of gasoline or diesel fuel carries downwind for a considerable distance. Be alert for an unusual odor—it may be the signal that a hazardous commodity has been released.
- If you see that a vehicle is on fire, or if you suspect that a dangerous material has been released or spilled, note the direction and velocity of the wind by observing flags, pennants, smoke, and so on. Remember that you will have to park upwind and uphill.
- Note the terrain. If fuel or another liquid has been released from a ruptured tank, you will need to park uphill from the crash site, as well as upwind (see Scansheet 22–1).

POSITIONING THE AMBULANCE

Parking the ambulance at the location of a sick or injured person may involve little more than positioning the vehicle in a driveway, along a curb, at the loading dock of an industrial plant, or in any other space provided for a vehicle. Parking at the scene of a vehicle accident may not be quite so easy.

Far too many ambulance drivers park their vehicles at accident scenes according to this formula: The closer the ambulance to the wreckage, the shorter the distance that equipment and people must be carried. This is not parking, this is merely stopping! Worse yet, it is stopping without regard for other vehicles that must use the road (including other emergency vehicles) and for any of a number of hazards that may have been produced by the accident.

Establishing the Danger Zone

Keep in mind that a "danger zone" exists around the wreckage at the site of every vehicle accident. The size of the zone depends on the nature and severity of accident produced hazards. In any case, an ambulance should never be parked within the danger zone.

When there are no apparent hazards:

- Consider the danger zone to extend for 50 feet in all directions from the wreckage. The ambulance will be away from broken glass and other debris, and it will not impede emergency service personnel who must work in or around the wreckage.

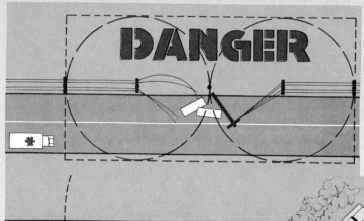

In accidents involving downed electrical wires and damaged utility poles, the danger zone should extend beyond each intact pole for a full span and to the sides for the distance that the severed wires can reach. Stay out of the danger zone until the utility company has deactivated the wires, or until trained rescuers have moved and anchored them.

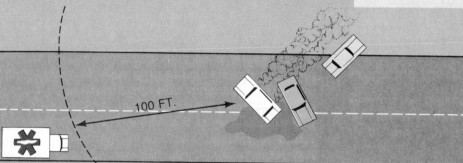

If no other hazards are involved—hazards such as dangerous chemicals or explosives—the ambulance should be parked no closer than 100 feet from a burning vehicle.

100 FT.

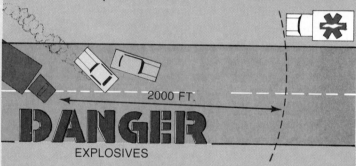

When hazardous materials are either involved in or threatened by fire, the size of the danger zone is dictated by the nature of the materials. If explosives are present, it may be necessary to park the ambulance 2000 feet from the accident.

2000 FT.

DANGER
EXPLOSIVES

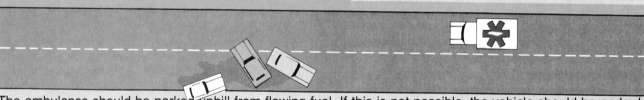

The ambulance should be parked uphill from flowing fuel. If this is not possible, the vehicle should be parked as far from the fuel flow as possible, avoiding gutters, ditches, and gullies that may carry the spill to the parking site.

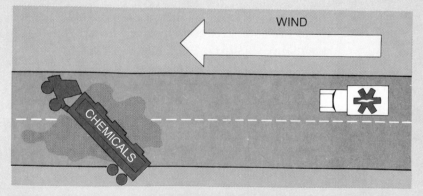

WIND

CHEMICALS

Leaking containers of dangerous chemicals may produce a health as well as a fire hazard. When chemicals have been spilled, whether fumes are evident or not, the ambulance should be parked upwind. If the hazardous material is known, seek advice from experts through the dispatcher or CHEMTREC (see Chapter 17).

- If using highway flares to protect the scene, make sure that the person igniting them has been trained as to the proper technique and wears some type of protective clothing. Many times a flare will sputter and hot pieces of phosphorus can splatter onto unprotected arms and clothing.
- Flares should have a wire flare stand on them rather than the older type with a spiked bottom. If you have the spiked type, after the flare has burned down and is out, remove the spike from the guardpost or asphalt so that it does not become a danger to either children or tires of passing vehicles.

When fuel has been spilled:

- Consider the danger zone to extend for a minimum of 100 feet in all directions from the wreckage. In addition to parking outside the danger zone, park upwind, if possible. Thus the ambulance will be out of the path of dense smoke if the fuel ignites. If fuel is flowing away from the wreckage, park uphill as well as upwind. If parking uphill is not possible, position the ambulance as far from the flowing fuel as possible. Avoid gutters, ditches, and gullies that can carry fuel to the ambulance. When personnel are available and conditions warrant it, have an EMT either divert the flow of fuel or form a dike using the hand shovel in your extrication tool kit. Then have that EMT stand by with a fire extinguisher until the arrival of the fire department. You should not use flares to protect the scene under these conditions; use small orange traffic cones during daylight operations and reflective triangles at night (see Scansheet 22–2).

When an accident vehicle is on fire:

- Consider the danger zone to extend for at least 100 feet in all directions even if the fire appears small and limited to the engine compartment. If fire reaches the vehicle's fuel tank, a resulting explosion could easily damage an ambulance parked closer than 100 feet.

When wires are down:

- Consider the danger zone as the area in which people or vehicles might be contacted by energized wires if they pivot around their points of attachment. Even though you may have to carry equipment and stretchers for a considerable distance, the ambulance should be parked at least one full span of wires from the poles to which broken wires are attached.

When a hazardous commodity is involved:

- Check the on-board hazardous material action guide for suggestions as to where to park, or request advice from an agency such as Chemtrec. In some cases you may be able to park 50 feet from the wreckage, as when no hazardous material has been spilled or released. In other cases you may be warned to park 2,000 feet or more from the wreckage, as when there is the possibility that certain high explosives may detonate. In all cases, park uphill and upwind from the wreckage when you discover that a hazardous material is present at an accident site. Park behind some manmade or natural barrier if possible.

Parking the Ambulance

There is usually no problem parking the ambulance at the location of a sick or injured person. The unit can be parked at the curb or in a driveway or at a loading platform. The parking task is not so easy at the scene of an accident, however (see Scansheet 22–3).

The only way to really ensure the safety of an ambulance at the scene of a vehicle accident is to park it completely off the roadway, as on a service road or in a driveway. To do so, however, will severely reduce or even negate the ability of flashing and revolving warning lights to warn approaching motorists before flares or other warning devices can be set out.

There are two schools of thought about positioning an ambulance or other emergency vehicle on a road leading to an accident site.

Some officials argue that the ambulance should be located beyond the wreckage (relative to the direction of traffic flow). However, most officials favor placing the unit at the edge of the danger zone between the wreckage and approaching vehicles. This is the best position to use the unit's warning lights, although it does not reduce the need for other warning devices. Moreover, the unit's headlights can be used for initial scene illumination at night.

Once the ambulance is parked, its emergency brake should be set and wheel chocks should be firmly wedged under the tires in such a way that forward movement will be retarded if the ambulance is struck from behind.

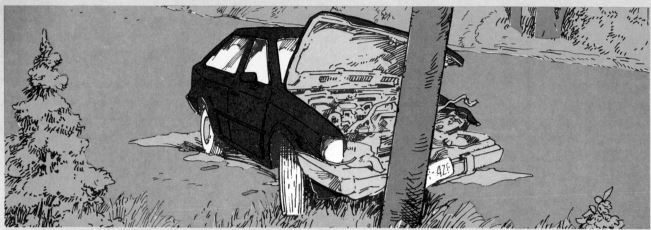

ACCIDENT VEHICLE: Car has crashed into pole. Note that no electrical wires are down.

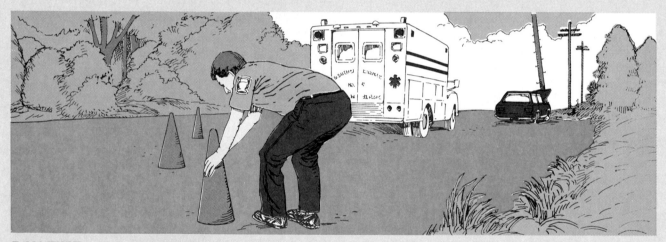

DAY TIME: EMT protects the scene with traffic triangles or cones.

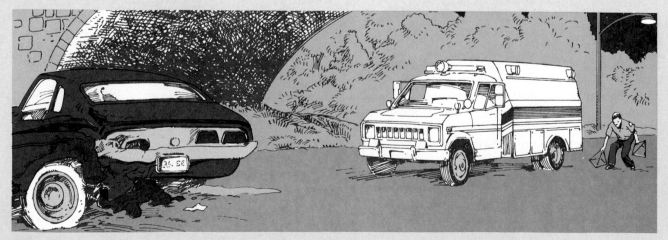

NIGHTTIME: EMT protects scene using reflective triangles.

SCAN 22—3 PARKING THE AMBULANCE

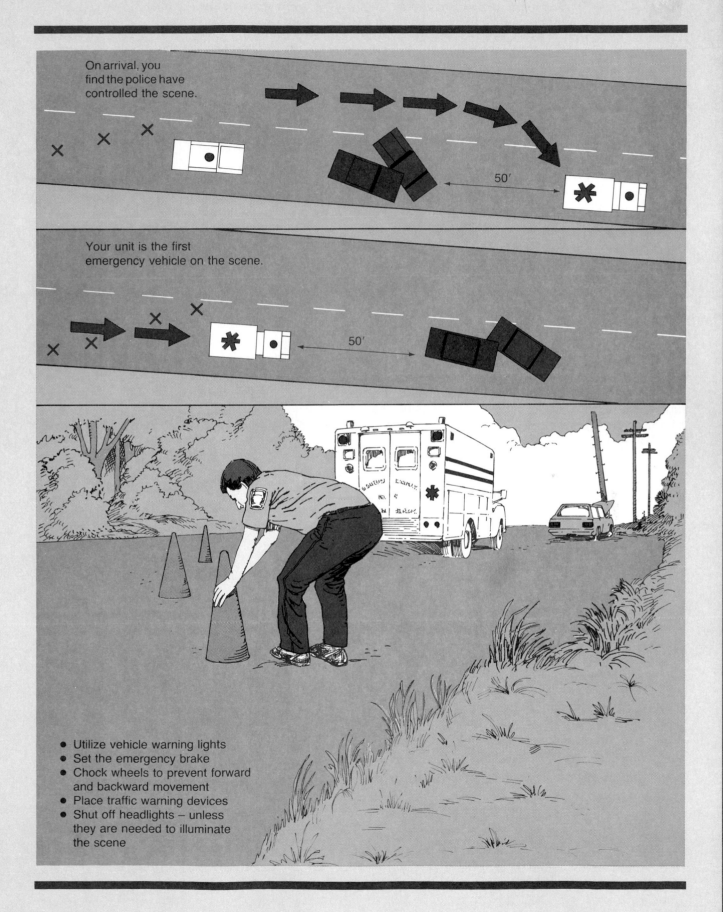

On arrival, you find the police have controlled the scene.

50'

Your unit is the first emergency vehicle on the scene.

50'

- Utilize vehicle warning lights
- Set the emergency brake
- Chock wheels to prevent forward and backward movement
- Place traffic warning devices
- Shut off headlights – unless they are needed to illuminate the scene

NOTE: Unless they are needed to illuminate the work area, the ambulance headlights should be turned off if the unit is parked facing oncoming traffic. Even low beams can cancel the effectiveness of flashing and revolving warning lights. Moreover, the headlights may confuse or even temporarily blind approaching motorists.

SUMMARY

In some areas of the country, citizen requests for assistance go directly to one-number emergency reporting centers where dispatchers control the movements of fire, ambulance, rescue, police, and other emergency service units.

In other areas, citizen requests go to either a fire or police dispatch center. Delays in alerting and subsequent delays in response are possible but are usually minimal because of cross-communication capabilities.

In still other areas, citizen requests can go to a small dispatch facility, the fire department, the ambulance service, the rescue squad, the police department, or even a place of business or someone's home. Valuable time is often lost because of the misdirection of calls.

EMS dispatchers should ask certain questions of a citizen requesting an ambulance for a sick or injured person. These questions should include:

- Do you have an emergency?
- What is the exact location of the (sick or injured) person?
- What is the nature of the emergency?
- Can you tell me the person's name and age?
- What is your name? What number are you calling from?
- Will you be at that number if I need more information?

Dispatchers should ask these questions of someone who is reporting a motor vehicle accident:

- What is the exact location of the accident?
- What number are you calling from?
- What is your name?
- How many and what kind of vehicles are involved?
- How many persons do you think are injured?
- Do the victims appear trapped?
- Is traffic moving?

- How many lanes are open?
- How far is traffic backed up?
- Are any of the vehicles on fire?
- Are any of the vehicles leaking fuel?
- Are any electrical wires down?
- Do any of the vehicles appear unstable? Is any vehicle on its side or top?
- Does any vehicle appear to be carrying a hazardous cargo?

Information transmitted to the ambulance service should be as complete as the information gathered.

A person who aspires to be an ambulance driver should follow a number of steps to prepare for the first run:

- Attend a formal emergency vehicle driver's course that includes both classroom and in-vehicle instruction.
- Learn the laws that regulate the operation of emergency vehicles within his state.
- Learn when to drive an ambulance, and when not to drive.

During an ambulance run, a good driver:

- Properly uses the audible and visual warning devices.
- Is prepared to employ special driving skills during inclement weather.
- Is prepared to share the road with other drivers.
- Is prepared to drive at night.
- Is ready to cope with sudden mechanical problems.
- Appreciates how certain factors affect response.
- Is prepared to select an alternate route.
- Drives defensively and avoids accidents.

During a response to the scene of a motor vehicle accident, the attending EMT should make observations and take steps to ensure a safe trip. Thus the operator can concentrate on the driving task.

As the ambulance leaves quarters and during the response, the attending EMT should:

- Confirm the location of the accident with the dispatcher.
- Ask whether there are any further details.
- Listen for other units on the radio.
- Listen for status reports.

- Picture in his mind the location of rescue equipment on the ambulance.
- Listen and look for other emergency service units approaching from side streets.

As the ambulance approaches the scene, the attending EMT should:

- Look for signs of an accident-related power outage.
- Observe traffic flow.
- Look for smoke in the direction of the accident scene.

When the ambulance is within sight of the accident scene, the attending EMT should:

- Look at the accident vehicles and assess the mechanisms of injury.

As the ambulance nears the wreckage, the attending EMT should:

- Look for accident victims on or near the road.
- Look for smoke that might not have been seen at a distance.
- Look for broken utility poles and downed wires.
- Be alert for persons walking along the side of the road toward the accident scene.
- Watch for the signals of police officers and other emergency service personnel.

- Sniff for odors characteristic of hazardous materials.
- Note the wind direction if a hazardous material has been spilled or released.
- Note the terrain.

A danger zone should be established around every motor vehicle accident site. When there are no apparent hazards, the danger zone should extend for 50 feet in all directions from the wreckage. When fuel has been spilled, the minimum danger zone should extend for 100 feet in all directions. When an accident vehicle is on fire, the minimum danger zone should extend for 100 feet in all directions. When wires are down, the danger zone should include the area in which persons or vehicles might be contacted by broken wires if they rotate around their point of attachment. When a dangerous commodity has been spilled or released, the danger zone should be established on the basis of advice from a hazardous materials action guide or other competent authority.

Most ambulance officials favor parking an ambulance at the edge of the danger zone between the wreckage and approaching traffic. Thus the unit's flashing and revolving lights will warn oncoming motorists and its headlights will illuminate the accident scene.

When the ambulance is parked facing approaching traffic, the headlights should be turned off unless they are needed to illuminate the wreckage. Headlights can cancel the effectiveness of warning lights, and they can temporarily blind approaching motorists.

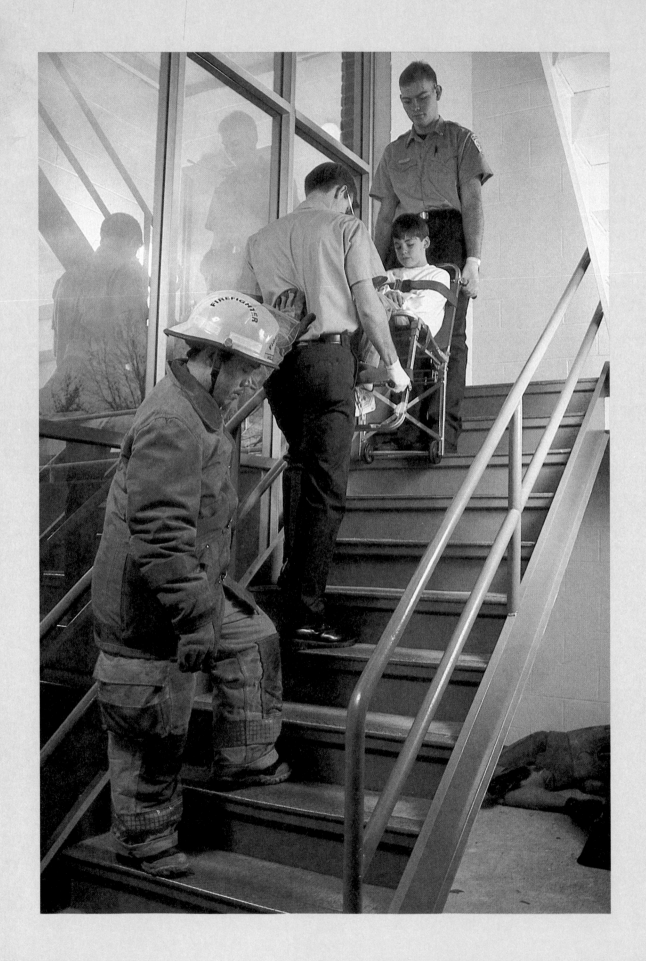

Transferring Patients to the Ambulance

OBJECTIVES   As an EMT, you should be able to:

1. List THREE situations that may necessitate the emergency evacuation of a sick or injured person before emergency care procedures can be completed. (p. 565)

2. List FOUR nonhazard situations when it may be necessary to move a sick or injured person before emergency care procedures can be completed. (p. 565)

3. List FIVE one-rescuer carries that can be used to move nonambulatory persons from dangerous environments. (p. 566)

4. List SIX one-rescuer drags that can be used to evacuate persons who cannot be assisted or carried from a dangerous environment. (p. 568)

5. State which emergency moves provide some support for a patient's spine and extremities. (p. 566)

6. List THREE techniques that two rescuers can employ to evacuate nonambulatory persons from dangerous environments. (p. 566)

7. Identify these patient-carrying devices:
   • Wheeled ambulance stretcher (p. 570)
   • Portable ambulance stretcher (p. 570)
   • Stair chair (p. 570)

• Scoop stretcher (orthopedic stretcher) (p. 571)
• Long spine board (p. 571)
• Basket stretcher (p. 571)

8. State what patient-carrying device (or devices) should be used in each of the following situations, assuming that the person does not have a spinal injury:
   • when movement to the ambulance is unrestricted (p. 571)
   • when the patient must be removed from a confined space, moved through a narrow opening, or carried along a narrow hallway (p. 571)
   • when the person must be carried down stairs (p. 571)
   • when the person must be moved from one level to another by rope or ladder (p. 571)
   • when the person must be carried over debris or rough terrain, or moved uphill. (p. 571)

9. State what patient-carrying device (or devices) should be used in each of the following situations, assuming that the person has a spinal injury:

- when the person is on the ground or the floor of a structure (p. 571)
- when the person is on a seat or the floor of a vehicle (p. 571)
- when the person is seated in a vehicle and

is immobilized on a short spine board or in a vest (p. 571)
- when the person must be moved from one level to another. (p. 571)

SKILLS   As an EMT, you should be able to:

1. Perform the following:
   - One-rescuer assist
   - Piggyback carry
   - Cradle carry
   - Pack-strap carry
   - Fireman's carry
   - Shoulder drag
   - Foot drag
   - Fireman's drag
   - Incline drag
   - Blanket drag
   - Clothes drag
2. As an EMT working with a partner, you should be able to evacuate sick or injured persons from dangerous environments by means of:
   - Two-rescuer assist
   - Two-rescuer extremities carry
   - Two-rescuer chair carry
3. As an EMT working with a partner, you should be able to prepare each of the following patient-carrying devices for use, transfer a patient to the device, properly position the patient on the device, cover the patient, secure the patient,

move the patient to the ambulance on or in the device, and load the patient into the ambulance.
   - Wheeled ambulance stretcher
   - Portable ambulance stretcher
   - Stair chair
   - Scoop stretcher
   - Long spine board
   - Basket stretcher
4. As an EMT working with a partner and assistants, you should be able to:
   - Safely move a conscious or unconscious patient, free of fractures of the extremities, using a three rescuer carry
   - Safely move an ambulance stretcher, long spineboard, or stair chair down a flight of stairs
   - Safely raise a patient to your knees so that he can be placed into a basket-type stretcher
   - Safely move a stretcher over debris or rough terrain.
   - Safely move a stretcher uphill by at least two means when walking up the hill is impossible

---

EMERGENCY EVACUATION PROCEDURES

On most ambulance runs you will be able to reach a sick or injured person without difficulty, assess his condition, carry out emergency care procedures where he lies, and then transfer him to the ambulance. You will not always work under the best of conditions. At times you will have to work in darkness, in the rain, and when it is cold, but you will be expected to provide on-the-spot care nonetheless.

Unfortunately, there will be times when circumstances will necessitate your moving an injured person before you can dress and bandage wounds or splint fractures, perhaps even before you can initiate basic life support efforts. In fact, there may be

times when you will have to move a person before you can even assess his condition.

Emergency and Nonemergency Moves

There are three types of moves used at the emergency scene. Dangers at the scene may require you to move a patient quickly, perhaps prior to assessment and care. This type of move is an **emergency move.** There are also **nonemergency moves,** like the moving of a patient to a cooler environment when he has apparent heat cramps. The third move is when you take the patient from the scene to the ambulance for transport. This type of move is called a **transfer.**

When To Move a Patient

There are times when you must move a patient quickly, using an emergency move. This type of move may have to take place before assessment can begin or be completed. The patient may need basic life support, wound care, or splinting of fractures; however, the move must still be made without delay. An emergency move should take place when:

- *The scene is hazardous*—Hazards may make it necessary to move a patient quickly in order to protect you and the patient. This may occur when the emergency scene involves uncontrolled traffic, fire or threat of fire, possible explosions, possible electrical hazards, toxic gases, or radiation.
- *Care requires repositioning*—You may have to move a patient to a hard, flat surface to provide CPR, or you may have to move a patient to reach life-threatening bleeding.
- *You must gain access to other patients*—You may have to quickly move an assessed patient with minor problems to reach a patient who needs life-saving care. This is seen most often in motor vehicle accidents.

It may become necessary to perform a nonemergency move of a patient. Such a move may be called for when:

- *Factors at the scene cause patient decline*—If a patient is RAPIDLY declining due to heat or cold, he may have to be moved. Should the patient appear to be allergic to something at the scene, he may have to be moved to reduce the chances of developing anaphylactic shock.
- *You must reach other patients*—When there are other assessed patients at the scene requiring care for life-threatening problems, you may have to move another patient to have the space needed to provide care. The patient being moved may need certain care procedures to avoid additional pain and injury before being moved.
- *Care requires moving the patient*—This is usually seen in cases where there are no injuries or severe medical problems. Problems due to extreme heat or cold (heat cramps, heat exhaustion, hypothermia, and frostbite) are good examples.

- *The patient insists on being moved*—You are not allowed to restrain a patient. Explain to the patient why he should not move or be moved. If he tries to move himself, you may have to assist him. A patient may become so insistent that stress worsens his condition. If this type of patient can be moved, and the move is a short one, you may have to move him in order to reduce the stress and provide care.

Nonemergency moves should be carried out in such a way as to prevent additional injury to the patient and to avoid discomfort and pain. The following rules are to be followed for a nonemergency move:

1. The patient should be conscious.
2. The patient assessment should be completed.
3. All vital signs should be within normal range and stable.
4. There should be no serious bleeding or wounds.
5. There must be ABSOLUTELY no signs of spinal injury, no injuries associated with spinal injury, and the mechanism of injury should not indicate any chances of such an injury.
6. All fractures must be immobilized or splinted.

Lifting Techniques

You must use the correct lifting techniques in order to avoid lower back and knee injuries. Utilizing the rules of correct lifting also will help you maintain your balance and help prevent a fall that could injure you and your patient. When you must lift a patient, you should:

1. Think through the move before attempting it. Know what you are going to do and how to prevent possible difficulties.
2. Do not attempt to lift or lower someone if you cannot handle and control the weight.
3. Always begin the move from a balanced position and stay aware of your balance. The loss of balance can cause serious injuries to you and the patient.
4. Make certain that you initially have good, firm footing and can maintain this throughout the lift.
5. Lift with your legs, not your back. Bend your

knees, keeping one foot slightly in front of the other. Keep your back straight as you lift with your legs.

6. Stay aware of your breathing. You do not want to lift and carry a patient while holding your breath.

7. When possible, keep your back straight when carrying a patient.

Types of Moves

None of these moves protects the patient's spine or provides adequate protection for unsplinted fractures. In an emergency move, you will have to use the most efficient method for the amount of time you have to move the patient. The most commonly used moves include:

- *One-Rescuer Moves*

  One-Rescuer Assist—patient is conscious and can walk with assistance.

  Piggyback Carry—patient is conscious, can stand, and has no fractures of the extremities.

  Cradle Carry—patient may be conscious or unconscious.

  Fireman's Carry—conscious or unconscious patient with no fractures of the extremities.

  Pack Strap Carry—this does not require any equipment. Use on the conscious patient with no fractures of the extremities.

  One-Rescuer Drags—conscious or unconscious patient with no fractures of the body part being held during the drag. The blanket drag offers some support for the spine and extremities.

- *Two-Rescuer Moves*

  Two-Rescuer Assist—patient is conscious and can walk with assistance.

  Extremity Carry—conscious or unconscious patient with no fractures of the extremities.

  Fireman's Carry with Assist—conscious or unconscious patient with no fractures of the extremities.

- *Three-Rescuer Move*

  Three-Rescuer Carry—conscious or unconscious patient, free of fractures of the extremities.

The most common emergency moves are presented in Scansheets 23–1 through 23–3. All these can be used for nonemergency moves, depending on the situation. If the rules for a nonemergency move are met, the one- or two-rescuer assist should be practical to use. A cradle carry or two-rescuer extremity carry may be useful in some cases.

If it is necessary to use a three-rescuer carry, use the following steps:

- Prior to movement, cross the patient's arms onto his chest and tie at the wrists using a soft bandage.

- Each rescuer kneels on the knee toward the patient's feet. The EMT at the head of the patient slides one arm under the patient's head and shoulders, supporting the head. The other arm is under the patient's upper back. The middle EMT slides one arm under the patient's waist and his other arm under the patient's hips. The EMT at the patient's legs places one arm under the patient's knees and one arm under the patient's ankles.

- The head-end rescuer directs all rescuers to lift patient to their knees.

- The head-end rescuer directs all rescuers to move to a standing position.

- On another signal, all rescuers roll the patient to their chests.

- Movement of the patient can take place either by the rescuers walking forward or by sidestepping.

TRANSFERRING THE PATIENT

Usually the transfer of a sick or injured patient involves little more than placing the patient on the wheeled ambulance stretcher and moving it a short distance to the ambulance. The process becomes more complicated when you believe the patient may have spinal injuries. For such cases, extrication collars and spine boards become part of the process. If a traction splint has been applied to a patient, special care must be taken to ensure that the splint will continue to immobilize the extremity and no additional injury occurs to the patient.

Transfer to the ambulance is accomplished in four steps, regardless of the complexity of the operation. The steps include:

1. Selecting the proper patient-carrying device.
2. Packaging the patient for transfer.
3. Moving the patient to the ambulance.
4. Loading the patient onto the ambulance.

SCAN 23–1 EMERGENCY MOVES—ONE RESCUER

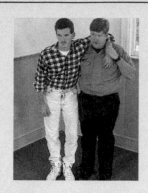

THE ONE RESCUER ASSIST

Place patient's arm around your neck, grasping his hand in yours. Place your other arm around patient's waist. Help patient walk to safety. Be prepared to change movement technique if level of danger increases.

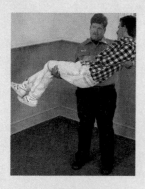

THE CRADLE CARRY

Place one arm across patient's back with your hand under his far arm. Place your other arm under his knees and lift. If patient is conscious, have him place his near arm over your shoulder.

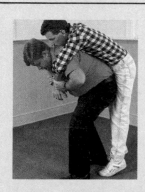

THE PACK STRAP CARRY

Have patient stand—turn your back to him, bringing his arms over your shoulders to cross your chest. Keep his arms straight as possible, his armpits over your shoulders. Hold patient's wrists, bend, and pull him onto your back.

THE PIGGY BACK CARRY

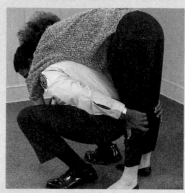

Assist the patient to stand. Place her arms over your shoulder so they cross your chest. Bend over and lift patient. While she holds on with her arms, crouch and grasp each thigh. Use a lifting motion to move her onto your back. Pass your forearms under her knees and grasp her wrists.

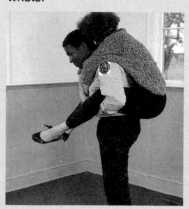

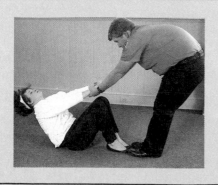

THE FIREMAN'S CARRY

Place your feet against her feet and pull patient toward you. Bend at waist and flex knees. Duck and pull her across your shoulder, keeping hold of one of her wrists. Use your free arm to reach between her legs and grasp thigh. Weight of patient falls onto your shoulders. Stand up. Transfer your grip on thigh to patient's wrist.

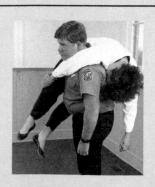

SCAN 23–2 EMERGENCY MOVES—ONE RESCUER DRAGS

CAUTION: Always pull in direction of long axis of patient's body. Do not pull patient sideways. Avoid bending or twisting the trunk if at all possible.

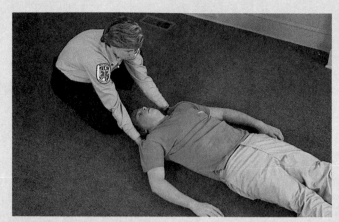

THE SHOULDER DRAG

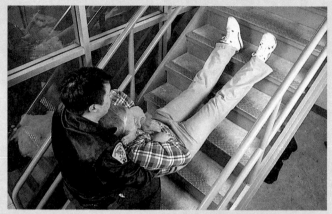

THE INCLINE DRAG . . . Always head first

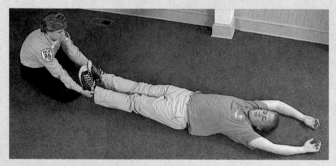

THE FOOT DRAG

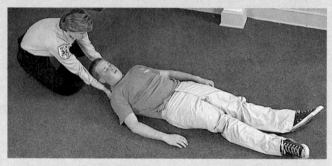

THE CLOTHES DRAG

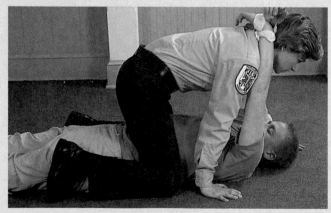

THE FIREMAN'S DRAG Place patient on his back and tie hands together with something that will not cut into his skin. Straddle the patient, facing his head; crouch and pass your head through his trussed arms and raise your body. This will in turn raise patient's head, neck, and upper trunk. Crawl on your hands and knees, dragging the person. During the drag, keep the patient's head as low as possible.

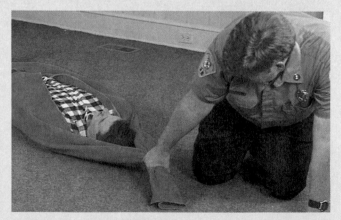

THE BLANKET DRAG Gather half of the blanket material up against the patient's side. Roll the patient toward your knees so that you can place the blanket under him. Gently roll the patient back onto the blanket. During the drag, keep the patient's head as low as possible.

SCAN 23—3 EMERGENCY MOVES— 2-RESCUER

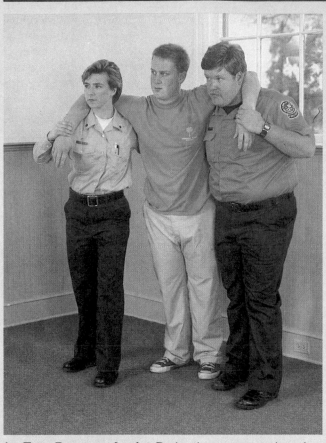

1 Two-Rescuer Assist Patient's arms are placed around shoulders of both rescuers. They each grip a hand, place their free arms around patient's waist and then help him walk to safety.

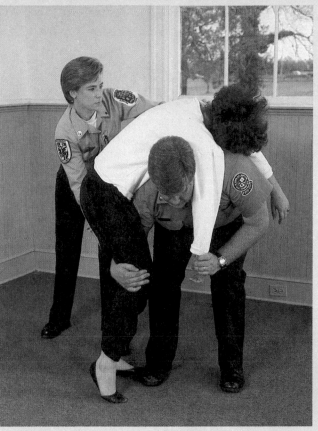

2 Fireman's Carry with Assistance Have someone help lift patient. The second rescuer helps to position the patient.

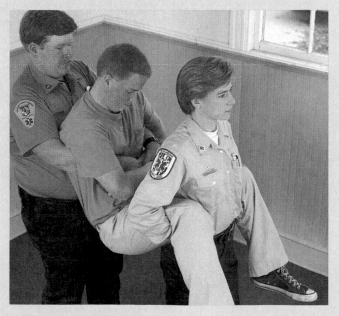

3 The Two-Rescuer Extremity Carry Place patient on back, with knees flexed. Kneel at patient's head— place your hands under his shoulders. Helper stands at patient's feet and grasps his wrists. Helper lifts patient forward while you slip your arms under patient's armpits and grasp his wrist. Helper can turn, crouch down, and grasp patient's knees. Direct helper so you both stand at the same time and move as a unit when carrying patient.

Conventional Patient-Carrying Devices

Ambulances generally are provided with a number of different patient-carrying devices (Figure 23–1):

- The *wheeled ambulance stretcher* may be a one-, two- or multilevel device. Most can be adjusted so that a patient can be transported flat, in a seated or semiseated position with or without the knees flexed, or in the Trendelenburg position (the head end of the stretcher tilted down).

- A *portable ambulance stretcher* is usually carried so that a second nonambulatory pa-

tient can be carried in an ambulance. It becomes a necessity when space limitations or other factors prevent the transfer of a sick or injured person on the wheeled stretcher. Some portable stretchers are simply tubular metal frames with canvas or coated fabric bottoms and foldaway wheels and legs. Some models fold into easily stored units, and some have adjustable backrests.

- A *stair chair* is useful when a person must be carried down stairs or through hallways too narrow for conventional stretchers. This device is not recommended for use with unconscious or disoriented patients. Some stair chairs can be converted into full-length portable stretchers.

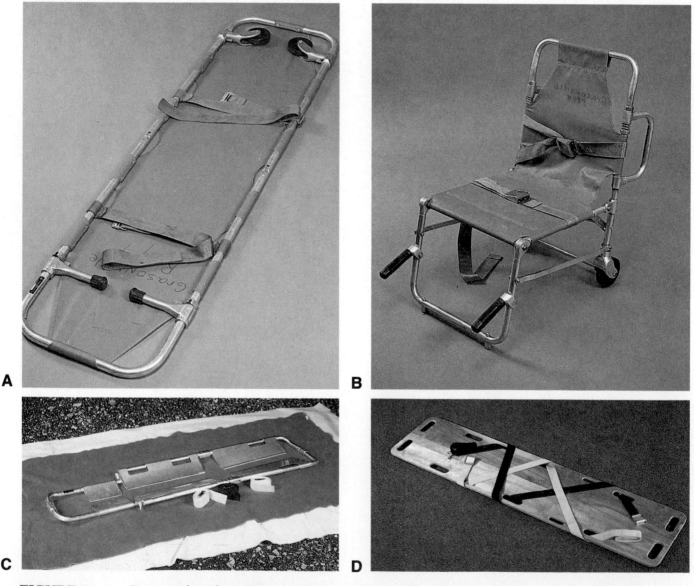

A   **B**   **C**   **D**

FIGURE 23–1. Conventional patient carrying devices, all with straps for securing patient to the device: **(A)** a portable ambulance stretcher; **(B)** a stair chair; **(C)** a scoop stretcher or orthopedic stretcher; **(D)** a long-spine board.

- A *scoop stretcher* (orthopedic stretcher) can be used to pick up a seriously injured person with a minimum of body movement. To use this type of stretcher effectively, you must have access to the patient from all sides. The scoop stretcher is not designed to be used as a primary spine immobilization device for suspected spinal injuries.
- A *long spine board* allows for the safe pickup and movement of a person with a suspected spinal injury. Some models are used with standard 9-foot straps; others have pins to which special straps can be quickly clipped. A number of head-restraint devices can be used with conventional wood spine boards.
- A *basket stretcher* is usually the device of choice when a sick or injured person must be moved from one level to another by ladder or rope. Newer model wire or plastic basket stretchers are usually provided with four-point bridles, security straps, and adjustable foot rests.

Selecting the Proper Patient-Carrying Device—No Spinal Injury

Almost any of the conventional patient-carrying devices can be used to transfer a patient who has no spinal injury. Selection of the device is usually influenced by the condition of the pathway from the patient's location to the ambulance.

- Use the wheeled ambulance stretcher when movement to the ambulance is unrestricted.
- Use the portable ambulance stretcher, a stair chair, a scoop stretcher, or a long spine board when a person must be removed from a confined space, moved through a narrow opening, or carried through a narrow hallway.
- Use a stair chair when it is impossible to carry a person down stairs on a stretcher and when an elevator is too small for a stretcher.
- Use a basket stretcher to move a person from one level to another by rope or ladder.
- Use a basket stretcher when a person must be carried over debris, rough terrain, or uphill.

Selecting the Proper Patient-Carrying Device—Possible Spinal Injury

When a person has a possible spinal injury, the patient-carrying device must provide straight-line neck and back immobilization. Selection of the device will be influenced by the location of the person and how the person must be moved.

- Use a long spine board or a scoop stretcher when a spine-injured person is on the ground or the floor of a structure. In certain circumstances, it may be necessary to use a scoop stretcher for the initial short distance transfer of the patient to a long spine board. Once immobilized on the board, the patient can be carried directly to the ambulance or secured to the cot and wheeled there.
- Use a rope sling to pull a patient onto a long spine board from a position on the seat or floor of a vehicle or from under a vehicle. If the person is on the floor and working space can be created by removing or displacing the seat (or seats), it may be possible to lift him from the vehicle on a scoop stretcher and then transfer the patient to a long spine board.
- Use a long spine board to immobilize a person who has been immobilized with a short spine board or vest (e.g., K.E.D.). The board can then be placed on the wheeled stretcher or in a basket stretcher, or it can be carried directly to the ambulance, depending on circumstances.
- Use a long spine board to immobilize the person and then secure the board and patient in a basket stretcher when a spine-injured person must be moved from one level to another and movement cannot be made over stairs or by elevator. Then move the stretcher by rope or ladder.

Packaging and Securing the Patient

Packaging refers to the sequence of operations required to ready the patient to be moved and to combine the patient and the patient-carrying device into a unit ready for transfer. A sick or injured patient must be packaged so that his condition is not aggravated. Necessary care for wounds and fractures should be completed. Impaled objects must be stabilized. All dressings and splints must be checked before the patient is placed on the patient-carrying device. The properly packaged patient is covered and secured to the patient-carrying device.

Covering the Patient

Covering a patient helps to maintain body temperature, prevents exposure to the elements, and helps assure privacy. A single blanket or perhaps just a sheet may be all that is required in warm weather. A sheet and blankets should be used in cold weather. When practical, cuff the blankets under the patient's chin, with the top sheet outside. Do not leave sheets and blankets hanging loose. Tuck them under the mattress at the foot and sides of the stretcher. In wet weather, a plastic cover should be placed over the blankets during transfer. This can be removed once in the ambulance to prevent the patient from overheating.

If a scoop-style stretcher is used, you will have to fold a blanket once or twice lengthwise and carefully tuck the blanket under the patient. Cover the patient as best you can, place the patient and scoop-style stretcher on a wheeled ambulance stretcher, and then apply full covering. The same directions apply when using the long spine board. Do not move a patient with possible spinal injury in order to tuck in a blanket.

When a basket stretcher is used, line the basket with a blanket prior to positioning the patient. If this is not done, cover the patient as you would in the case of the scoop-style stretcher.

A patient being transferred on a stair chair should be covered. Have the patient sitting upright with his hands folded over his lap and his legs together. Drape a sheet and then a blanket over the patient's body and shoulders. Carefully tuck in the sheet and blanket all around.

In cold or wet weather cover the patient's head, leaving the face exposed. If the nature of the patient's injuries allows you to do so:

1. Place a towel flat under the patient's head.
2. Pull the outermost edge of the towel up and over the patient's head so that it covers the forehead, but not the eyes.
3. Draw the corners of the towel diagonally to the patient's chest, allowing the towel to drape each side of the patient's head (Fig. 23-2).

Many of today's devices used for the transfer and transport of patients should have a minimum of three straps holding the patient securely to the device. The first strap should be at the chest level, the second at the hip or waist level, and the third on the lower extremities. Sometimes there is a fourth strap used if those at the chest area are crossed, in which case two are needed.

All patients, including those receiving CPR, must be secured to the patient-carrying device before you attempt to transfer them to the ambulance.

If your patient is not on a carrying device (i.e., spineboard) and is just on the ambulance stretcher, some states, as a matter of policy, require shoulder

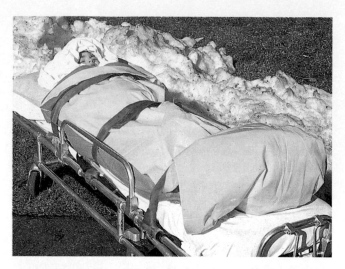

FIGURE 23–2. Covering the patient during normal, wet, or cold weather conditions.

harnesses that secure the patient to the stretcher to prevent him from being catapulted from the patient area through to the driver's compartment as a result of a sudden stopping of the ambulance.

The Wheeled Ambulance Stretcher

This is the most commonly used patient-carrying device. The principles of transfer that apply to this device also apply in general to all others.

Preparing the Stretcher

Elevate the stretcher to bed-level if it is a two-level or multilevel device. Unfasten the safety straps; tuck them under the mattress or otherwise make sure they do not become tripping hazards. Lower the rail on the loading side of the stretcher. Remove the blankets and the top sheet; place them on a clean surface nearby. Place the pillow in the appropriate position.

Transferring the Patient

In some cases, a patient may stand and help place himself on the stretcher. When the patient with *no* spinal injury is in a vehicle, wreckage, or debris, you may have to adapt a standard patient moving technique to transfer him to the stretcher. An example would be to modify the cradle carry for someone seated and turned sideways in the front of an automobile. The patient *with* spinal injury should be secured to a long spine board before being transferred to the stretcher. The long board and the secured patient are lifted as a unit and secured to the wheeled ambulance stretcher.

The transfer of a bed-level or ground-level patient may require you to use special lifting techniques. There are two techniques commonly used to transfer the bed-level patient to a wheeled ambulance stretcher: **the direct carry method and the draw sheet method.** For the transfer of a ground-level patient, **a modified direct carry method** is used. These methods are shown on Scansheet 23–4a and b. Regardless of the method used, protect yourself. Do not position yourself too far from the patient and do not strain to lift the patient. You must protect yourself from lower back strain and hernia. Also, you must be certain not to lose your balance and possibly injure yourself, your partner, or the patient.

Covering and Securing the Patient

As noted earlier, all patients should be covered and secured to the patient-carrying device. A top sheet and blankets, as required by weather, are to be applied over the patient's body. The side rails should be locked in the up position and the body straps should be fastened.

Moving and Loading the Patient

Regardless of the method used to move a patient, you and your partner should walk naturally at a smooth, fairly slow pace.

Use the pull handles to roll and maneuver the stretcher. Roll the stretcher at a safe, constant speed. Turn corners slowly and squarely to minimize discomfort to the patient. Lift the stretcher over thresholds and rugs. Use caution when maneuvering the stretcher; bumps from a wheeled stretcher can cause unsightly and costly damage to walls and furniture. Roll the stretcher to within 3 feet of the ambulance loading door.

The wheeled stretcher can be carried by the end carry method or the side carry method. The **end carry** is most widely used, with the **side carry** used to load the patient into the ambulance. The side carry technique of carrying and loading a patient secured to a wheeled ambulance stretcher is shown in Scansheet 23–5.

Folding Stair Chairs

These devices are useful for narrow corridors, narrow doorways, small elevators, and for taking a patient up or down stairs. *They should not be used for patients who are unconscious or disoriented. They should not be used when a patient has a possible spinal injury or fractures of the lower extremities.* When a folding stair chair is not available, a strongly constructed desk chair may be used to move the patient.

Preparing a Stair Chair

The chair is unfolded and secured by positive locking devices (not on all chairs). The safety straps are unfastened and positioned so that they do not become tripping hazards. Sheets and blankets should not be draped over the chair prior to positioning the patient.

Transferring the Patient

The direct carry method can be modified when a bed-level patient must be moved into a stair chair. The first part of the technique is the same as for transfer of a patient to a wheeled stretcher. When it is time to move the patient from the bed, however, the foot-end EMT slides his arm under the patient's thighs rather than under the midcalf. This maneuver allows the lower part of the patient's legs to drop down into a sitting position as he is eased into the chair.

When transferring a ground-level patient, a modification of the direct carry method can be used. There also are two other methods that can be used effectively.

The Extremity Transfer This technique can be used to move a patient from the floor or ground to a stair chair or to any other patient-carrying device, for that matter. This method is not to be used, however, when the patient has a spinal injury or extremity fractures. (Figure 23–3.)

1. One EMT assumes a head-end position, while the other EMT takes the foot-end position.
2. The EMTs assist the patient to a sitting position.
3. The head-end EMT reaches under the patient's armpits and grasps the patient's wrists, holding the arms to the patient's chest.
4. The foot-end EMT flexes the patient's knees and slides his hands into position under the knees.
5. Simultaneously, on the command of the head-end EMT, both EMTs move to a standing position, lifting the patient.
6. They carry the patient to the chair and lower him onto it.
7. The patient is draped with a sheet and blanket placed over his body and shoulders.
8. The patient is secured to the chair with three straps. One is fastened around the chest and the back of the chair. A second strap is placed across the thighs and around the seat of the

SCAN 23—4 WHEELED AMBULANCE STRETCHERS—TRANSFERRING THE PATIENT

The Bed-level Patient: Direct Carry Method

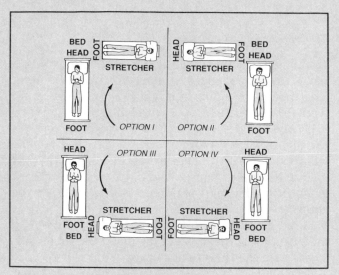

Stretcher is placed at 90° angle to bed, depending on room configuration.

1

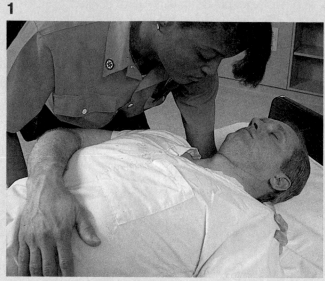

The head-end EMT cradles patient's head and neck by sliding one arm under patient's neck to grasp shoulder.

2

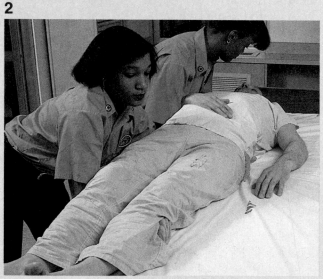

Foot-end EMT slides one arm under the patient's sacrum and moves her arm from under patient's knees to a position under mid-calf area. Head-end EMT places her free arm under small of patient's back.

3

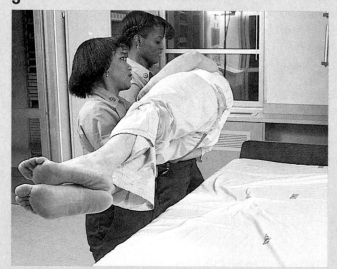

EMTs slide patient to edge of bed and bend toward him with their knees slightly bent. They curl patient to their chests and return to a standing position. The patient is lifted, cradled in their arms.

NOTE: If wheeled stretcher is a single-level unit, EMTs will have to stop one step from stretcher. Step forward with left foot and bend right knee to the floor. Each EMT should swing his left knee to a position outside his left arm. Both EMTs can now roll forward and place patient gently onto mattress.

Bed-Level Patient: Draw Sheet Method

1

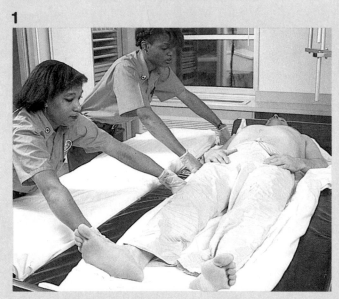

Bottom sheet of bed is rolled from both sides of bed toward patient. The stretcher, with its rails lowered, is placed parallel to bed, touching side of bed.

2

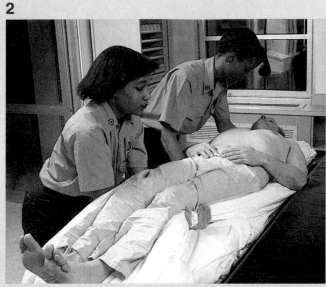

EMTs pull on drawsheet to move patient to side of bed. They each use one hand to support patient while they reach under him to grasp drawsheet. EMTs simultaneously draw patient onto stretcher.

Transferring the Ground-Level Patient

1

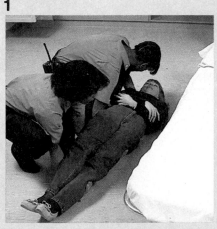

Stretcher is set in its lowest position and placed on opposite side of patient. EMTs drop to one knee, facing patient. Rescuer's arms are positioned as they are for a direct carry.

2

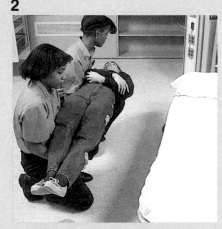

EMTs lift patient to their knees.

3

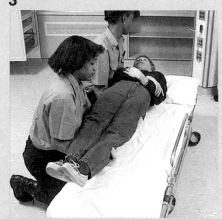

They stand and carry patient to stretcher, drop to one knee, and roll forward to place patient onto mattress.

SCAN 23–5 WHEELED AMBULANCE STRETCHERS—MOVING AND LOADING PATIENT

Loading the Ambulance

1

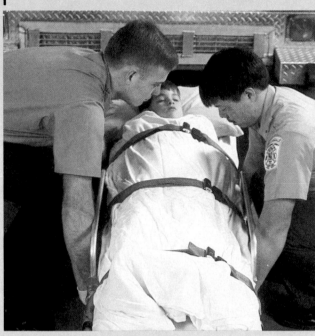

Make sure stretcher is locked in its lowest level before lifting onto the ambulance. EMTs should position themselves on opposite sides of stretcher, bend at the knees, and grasp lower bar of stretcher frame.

2

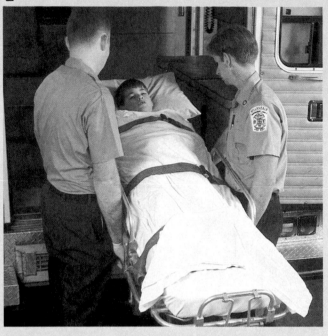

Both EMTS come to a full standing position with their backs straight. Oblique stepping movements are used to move stretcher onto the ambulance.

3

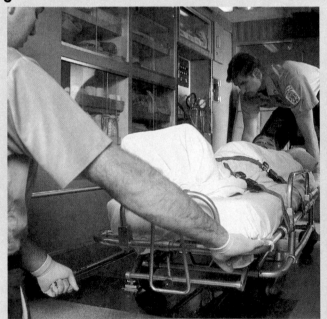

Stretcher is moved into securing device.

4

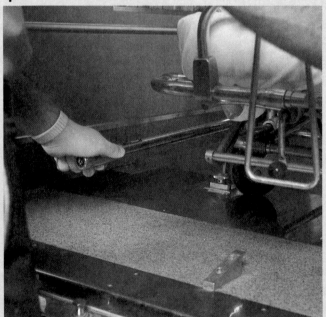

Make certain both forward and rear catches are engaged to hold stretcher.

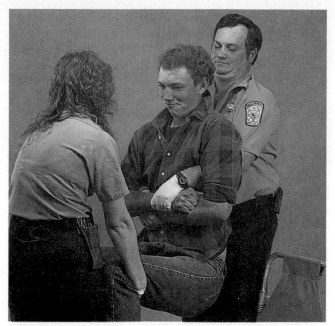

A. The EMTs assist the patient to a sitting position. On the signal from the head-end EMT, both lift the patient.

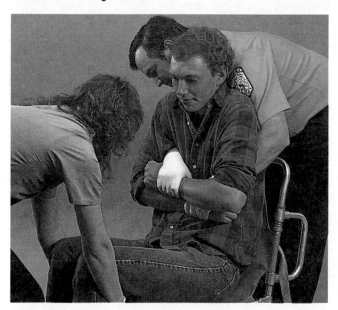

B. The EMTs lower the patient into the chair. Then the patient is secured and ready for transfer.

FIGURE 23–3. Extremity transfer to a stair chair.

chair. The third is fastened around the patient's legs and the lower portion of the chair.

Moving a Stair Chair

A loaded stair chair is fairly easy to carry and maneuver, especially if the chair is on wheels. As with the ambulance stretcher, stair chairs should be rolled

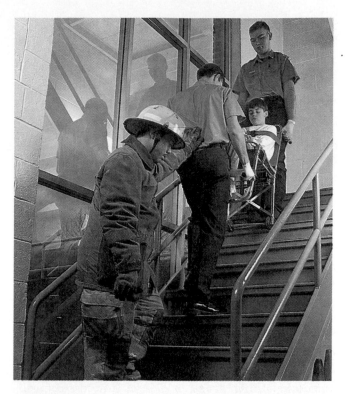

FIGURE 23–4. Moving a stair chair down steps.

whenever possible; this reduces the risk of back strain for the EMTs and injury to the patient. The following procedure is suggested when a stair chair must be carried over level ground.

When the chair and patient are to be moved, one EMT must be behind the chair to tilt the chair back. This must be done carefully if the chair has wheels. The other EMT should stand at the patient's feet, with his back to the patient. As the chair is tilted back, he should crouch and grasp the chair by its legs. The two EMTs should lift the chair simultaneously and carry the patient to the wheeled stretcher. The patient should be transferred to the wheeled stretcher as soon as possible and before he is loaded onto the ambulance.

If the patient and chair must be carried down stairs, the foot-end EMT should face the patient while carrying the chair. A third person should support the foot-end EMT while the chair is being moved down the steps. If the chair has wheels, they should not be allowed to touch the steps.

Scoop-Style (Orthopedic) Stretchers

The scoop-style stretcher can be used to lift and carry most patients; however, *in cases of possible spinal injury*, it should be used only to transfer a patient to a long spine board. A scoop-style stretcher should not be used to transport a patient with a possible spinal injury.

Preparing the Patient with Possible Spinal Injury

An extrication or rigid collar should be secured to the patient as soon as possible. Someone should continue to support the head after the collar is applied and throughout the stretcher application procedure. The patient should be placed in a supine position, as anatomically straight as possible. His arms should be secured in place, with a cravat bandage applied to hold the wrists together (Figure 23–5).

Preparing the Stretcher

ALWAYS adjust the length of the stretcher to fit the height of the patient. Separate the stretcher halves and place one half on each side of the patient. If the stretcher is the folding type, make sure the pins are properly set.

Applying the Stretcher

Slide the stretcher halves under the patient one at a time. This may be difficult since the stretcher may snag on clothing, grass, or debris. If necessary, roll the patient as a unit to either side to allow for proper positioning of the parts. Mate the latch parts and make certain that the stretcher halves are securely locked together. Latching should be done from head to feet. Adjust the head support.

Covering and Securing the Patient

The patient is covered with a blanket folded to size. A rolled blanket or a commercial head restraint is placed on each side of the patient's head and the head is secured to the stretcher by a cravat. Then the stretcher straps are fastened across the chest, hips, and legs.

The Velcro at the head end of folding scoop-style stretchers may not remain secure. To guard against this, tape the patient's head or tie securely with a cravat.

Moving the Patient

Lift the scoop-style stretcher by the end-carry method. The patient should be moved to a long spineboard as soon as possible. The patient and long spine board should be secured as a unit to the wheeled ambulance stretcher by using three straps.

Basket Stretchers

WARNING: Do NOT attempt to move a patient in a basket stretcher by rope or ladder unless you have

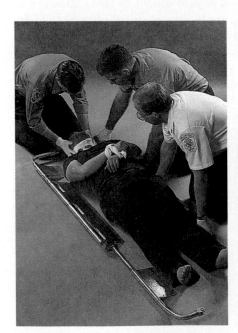

A. One EMT carefully supports the patient's head while half of the stretcher is positioned.

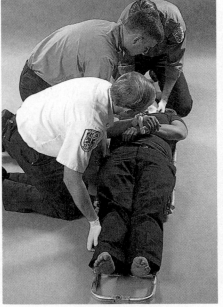

B. The stretcher halves are securely locked together, and the head support is properly positioned.

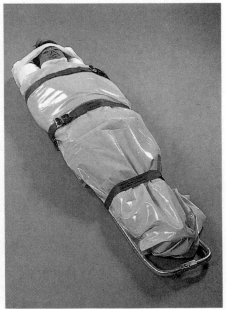

C. A patient properly positioned, covered, and secured on a full spine board or a scoop stretcher.

FIGURE 23–5. Applying the scoop-style stretcher and covering and securing the patient for transport.

been specifically trained in the techniques used for such moves.

The basket stretcher can be used to move patients from one level to another or over rough terrain. The basket should be lined with blankets prior to positioning the patient.

Transferring the Patient to the Stretcher

If the patient has no spinal injury, modifications of the direct carry and extremity transfer methods can be used by two EMTs to transfer a bed-level or ground-level patient to a basket stretcher. The draw sheet method also can be used to transfer a bed-level patient who has no spinal injury, provided the draw sheet can support the patient's weight while he is being lowered into the stretcher hammock-style.

Two additional techniques may be used to transfer a floor- or ground-level patient to a basket stretcher when he is heavy or when two EMTs cannot accomplish the transfer by themselves. Each technique requires additional personnel, however.

The Three-Rescuer Lift   This is a modification of the lift that was used for the three-rescuer carry noted earlier. Prior to movement, cross the patient's arms onto his chest and tie at the wrists using a soft bandage. Each rescuer kneels on the knee toward the patient's feet. The EMT at the head of the patient slides one arm under the patient's head and shoulders, supporting the head. The other arm is under the patient's upper back. The middle EMT slides one arm under the patient's waist and his other arm under the patient's hips. The EMT at the patient's legs places one arm under the patient's knees and one arm under the patient's ankles. Once the patient is brought to knee level, he can be lowered into the basket stretcher.

The Blanket Lift   In this procedure, the blanket serves as the basket liner as well as the lifting mechanism. This lift can be done with four rescuers; however, it is best done with five. Four people can do the lifting, while the fifth one positions the stretcher. The procedure for placing the patient on the blanket is:

- Gather half of the blanket material up against the patient's side.
- Roll the patient toward your knees so the blanket can be placed under the patient.
- Gently roll the patient back onto the blanket.
- With two rescuers on each side, grasp the edge of the blanket and roll it in toward the patient.

- Lifting by the rolled edges of the blanket, the patient is brought to knee-level while the fifth rescuer positions the stretcher.

Long Spine Boards

There are a number of patient-carrying devices that can be used to carry injured persons away from wrecked vehicles. Rather than focus attention on appliances that might be carried on some ambulances but not others, we will discuss patient removal tasks with the one patient-carrying device that is carried on most ambulances in this country—the long spine board.

Moreover, we will show you how it can be used in conjunction with the rope sling, one of the most versatile (and least expensive) tools that can be carried on an ambulance.

A proper rope sling results when the ends of a 20-foot length of 1-inch nylon rope are joined in a long splice. The rope is soft, and when the sling is properly applied, there is very little downward pressure on a person's chest. Nonetheless a sling would not be used to remove a person who has chest injuries.

A rolled sheet can be used effectively as a sling. A strap should be used only when there is nothing else available; a strap can dig into a person's underarms. A small-diameter rope or wire should never be used as a sling.

The basic procedures for using the long spine board were presented in Chapter 11. Here, we will consider some of the transfers that may be used when it is not possible to log-roll the patient.

Transferring a Patient with a Rope Sling

In some accident situations, it may not be possible for rescuers to position themselves around a patient during the transfer effort. He may be under a vehicle or a piece of machinery or in a pocket of debris. A 1-inch-diameter rope sling or loop can be used to great advantage in situations like these. Rope slings are especially efficient when there are only two EMTs (Fig. 23–6).

1. Manually stabilize the head and neck, and apply an extrication or rigid collar. The head and neck are manually stabilized until the patient is secured to the long spine board.
2. Slip the rope sling over the person's chest and under his arms.
3. If the sling is adjustable, slide the steel rings down the rope. Position them as close to the

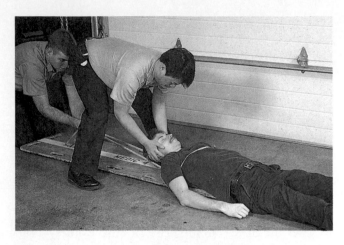

FIGURE 23–6.   Moving a patient onto a long spine board using a rope sling.

person's head as possible. This will assure that a straight pull is made, and the doubled rope will help to support the person's head.

4. As you slightly raise the person's head and shoulders, have your partner slide the end of the board under them.

5. Exert a smooth, steady pull on the rope to move the person onto the board. Keep your hands as low to the board as you can to assure that the person's spine is kept straight.

6. Continue to pull on the rope until the person is completely on the board.

It may be necessary to angle the board slightly to move the patient onto it, for example, when an accident victim must be pulled through the window of an overturned car. The door frame and the curved portion of the roof will prevent a straight pull.

Transferring a Patient from under the Dashboard of a Vehicle

An accident victim may be found between the front seat and the dashboard. If proper tools are available, the front seat should be removed or displaced to the rear while the patient is protected. Working room is thus provided, and the patient can be moved directly onto a long board without difficulty. It also may be possible to lift him with a scoop stretcher.

If tools are unavailable to remove or displace the seat, the patient can be transferred to a seat-level long board by four persons. Rescuers should first force both front doors of the vehicle beyond their normal range of motion to provide an unobstructed work area on each side.

1. One rescuer (usually one of the EMTs) takes up a position at the patient's head. While

he maintains an open airway and applies manual traction by the jaw-thrust, the other EMT applies an extrication collar.

2. After applying the collar, the second EMT positions himself outside the vehicle at the patient's feet.

3. Two other rescuers climb into the area behind the front seat, and reach over and grasp his clothing at the shoulder, chest, waist, and thigh. If the patient is in a tight garment that cannot be easily grasped, the rescuers reach over and place their hands under the patient's body.

4. On a signal from the head-end EMT, all rescuers lift the patient, keeping his back and legs against the front of the seat. If any spinal injury is suspected, extreme care must be used to move the patient as a unit.

5. They slide the patient onto the long board in a face-up position, secure him, and remove the patient from the vehicle.

Transferring a Patient from between the Front and Rear Seats of a Vehicle

This technique is essentially the same as the one just described. In this case, however, the two assisting rescuers lean over the back of the front seat to lift the patient onto a board laid on the rear seat.

Moving Stretchers Over Debris or Rough Terrain

Debris and rubble (such as that produced by a building collapse) and rough terrain may prevent the easy movement of a stretcher from the point of care to the ambulance.

Six persons should carry a stretcher when debris or rough terrain makes walking difficult. If one person stumbles, it is not likely that the others will drop the stretcher.

In extreme situations when walking with a stretcher is virtually impossible, it may be necessary for the six (or more) persons to stop at the obstacle or debris and have two or more rescuers go to the opposite side of the debris, ready to receive the stretcher as it is passed to them. (Remember, when passing a stretcher from hand to hand from one rescuer to another, it is imperative to keep the stretcher at shoulder height. In this manner, no one is straining to keep the stretcher level. Also keep the patient's head uphill and the stretcher as level as possible.)

As the stretcher passes from hand to hand, the two rearmost rescuers drop from the end of the line and move to the head. Progress of the stretcher can be halted at any point to enable someone to get sure footing. When the stretcher is once again on level ground, the six-rescuer carry can continue. The procedure is known as the six-rescuer shift.

Moving a Stretcher Uphill

In off-road vehicle accident situations, it may be impossible for two, four, or even six persons to climb a hill with a stretcher. There are several other ways by which the uphill transfer of a stretcher can be accomplished, however.

Hand-to-Hand Movement

If there are sufficient emergency service personnel and bystanders available at the scene and the distance is not great, two lines of persons can be formed between the foot and the top of the hill. The helpers remain in place while they pass the stretcher from hand to hand.

The Six-Person Shift

When personnel are limited, six persons can transfer a stretcher uphill in the same manner described for moving a stretcher over debris and rough terrain. As the stretcher passes from their hands, the rearmost persons move to the head of the line. The leapfrogging continues until the stretcher is at the top of the hill.

Guide Ropes

Two ropes can be used to advantage when a hill is so slippery that a stretcher cannot be carried safely. The ropes are secured to strong anchor points 6 feet apart and about 4 feet from the ground. The rope is tossed or carried downhill, and the ends are secured to trees or other anchor points or held by one or two individuals. Thus two parallel handlines are formed. Proper positioning of the ropes is important. If the ropes are too close to the ground, the stretcher bearers will have to stoop as they reach the top of the hill. If the upper anchor points are too far apart, the stretcher bearers will have to relinquish their grip on the ropes before they reach safe ground.

Once the lines are in place, four or six persons can pull themselves up the hill with one hand while pulling the stretcher along with the other hand. If one bearer stumbles, the others can stop and wait in place while he regains his footing.

When the hill is both slippery and steep, the stretcher can be pulled uphill by a third line manned by personnel at the top of the incline (e.g., truck drivers, police officers, or firefighters). Four or six

rescuers will still be needed to support the stretcher but, by keeping a slow steady pull on the hauling line, the task will be much easier.

- The third line should be tied off at an anchor point at the top of the hill between the two guide lines.
- A single pulley is attached to the head of the stretcher.
- The hauling line is placed through the pulley and brought back to the top of the hill.
- The hauling line is now threaded through a second single pulley, which is anchored at the top of the hill next to the initial anchor point.
- On the given signal, when all personnel are ready, the stretcher with rescuers can be pulled up the steep incline.
- Use this method only if pulleys are available from a rescue unit.

The above-listed procedures are those to be used for moving a stretcher uphill.

Special Transfer Devices

In concluding this chapter showing the various patient transfer devices used by today's ambulance services, we would be remiss if we did not mention some of the additional stretchers used by many EMTs in the field.

- *Miller board*—used by many EMTs where a full spine board is needed when using a wire basket stretcher that has leg dividers. Also used in recovery from water accidents.
- *Reeves stretcher*—a canvas or synthetic rubberized material that has wooden slats sewn into pockets. It has six large lifting and carrying handles (three on each side), making this a good stretcher for narrow and restricted hallways such as are found in mobile homes.
- *Reeves sleeve*—an envelope configuration into which a regular long spine board can be inserted. There are tabs with quick-hitch straps that encapsulate the patient, making him secure in almost any position in which you might need to carry him.
- *SKED*—a device that comes rolled in a package. When opened, this stretcher can be quickly assembled and used to rescue someone from a given height, snow, or water emergency.

SUMMARY

It will be necessary for you to quickly evacuate a sick or injured person from a building or other location whenever his life and yours are threatened by fire, explosion, building collapse, electrocution, smoke, toxic fumes, or radiation.

You may have to evacuate injured persons quickly from vehicle accident locations when lives are threatened not only by accident-produced hazards but also by passing cars.

Exposure to a life-threatening hazard is not the only situation that may necessitate your moving a sick or injured person before you can accomplish emergency care procedures. You may have to move someone simply because there is no room for you to carry out patient care activities. Or you may have to move a lesser-injured person in order to reach someone who may die unless life-saving care is provided without delay.

Do not just rush in, grab a person by the clothes or extremities, and drag him from the hostile environment, however. Choose an evacuation technique that will be least harmful.

If the person can stand and walk, simply assist him to a safe place.

If there are no indications of extremity or spinal injury, use a piggyback carry to move a conscious person and the cradle carry or one of the pack-strap carries to move an unconscious person.

One of a number of drags can be used to move a person who cannot be either assisted or carried:

- Use the shoulder drag or foot drag when a quick movement is essential.
- Use the fireman's drag when you must move a person along a smoke-filled hallway. Your face will be at the level where the air is likely to be clear.
- Use the incline drag to move a person down a stairway when there is no indication of fractures or spinal injury.
- Use the blanket drag when it is absolutely necessary to move a person who has extremity fractures or a suspected spinal injury quickly. Keep the spine and extremities in a straight line, and drag the person with his head as close to the floor as possible.
- Use the clothes drag to move a person when a blanket is not available and rapid evacuation is essential.

A number of two-rescuer techniques can be used to move persons who have neither fractured extremities nor a spine injury:

- Assist an ambulatory person from a hostile environment by supporting him between you and your partner.
- Use either the two-rescuer extremities carry or the chair carry when you must quickly move a person through a narrow opening or along a narrow hallway.

Use any of a variety of patient-carrying devices when emergency evacuation is not necessary. The devices that are usually carried on an ambulance are the wheeled ambulance stretcher, a portable ambulance stretcher, a stair chair, a scoop stretcher, a long spine board, and, if space permits, a basket stretcher.

When your patient does not have a spinal injury, select a carrying device with regard to the pathway from the point of care to the ambulance:

- Transfer him to the ambulance on the wheeled stretcher when movement is unrestricted.
- Use a portable stretcher, stair chair, scoop stretcher or long spine board when the person must be removed from a confined space, moved through a narrow opening, or carried through a narrow hallway.
- Use a stair chair when it is not possible to move a patient down stairs on a stretcher and when a person must be moved in an elevator that is too small for a stretcher.
- Use a basket stretcher when a person must be moved from one level to another by rope or ladder, or when a person must be moved over debris or rough terrain or uphill.

When your patient has a spinal injury, select a carrying device suited to his location and situation:

- Use a scoop stretcher secured to a long spine board to move the person from the ground or floor of a structure.
- Use a rope sling to pull a person onto a long spine board from the seat or floor of a vehicle. If the person is on the floor and the seats can be removed or displaced, it may be possible to lift the person from the vehicle on a scoop stretcher.
- Once a person has been immobilized on a short spine board or vest, he can be pivoted onto a long spine board and carried from the wreckage.
- When a spine-injured person must be moved from one level to another, first immobilize him on a long spine board. Secure the board

in a basket stretcher, and then lower the stretcher by rope or slide it down the beams of a ladder.

The procedure for transferring a sick or injured person to an ambulance on a patient-carrying device usually includes these steps: preparing the stretcher, transferring the patient to the stretcher, properly positioning the patient on the stretcher, covering the patient, securing the patient, carrying or wheeling the stretcher to the ambulance, and loading the stretcher in the ambulance.

Four to six rescuers should carry a stretcher over rough terrain. If one person stumbles, the others will be able to support the stretcher while he regains his footing.

When walking over rubble or debris is impossible, have six or more rescuers pass the stretcher from hand to hand while they "leapfrog" from the rear of the line to the head.

When a stretcher must be moved uphill and there is sufficient personnel, two lines of rescuers can pass the stretcher from hand to hand if the hill is not steep and the distance is not great. When personnel are limited, six people can move the stretcher in the manner suggested for moving a stretcher over debris.

When the hill is slippery, stretcher bearers can pull themselves and the stretcher uphill with ropes attached to anchor points at the top and bottom of the hill.

When the hill is both steep and slippery, rescuers at the top of the hill can pull the stretcher up with a third line while bearers support the stretcher.

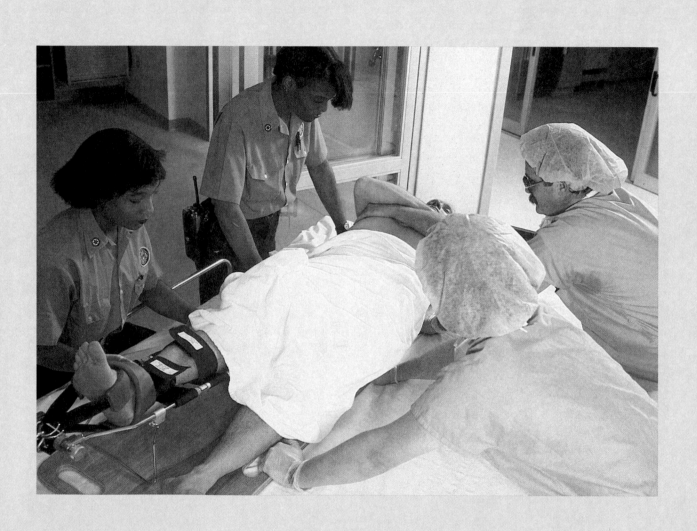

Transporting the Patient to a Hospital

OBJECTIVES   As an EMT, you should be able to:

1. List TWELVE steps for preparing a sick or injured person for transportation to a medical facility. (pp. 586–587)
2. List TEN activities in which the attending EMT may have to engage during the transportation of a sick or injured person to a medical facility. (pp. 588–589)
3. List EIGHT essential elements of ambulance-hospital radio communication. (pp. 589–591)

4. Describe the procedure for caring for a patient who goes into cardiac arrest during transportation. (p. 589)
5. Describe an orderly procedure for transferring a patient to the care of emergency department personnel. (pp. 591–593)

SKILLS   As an EMT, you should be able to:

1. Prepare a patient for transportation in the ambulance.
2. Monitor a patient's vital signs during transportation.
3. Adjust bandages and splints as necessary to

ensure that circulation is not impaired during transportation.
4. Relay accurate and meaningful information by radio to emergency department personnel.
5. Complete an orderly patient transfer.

PREPARING THE PATIENT FOR TRANSPORT

A common practice in the not-too-distant past was for ambulance attendants to load a sick or injured person into the patient compartment of an ambulance and then climb onto the front seat for the trip to a hospital. Too many times patients, even seriously ill or injured ones, were left to fend for themselves during transit.

Activities during this phase of an emergency care effort include far more than just transportation. A series of tasks must be undertaken from the time a patient is loaded into the ambulance until he is handed over to emergency department personnel. Not the least of these tasks is continuation of the emergency care measures initiated on first contact with the patient.

There are 12 steps that may be required to prepare a person for transport once he is in the ambulance.

Step 1: Secure the Cot in Place in the Ambulance

Your first efforts should be to ensure that the patient is safe during the trip to the hospital. Before closing the door, and certainly before signaling the driver to move, make sure that the cot is securely in place.

Patient compartments are equipped with positive locking devices that prevent the wheeled ambulance cot from moving about while the ambulance is in motion. It is unlikely, but in your haste you may engage the forward part of the cot in the hook of the fastener bar and fail to engage the rear hook completely. The fact that the cot is not secure might go undetected until the ambulance moves. An unfastened stretcher can create havoc in the patient compartment, and both you and your patient can be injured before the ambulance can be brought to a stop.

Step 2: Properly Position the Patient

The need to move a patient from an upper floor or over rough terrain requires that he be firmly secured to a stretcher. Even an uncomplicated movement of the wheeled ambulance stretcher for a short distance may have to be accomplished with the patient in the supine position. This does not mean, however, that he must be transported to the hospital while in that position. On the contrary, positioning should be dictated by the nature of his illness or injury.

If he was not transferred to the ambulance in that position:

- Shift an unconscious patient, or one with a low level of awareness, into a position that will promote maintenance of an open airway and the drainage of fluids.
- Position the security straps so the patient will be secure in this position during transportation.

Step 3: Allow for Respiratory or Cardiac Complications

A patient with a heart condition or respiratory difficulty should be transported in the position that allows him to breathe freely. Adjust the stretcher accordingly.

If the patient is likely to develop cardiac arrest, position a short spine board or CPR board between him and the ambulance cot prior to starting on the trip to the hospital. Then if he does go into arrest, there will be no need to locate and position the board. Riding on a hard board may not be comfortable for a patient, but it is better that he suffer temporary discomfort than permanent injury or even death from delayed resuscitation efforts.

Step 4: Adjust Security Straps

Security straps applied when a patient is being prepared for transfer to the ambulance may tighten unnecessarily by the time he is loaded into the patient compartment.

Adjust straps so they still hold the patient safely in place but are not so tight that they interfere with circulation or respiration or cause pain.

Step 5: Loosen Constricting Clothing

As with straps, clothing may interfere with circulation and breathing. Loosen ties, belts, and open any clothing around the neck. Straighten clothing that is bunched under safety straps. Remember that clothing bunched at the crotch may be painful to the patient. Before you do anything to rearrange the clothing of a patient, however, tell him or her what you are going to do and why.

Step 6: Ensure an Open Airway and Adequate Air Exchange

Ascertain that a conscious patient is breathing without difficulty once you have positioned him on the stretcher. If the patient is unconscious with an airway in place, make sure he has an adequate air exchange once you have moved him into position for transport.

Step 7: Check Bandages

Even properly applied bandages can loosen during transfer to the ambulance, especially if there is considerable body movement. Check each bandage to see that it is secure.

Do not consider the problem of a loosened bandage lightly. Severe bleeding can resume when the pressure from a bandage is removed from a dressing, and if the wound site is covered with a sheet or blanket, bleeding may go unnoticed until the patient develops shock or is delivered to the hospital.

Step 8: Check Splints

Immobilizing devices can also loosen during transfer to the ambulance. Inspect the bandages or cravats that hold board splints in place. Test air splints with your fingertip to see that they have remained properly inflated during the transfer procedure. Inspect traction devices to ensure that proper traction is still maintained.

Check the splinted limb for distal pulse, skin color and temperature at the fingertips or toes, capillary refilling, and neurologic activity.

Remember that the safe adjustment of splinting devices is virtually impossible when an ambulance is pitching about during the trip to a hospital.

Step 9: Determine and Record Vital Signs

Once you have properly positioned the patient and adjusted straps, clothing, and bandages, measure and record his vital signs. Keep in mind that an accurate measurement of vital signs may not be possible if the trip to the hospital is particularly rough.

Step 10: Load a Relative or Friend Who Must Accompany the Patient

As a matter of policy, many ambulance services will not allow a relative or friend to accompany a sick or injured person to a hospital. In some instances, the practice is prohibited by the ambulance service's insurance company.

Consider these guidelines if your service does not prohibit the transportation of a relative or friend with a sick or injured person: First, encourage the person to seek alternate transportation, if such is available. If there is just no other way that the relative or friend can get to the hospital, allow him to ride in the passenger's seat in the driver's compartment—not in the patient's compartment where he may interfere with your activities. Make certain the person buckles his seat belt.

Step 11: Load Personal Effects

If a purse, briefcase, overnight bag, or other personal item is to accompany the patient, make sure it is placed and properly secured in the ambulance. If you load personal effects at the scene of a vehicle accident, be sure to tell a police officer what you are taking.

Step 12: Reassure the Patient

Apprehension often mounts in a sick or injured person after he is loaded in an ambulance. Not only is he held down by straps in a strange, confined space, but he may also be suddenly separated from family members and friends who have comforted him to this point.

Say a few kind words and offer a reassuring hand. Remember that a favorite toy such as a teddy bear can do much to calm a frightened child. Many ambulance units carry a sanitized, soft or padded brightly colored toy in a compartment just for frightened children. It is difficult at best to get information from a young child whose parents may have been injured and transported in another ambulance. Small children don't, as a rule, carry identification and you are a complete stranger in a hostile environment.

The crash scene, confusion, noise, injuries, possibly pain, disappearance of a parent, EMTs caring for injuries and gathering much needed information all lead to a hectic experience for a child. A female EMT or police officer may be helpful. Sometimes young children feel more comfortable talking to a woman. A smile and calm reassuring tone of voice are something that cannot be learned from a textbook, and they may be the most critical care needed by the frightened child (Figure 24–1).

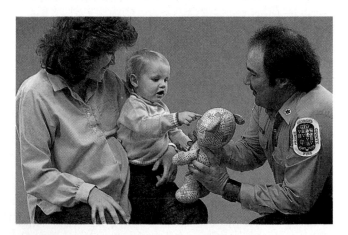

FIGURE 24–1. Reassuring the child patient with a teddy bear.

When you are satisfied that the patient is ready for transportation, signal the driver to begin the trip to the hospital.

CAUTION: Under no circumstances should you allow smoking in either the patient's compartment or the driver's compartment while oxygen is being administered. Oxygen itself is not flammable; it does, however, cause other combustible materials to burn vigorously. High concentrations of oxygen can develop in voids between articles of clothing and even under the cot linens and blankets. If a chance spark ignites clothing or bedding, the results can be disastrous. Weather permitting, ventilate the patient compartment well while oxygen is being delivered.

CARING FOR THE PATIENT WHILE EN ROUTE TO THE HOSPITAL

Seldom will you be able to merely ride along with your patient. You may have to undertake a number of activities on the way to the hospital.

Step 1: Continue to Provide Emergency Care as Required

If life-support efforts were initiated prior to loading the patient into the ambulance, they must be continued during transportation to the hospital.

Maintain an open airway, resuscitate, administer to the patient's needs, provide emotional support, and do whatever else is required, including updating your findings from the initial patient assessment effort.

Step 2: Compile Additional Patient Information

If the patient is conscious and emergency care efforts will not be compromised, record patient information.

Compiling information during the trip to the hospital serves two purposes. First, it allows you to complete your report. Second, supplying information temporarily takes your patient's mind off his problems. Remember, however, that obtaining patient information is not an interrogation session. Ask your questions in an informal manner.

Step 3: Continue Monitoring Vital Signs

Keep in mind that changes in vital signs indicate a change in a patient's condition. For example, a drop in blood pressure may signify deepening shock.

Record vital signs on your report form and be prepared to relate changes in vital signs to an emergency department staff member as soon as you reach the medical facility.

Step 4: Radio Patient Information to the Medical Facility

Effective radio communications are described at the end of this section.

Step 5: Check Bandages

Even though you checked bandages after loading the patient into the ambulance, check them again while in transit. Shifting of the patient in response to swaying of the ambulance may have caused bandages to loosen (or tighten). Adjust them as required. If dressings and bandages become blood soaked, add fresh ones in a continuing effort to control bleeding. Remember that under no circumstances should you replace blood-soaked dressings and bandages with fresh ones.

If the fingers and toes of bandaged extremities become cool and blue tinged, loosen the bandage slightly; it may be interfering with circulation. Be careful not to disturb any impaled object while checking and adjusting bandages.

Step 6: Check Splints

Make both a visual and manual check to ensure that splinting devices have not shifted. Make adjustments if necessary. Ensure that circulation and nerve functions are not impaired. Check distal pulse, capillary refill, skin temperature and color, and neurologic activity.

Step 7: Collect Vomitus if the Patient Becomes Nauseated

If he is not already in position, arrange the patient so that the chance of him aspirating vomitus is minimized. Be prepared to apply suction. Place an emesis basin, bag, or pail by his mouth. When he has finished vomiting, place a towel over the container and deliver it to emergency department personnel when you hand over the patient. Examination of the vomitus may be important to treatment and therapy, especially in cases of poisoning.

Step 8: Talk to the Patient, but Control Your Emotions

Continued conversation is often soothing to a frightened patient. Occasionally, however, conversation may be difficult for you. Your patient may be a reeking, incoherent alcohol abuse victim, or a reckless driver who struck and killed a child before wrecking his own vehicle, or a drug addict with a life style completely alien to yours.

Regardless of the situation, do not allow your emotions or personal feelings to overshadow professional ethics and interest in your patient's welfare. If you find it difficult to converse in an ordinary manner, at least assure your patient that everything possible is being done to help him and that he will soon be at a medical facility.

Step 9: Advise the Driver of Changing Conditions

No one likes a "back seat" driver. However, there will be times when you must ask the driver to adjust speed or alter his driving technique to suit the needs of your patient.

If, on the one hand, what began as a routine transport develops into an emergency run, you will have to ask the driver to accelerate. On the other hand, if you think that swaying because of high speeds and uneven streets is detrimental to a patient's condition, have the driver slow down or take an alternate route.

While the driver of an ambulance is responsible for his vehicle and the passengers carried in it, it is your responsibility to care for sick and injured persons; thus the driver should operate the ambulance according to your suggestions.

Step 10: If the Patient Goes into Cardiac Arrest, Have the Driver Stop the Ambulance and Initiate CPR

If cardiac arrest develops, have the driver stop the ambulance while you initiate CPR. Signal the driver to start up again once you have established CPR. Make certain that the emergency department is made aware of the arrest.

If you routinely position a rigid device between the back of high-risk patients and the cot mattress, you have only to drop the cot back to a horizontal position and start CPR. If not, you must position an object like a short spine board or CPR board so that chest compression efforts will be effective.

RADIO COMMUNICATIONS DURING TRANSPORT

While ambulances have been equipped with two-way radios for quite some time, intercommunication capabilities were generally limited to dispatch centers and ambulances. If ambulance personnel needed to discuss anything with hospital staff members, it usually had to be done through a third party over a combination of telephone and radio links. The proce-

dure was time consuming and error prone. With the development of efficient emergency medical service communication systems, however, EMTs now have the capability to talk directly with emergency department personnel.

Numerous protocols have been developed for ambulance-hospital radio communications. To be effective, radio messages from ambulances to hospitals should be brief but complete and transmitted without often-misunderstood and confusing codes.

An informational message from an EMT should include:

- Hospital identification
- Ambulance designation
- Brief description of what happened
- Facts learned during the subjective interview
- Facts learned during the objective examination
- What injuries or medical problem you suspect
- Emergency care provided thus far
- Your estimated time of arrival at the medical facility

Step 1: Identify the Hospital in Your Initial Call

"Mercy Hospital . . ."

Complex EMS communication systems may have many hospitals in the network. Make sure that your message is immediately received by the proper hospital by identifying that facility at the start of your message.

Step 2: Identify Your Unit

". . . this is ambulance Adam one three."

Obviously there cannot be effective point-to-point communication unless both the message originator and the receiver are identified. Identify your unit, making sure that you clearly enunciate letters and numerals, thus minimizing misunderstanding. Keep in mind that persons who do not use two-way radios routinely often confuse words and phrases, especially when radio traffic or noise is considerable. For example "fifteen" may be mistaken for "sixteen." When there is a chance that your unit designation will be misunderstood, use the phonetic alphabet and enunciate each numeral separately.

The phonetic alphabet is shown in Table 24–1.

Table 24–1. THE PHONETIC ALPHABET

A	Adam	H	Henry	O	Ocean	V	Victor
B	Boston	I	Ida	P	Paul	W	Walter
C	Charlie	J	John	Q	Queen	X	X-ray
D	David	K	King	R	Robert	Y	Young
E	Edward	L	Lincoln	S	Sam	Z	Zebra
F	Frank	M	Mary	T	Tom		
G	George	N	Nora	U	Union		

At this point give someone at the hospital the chance to answer your call.

Step 3: Give a Brief Description of What Happened

"We are transporting a man who has fallen approximately 20 feet from a ladder onto a concrete floor."

Remember that you have been taught to consider the mechanisms of injury when assessing an accident victim. When you briefly but accurately describe the incident to which you have responded, emergency department personnel can often visualize the mechanisms of injury.

Just as you were able to surmise that the man could have suffered long bone fractures, a head injury, a spinal injury, or abdominal insult by observing the mechanisms of injury, so, too, can emergency department personnel make an intelligent guess when you describe the incident to them.

Step 4: State What You Learned in the Subjective Interview

"The patient is a 34-year old male who complains of a headache and severe pain in the right leg. He was unconscious for a short time following the fall. He is a patient of Dr. Robert Johnson."

Do not waste time transmitting negative information such as "the patient is not taking medication" or "the patient has no known allergies." Hospital personnel will generally assume that if such information is not transmitted, nothing has been learned.

Step 5: State What You Learned From the Objective Examination

"The patient appears to be confused and is obviously in pain. Vital signs are BP 140 over 90, pulse 86 and strong, respirations 26 and normal. Positive findings are a contusion of the back of the head and swelling and point tenderness over the right femur."

Start with your assessment of the patient's overall condition, follow with vital signs and then relate any positive findings from your objective examination.

When an accident victim has suffered multiple injuries, recite the major ones; do not bother with minor injuries, such as cuts and bruises.

Step 6: Report What Injuries or Medical Problems You Suspect

"I suspect a fracture of the right femur and concussion."

The verb "suspect" does not cast doubt on your ability to assess a sick or injured person's condition. It simply underlines the fact that your assessment is tentative, based on observations made at the scene of the accident. EMTs are often criticized for making a "final diagnosis" at the time they arrive on the scene, only to have it proved wrong when the patient is examined at the medical facility.

When this happens, many EMTs become reluctant to transmit *any* conclusions about a patient's condition, lest they be criticized by the emergency department staff.

Step 7: Report What You Have Done for the Patient

"We have applied a traction splint and are providing 6 liters of oxygen."

Again there is little need to relate what has been done for minor injuries, such as the application of a bandage to a small wound.

Step 8: Give Your Estimated Time of Arrival at the Medical Facility

"We will arrive at your location in approximately ten minutes."

Knowing when you will reach the hospital with the patient will often be of little consequence to the emergency department staff, since most emergency departments are ready to receive patients at any time. But when you have a patient in critical condition and when the department is crowded with other patients, knowing the time of arrival allows staff members to seek additional help, gather specialized equipment, and clear a treatment area.

Now . . . look at the entire message.

"Mercy Hospital, this is ambulance Adam one three.

We are transporting a man who has fallen approximately 20 feet from a ladder onto a concrete floor. The patient is a 34-year old male who complains of a headache and a severe pain in the right leg. He was unconscious for a short time after the fall. He is a patient of Dr. Robert Johnson. The patient appears confused and is obviously in pain. Vital signs are BP 140 over 90, pulse 86 and strong, respirations 26 and normal. Positive findings are a contusion of the back of the head and swelling and point tenderness over the right femur. I suspect a fractured femur and a concussion.

We have applied a traction splint and are providing 6 liters of oxygen. We will arrive at your location in approximately ten minutes."

Thus in about 45 seconds you can transmit a wealth of information about a sick or injured person, information that will help emergency department personnel plan a course of definitive care even before they see the patient.

If your patient has an injury or illness that requires special emergency care procedures (as in cases of poisoning), request advice from the emergency department by radio.

TRANSFERRING THE PATIENT TO THE CARE OF EMERGENCY DEPARTMENT PERSONNEL

Definitive emergency care can no longer be delivered by an individual; it must come from a well-educated and competent team of emergency medical technicians, nurses, physicians, administrators, and allied health personnel. Although the responsibilities of each team member may vary, each person plays an important part; failure of any team member to do his job may mean the difference between rehabilitation and disability, a short-term or long-term hospital stay, even life or death to the victim of a sudden illness or injury. It is therefore critical that all personnel responsible for some facet of life support and emergency care provide optimum service at all times and in complete harmony with other persons within the system.

Steps in Patient Transfer

It is usually the emergency department nurse to whom the EMT most directly relates, either through the ambulance–hospital radio communication system or in face-to-face contact in the hospital. The following are steps that you might take to see that the transfer of a patient to the care of emergency department personnel is accomplished smoothly and without incident. Brief as it may be, the transfer is a crucial step during which your primary concern must be the continuation of patient care activities.

The steps of the transfer are illustrated in Scan 24–1.

Step 1: In a Routine Admission Situation or When an Illness or Injury is Not Life-threatening, Check First to See What Is to Be Done with the Patient

If emergency department activity is particularly hectic, as it is when several seriously injured accident victims are admitted at the same time, it might be better to leave your patient in the relative security and comfort of the ambulance while you determine where he is to be taken. Otherwise the patient may be subjected to distressing sights and sounds and perhaps be in the way. Under no circumstances should you simply wheel a nonemergency patient into a hospital and place him on a bed or a gurney and leave him! This is an important point. Unless you transfer care of your patient directly to a member of the hospital staff, you may be open to a charge of abandonment.

Keep in mind that staff members may be treating other seriously ill and injured persons, so suppress any urge to demand attention for your patient. Simply continue emergency care measures until someone can assume responsibility for the patient. Remember, this is what you have been trained to do. When properly directed, transfer the patient to a bed or gurney.

Step 2: Assist Emergency Department Staff Members as Required

All EMTs can and should participate in the early emergency department care of sick and injured persons. Even when the emergency department staff has taken over completely, it is often beneficial for the EMTs to remain in the area to be of assistance. The experience not only promotes better patient care but also fosters improved communication and understanding between EMTs and emergency department personnel. Also important is the fact that working with the staff gives an EMT the opportunity to learn more about definitive care procedures while the staff can evaluate the EMT's abilities.

SCAN 24–1 TRANSFERRING THE PATIENT

1

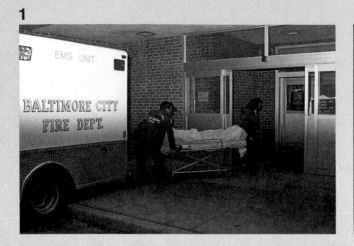

Transfer the patient as soon as possible. In a routine admission or when an illness or injury is not life-threatening, first check to see what is to be done with the patient. An EMT should remain with the patient until transfer is complete.

2

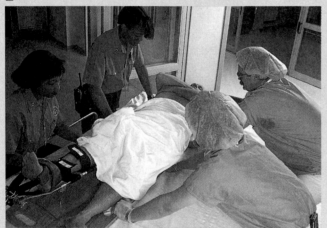

Assist the emergency department staff as required.

3

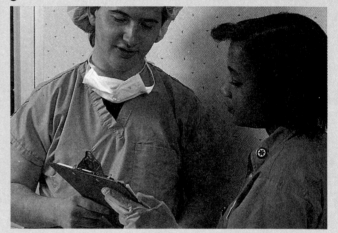

Transfer patient information.

4

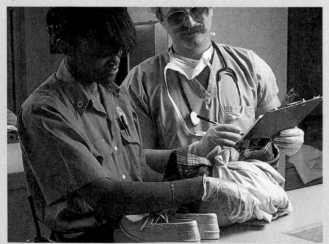

Transfer the patient's personal effects.

5

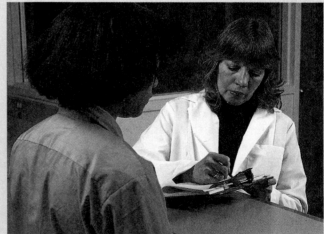

Obtain your release from the hospital.

Step 3: As Soon as You Are Free from Patient Care Activities, Transfer Patient Information

Either verbally or by written report (or, better yet, by both means), transfer to a staff member the information that you have compiled about your patient and his illness or injury. Remember to relate any changes in the patient's condition and level of consciousness that you noted during initial emergency care and subsequent transportation activities.

Step 4: Transfer the Patient's Personal Effects

If a patient's valuables or other personal effects were entrusted to your care, transfer them to a responsible emergency department staff member and have that person give you a written receipt. Often space is provided on the ambulance report form for this purpose. Although the procedure may be a nuisance for staff members, it gives you a measure of protection from a charge of theft.

Step 5: Obtain Your Release from the Hospital

This task is not as formal as it sounds. Simply ask the emergency department nurse or physician if your services are still needed. In rural areas where not all hospital services are available, it may be necessary to transfer a seriously ill or injured person to another medical facility. If you leave and have to be recalled, valuable time will be lost.

On the other hand, a person's condition may be such that he will not be admitted to the hospital and you may have to take him home. If you are recalled in this case, it is your time that is taken up.

SUMMARY

Prepare a sick or injured person for transportation to a medical facility by securing the cot, properly positioning the patient, allowing for respiratory or cardiac complications, adjusting constricting straps, loosening constricting clothing, ensuring an open airway, checking bandages, checking splints, determining and recording vital signs, loading a relative or friend, loading personal effects, and reassuring the patient.

During transportation, continue life-support efforts as required, compile additional patient information if possible, radio patient information to the medical facility, check bandages, check splints, administer CPR if the patient goes into cardiac arrest, collect vomitus if the patient becomes nauseated, talk to the patient, and advise the driver of changing conditions.

When you radio patient information to the medical facility, be sure to include (1) the hospital identification, (2) the ambulance designation, (3) a brief description of what happened, (4) facts learned from the subjective interview, (5) facts learned from the objective examination, (6) what injuries or medical problem you suspect, (7) the emergency care provided, and (8) your estimated time of arrival at the facility.

Ensure the smooth transfer of patient care to the hospital staff by first checking to see what is to be done with the patient, then assisting emergency department staff members, transferring accurate patient information, transferring personal effects, and checking to see if you are still needed before leaving the hospital.

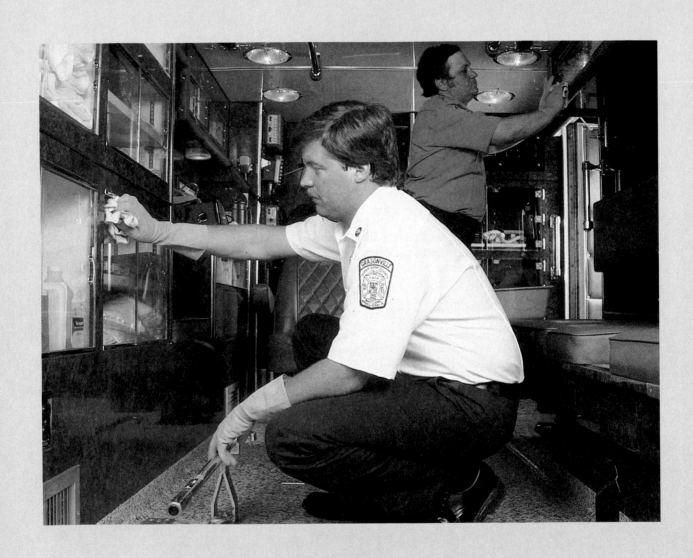

Terminating
the Run

OBJECTIVES   As an EMT, you should be able to:

1. List activities that should be undertaken at a medical facility to make the ambulance ready for immediate service. (p. 596)

2. Describe the decontamination procedure that might be followed during the return to quarters when a person with a communicable disease

was transported or when the patient compartment has a disagreeable odor. (pp. 598–601)

3. List activities that should be undertaken in quarters to make the ambulance and equipment ready for service. (pp. 598–601)

SKILLS   As an EMT, you should be able to:

Carry out procedures that will prepare the ambulance and its equipment for service when you are at the hospital, enroute to quarters, and in quarters.

An ambulance run is not really over until the personnel and machines that comprise the prehospital emergency care delivery system are ready for the next response.

The functions of EMTs in this final phase of activity include more than just changing the stretcher linen and cleaning the ambulance. A number of tasks must be accomplished at the hospital, during the return to quarters, and after arrival at the station.

ACTIONS THAT CAN BE TAKEN AT THE HOSPITAL

Activities should be directed toward making the ambulance ready to respond should another call be received before the unit can return to quarters. Time, equipment, and space limitations preclude vigorous cleaning of the ambulance while it is parked at the hospital. However, you should make every effort to quickly prepare the vehicle for the next patient (Figure 25–1).

1. Quickly clean the patient compartment while wearing rubber gloves according to Centers for Disease Control (CDC) guidelines.
   - Clean up blood, vomitus, and other body fluids that may have soiled the floor, and wipe down any equipment that has been splashed.
   - Remove and dispose of trash such as bandage wrappings, contaminated dressings, open but unused dressings, and similar items.
   - Sweep away caked dirt that may have been tracked into the patient compartment. When the weather is inclement, sponge up water and mud from the floor.
   - Use a deodorizer to neutralize odors of vomit, urine, and feces. Various sprays and concentrates are available for this purpose.
2. Prepare respiratory equipment for service.
   - Clean and disinfect nondisposable used bag-valve-mask units, oxygen masks, nasal cannulae, and other parts of respiratory-assist and inhalation therapy devices to keep them from becoming reservoirs of infectious agents that can easily contaminate the next patient.
   - Place used disposable items in a plastic bag and seal it. Replace the items with similar ones carried in the ambulance as spares.
3. Replace expendable items.
   - Replace expendable items from hospital storerooms on a one-for-one basis—items such as sterile dressings, bandaging materials, towels, disposable masks, caps and gowns, latex gloves, sterile water, and intravenous solutions.
   - Do not take advantage of this exchange program. Keep in mind that the constant abuse of a supplies replacement program usually leads to its discontinuation. At the very least, abuse places a strain on ambulance–hospital relations.

4. Exchange equipment according to local policy.
   - Exchange items such as splints and spine boards. Several benefits are associated with an equipment exchange program: there is no need to subject patients to injury-aggravating movements just to recover equipment, crews are not delayed at the hospital, and ambulances can return to quarters fully equipped for the next response.
   - When equipment is available for exchange, quickly inspect it for completeness and operability. Parts are sometimes lost or broken when an immobilizing device is removed from a patient and if persons caring for the patient are not completely familiar with the device, loss or damage goes unnoticed.
   - If you do find that a piece of equipment is broken or incomplete, notify someone in authority so the device can be repaired or replaced. Remember that the next EMT to exchange equipment may not be as thorough in his examination as you are. He may take an item that will be useless when needed.
5. Make up the ambulance cot.

Making up the Ambulance Stretcher

The following procedure is one of many that can be used to make up a wheeled ambulance stretcher.

- Remove unsoiled blankets and place them on a clean surface.
- Remove the pillow case and place the pillow on a clean surface.
- Remove all soiled linen and place it in the designated receptacle.
- Raise the stretcher to the high-level position, if possible; this makes the procedure easier. The stretcher should be flat.
- Lower the side rails and unfasten straps.
- Clean the mattress surface with an appropriate detergent if necessary.
- Turn the mattress over; rotation adds to the life of the mattress.
- Center the bottom sheet on the mattress and open it fully. If a full-sized bed sheet is used, first fold it lengthwise.

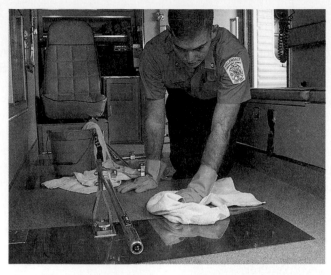

A. Clean the ambulance interior as required.

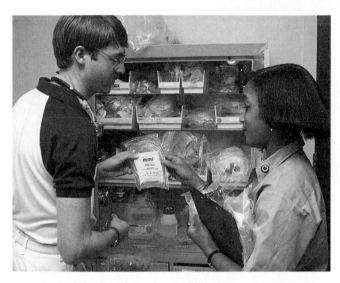

B. Replace respiratory equipment as required.

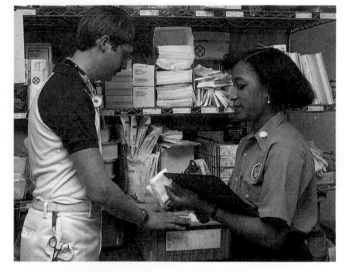

C. Replace expendable items according to local policies.

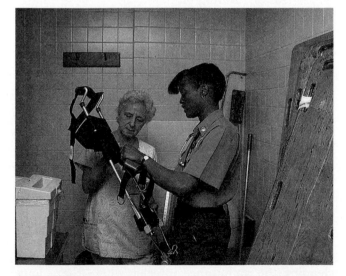

D. Exchange equipment according to local policies.

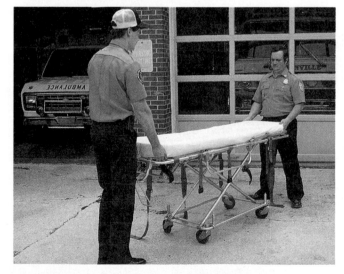

E. Make up the wheeled stretcher.

FIGURE 25–1. Actions that can be taken at the hospital.

- Tuck the sheet under each end of the mattress; form square corners and then tuck under each side.
- Place a disposable pad, if one is used, on the center of the mattress.
- Place the slip-covered pillow lengthwise at the head of the mattress.
- Open the top sheet fully; fold it lengthwise first; then fold it in half and place it at the foot of the mattress.
- Fully open the blanket. If a second blanket is used, open it fully and match it to the first blanket. This task should be done with an EMT at each end of the stretcher.
- Fold the blanket(s) lengthwise to match the width of the stretcher; fold one side first, then the other.
- Tuck the foot of the folded blanket(s) under the foot of the mattress.
- Tuck the head of the folded blanket(s) under the head of the mattress.
- Buckle the safety straps and tuck in excess straps.
- Raise the side rails and foot rest.
- Use the securing strap to hold the pillow.

The stretcher is now ready for the next patient. It must be reemphasized that this is one of many techniques for preparing a wheeled ambulance stretcher for service. Whatever the method, it should meet the following objectives:

- All linens, blankets, and pouches should be stored neatly on the stretcher.
- Preparation for the next call should be done as soon as possible.
- All linen and blankets should be folded or tucked so that they will be contained within the stretcher frame.
- Replace the cot in the ambulance.
- Check for equipment left in the hospital. Make sure that any nondisposable patient care items have been replaced.

ACTIONS THAT CAN BE TAKEN WHILE EN ROUTE TO QUARTERS

Emphasis should be on a safe return. An ambulance driver may practice every suggestion for safe vehicle operation while en route to the hospital and then totally disregard those suggestions during the return to quarters. Defensive driving must be a full-time effort.

1. Radio the dispatcher that you are returning to quarters and that you are available (or not available) for service.
   - Valuable time is lost if a dispatcher has to locate and alert a back-up ambulance when he does not know that a ready-for-service unit is on the road. Be sure that you notify the dispatcher if you stop and leave the ambulance unattended for any reason during the return to quarters.
2. Air the ambulance if necessary.
   - If the patient just delivered to the hospital has a communicable disease, or if it was not possible to neutralize disagreeable odors while at the hospital, make the return trip with the windows of the patient compartment partially open, weather permitting. If the unit has sealed windows, use the air-conditioning or ventilating system to air the patient compartment.
3. Refuel the ambulance.
   - Local policy usually dictates the frequency with which an ambulance is refueled. Some squads require the driver to refuel after each run regardless of the distance traveled. In other squads the policy is to refuel when the gauge reaches a certain level. At any rate the fuel should be at a level that the ambulance can respond to an emergency and then to a medical facility without fear of running out.

ACTIONS THAT CAN BE TAKEN WHEN IN QUARTERS

When you return to quarters, there are many activities that need to be completed before the ambulance can be placed in service, and before it is ready for another call.

With the emphasis today on protection from AIDS and other diseases, you need to take every precaution to protect yourself. It is essential that, while handling contaminated linen, cleaning the equipment, handling the respiratory equipment and cleaning the ambulance interior where there may be many hidden nooks and crannies where the patient's blood or body fluids could be, you wear suitable gloves as a precaution.

1

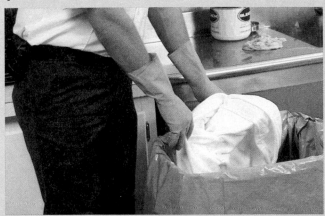

Place dirty linens in a sealable hamper.

2

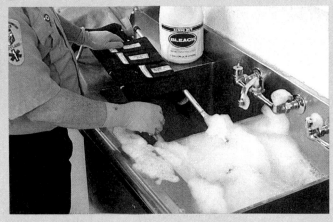

Remove and clean patient care equipment as required.

3

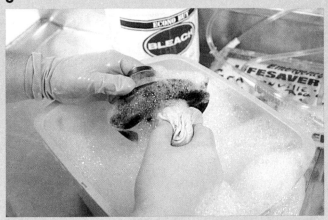

Clean and sanitize respiratory equipment as required.

4

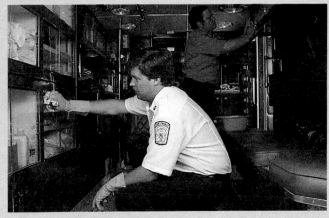

Clean and sanitize the ambulance interior as required. Any devices or surfaces which have come into contact with patient or his fluids must be cleaned with germicide.

5

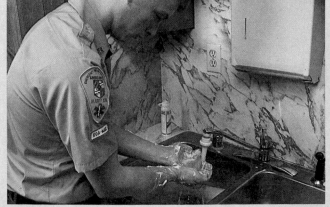

Wash thoroughly. Change soiled clothing. If exposed to communicable disease, this is first activity.

6

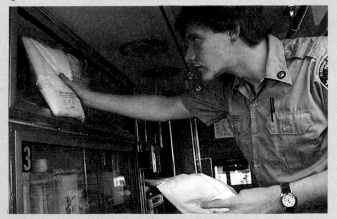

Replace expendable items as required.

(Scan continues on next page.)

7

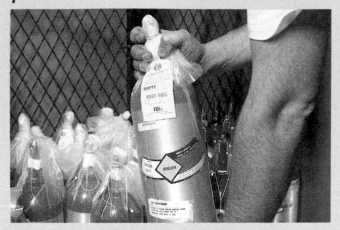

Always refill oxygen and air cylinders.

8

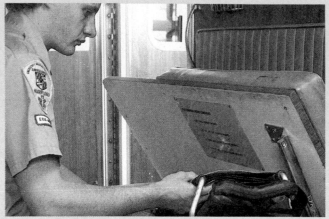

Replace patient care equipment as needed.

9

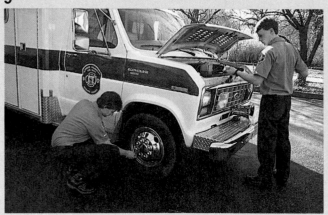

Maintain ambulance as required. Report problems that will take vehicle out of service.

10

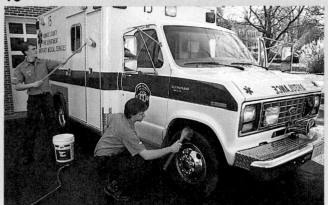

Clean the ambulance exterior as needed.

11

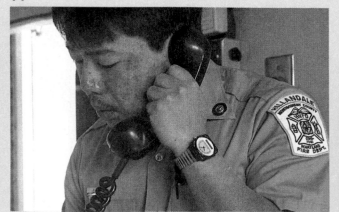

Report the unit ready for service.

12

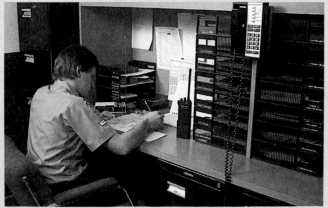

Complete any unfinished report forms as soon as possible.

Now you are ready to complete your cleaning and disinfecting chores (Scan 25–1):

1. Place soiled linens in a sealable container.
2. Clean any equipment that touched the patient.
   - Brush stretcher covers and other rubber, vinyl, and canvas materials clean, then wash them with soap and water.
3. Clean and sanitize used nondisposable respiratory-assist and inhalation therapy equipment in the following manner:
   - Disassemble the equipment so that all surfaces are exposed.
   - Fill a large plastic container with a surgical soap and water solution. Follow directions on the label of the soap container to ensure a proper concentration.
   - Soak the items for 10 minutes or as directed.
   - Clean the inner and outer surfaces with a suitable brush. Inner surfaces can be cleaned with a small bottle brush, while outer surfaces can be cleaned with a hand or nail brush. Make sure all encrusted matter is removed.
   - Rinse the items with tap water.
   - Soak the items in a germicidal solution. An inhalation therapist at a local hospital can suggest a germicide suitable for respiratory equipment. Follow directions for dilution, safe handling, and soaking time. Rubber gloves are recommended when using some germicides.
   - After the prescribed soaking period, hang the equipment in a well-ventilated clean area and allow it to dry for 12 to 24 hours.
4. Clean and sanitize the patient compartment.
   - Use a germicide to clean any fixed equipment or surfaces contacted by the patient or splashed with body fluids.
5. Prepare yourself for service.
   - Wash thoroughly, paying attention to the areas under your fingernails. Remember that contaminants can collect there and become a source of infection not only to you but also to the persons whom you touch.
   - Change soiled clothes. Clean contaminated clothing as soon as possible, especially if you were exposed to someone with a communicable disease.

6. Replace expendable items with items from the unit's storeroom.
7. Refill oxygen cylinders even if only a small volume of gas was used.
8. Replace patient care equipment.
9. Carry out postoperation vehicle maintenance procedures as required.
   - Check fluid levels, tire pressures, warning devices, lights, and so on. If you find something wrong with the vehicle, correct the problem or make someone in authority aware of it.
10. Clean the vehicle.
    - A clean exterior lends a professional appearance to an ambulance.
    - Check the vehicle for broken lights, glass and body damage, door operation, and other parts that may need repair or replacement.
11. Report the unit ready for service.
12. Complete any unfinished report forms as soon as possible.

SUMMARY

Termination activities begin at the hospital, continue during the return to quarters, and end when the ambulance is in quarters and completely ready for service. Disposable gloves should be worn by EMTs during any cleaning operation.

Before leaving the hospital, clean the interior of the ambulance as necessary. Wipe blood, vomitus, and body fluids from the floor, equipment, and compartment surfaces. Remove any trash generated during the patient care effort. Replace disposable masks and other expendable items and exchange equipment according to local policy. Make up the ambulance stretcher.

Radio the dispatcher that you are returning to quarters and that you can (or cannot) respond to calls. Air the ambulance (if necessary, and weather permitting) during the return to quarters. Refuel the ambulance, if necessary.

When in quarters, dispose of soiled linens, clean patient care and respiratory equipment, replenish oxygen cylinders, clean and sanitize the patient compartment, replace expendable items and patient care equipment, maintain and clean the ambulance, care for yourself, complete the report, and report the ambulance ready for service.

3236414

MARYLAND AMBULANCE INFORMATION SYSTEM (FORM 4)

PATIENT _____ INCIDENT NUMBER _____ CENSUS BOX _____ DATE _____

ADDRESS _____ INCIDENT LOCATION _____ CALL RECD _____

DRV (1)	ID #	CALL RCD	DPT STA	ARV LOC	DPT LOC	ARV HOS	DPT HOS	RTN STA	AMB #
EMTP ○ IVT ○	0123456789								
CRT ○ EMTA ○	0123456789								
PIL ○ ARC ○	0123456789								
E/M ○ OTHR ○	0123456789								

ATD (2)	ID #
EMTP ○ IVT ○	0123456789
CRT ○ EMTA ○	0123456789
ATT ○ ARC ○	0123456789
E/M ○ OTHR ○	0123456789

ATD (3)	ID #	CTY	DATE	RCE	AGE
EMTP ○ IVT ○	0123456789				
CRT ○ EMTA ○	0123456789			B	
ATT ○ ARC ○	0123456789			W	
E/M ○ OTHR ○	0123456789			O	

PUPILS
EQL ○ NR ○ CTL ○
DIL ○ CST ○
NEQ ○ LL ○ RL ○

COMA SCORE
EYE ① ② ③ ④
MOT ① ② ③ ④ ⑤ ⑥
VRB ① ② ③ ④ ⑤

ILL/EMER
AIR OB ○ DROWN ○ RESPIR ○
BEHAV ○ DRUG ○ SEIZRE ○
BURN ○ GI ○ SHOCK ○
CARDC ○ HEMOR ○ SM INH ○
CH PN ○ HSPCE ○ STING ○
CVA ○ INTRN ○ TRAUMA ○
DIABT ○ MATRN ○ OTHER ○
DOA ○ POISON ○

SEX M ○ F ○

VITALS TIME 1 / **VITALS TIME 2**
SYS DIA PUL RES | SYS DIA PUL RES

CARE
AIRWY ○ SP IMB ○ TRNPRT ○
BL DRW ○ SPLINT ○ OTHER ○
CD PCK ○ OXYG ○
CN BLD ○ CPR ○ (S) (F)
CRS IN ○ CPR MCH ○ (S) (F)
EXTRIC ○ DFIB ○ (S) (F) ① ② ③
OB DEL ○ EOA ○ ① ② ③
RESTRN ○ MAST ○ ① ② ③
MN VTL ○ ① ② ③

LOCATION AND INJURY TYPE
ABRA / AMPU / BURN / CONT / CRSH / DISL / FRAC / GNST / LACR / PUNC / STAB
HEAD ○ FACE ○ EYE ○ NECK ○ CHST ○ BACK ○ ABDM ○ GEN ○ ARM ○ LEG ○ HAND ○ FOOT ○

EKG ① ② ③

MEDS
VFIB (F) (L) | LIBO ① ② ③
CRSE (F) (L) | LIDP ① ② ③
FINE (F) (L) | EPIV ① ② ③
VTCH (F) (L) | EPSQ ① ② ③
AS (F) (L) | ATRO ① ② ③
PVCS (F) (L) | SOBI ① ② ③
SB (F) (L) | NARC ① ② ③
AVB (F) (L) | D50 ① ② ③
PAT (F) (L) | NITR ① ② ③
ST (F) (L) | MS ① ② ③
SVT (F) (L) | CAL ① ② ③
SR (F) (L) | OTHR ① ② ③
OTHR (F) (L)

IV ATTS: 1 ○ 2 ○ R ○
IV SUCC: 1 ○ 2 ○ 0 ○

IV SOLUTIONS
R/L ○
D5W ○
NS ○
D5½NS ○

RADIO
GOOD ○ FAIR ○
POOR ○
NO CONTACT ○

CNSLT HOSP: 0123456789

RECV. HOSP: 0123456789

TRANSPORT BY
AMBU ○
HELIC ○
REFSD ○
NONE ○
FALSE ○
CANCL ○

TYPE OF CALL
VEHIC ○ MOTCY ○
INDUS ○ PEDES ○
REC ○ OTHER ○
ASSLT ○ ROUTN ○
MED ○ TRSFR ○
MULT PATIENTS ○
ADDIT NAR. ○
EXCEP. CALL ○

HOSP CHOSEN
CLOSE ○ RERTE ○ CNSLT ○
PROCL ○ OTHER ○
PHYSICIAN _____

MILEAGE
FINISH _____
START _____
TOTAL _____

TOTAL MILES
0123456789
0123456789
0123456789

HOSP. SIG.

PRIORITY ① ② ③ ④

MAKE NO MARKS IN THIS AREA

COMMENTS

COMPLETED BY

CALL NUMBER

_____
_____
_____
_____

3236414

NCS Trans-Optic® EP01-26674:321   A9102

DO NOT WRITE BELOW THIS LINE

MIEMSS COPY

Communications and Reports

OBJECTIVES As an EMT, you should be able to:

1. Define "communication." (p. 604)
2. List FOUR ways to improve your oral communication skills. (p. 604)
3. State the FOUR basic components of an emergency communications system. (p. 604)
4. List at least FOUR ways in which this communications system may be expanded. (p. 604)

5. Give TEN rules to follow in regard to ambulance radio communications. (p. 605)
6. State when you can use codes in a radio communication. (p. 605)
7. List the information that can be gained from an accurate and complete ambulance run report. (pp. 605–607)

SKILLS As an EMT, you should be able to:

1. Present oral reports in a calm professional manner.

2. Conduct proper radio communications.
3. Complete all reports required by your system.

COMMUNICATION

In emergency care, communication means more than radio transmissions. Being able to talk with people is an important trait of an EMT. You must be able to talk with bystanders at the scene so that they will give you information and let you take charge. An efficient patient assessment may depend on your ability to ask a patient questions and listen to his statements. Personal interaction is one of the most important things in gaining patient confidence; it is the main approach that you take when dealing with patients having stress reactions, emotional emergencies, or psychological emergencies.

Your ability to communicate with others is very important when interacting with the members of the EMS System. On a typical ambulance run, you may have to talk with the dispatcher, other members of the ambulance crew, First Responders, other EMTs responding to the scene, and the emergency department staff. You must be able to speak clearly and calmly, using the correct terminology to allow for effective oral communication.

You also must be able to listen to others. The ability to listen to others so that they have confidence in you as a member of the patient care team is a major skill you must develop as an EMT.

To improve your skills in oral communications while on duty:

- Use correct terminology whenever possible. Do not use layperson's terms or slang.
- Do not use a term unless you know its meaning.
- Use complete sentences when you speak.
- Speak calmly using a neutral tone.

In addition to oral communications skills, you will have to develop written skills as they apply to your duties as an EMT. Just as listening is an important part of oral communication, reading is a major element in written communications skills. Make certain that you read reports and memoranda. Too many people scan over documents, missing important information.

Your written reports are very important. Make certain that they are filled in correctly, they are complete and accurate, and the correct terminology has been used.

RADIO COMMUNICATIONS

We have covered radio communications between the EMT and the dispatcher, and the ambulance and the emergency department. We also have stressed that you should make use of radio communications with the dispatcher to obtain the help you need at an accident, or when hazardous materials are at the scene. In this chapter, the radio communications system and some general considerations about its use will be covered.

The Emergency Communications System

The basic communications system includes:

- Dispatcher base station
- Ambulance transmitter/receiver
- Emergency department remote center
- Telephone line backup

With these components, the ambulance can send and receive messages from the dispatcher and the emergency department.

This system can be expanded in many ways to include:

- Portable transmitter/receivers—to allow EMTs at the scene to communicate with each other and to send and receive messages while they are at the scene but away from the ambulance.
- Ambulance repeater stations—to retransmit between the two-way radio and the portable units.
- Biotelemetry—to send to the emergency department an electrocardiogram (ECG) while it is being taken at the scene.
- Telephone patches—done via the dispatcher base station to allow radio communications to be connected with telephones.

Ambulance Communications Procedures

The Federal Communications Commission has allocated certain frequencies for emergency medical use. They have ruled, "Except for test transmissions, stations licensed to ambulance operators or rescue squads may be used only for the transmission of messages pertaining to the safety of life or property and urgent messages necessary for the rendition of an efficient ambulance or emergency rescue service." This means that you are to use the ambulance radio for official use only. Your calls are to relate to your duties and they are to be carried out in a professional manner.

When using the radio:

- Do not try to transmit if other EMS personnel are using the channel or the dispatcher is sending to you.
- Speak into the microphone using normal voice volume. Keep the tone of your voice neutral, and slow down your rate of speech.
- Speak clearly, making an effort to pronounce each word distinctly.
- Be brief, using the correct terms and phrases needed to make your messages understood. Know what you are going to say before you press the transmit key.
- Avoid using codes and abbreviations, unless they are part of your system and will be understood by the person receiving the message.
- Receive a full message from the sender. Do not attempt to cut him off so that you can send.
- Do not use slang or profanity.
- Do not use individual's names. Use unit, dispatch, and hospital identifications.
- Politeness is understood to be part of every radio transmission. Do not use "please," "thank you," and other such terms.
- If you do not understand something that is said while receiving, ask for a repeat. Never pretend to understand what was said.

Codes

Many EMS systems use some form of code in their radio communications. DO NOT use a code unless

Table 26–1. EXAMPLES FROM THE 10-CODE

10–1	Signal weak
10–2	Signal strong
10–3	Stop transmitting
10–4	Affirmative
10–7	Out of service
10–8	In service
10–9	Repeat
10–10	Negative
10–17	En route
10–18	Urgent
10–20	Location
10–22	Disregard
10–26	Estimated time of arrival
10–30	Danger
10–33	Emergency (help)

it is part of your system. If the code is not used by the emergency department, then you have wasted time and a transmission.

One of the most popular codes being used is the "10-Code." Efficient use of this code helps to reduce transmission time. The codes from 10–1 to 10–34 should not be altered. Codes 10–35 to 10–39 are reserved. Codes from 10–40 and up can be used according to local assignment.

REPORTS

Reports can be oral or written. When you radio the emergency department from the scene or during transport, this is an oral report. Upon arrival at the medical facility, you will be giving an oral report to the emergency department staff. Your report is to be brief, yet accurate and complete, and presented in a calm professional manner. The information you give in oral reports becomes part of the patient's medical record.

Written reports are very important in an EMS system. They help to keep track of patient information, provide the emergency department with information, serve as part of the patient's medical record, and supply information on personnel and equipment usage and needs.

One thing that you must bear in mind is that your written report becomes a legal record that can be used in a court of law if ever needed. It is very

EMS

EMS REGION II
STATE OF NEW HAMPSHIRE
STANDARD EMERGENCY PATIENT RECORD

First Responder: _____

FR Time Out: _____:_____

FR On Scene: _____:_____

Town of Incident: _____

Incident Location: _____

Patient Name: _____

Address: _____

Next of Kin: _____

Address: _____

Patient's Home Phone #: _____

Patient's S.S. #: _____

M.V. Accident?: _____ Y _____ N

Time Dispatched: _____:_____

Amb Time Out: _____:_____

Amb On Scene: _____:_____

En Route: _____:_____

At Hosp: _____:_____

In Service: _____:_____

Trauma Score: _____

Mileage: _____

Gas Usage: _____

Code Toned Out: _____

Ambulance Service: _____

Response Unit: _____

Patient Status: _____

Date: ___/___/___

Age: _____

Sex: _____

Receiving Hospital: _____

M.D.: _____

Pt. #: _____

Incident: _____

Pt. D.O.B.: _____

For BEMS Use Only

Town Code _____

Amb Code _____

Hosp. Code _____

Chief Complaint & History (or Mechanisms of Injury): _____
_____
_____
_____
_____
_____

Observations: _____
_____
_____
_____
_____
_____
_____
_____
_____

For E.R. Use Only

☐ Admitted

☐ Transferred to

☐ Released

☐ Expired

Type of Illness/Injury

☐ 1. Trauma

☐ 2. Burn

☐ 3. Cardiac

☐ 4. Neonate

☐ 5. Behavioral

☐ 6. Poison

☐ 7. Spinal Cord

☐ 8. Head

☐ 9. Respiratory

☐ 10. Other

Pulse: _____

Rhythm: _____ Reg.

Time Vitals _____ Irreg.

Were Taken: Strength: _____ Weak

_____ Strong

Respirations: _____

Rhythm: _____ Reg.

_____ Irreg.

Type: _____ Normal

_____ Labored

Blood Pressure

/

Pupils:

_____ Equal

_____ Unequal

_____ Fixed, Dilated

_____ Constricted

_____ Responsive

_____ Unresponsive

BLS & ALS Procedures	Time
☐ CPR (Layperson)	_____:_____
☐ CPR (service)	_____:_____
☐ EOA	_____:_____
☐ MAST	_____:_____
☐ Cardiac Monitor	_____:_____
☐ I.V.	_____:_____
☐ Drugs	_____:_____

Color:

_____ Cyanotic

_____ Pale

_____ Flushed

_____ Normal

Skin Temperature:

_____ Hot

_____ Cold

_____ Normal

Moisture:

_____ Dry

_____ Moist

_____ Nomal

Mental Status:

_____ A - Alert

_____ V - Responds to Verbal Stimulus

_____ P - Responds to Painful Stimulus

_____ U - Unresponsive

Medic Alert: _____ **Allergies:** _____

Medications: _____

Treatment Given: _____
_____
_____
_____
_____
_____

**Additional Vitals:

Time	Pulse	Resp.	BP
_____:			/
_____:			/
_____:			/
_____:			/

Refusal of Care / Transport _____

Witness: _____

Reporting Attendant's Signature

Additional Information: _____
_____
_____

Other Attendants: _____

E.T.A. _____

Insurance Nos.: _____
_____
_____

Report by Radio Only the Information in Bold Type. Report ** Only if Changed.

White-Ambulance   Yellow-State   Pink-Hospital   Goldenrod-Local Option

FIGURE 26–1a. EMS New Hampshire Patient Record.

CRAMS SCORE

(ONCE SCORED AT THE SCENE, NEVER RESCORE TO A HIGHER VALUE LATER.)

CIRCULATION

NORMAL CAPILLARY REFILL & BP OVER 100	2
DELAYED CAPILLARY REFILL OR BP 85-99	1
NO CAPILLARY REFILL OR BP UNDER 85	0

RESPIRATION

NORMAL RATE & EFFORT	2
ABNORMAL LABORED, SHALLOW OR RATE OVER 35	1
ABSENT	0

ABDOMEN / THORAX

ABDOMEN & THORAX NOT TENDER	2
ABDOMEN OR THORAX TENDER	1
ABDOMEN RIGID, THORAX FLAIL OR DEEP PENETRATING INJURY	0

MOTOR

NORMAL IN OBEYING COMMANDS	2
RESPOND ONLY TO PAIN - NO POSTURING	1
POSTURES OR NO RESPONSE	0

SPEECH

NORMAL & ORIENTED	2
CONFUSED OR INAPPROPRIATE	1
NONE OR UNINTELLIGIBLE SOUNDS	0

TOTAL _____

PT. NAME _____ DATE __/__/__

AMBULANCE: PLEASE LEAVE TRAUMA SCORE CARD
ATTACHED TO YELLOW HOSPITAL COPY FOR E.D. USE.

FIGURE 26–1b. CRAMS Score (Circulation, Respiration, Abdomen /Throat, Motor, Speech)

important that everything on the form or report be filled out completely. Spelling must be checked, times must agree, signatures needed must be acquired. Your observations at the scene, the surroundings when you arrived, what the witnesses had to say—everything must be validated and documented for any future need. If you don't write it down, you have no proof that it happened.

If something about the injury does not match the mechanics of injury or the lack of it, the proper authorities (i.e., police) must be made aware for them to possibly follow up with an investigation. If you suspect that a crime has been committed, note this on your report. No matter how minor something may seem at the time, it may become very important weeks or even months later if insurance companies or other agencies question the event. Don't take chances. Validate everything that seems important to you at the time.

Written reports may include:

- Patient assessment and care forms (also called field or street forms)
- Special assessment forms (e.g., neurologic)
- Ambulance run reports
- Release forms when consent is not granted
- Vehicle inspection forms

Many systems have combined most of these forms so that one report will cover all the needed information. Figures 26–1 and 26–2 are examples of the types of form EMTs will be expected to fill out. Those that have a minimum of small squares to check off while in the moving ambulance are the easiest to fill out (Figs. 26–1a and b, and 26–2). Other forms with small squares to check off and shaded areas are difficult to read at best, but, in the patient area with the lights either dimmed or running the overhead blue compartment lights, they are almost impossible to fill out accurately (Fig. 26–3a and b). Regardless of the forms used by your system, you will be asked to provide information that is required by all systems. Someone reading your report will be able to tell:

- An ambulance run occurred and the date it occurred
- If it was an emergency run
- Who ordered the run (e.g., the dispatcher)
- Who made the run
- Time out of quarters
- Location of the scene and arrival time
- Assessment of the patient
- Care rendered
- Changes in the patient's condition
- Time leaving the scene
- Destination and time of arrival
- A transfer was completed
- Time back in quarters

Remember, the report must be accurate and complete, using the proper terms (correctly spelled). The report should be completed in quarters, as soon as possible.

SUMMARY

Communication involves both oral and written skills.

In all communications involving EMT duties, be brief yet accurate and complete. Use the correct terminology, written or spoken, so that it can be understood. Communicate orally in a calm professional manner.

The basic components of an EMS radio communications system are the dispatcher base station, the ambulance transmitter/receiver, and the emergency department remote center. Telephone backup should be part of the system.

Radio communications should be limited to offi-

KEENE FIRE DEPARTMENT
EMERGENCY MEDICAL SERVICES
DEFIBRILLATION REPORT

PATIENT'S NAME: _____ DOB: __/__/__ AGE:_____

AMBULANCE RUN #:_____
VITAL SIGNS UPON ARRIVAL:

PULSE: _____ RESPIRATIONS: _____ B/P:__/___

CPR STARTED BY:_____ bystander _____ service TIME:_____

L.O.C. A _____ (alert)
         V _____ (verbal)
         P _____ (painful)
         U _____ (unresponsive)

DEFIBRILLATORY INTERVENTION

SHOCK 1:   RHYTHM: _____ TIME: _____ : _____

       POST SHOCK VITALS:
              PULSE: _____ RESPIRATIONS: _____ B/P: _____

SHOCK 2:   RHYTHM: _____ TIME: _____ : _____

       POST SHOCK VITALS:
              PULSE: _____ RESPIRATIONS: _____ B/P: _____

SHOCK 3:   RHYTHM: _____ TIME: _____ : _____

       POST SHOCK VITALS:
              PULSE: _____ RESPIRATIONS: _____ B/P: _____

NARRATIVE:

_____

_____

_____

_____

TIMES:

OUT: _____   IN: _____

ON SCENE: _____   CODE 9: _____

ENROUTE: _____   AT HOSP: _____

EMT-D: _____

ATTENDANTS: _____

_____

EQUIPMENT USAGE: (show quantity)

Monitor electrodes   _____

Defib electrodes   _____

ECC Paper   _____

Micro cassette   _____

FIGURE 26–2. Defibrillation Report, Keene, N.H., Fire Department.

Prehospital Care Report

USE BALL POINT PEN ONLY.

M D Y

DATE   RUN NO

Press Down Firmly. You're Making 4 Copies.

AGENCY CODE   VEH. ID

Name	Agency Name	MILEAGE		USE MILITARY TIMES

Name

Address

Ph #

A G E   D O B M   D   Y   S E X ☐ M ☐ F

Physician

Next of Kin

Agency Name

Call Location

CHECK ONE   ☐ Residence ☐ Health Facility ☐ Farm ☐ Indus. Facility
☐ Other Work Loc. ☐ Roadway ☐ Recreational ☐ Other

Call Origin

Dispatch Information

CALL TYPE AS REC'D.
☐ Emergency
☐ Non-Emergency
☐ Stand-by

INTERFACILITY TANSFER
☐ Yes
TYPE OF TRANSFER
☐ BLS ☐ ALS

MILEAGE
END
BEGIN
TOTAL

HOSPITAL COMMUNICATIONS
☐ Yes ☐ Directly ☐ Thru Dispatch
☐ VHF ☐ UHF ☐ Phone
☐ No ☐ Communication Difficulties

USE MILITARY TIMES
CALL REC'D
ENROUTE
AT SCENE
FROM SCENE
AT DESTIN
IN SERVICE
IN QUARTERS

MECHANISM OF INJURY
☐ MVA (complete seat belt section)   ☐ Fall of ____ feet ☐ GSW ☐ Other
☐ Struck by vehicle   ☐ Unarmed assault ☐ Knife ☐ _____

☐ Extrication required _____ minutes

Seat belt used?
☐ Yes ☐ No ☐ Unknown

Seat Belt Use
Reported By ☐ Crew ☐ Patient
☐ Police ☐ Other

CHIEF COMPLAINT   SUBJECTIVE ASSESSMENT

PRESENTING PROBLEM

☐ Airway Obstruction
☐ Respiratory Arrest
☐ Respiratory Distress
☐ Cardiac Related (Potential)
☐ Cardiac Arrest

☐ Allergic Reaction
☐ Syncope
☐ Stroke/CVA
☐ General Illness/Malaise
☐ Gastro-Intestinal Distress
☐ Diabetic Related (Potential)
☐ Pain _____

☐ Unconscious/Unresp.
☐ Seizure
☐ Behavioral Disorder
☐ Substance Abuse (Potential)
☐ Poisoning (Accidental)

☐ Shock
☐ Head Injury
☐ Spinal Injury
☐ Fracture/Dislocation
☐ Amputation

☐ Other _____

☐ Multiple Trauma
☐ Trauma-Blunt
☐ Trauma-Penetrating
☐ Soff Tissue Injury
☐ Bleeding/Hemorrhage

☐ OB/GYN
☐ Burns
Environmental
☐ Heat
☐ Cold
☐ Hazardous Materials
☐ Obvious Death

PAST MEDICAL HISTORY

☐ Hypertension ☐ Stroke
☐ Seizures   ☐ Diabetes
☐ COPD   ☐ Cardiac
☐ Allergy   ☐ Other (List)
☐ Medication

VITAL SIGNS

	TIME	RESP	PULSE	B.P.	LEVEL OF CONSCIOUSNESS	GCS	TS	R	PUPILS	L	SKIN
		Rate: ☐ Regular ☐ Shallow ☐ Labored	Rate: ☐ ☐ Regular ☐ Irregular		☐ Alert ☐ Voice ☐ Pain ☐ Unresp.				Normal Dilated Constricted Sluggish No-Reaction		☐ Unremarkable ☐ Cool ☐ Pale ☐ Warm ☐ Cyanotic ☐ Moist ☐ Flushed ☐ Dry ☐ Jaundiced
		Rate: ☐ Regular ☐ Shallow ☐ Labored	Rate: ☐ ☐ Regular ☐ Irregular		☐ Alert ☐ Voice ☐ Pain ☐ Unresp.				Normal Dilated Constricted Sluggish No-Reaction		☐ Unremarkable ☐ Cool ☐ Pale ☐ Warm ☐ Cyanotic ☐ Moist ☐ Flushed ☐ Dry ☐ Jaundiced
		Rate: ☐ Regular ☐ Shallow ☐ Labored	Rate: ☐ ☐ Regular ☐ Irregular		☐ Alert ☐ Voice ☐ Pain ☐ Unresp.				Normal Dilated Constricted Sluggish No-Reaction		☐ Unremarkable ☐ Cool ☐ Pale ☐ Warm ☐ Cyanotic ☐ Moist ☐ Flushed ☐ Dry ☐ Jaundiced

OBJECTIVE PHYSICAL ASSESSMENT

☐ Physical Findings Unremarkable

Head/Neck Upper Extr. Chest/Back Abd/Pelvic Lower Extr.

1) Pain
2) Wound
3) Fracture/Disloc. Open
4) Fracture/Disloc. Closed
5) Bleeding/Hemorrhage
6) Loss of Motion/Sensation
7) Sprain/Strain
8) Burn ___ Deg ___ %
9) Internal

COMMENTS

TREATMENT GIVEN   MEDICAL CONTROL INFORMATION   Insurance Data

☐ Airway Cleared
☐ Oral airway
☐ Esophageal Obturator Airway/Esophageal Gastric Tube Airway (EOA/EGTA)
☐ Endo Tracheal Tube (E/T)
☐ Oxygen Administered @ _____ L.P.M., Method _____
☐ Suction Used
☐ Artificial Ventilation Method _____
☐ C.P.R. in progress on arrival by: ☐ Citizen ☐ Firefighter ☐ Police Officer
☐ C.P.R. Started @ Time ▶ _____   Time from Arrest Until C.P.R. ▶ _____ Minutes
☐ EKG Monitored (Attach Tracing) [Rhythm(s) _____]
☐ Defibrillation/Cardioversion No. Times _____ With _____ Watt/Sec.

☐ Medication Administered (Use Continuation Form)
☐ IV Fluid _____ No. of Established ___ No. Of Attempts ___
☐ Mast Inflated (Time Inflated: _____)
☐ Bleeding/Hemorrhage Controlled (Method Used: _____)
☐ Spinal Immobilization by ☐ Neck ☐ Back
☐ Limb Immobilized by ☐ Fixation ☐ Traction
☐ (Heat) or (Cold) Applied
☐ Vomiting Induced @ Time _____ Method _____
☐ Restraints Applied, Type _____
☐ Baby Delivered @ Time _____ In County _____
    ☐ Alive ☐ Stillborn ☐ Male ☐ Female
☐ Other _____

DISPOSITION (See list)   DISP. CODE   CONTINUATION FORM USED   Yes

CREW

IN CHARGE	DRIVER'S NAME	NAME	NAME
☐ EMT ☐ AEMT #	☐ EMS-FR ☐ EMT ☐ AEMT #	☐ EMS-FR ☐ EMT ☐ AEMT #	☐ EMS-FR ☐ EMT ☐ AEMT #

FIGURE 26–3. Prehospital Care Report: (a) front; (b) back.

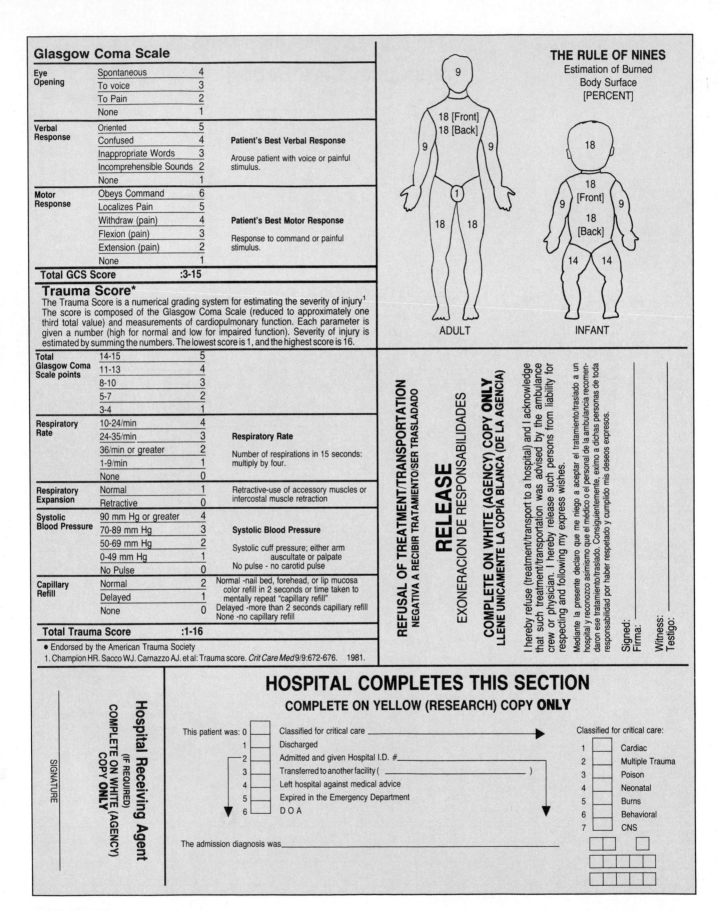

Glasgow Coma Scale

Eye Opening	Spontaneous	4
	To voice	3
	To Pain	2
	None	1

Verbal Response	Oriented	5	**Patient's Best Verbal Response**
	Confused	4	
	Inappropriate Words	3	Arouse patient with voice or painful stimulus.
	Incomprehensible Sounds	2	
	None	1	

Motor Response	Obeys Command	6	**Patient's Best Motor Response**
	Localizes Pain	5	
	Withdraw (pain)	4	
	Flexion (pain)	3	Response to command or painful stimulus.
	Extension (pain)	2	
	None	1	

Total GCS Score :3-15

Trauma Score*

The Trauma Score is a numerical grading system for estimating the severity of injury[1] The score is composed of the Glasgow Coma Scale (reduced to approximately one third total value) and measurements of cardiopulmonary function. Each parameter is given a number (high for normal and low for impaired function). Severity of injury is estimated by summing the numbers. The lowest score is 1, and the highest score is 16.

Total Glasgow Coma Scale points	14-15	5	
	11-13	4	
	8-10	3	
	5-7	2	
	3-4	1	

Respiratory Rate	10-24/min	4	**Respiratory Rate**
	24-35/min	3	
	36/min or greater	2	Number of respirations in 15 seconds: multiply by four.
	1-9/min	1	
	None	0	

| Respiratory Expansion | Normal | 1 | Retractive-use of accessory muscles or intercostal muscle retraction |
| | Retractive | 0 | |

Systolic Blood Pressure	90 mm Hg or greater	4	**Systolic Blood Pressure**
	70-89 mm Hg	3	
	50-69 mm Hg	2	Systolic cuff pressure; either arm auscultate or palpate
	0-49 mm Hg	1	No pulse - no carotid pulse
	No Pulse	0	

Capillary Refill	Normal	2	Normal -nail bed, forehead, or lip mucosa color refill in 2 seconds or time taken to mentally repeat "capillary refill"
	Delayed	1	Delayed -more than 2 seconds capillary refill
	None	0	None -no capillary refill

Total Trauma Score :1-16

● Endorsed by the American Trauma Society
1. Champion HR. Sacco WJ. Carnazzo AJ. et al: Trauma score. *Crit Care Med* 9/9:672-676. 1981.

THE RULE OF NINES
Estimation of Burned
Body Surface
[PERCENT]

ADULT

INFANT

REFUSAL OF TREATMENT/TRANSPORTATION
NEGATIVA A RECIBIR TRATAMIENTO/SER TRASLADADO

RELEASE
EXONERACION DE RESPONSABILIDADES

COMPLETE ON WHITE (AGENCY) COPY ONLY
LLENE UNICAMENTE LA COPIA BLANCA (DE LA AGENCIA)

I hereby refuse (treatment/transport) to a hospital) and I acknowledge that such treatment/transportation was advised by the ambulance crew or physician. I hereby release such persons from liability for respecting and following my express wishes.

Mediante la presente declaro que me niego a aceptar el tratamiento/traslado a un hospital y reconozco asimismo que el médico o el personal de la ambulancia recomendaron ese tratamiento/traslado. Consiguientemente, eximo a dichas personas de toda responsabilidad por haber respetado y cumplido mis deseos expresos.

Signed: Firma:

Witness: Testigo:

HOSPITAL COMPLETES THIS SECTION
COMPLETE ON YELLOW (RESEARCH) COPY ONLY

This patient was:
0 Classified for critical care
1 Discharged
2 Admitted and given Hospital I.D. #
3 Transferred to another facility ( )
4 Left hospital against medical advice
5 Expired in the Emergency Department
6 D O A

The admission diagnosis was

Classified for critical care:
1 Cardiac
2 Multiple Trauma
3 Poison
4 Neonatal
5 Burns
6 Behavioral
7 CNS

Hospital Receiving Agent
(IF REQUIRED)
COMPLETE ON WHITE (AGENCY) COPY ONLY

SIGNATURE

FIGURE 26–3. *continued*

cial use. Keep your transmission as brief as possible. Make sure you know what you are going to say before you go on the air. Make your transmission as accurate as possible.

Do not interrupt someone else using the channel or the dispatcher. Remember to wait for the person who is transmitting to finish before you start your own transmission.

Use codes only if they are part of your system and the person receiving knows the code.

Make your written reports accurate and complete, and finish them as soon as possible. Use correct terminology in your reports; the patient information in your report becomes part of the patient's medical record.

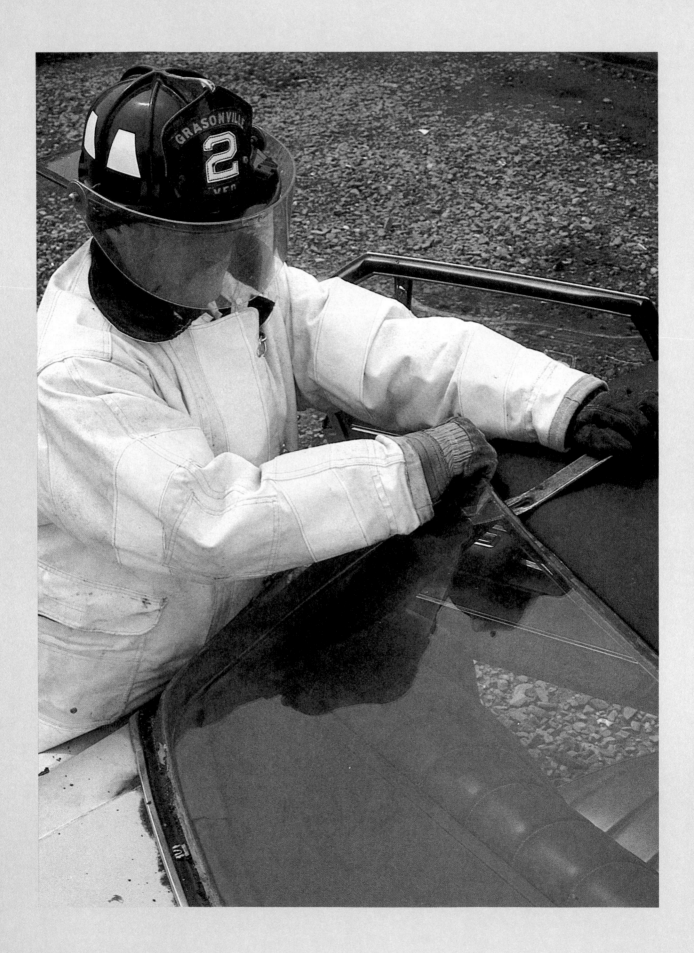

Vehicle Rescue

INTRODUCTION

As you progress through your career as an Emergency Medical Technician, you will undoubtedly hear repeated use of the term, *Golden Hour*. Military medical personnel discovered during the Korean conflict that if a seriously wounded individual could be delivered into the hands of specially trained surgical personnel within an hour of the time of injury—the Golden Hour—the chance of that person surviving was reasonably high. The Golden Hour concept was further developed during the Vietnam war through the use of trained medics and aeromedical evacuation. The concept became popular in the civilian EMS community when Dr. R Adams Cowley of the University of Maryland created the Shock Trauma Center in Baltimore. Today, if a seriously injured person can be transported to a trauma center within an hour of the occurrence of an accident, the chance for survival is high.

There are no pauses in the Golden Hour. Once the clock starts, it doesn't stop. It doesn't stop while a witness to an accident seeks a phone. It doesn't stop while an operator at an emergency reporting center elicits and records information about the accident, and it doesn't stop while a dispatcher alerts the appropriate emergency service organizations.

The clock doesn't stop while volunteer EMTs respond to the ambulance garage from their homes and workplaces, nor does it stop while an ambulance is responding to the location of the accident. If the accident has resulted in entrapment, the clock doesn't stop while the lead EMT assesses the situation and decides on a course of action, and it doesn't stop during the rescue effort that follows. From the moment that an accident occurs, time marches on, and as the minutes of the Golden Hour slip away, so do the chances that a seriously injured person will fully recover.

While there may be nothing that you can do as an EMT to reduce the notification, alerting, dispatching, and response times associated with accident calls, or the time it takes to transport an injured person to a medical facility, there is much you can do to reduce the time it takes to manage hazards and then reach, disentangle, and remove accident victims from mechanisms of entrapment.

Don't think that these four activities are all there is to vehicle rescue, however. Vehicle rescue is a system of dozens of operations included in 12 identifiable phases of activity.

The 12 Phases of Vehicle Rescue

Asked to define *vehicle rescue*, the average EMT will probably respond something like this: "Vehicle rescue is the extrication of injured persons from accident vehicles." This is not an unusual response. The terms *vehicle rescue* and *extrication* are synonymous in the minds of many EMS personnel because training programs, textbooks, magazine articles, and audiovisual materials have conditioned them to think that way.

Extrication is defined as the disentanglement of a person from a predicament, and the definition does seem to characterize a vehicle rescue effort. However, extrication or, better yet, disentanglement is but one of 12 phases of activity that EMS and other emergency service personnel may have to undertake to accomplish the safe and efficient removal of an accident victim from the dangerous environment of an accident scene.

Following are the events that may occur from the time an ambulance crew or rescue squad finishes with one accident call until the time it finishes with the next.

- **PHASE 1—PREPARING FOR RESCUE OPERATIONS.** This is an indefinite period during which the unit prepares for the next accident response. Equipment is maintained, supplies are checked, officers and squad members continue their training, and the vehicle is kept ready for service.

- **PHASE 2—RESPONDING TO THE ACCIDENT LOCATION.** This phase of a vehicle rescue operation begins when a call for help is received, continues while the unit responds to the accident location, and ends when the unit is safely parked with regard to traffic and hazards.

- **PHASE 3—ASSESSING THE SITUATION.** The lead EMT examines the scene and notes such things as the number and types of vehicles involved, the mechanisms of entrapment, the number of people injured and the extent of their injuries, and hazards that the accident has produced. The EMT matches what has to be done to the on-scene capabilities and calls for help as required.

- **PHASE 4—REACHING OFF-ROAD WRECKAGE.** When an accident occurs in an urban or suburban area, EMTs may have only to walk a short distance from the ambulance to the damaged vehicles. In rural areas, EMTs may have to use special techniques to reach accident vehicles that are at the bottom of hills too steep to descend without assistance.

- **PHASE 5—MANAGING ACCIDENT-RELATED HAZARDS.** During this phase of activity, rescuers eliminate or manage a variety of traffic and nontraffic hazards so that rescue and patient care activities can be carried out safely.

- **PHASE 6—GAINING ACCESS TO TRAPPED OCCUPANTS.** Rescuers make openings in the wreckage so they can initiate life-saving efforts.

- **PHASE 7—CARING FOR LIFE-THREATENING CONDITIONS.** When an ambulance crew is working alone at the scene of a vehicle accident, EMTs must care for life-threatening injuries before they can carry out disentanglement and removal operations. When they are working in concert with rescue squad personnel, EMTs can start patient care activities at the start of this phase and continue them without interruption until the injured persons are delivered to medical facilities.

- **PHASE 8—DISENTANGLING TRAPPED PERSONS.** This phase of a vehicle rescue operation has three parts. First, rescuers protect the victims. Next, rescuers expand existing openings in the wreckage or create new ones through which the injured persons can be removed. Then rescuers remove mechanisms of entrapment from around the victims.

- **PHASE 9—PACKAGING THE INJURED PERSONS.** When mechanisms of entrapment are out of the way, rescuers "package" the occupants; that is, they dress wounds and immobilize body parts so that injuries will not be aggravated while the victims are being removed from the vehicle.

- **PHASE 10—REMOVING INJURED PERSONS FROM THE WRECKAGE.** During this phase of activity, rescuers carefully remove the injured persons from the accident vehicles and secure them to full-body immobilization devices.

- **PHASE 11—TRANSFERRING INJURED PERSONS TO THE AMBULANCE.** In urban and suburban areas, rescuers may have to do nothing more than carry a stretcher or wheel the ambulance cot a few feet from the wreckage to the ambulance. When accident vehicles are off the road in a rural area, rescuers may have to employ special equipment to move injured persons up a steep hill, from the bottom of a ravine, or across a body of water.

• **PHASE 12—TERMINATING THE OPERATION.** The final phase of a vehicle rescue operation begins when all the injured persons have been transferred to ambulances, and ends when the system of people and equipment known as the ambulance crew or the rescue squad is once again ready for service.

Your Role As an EMT in Vehicle Rescue Operations

How many of these phases of activity you will participate in as an EMT will depend on the role that your EMS unit plays in community vehicle rescue operations.

If you live in an area where the ambulance responds to accident locations simultaneously with a rescue unit and fire apparatus, you may never be called on to perform rescue operations. You and a partner on the ambulance will probably begin patient care efforts as soon as injured persons are accessible, and it will be your job to continue those efforts during subsequent disentanglement, removal, and transfer operations. This is usually the situation in urban areas that have full-time emergency services and in suburban areas where fire, ambulance, and rescue services are all provided by the same volunteer fire department.

If you are employed by a private or municipal ambulance service in a community that has a volunteer fire department, there will undoubtedly be times when you will arrive at locations of vehicle accidents before the rescue squad. An ambulance with full-time personnel is usually able to respond to an accident scene within seconds of the receipt of a call for help, while volunteers must respond first to the fire station and then to the scene. As you can imagine, lives can be saved if the ambulance is equipped and the EMTs are trained to at least manage hazards and gain access to seriously injured persons while the rescue unit is responding.

If you are a member of an ambulance service in a rural area where the local fire department does not have rescue capabilities, and properly equipped and trained rescue units must travel considerable distances to reach accident locations, you may be called on to carry out all phases of vehicle rescue.

EMT candidates cannot be trained for all 12 phases of vehicle rescue in the small time slot usually provided in basic training courses. What prospective EMT's can learn in a short time are the techniques of hazard management, gaining access, and disentanglement that are most often used during vehicle rescue operations. The following four sections have been written with that goal in mind.

As you read through the rest of this chapter, you must be aware that the supplies and equipment listed and described in Section One are not the only items that might be carried on an ambulance that responds to vehicle accidents. Nor are the procedures that are included in Sections Two through Four the only ways of accomplishing the dozens of tasks that might be required during vehicle rescue operations. They are representative of what might be accomplished by the crew of an ambulance that has what should be considered minimal equipment.

What you actually do in the way of vehicle rescue will depend on the level of your training, how well your ambulance is equipped, and the restraints imposed by local policies and protocols.

Whatever your responsibilities for vehicle rescue may be, remember that proficiency does not result from reading textbooks. While reading will make you aware of theory and practice, it is learning skills under the direction of a competent instructor and practicing those skills under the supervision of an experienced officer that will make you a proficient EMS rescuer. After you complete your EMT course, avail yourself of every opportunity to attend formal vehicle rescue courses, especially those that are specially designed for EMS personnel.

SECTION ONE
Equipment for Vehicle Rescue

OBJECTIVES As an EMT trained in vehicle rescue procedures, you should be able to:

1. List at least seven ways in which EMS personnel can be injured at the locations of vehicle accidents. (pp. 616–617)
2. List at least four human factors that increase the potential for an EMT being injured during vehicle rescue operations. (p. 617)
3. List at least seven unsafe acts that can result in injury to an EMT during vehicle rescue operations (p. 617)
4. State the unsafe act that contributes most to the injury of EMS personnel during accident scene activities. (p. 617)

5. List items that should be worn by EMS personnel for personal protection during vehicle rescue operations. (pp. 617–618)

6. List items that should be carried on an ambulance for protection against infectious agents during vehicle rescue, patient care, and postrun equipment-cleanup operations. (p. 619)

7. List supplies and equipment that should be carried on an ambulance for each of the following categories of vehicle rescue operations:
   • Safeguarding accident victims (p. 620)
   • Hazard management (pp. 620–621)
   • Warning and signaling (p. 621)
   • Illumination (p. 621)
   • Gaining access and disentanglement (p. 621)

   • Lifting, lowering, and pulling (p. 622)
   • Removing injured persons from mechanisms of entrapment (p. 623)

8. List at least nine hazard management procedures that can be accomplished with the supplies and equipment that are listed and described in this section. (p. 623)

9. List at least nine gaining-access procedures that can be accomplished with the supplies and equipment that are listed and described in this section. (pp. 623–624)

10. List at least six disentanglement procedures that can be accomplished with the supplies and equipment that are listed and described in this section. (p. 624)

SKILLS   As an EMT trained and equipped for vehicle rescue procedures, you should be able to:

1. Identify and use the supplies and equipment available on your ambulance for vehicle rescue operations.

SUPPLIES AND EQUIPMENT

As an EMT who will be performing rescue procedures as well as taking care of injured persons, you should be able to identify supply items, tools, and appliances that you can use to manage hazards, gain access to the occupants of accident vehicles, and disentangle trapped persons.

There are hundreds of items that might be carried on an ambulance for vehicle rescue operations, ranging from simple hand tools to complex powered tools. What is actually carried depends on factors such as available space on the ambulance and perceived need.

Following are supplies and equipment that might be carried on a Type I ambulance that operates in a service area where a properly equipped rescue squad, search and rescue unit, or rescue-equipped fire apparatus is not likely to arrive at the location of a vehicle accident until well after the arrival of the ambulance. Depending on the space available and your service's responsibilities for rescue, your ambulance may have more or less equipment.

Keep in mind that the items listed can be used not only for vehicle rescue activities, but also for gaining access to locked structures, disentanglement

from machinery, and other nonvehicle rescue activities in which EMS personnel may become involved.

Protective Equipment for Ambulance Personnel

It's amazing that the EMTs and paramedics who do so much for sick and injured people often have little regard for their own safety, but it's true. Newspapers, TV news broadcasts, and magazine photos often show EMS personnel operating at accident locations with nothing more than ordinary clothes to protect them. Consider some of the things that make accident locations dangerous workplaces for EMTs:

• Shards and fragments of broken glass, metal, and plastic debris with jagged edges and sharp-pointed objects are mechanisms of injury that can abrade, puncture, lacerate, incise, and even avulse unprotected body parts.

• Flying particles of glass, metal, and even paint can enter unprotected eyes during rescue efforts.

- An unstable vehicle can topple onto and crush rescuers.
- Smoke, toxic gases, noxious fumes, and dusts can enter unprotected respiratory tracts.
- Contact with energized conductors can result in lethal electrocution.
- Flames, radiant heat, exhaust pipes, catalytic converters, and other hot objects can burn unprotected skin surfaces, as can a multitude of dangerous chemicals.
- Powerful rescue tools can exert twisting forces sufficient to break bones; even forceful contact with simple hand tools can result in injury to unprotected body parts.

The elements can also contribute to a hazardous accident scene environment. Rain and snow make tools and vehicle surfaces slippery, and ice makes road surfaces treacherous. Heat and cold can adversely affect a rescuer's performance.

Mechanisms of injury and the elements are not the only threats to personal safety at accident locations, however. A number of human factors can increase the potential for injury:

- A poor attitude toward personal safety
- Little or no training in rescue procedures, or poor training
- A lack of skill in tool use
- Physical problems that prevent a rescuer from performing strenuous operations

---

Unsafe and improper acts also cause injuries at accident locations, as when rescuers:

- Fail to eliminate or control hazards
- Fail to select the proper tool for a particular task
- Use improper or unsafe tools
- Work at an unsafe speed
- Fail to recognize mechanisms of injury and unsafe surroundings
- Improperly lift heavy objects
- Deactivate safety devices designed to prevent injury

WARNING: The unsafe act that contributes most to accident scene injuries is the failure to wear protective gear during rescue operations.

EMS personnel are more likely to be injured during rescue operations than firefighters or squad members for two reasons. First, EMTs must work without the benefit of protective gear if it is not provided for them. Second, EMS personnel seldom learn the value of protective gear during training activities.

While there is not much you can do as an EMT to reduce the number of injury-producing mechanisms or control the elements at accident scenes, there is a great deal you can do to reduce the potential for personal injury. Learn the value of protective gear, acquire some if none is provided, and use it!

Figure 27-1 shows two EMTs dressed for rescue operations. The EMT on the left is dressed for a wide range of hazard management, gaining access, and disentanglement operations. The EMT on the right is dressed for situations where exposure to accident-related hazards is minimal.

Good head protection is essential. Trendy baseball caps, uniform hats, and wool watch caps do little other than to identify the wearer as a member of an emergency service, keep the wearer's head warm during cold weather periods, and protect it from sunlight during warm weather.

- The **rescue helmet** protects the EMT from water, impact, penetration, laceration, heat, cold, and contact by dangerous materials. This particular model does not have the rear brim that often makes a firefighter's helmet unsuitable in tight spaces.
- The **construction hard hat** is favored by many EMTs because of its light weight and compact design. A hard hat should have a

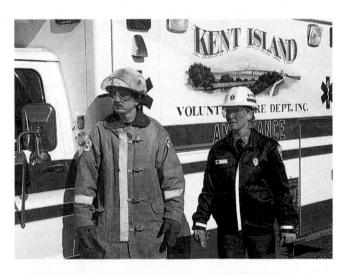

FIGURE 27–1. Supplies and Equipment for Personal Protection: The EMT at the left is dressed for maximum protection. The EMT at the right is dressed for times when exposure to accident-produced hazards is minimal.

full suspension and a secure chin strap. A plastic "bump cap" of the type worn by butchers and warehouse workers should not be worn during rescue operations; it does not provide adequate protection.

Regardless of the type, a helmet should be brightly colored, and it should have reflective stripes and lettering for maximum visibility day and night. Also, it should have a star of life affixed to each side to identify the wearer as an EMS provider.

Good eye protection is vitally important. The hinged plastic helmet shield that many rescuers rely on does not provide adequate eye protection during aggressive rescue operations. Depending on the type of shield used, flying particles of debris can strike the wearer's eyes from underneath or from the side.

- **Safety goggles** afford the EMT a full field of vision and wrap-around protection; the soft vinyl frame conforms to the contours of the wearer's face. Goggles should protect the wearer's eyes not only from flying solid particles, but also from dust and chemicals. The goggles should have indirect venting to keep them fog free.

If you decide to wear safety goggles for eye protection, resist the temptation to store them around your helmet. The head band will lose its elasticity.

- **Safety glasses** protect the wearer's eyes from impact and flying objects if they have large lenses and side shields. Yellow safety glasses are especially good for rescue operations. They make objects appear remarkably sharp on dull days or in low-light situations.

An EMT will often take steps to protect his scalp, skull, eyes, ears, and hands during a rescue operation and leave his upper body virtually unprotected. A lightweight jacket, a uniform shirt, or a T-shirt does little to protect the wearer from jagged edges and pointed pieces of debris.

- The **turnout coat** affords several levels of upper body protection against radiant heat, sharp-edged and pointed objects, and the elements. A bright color and reflective lettering and stripes make the wearer highly visible during night and day. A short coat is less cumbersome when it is necessary to work in tight spaces.
- While an **EMS** or **rescue jacket** does not have the protective features of a turnout coat, it will protect the wearer from the elements and minor injury that might occur during other than gaining access and disentanglement operations.

Thick leather gauntlets and some so-called "firefighter's gloves" are so bulky that they prevent the manual dexterity that is important during rescue operations. On the other hand, some fabric "garden" gloves are so thin that they offer no protection at all.

- Lightweight **leather gloves** protect the hands while allowing good manual dexterity.

Because of the hazardous situations in which they often have to work, EMS personnel should give the same consideration to lower body protection as to protection for the upper body.

- **Turnout pants** protect the wearer from radiant heat and sharp and pointed mechanisms of injury, although they sometimes make moving about in confined spaces difficult. The cuffs should be wide enough for the pants to be pulled over work shoes if they will not be worn with **short rubber boots.**
- **Fire-resistant trousers or coveralls** offer good protection from flames and radiant heat, but they do little to shield the wearer from other mechanisms of injury.

While they are easy to put on and while they keep the feet dry, firefighter's boots are heavy and bulky, and unless they are the correct size, they offer little foot and ankle support.

- **High-top work shoes** have several advantages. They can be worn all the time as part of the uniform. The extended tops protect the ankles. Steel caps protect the toes from impact by a falling object, and steel inserts protect the soles of the feet from sharp-pointed objects.

Full-length boots can be worn during vehicle rescue operations. Better quality boots have steel toe caps, arch protectors, and shin guards. If boots are your choice for foot protection, be sure to wear them pulled all the way up during rescue operations. The cuffs that result when boots are worn with the tops only partly pulled up become repositories for glass and metal particles. When the tops are pulled up and debris falls into the foot compartment, just a few steps can result in incapacitating foot injuries.

While they are not personal protection items in the strictest sense of the word:

- **Ice cleats** prevent dangerous falls when an EMT must work on ice-covered roads.

Every ambulance should be equipped with respiratory protection whenever crew members may have to work in oxygen-deficient structures, smoke-filled structures such as buildings on fire, and high-temperature environments such as boiler and heater rooms.

- The **self-contained breathing apparatus** affords the EMT complete respiratory protection in oxygen-deficient and toxic atmospheres, as when a hazardous commodity has been spilled or released at the scene of a vehicle accident.

There are other items that an EMT can use for personal protection, many of which can be carried in the pockets of a turnout coat.

- The **fluorescent and reflective vest** makes an EMT highly visible when it is necessary to work near active traffic lanes at accident locations.
- A **Nomex™ hood** of the type favored by firefighters will protect the wearer not only from radiant heat, but also from cold. A one-size-fits-all hood can be carried in a turnout coat pocket.
- A **dust respirator** filters dangerous dusts that are often a problem when a truck carrying cement, grain, or another finely divided material has been involved in an accident.
- A **thermal mask** will prevent the inhalation of extremely cold air during cold weather operations.
- A personal **flashlight** reduces the potential for injury when it is used to illuminate dangerous work areas.
- A **high-intensity Cyalume®** Lightstick will provide emergency illumination when a flashlight fails or when light is needed while working in a dangerous atmosphere.
- A quality **pocket knife** should be carried not so much for rescue operations, but for survival measures.

Because of size differences, personal preferences for equipment, space limitations on the ambulance, and the chance that gear will be damaged if it is stored for long periods of storage in a compartment, each EMT should have his or her own personal set of protective gear. A commercially available nylon fabric bag can easily contain all the items listed above. It can be easily transferred from a personal vehicle to the ambulance at the beginning of a tour of duty, carried in any convenient space, and removed from the ambulance at the end of the tour.

Supplies and Equipment for Protection Against Infectious Agents

EMS personnel who assist in vehicle rescue operations must consider the problem of infectious agents very seriously. Every accident victim should be looked on as possibly carrying an infectious disease. Accordingly, every rescuer should wear barrier protection any time he or she is likely to be exposed to an accident victim's blood or body fluids and wastes during and after rescue operations. In addition to the protective clothing listed and described thus far, three more items should be carried with personal protective gear.

- **Medical grade latex gloves** should be worn for all patient care activities that may result in contact with an accident victim's blood and/or body fluids.
- A **medical grade face mask** should be worn when blood and/or body fluids might be splashed in the eyes, nose, or mouth.
- **Midweight plastic or rubber gloves** should be worn for nonpatient care activities that may involve handling items contaminated with an accident victim's blood or body secretions and when cleaning equipment after a rescue operation.

Protection against infectious agents should not be limited to wearing barrier devices at the locations of accidents where blood and body fluids are present. EMS personnel—indeed, all emergency service personnel who come into contact with injured people—should have cuts, abrasions, insect bites, and other breaks in the skin covered with adhesive compresses or small dressings before reporting to work.

Supplies and Equipment for Safeguarding Accident Victims

It's bad enough when accident victims are lacerated, incised, abraded, punctured, twisted, bent, broken, or crushed as the result of a motor vehicle accident. Shielding victims with some inexpensive devices and exercising care during gaining access and disentanglement operations will minimize the chance that the victims will suffer additional injuries.

- An **aluminized rescue blanket** can be used to protect the occupants of an accident vehicle from radiant heat when the vehicle is on fire or when an adjacent accident vehicle is burning. This type of blanket also serves well to shield accident victims from the elements and, to a degree, from flying particles of glass and metal that are generated during rescue operations.
- A **lightweight vinyl-coated paper tarpaulin** can be used to protect accident victims from the elements and debris when there is no danger of fire.
- The **wool blankets** that are a part of the ambulance inventory will protect accident victims from the cold.
- **Disposable paper blankets** should be used to protect accident victims from cold whenever glass must be broken near them. Glass particles are just about impossible to remove from wool blankets.
- The **short wood spine board** that is part of the ambulance inventory can be used to shield an accident victim from contact with tools or debris.
- **Hard hats, safety goggles, industrial hearing protectors, disposable dust masks,** and **thermal masks** (in cold weather areas) will protect accident victims' head, eyes, ears, and respiratory passages.

Supplies and Equipment for Hazard Management

Any of a number of hazards may be present at the location of a vehicle accident, including fire, smoke, noxious fumes, toxic gases, darkness, slippery surfaces, electrical conductors, water, unstable vehicles or other mechanisms of entrapment, the threat of an explosion, spectators, traffic, and more. Since these hazards threaten not only accident victims but also the people who respond to them, an ambulance should have items that can be used to control the more frequently produced hazards.

- A **20-pound A:B:C: dry chemical fire extinguisher** should be available for extinguishing minor fires involving ordinary combustible materials, flammable liquids, and electrical equipment.
- A **2½-gallon pressurized water fire extinguisher** should be available for use on

upholstery and other ordinary combustible materials.
- The two **wheel chocks** that are carried on the ambulance can be used to prevent the forward or rearward movement of an accident vehicle.
- A pound of **duct sealant** or a sealant designed specially for hazardous material containers should be carried for times when it is necessary to seal a minor leak in an accident vehicle's fuel tank.
- Twelve **golf tees** should be carried for sealing an accident vehicle's severed fuel lines. The duct sealant and golf tees can be kept in a plastic food container.
- An **adhesive spray or 2-inch tape** can be used to minimize the spread of glass fragments when an accident vehicle's windows must be broken close to occupants. Duct tape can also be used to cover the sharp ends of severed roof pillars and sharp sheet metal edges.
- **7 × 50 "armored" binoculars** and a **hazardous material guide** should be on every ambulance for identifying hazardous materials present at vehicle accident locations.
- **Cat litter** is excellent for making an icy or wet road slip resistant. A gallon plastic jug of cat litter covers a wide area.
- A **folding pointed-blade shovel** can be used to remove granular debris from around an accident victim.
- A **folding tree saw** is handy when tree branches must be removed from around a trapped person in an off-road accident situation.
- **Battery pliers** are the best tool for disconnecting a vehicle's battery from the electrical system.
- Various lengths of **split 1½-inch fire hose** can be used to protect rescuers and accident victims from sharp sheet metal edges.
- Short **unsplit sections of 2½-inch fire hose** (or larger) can be slipped over the sharp stubs of roof pillars when an accident vehicle's roof is folded back and removed.
- **Heavy-duty rubber cargo straps with S-hooks** are handy for a variety of tasks, including holding cribbing and jacks in place, securing doors in their wide-open position, and preventing the blow back of folded roof sections.
- Twenty pieces of **2 by 4 by 18-inch wood cribbing** (or more if space permits) should be available for stabilizing accident vehicles

and other mechanisms of entrapment. Cribbing can be easily stored and carried in a square plastic milk jug container.

- Twelve **2 by 4 by 12-inch hardwood wedges** should be in the inventory for holding door frames open, changing the direction of cribbing, and so on.

Supplies and Equipment for Warning and Signaling

Because of their patient care responsibilities, EMS personnel seldom become involved in extensive traffic control activities. This does not mean that ambulances should not be equipped with basic warning and signaling devices, however.

- Twelve **30-minute flares with wire stands** can be used for traffic control day or night.
- Twelve **red Cyalume® Lightsticks** for traffic control, especially at locations where fuel has been spilled.

Supplies and Equipment for Illumination

Adequate illumination of work areas and accident vehicle interiors is important. Victims and emergency service personnel can be injured when attempts are made to carry out critical rescue operations in the dark. If the ambulance has a 110-volt power supply:

- Two **300- or 500-watt floodlights with stands** should be carried for even illumination of work areas.
- A **100-foot, heavy-duty 3-wire extension cord terminating in a junction box** will carry power to lights and tools.
- A **12-volt trouble light with a 50-foot cord and battery clips** can be used to quickly illuminate an accident vehicle while other lights are being set up. Power for the trouble light can often be drawn from the vehicle's battery.
- Twelve **high-intensity white Cyalume® Lightsticks** should be carried on the ambulance for emergency illumination and safe lighting in a flammable atmosphere.
- Two **battery-powered or rechargeable hand lights** should be available for the illumination of work areas when other lighting is not immediately available.

Hand Tools for Gaining Access and Disentanglement

It's an unfortunate commentary on our times when an EMT throws up his hands in despair and cries that he cannot carry out a rescue operation because of a lack of special equipment. There are two reasons why an otherwise rational person might act in this manner. The basic EMT training program may not have prepared him to cope with an accident situation, and many exposures to printed matter and television may have left him with a feeling of inadequacy—a feeling that he cannot rescue people because he does not have either sophisticated equipment or the knowledge of special techniques.

It may be too obvious to require mentioning, but when you think of your responsibilities for rescue at the scene of an accident, think positively! Experiences have shown that in the majority of accident situations studied, access to trapped persons was gained quickly and disentanglement was accomplished with simple hand tools. So if your unit is one that often arrives at accident locations before other emergency service units, don't be discouraged. Remember that you can cope with almost any entrapment situation with basic tools, basic techniques, and an "I can make do with what I have" attitude.

The inventory of a rescue ambulance should include:

- An **8-inch and a 12-inch adjustable wrench** for general disassembly operations.
- **Combination aircraft snips** for cutting sheet metal and seat belts.
- Two **3- or 4-pound drilling hammers** for use with metal-cutting tools and for other operations in which striking force is needed.
- An **awl with a steel shank** for unlocking vehicle doors with a minimum of effort and damage.
- A **manual or spring-loaded center punch** for breaking tempered glass windows.
- A **noose tool** for opening doors that have an accessible mushroom-head or straight-shank lock knob.
- Three **hacksaw frames fitted with an 18-teeth-per-inch high-speed shatterproof blade** for severing metal components.
- Two **linoleum knives** for removing gasket-mounted windshields, for cutting vehicle headliners and upholstery, and for other cutting operations.
- **Ten-inch locking-type pliers** for facilitating grasp and for breaking away the plastic covering of steering wheels.

- **Ten-inch water pump pliers** for facilitating grasp.
- **Eight-inch side cutting pliers** for cutting wiring and severing seat springs and for other cutting operations.
- Two **12- to 15-inch multipurpose flat pry bars** for prying trim from around vehicle windows, for prying open doors, and for other prying operations when a larger tool is neither suitable nor indicated.
- A **panel cutter** for making openings in sheet-metal panels.
- A **2- by 18-inch ripping chisel** for severing metal components, especially a vehicle's door lock and latch mechanisms. A ripping chisel can also be used to make openings in sheet-metal panels.
- An **8-inch and a 12-inch flat blade, square shank screwdriver** for general disassembly operations. The larger of the screwdrivers is also an excellent tool for making openings in sheet-metal panels.
- A **10-inch and a 6-inch Phillips screwdriver** for general disassembly operations. A Phillips screwdriver can also be used to break tempered glass windows when another pointed tool is not available.
- A **10-inch cabinet blade screwdriver with a 3/16-inch tip** for unlatching trunk lids after an opening has been made in the deck.
- Four **windshield knives** for removing adhesive-mounted windshields and rear windows. Two knives should have a conventional blade. The other knives should have a long blade for windows with wide adhesive strips.
- A **utility knife with a retractable blade** (razor knife) for cutting upholstery, head liners, soft dash components, and the like.
- Two **spray containers of lubricant** for hacksaw operations. Any cutting oil can be used; however, using a soap-and-water solution will minimize the chance of contaminating open wounds with a petroleum product when cutting must be done close to an accident victim.
- An **ax-style, combination forcible entry tool** for cutting, striking, and prying operations. The extendable handle provides added leverage.
- A **spare parts kit** that contains hacksaw blades and replacement blades for the panel cutter, the utility knife, and the windshield knives. These blades are all field replaceable.

Long-Handled Tools for Gaining Access and Disentanglement

- A **36- or 42-inch bolt cutter with hardened steel jaws** for severing lock shackles, steering wheels, and other round or tubular metal components.
- A **36- or 42-inch combination forcible entry tool** for prying, lifting, and displacing operations when leverage is needed.
- A **6-pound flat head fire ax** for removing a section of a windshield that cannot be removed by conventional means, for making an opening in a sheet-metal panel when another cutting tool is not available, and for clearing brush and wood debris from an accident vehicle.
- A **51-inch pinch bar** for prying, lifting, and displacing when leverage is needed.
- A **36-inch 8-pound sledgehammer** for striking operations.

Equipment for Lifting, Lowering, and Pulling

- A **chain or cable hand winch** rated for a minimum 2-ton pull for moving vehicle doors beyond their normal range of motion; for displacing steering columns, dash assemblies, and quarter panels; for stabilizing an unsteady vehicle; for separating accident vehicles; and for moving machinery, large pieces of cargo, and debris.
- A **rescue chain set** for use with the hand winch and for securing vehicle components. The set should include a 6- and a 12-foot chain, each having a working strength of 4,100 pounds, and each having a slip hook at one end and a ring and a grab hook at the other end.
- Two **Hi-Lift® jacks** for lifting and stabilizing operations. These jacks have a lifting capacity of 7,000 pounds and can be used with a rescue chain in the manner of hand winches.
- A 100-foot (or longer) length of **1/2-inch static kernmantle rope** that has a breaking strength of 9,000 pounds, for use as a lifeline.
- Two 50-foot (or longer) lengths of 3/8-inch static kernmantle ropes for other than lifeline uses.

Equipment for Removing Injured Persons from Mechanisms of Entrapment

- A **6-foot-diameter, 1-inch nylon rope sling** with a sliding choker, for pulling injured persons onto a long spine board or other rigid patient-carrying device with a minimum of body movement.
- A wood **long spine board with web straps** for full-body immobilization and for transporting an injured person to an ambulance.
- A **scoop-style stretcher** for lifting, immobilizing, and carrying injured persons.

STORING THE EQUIPMENT ON THE AMBULANCE

The supplies and equipment that are listed in this section are displayed next to a type I ambulance in Figure 27-2. People who are unfamiliar with rescue equipment are quick to ask how such an inventory can be stored. To prove that it can be done, Figure 27-2 shows all the items with one exception stored in the compartment. Including most of the items in *kits* makes storage easy. The briefcase that holds the binoculars and hazardous materials action

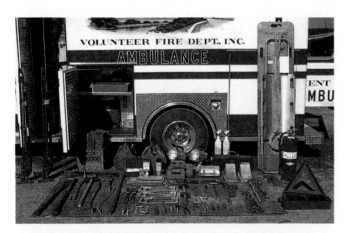

FIGURE 27–2. Supplies and Equipment for Vehicle Rescue Operations: The supplies and equipment that are listed in this section are laid out next to an ambulance that responds to areas where there is no rescue unit. With the exception of the crew's personal gear and the hazardous materials identification kit, all the supplies and equipment are stored in the open compartment.

guides is stored behind the driver's seat so it is easily accessible.

TASKS THAT CAN BE ACCOMPLISHED WITH THE SUPPLIES AND EQUIPMENT SHOWN

Equally surprising to many people is what can be accomplished by specifically trained EMS personnel with the supplies and equipment shown. In an effort to manage accident-related hazards, a two-person ambulance crew should be able to:

- Initiate traffic-control measures
- Initiate spectator-control measures
- Seal an accident vehicle's leaking fuel tank
- Plug an accident vehicle's leaking fuel lines
- Use a portable fire extinguisher to put out a fire under an accident vehicle or a fire in an accident vehicle's engine compartment, passenger compartment, or trunk
- Make a wet or icy road slip resistant
- Effectively light work areas on, in, and around an accident vehicle
- Stabilize an accident vehicle that is on its wheels, side, or roof
- Disable an accident vehicle's electrical system

To reach the occupants of an accident vehicle, the crew should be able to use the equipment shown to:

- Unlock and unlatch a vehicle's doors
- Force open jammed doors after they have been unlocked and unlatched
- Remove gasket-mounted and adhesive-mounted windshields and rear windows from accident vehicles intact
- Remove a section of an accident vehicle's windshield when the windshield cannot be removed intact
- Break an accident vehicle's tempered glass windows in such a way that the spread of fragments to the interior of the vehicle is minimal
- Use a long spine board to facilitate entry into an accident vehicle through window openings
- Enter a vehicle that is on its wheels, side, or roof when entry through door or window openings is not possible

- Open the trunk of a passenger car when the key is not available
- Lift the side of a vehicle to reach an injured person trapped underneath

To disentangle occupants from mechanisms of entrapment, the crew should be able to use the equipment shown to:

- Create unobstructed exitways in an accident vehicle by displacing doors beyond their normal range of motion
- Create working space in an accident vehicle by folding back or folding back a section of the roof or by removing the roof altogether
- Create working space in front of an injured driver by removing a portion of the steering wheel, removing the steering wheel altogether, or displacing or severing the steering column
- Displace an accident vehicle's pedals to free a driver's trapped foot
- Displace the front seat of an accident vehicle so that a person who is lying on the floor of the vehicle can be removed safely
- Displace the dash of an accident vehicle so a person who is on the floor against the firewall can be removed safely

Sections Two, Three, and Four of this chapter show how the supplies and equipment listed above can be used to accomplish these tasks.

SUMMARY

While many EMS personnel think of vehicle rescue as the extrication of injured persons from wreckage, vehicle rescue is a system of operations that may include 12 phases of activity, including:

- Preparing for rescue operations
- Responding to the accident location
- Assessing the situation
- Reaching off-road wreckage
- Managing accident-related hazards
- Gaining access to trapped occupants
- Caring for life-threatening conditions
- Disentangling trapped persons
- Packaging the injured persons
- Removing injured persons from the wreckage
- Transferring injured persons to the ambulance
- Terminating the operation

How many of these activities you will participate in as an EMT depends on the role that your EMS unit plays in vehicle rescue operations. If your ambulance is first on the scene of a vehicle accident and other emergency service units will be delayed in responding or if there is no rescue unit to respond at all, you and your partner may have to initiate traffic-control efforts, eliminate or manage hazards, gain access to vehicle occupants, initiate life-saving measures, disentangle trapped persons, remove injured persons from the wreckage, and transfer them to the ambulance.

When this is the case, a variety of items should be carried on the ambulance for safeguarding accident victims and providing hazard management, for warning and signaling, and illumination, and for gaining access, disentanglement, and patient removal operations.

As a trained EMT, you should be able to identify the supplies and equipment carried on the ambulance for vehicle rescue operations, know when and where to use the items, and be able to use them safely.

Ensure your personal safety at all times during rescue operations by wearing the appropriate protective gear.

SECTION TWO
Managing Accident-Related Hazards

OBJECTIVES: As an EMT trained in vehicle rescue procedures, you should be able to:

1. Describe the procedure for safely igniting road flares. (p. 626)
2. State the rule for placing flares to control the movement of vehicles past an accident location. (p. 626 and p. 628)
3. Describe the procedure for placing flares on a straight section of road. (p. 627)
4. Describe the procedure for placing flares ahead of a curved section of road. (p. 627)

5. Describe the procedure for placing flares on a hilly road. (p. 627)

6. Describe at least one procedure for controlling the movement of spectators at accident locations. (p. 628)

7. Describe a procedure that might be followed when wires are down at an accident location and the ambulance is not equipped with special devices for moving the wires. (p. 629)

8. Describe a survival procedure that might be followed when ground at an accident location is energized by a downed wire. (p. 630)

9. Describe a procedure that might be followed when a utility pole is broken at an accident location, but wires are intact. (p. 630)

10. Describe a procedure that might be followed when a pad-mounted transformer has been damaged by a vehicle. (p. 630)

11. Describe a procedure for extinguishing a fire in the engine compartment of an accident vehicle when the hood is open, when the hood is only partially open, and when the hood is closed. (p. 631)

12. Describe a procedure for extinguishing a fire under the dash or in the upholstery of an accident vehicle. (p. 631)

13. Describe a procedure for extinguishing a fire in the trunk of an accident vehicle. (p. 631)

14. Describe a procedure for extinguishing fuel that is burning under an accident vehicle. (p. 631)

15. Describe a procedure for plugging leaks in the fuel tank and fuel lines of an accident vehicle. (p. 633)

16. Describe two procedures for stabilizing an accident vehicle that is on its wheels after the wheels are chocked. (pp. 633–634)

17. State the advantage of stabilizing a vehicle that is on its side in a vertical position rather than in the position found. (p. 635)

18. Describe at least four procedures for stabilizing a vehicle on its side in the vertical position. (pp. 635–636)

19. State the danger that an overturned vehicle poses to rescuers when the roof pillars are intact. (p. 636)

20. Describe at least three procedures for stabilizing an overturned vehicle. (p. 636)

21. State the reason why it may not be a good practice to always cut or disconnect the battery cable(s) of an accident vehicle. (p. 637)

22. Describe a procedure for disconnecting a battery cable when disrupting an accident vehicle's electrical system is indicated. (p. 637)

SKILLS As an EMT trained and equipped for vehicle rescue procedures, you should be able to:

1. Safely ignite, position, and extinguish traffic control flares.

2. Take steps to safeguard victims, spectators, and emergency service personnel from electrical shock in each of the following accident situations:
   - When a utility pole is broken and wires are down
   - When a utility pole is broken but wires are intact
   - When a pad-mounted transformer has been struck by a vehicle

3. Take appropriate survival measures when on energized ground at an accident location.

4. Use the correct portable fire extinguisher to extinguish a fire in or under an accident vehicle.

5. Seal an accident vehicle's leaking fuel tank and/or fuel lines.

6. Stabilize an accident vehicle that is on its wheels.

7. Stabilize an accident vehicle on its side.

8. Stabilize an overturned accident vehicle.

9. Disable an accident vehicle's electrical system.

HAZARDS

When asked about hazards that might be encountered at the locations of motor vehicle accidents, untrained rescuers are likely to list those that are most common: fragments of broken glass and pieces of sharp-edged and sharp-pointed debris. While these things can inflict injury, seldom are they more than nuisances to be dealt with as a rescue operation progresses.

A number of other hazards can severely threaten the safety of accident victims, rescuers, and spectators, hazards such as downed wires and damaged electrical equipment, fire, spilled fuel, a slippery road, the weather, darkness, instability, and two hazards that are present at virtually every accident location: traffic and spectators.

Accident-related hazards must be managed, if not eliminated altogether, before any attempt is made to reach injured persons in damaged vehicles. Let's see how you and a partner on the ambulance might take care of a variety of hazards from the moment you leave the ambulance.

CONTROLLING THE MOVEMENTS OF VEHICLES

Accidents invariably produce some sort of traffic problems. If an accident occurs along a two-lane road, the roadway is often blocked by wreckage. At the very least, vehicles moving in both directions will have to use one lane. An accident on a four-lane highway can necessitate the merging of two or three lines of vehicles into one lane, with the result being a massive traffic jam. Even on a six-lane divided superhighway a relatively minor accident can cause a tremendous traffic problem.

There need be no physical impediment such as wreckage to create traffic jams. Massive backups often occur when curious drivers slow down as they pass an accident scene in order to see what has happened.

When there is a full emergency service response to an accident call, there are usually enough rescuers, firefighters, and police officers for traffic-control duties. But what about the situation in which an ambulance responds to an accident location alone or much ahead of other emergency service units?

Obviously, rescue and emergency care efforts have priority over all other activities when personnel on hand is limited. This does not mean that a two-person ambulance crew cannot initiate a basic traffic-control plan, however, such as channeling the movement of vehicles past the accident scene. Then if the road must be blocked or if a detour must be established, those efforts can be undertaken by other emergency service personnel.

The warning lights of your ambulance will serve as the first form of traffic control; however, you should position other warning devices as soon as possible. Adverse weather conditions, darkness, vegetation close to the road, and curved roadways may prevent approaching motorists from seeing the ambulance warning lights until they are too close to the danger zone to stop safely.

Using Flares for Traffic Control

Although some persons argue that flares are unsafe, they are still the best device for warning motorists of dangerous conditions. Moreover, several dozen flares can be carried behind the front seat of an ambulance, while battery-powered flashing lights take up valuable compartment space.

Igniting Flares

Using the following procedure, you will be able to ignite flares without being struck by molten sulfur.

- While you grasp the flare near the base with one hand, use your free hand to pull the tear strip away from the plastic cap and expose the scratching surface. Pull the cap from the body of the flare to expose the ignitor.
- Hold the flare in one hand and the cap in the other so that the scratching surface is positioned against the ignitor. While you hold the cap stationary, move the flare away from your body so that the ignitor rubs against the scratching surface. Repeat this operation if the flare does not ignite the first time.
- Keep the lighted flare away from your body as you position it on the wire stand or on the ground with the plastic holder in place.

Positioning Flares

If vehicular wreckage is blocking only one lane of a road, it is usually wise to channel traffic past the scene over the unblocked lanes. This should eliminate the buildup of vehicles that often results in a traffic jam that prevents the movement of emergency as well as other vehicles. Flares can be positioned quickly, but for them to be effective they must be placed according to plans such as those shown in Figure 27-3.

A number of factors must be considered when deciding how to set out a string of flares, including:

- Posted speed of the road
- Stopping distances required for vehicles traveling at the posted speed
- Volume of traffic
- Condition of the road surface
- Weather
- Character of the road (straight, curved, or hilly)

Posted speed (mph)	Stopping distance for that speed*		Posted speed (in feet)		Distance of the farthest warning device
20 mph	50 feet	+	20 feet	=	70 feet
30 mph	75 feet	+	30 feet	=	105 feet
40 mph	125 feet	+	40 feet	=	165 feet
50 mph	175 feet	+	50 feet	=	225 feet
60 mph	275 feet	+	60 feet	=	335 feet
70 mph	375 feet	+	70 feet	=	445 feet

* Distances are given for passenger cars.

A. Flares are positioned according to a formula that includes the stopping distance for that speed, and the posted speed in feet.

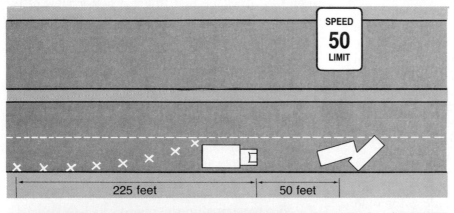

B. Flares positioned on a straight road. Approaching vehicles are moved into the correct lane before they reach the edge of the danger zone.

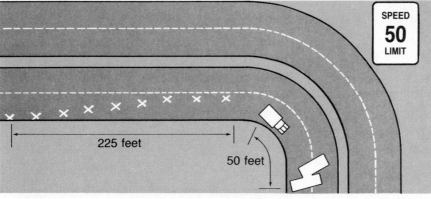

C. Flares positioned ahead of a curved section of road. The beginning of the curve is considered to be the edge of the danger zone.

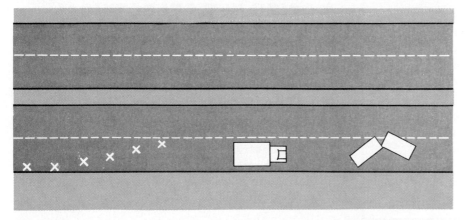

D. Flares are placed on a hill to slow vehicles and make them turn into the correct lane before they reach the top of the hill.

FIGURE 27–3. Positioning flares to control the movement of vehicles past accident scenes.

There is a basic rule for positioning flares: the farthest flare should be placed at a distance from the edge of the danger zone equal to the stopping distance for the road's posted speed plus the distance in feet equal to the posted speed. This ensures that when an approaching motorist traveling at the posted speed first sees the flare that is farthest from the danger zone, even though he may not see it until he is next to it, he will be able to stop his vehicle before it reaches the edge of the danger zone.

Be aware that the total distance given for the flare placement begins at the edge of the danger zone around the wreckage, not from the vehicles at the center of the zone. The typical danger zone is the area around the accident vehicles included in a circle with a radius of 50 feet. Remember that the danger zone may be considerably larger if certain hazards are present.

When an accident occurs on a curved portion of road, consider the start of the curve as the edge of the danger zone and set the flares out as you would on a straight road. Figure 27-3C shows how flares should be set out ahead of a curve.

When an accident occurs on a hill, one edge of the danger zone should be the crest of the hill. Thus vehicles traveling on the same side of the road as the accident vehicles will be slowed and in the correct lane by the time they reach the top of the hill.

Remember these points when you are placing flares:

- Do not throw flares out of the ambulance when it is moving.
- Position a few flares at the edge of the danger zone as soon as the ambulance is parked; they will supplement the ambulance warning lights.
- Take a handful of flares and walk toward the oncoming traffic. Ignite flares and position them in such a way that they will channel vehicles into the unblocked lane before they reach the danger zone. Position flares every 10 feet, if possible.
- Be sure to look for spilled fuel, dry vegetation, and other combustible materials before you ignite and position flares, especially along a side of the road.
- If the accident has occurred on a two-lane road, position flares in both directions.

When the highway is heavily traveled by large trucks, you would do well to extend the flare strings beyond the distances recommended on the chart.

Remember that the stopping distances for large trucks are much greater than for cars.

CONTROLLING THE MOVEMENTS OF SPECTATORS

Spectators at vehicle accident locations do more than just create problems for passing motorists. If they are allowed to wander freely, they can and will close in on the wreckage just to get a better view of the operation. In fact, they may get so close that they will interfere with the rescue and emergency care efforts.

Rescue squads have the personnel and equipment for crowd control; ambulances usually do not. This does not mean that you as an EMT cannot initiate some form of crowd-control measure.

- Quickly scan the bystanders for some apparently responsible persons such as truck and bus drivers or someone wearing a uniform. Ask if there are any off-duty emergency service personnel in the crowd.
- Ask the persons that you recruit to keep the crowd away from the danger zone. Give them a roll of barricade tape if you have one.

WARNING: The plan is simple, and it usually works! Be sure not to put the recruited personnel in unsafe positions, however, like near spilled fuel or an unstable vehicle. The use of non-public safety personnel must be allowed by your EMS System.

COPING WITH ELECTRICAL HAZARDS

The dangers of electricity at vehicle accident locations can be many and varied. Since local policies usually dictate what EMS personnel can and cannot do regarding the use of specialized equipment, included here are only suggestions for survival. **Under no circumstances should you attempt to move a downed wire with makeshift equipment.**

Keep in mind these points about accident-produced electrical hazards:

- High voltages are not as uncommon on roadside utility poles as people think. Wood poles sometimes support conductors of as much as 500,000 volts.

- In addition to primary and secondary power conductors, utility poles also support telephone and TV subscriber cables and conductors for fire alarm, street light, and traffic signal circuits.
- The bright, uninsulated guy wire that stabilizes a utility pole may not be the nonconductor you think it is. When a pole is broken, guy wires may be energized by severed or displaced conductors. In fact, every conductor supported by the pole may be carrying the highest voltage present.
- Voltages of primary and secondary conductors cannot be determined from the size of the wire and the number of stand-off insulators.
- The coverings of high-voltage conductors serve more to protect them from the weather than to insulate them.
- There is no way to tell the direction of current flow at any given time.
- Fuses do not always blow and circuit breakers do not always open when power distribution lines go to ground. The load must be greater than the rating of the safety device.
- The ground cable or the pole itself may be energized when a pole is broken or displaced as the result of an accident.
- There is no way to determine whether a downed conductor is energized without a testing device.
- Energized downed conductors may or may not arc to the ground.

There is no assurance that a dead wire at the scene of an accident will not become energized again unless it is cut or otherwise disconnected from the system. When an interruption of current is sensed in most power distribution systems, automatic devices restore the flow of current two or three times over a period of minutes.

WARNING: Ordinary personal protective clothing does not afford protection against electrocution.

Remembering these points along with the following procedures may keep you alive at the scene of an accident where unconfined electricity is a hazard.

Broken Utility Pole with Wires Down

Fortunately, a broken utility pole with wires down is not a common result of vehicle accidents. But when such a problem does exist, it usually is a threat to rescuers and victims alike and is a situation in which safe operations may not be possible until a power

company representative can disrupt the flow of current.

Let's say that you have arrived at the location of an accident and have discovered that a utility pole is broken and that wires are down. The ambulance is parked outside the danger zone recommended for such situations.

- Before you leave the ambulance, be sure that no portion of the vehicle, including the radio antenna, is contacting any sagging conductors adjacent to or across the road.
- When you leave the ambulance, determine the number of the nearest pole that you can safely approach in such a way that a severed wire will not contact you if the wire arcs and jumps.
- When you have the pole number, instruct your dispatcher to advise the power company of the exact location of the accident and the pole number.
- Order spectators from the danger zone.
- Discourage the occupants of the accident vehicles from leaving the wreckage even if the vehicle is not in direct contact with a downed wire. The wire may arc and contact the vehicle, or the ground near the vehicle may be energized.
- **Do not attempt to move any wires with wood poles, tools with wood handles, natural fiber ropes, or any other objects that might have a high moisture content, and most certainly do not attempt to move a downed wire with a metal tool or implement. In fact, do not attempt to move a downed wire at all unless you are specially trained and equipped with tools rated for voltages greater than those present.**
- Stand in a safe place until a representative of the power company can cut the wires or otherwise disconnect them from the power distribution system.
- Prevent spectators and nonessential emergency service personnel from entering the danger zone until the hazard has been eliminated.
- Prohibit traffic flow if vehicles must pass through the danger zone.

When you respond to an accident location in a rural area at night, you may not have a clue that a pole has been broken and a wire is down. You may approach the scene from the direction opposite the path that the accident vehicle took. There may not be any buildings or other structures nearby that, if unlighted, would alert you to a power outage. And the downed wire may not be arcing. Make it your policy to be extra careful whenever you are in a really dark area.

- As you walk from the ambulance to the accident vehicle, sweep the area ahead of you, to each side, and overhead with a beam of a powerful handlight. Remember that an energized conductor may be dangling just at head level.
- If you discover that a wire is down, leave the area in such a way that if the wire arcs and jumps, reel curl will move it away from you. Reel curl is the tendency for wires to coil when they are no longer under tension.

There may be a time, especially during wet weather operations, that you will not discover that a wire is down at an accident scene until you experience a phenomenon known as ground gradient. Voltage is greatest at the point where a conductor contacts the ground and then diminishes as the distance from the point of contact increases. That distance can be several inches or many feet. Being able to recognize ground gradient and knowing what actions to take when you do will probably save your life.

- Stop your approach to an accident vehicle immediately if you feel a tingling sensation in your legs and lower torso. This sensation signals that you are on energized ground and that current is entering one foot, passing through the lower part of your body, and exiting through your other foot. If you continue on, you chance being electrocuted!
- Do not simply turn and walk in a different direction. If the broken wire arcs and jumps closer to you, your body may complete a circuit on ground that is energized with lethal current.
- Turn 180 degrees and take one of two escape measures. Bend one leg at the knee and grasp the foot of that leg with one hand. Hop to a safe place on one foot. Or shuffle away from the danger area while keeping your feet close together. Either technique minimizes the chance that your body will complete a circuit with energized ground.

Broken Utility Pole with Wires Intact

A broken utility pole, but one with wires intact, is not a situation to be considered lightly. Conductors

that are supporting a 1,000-pound (or heavier) utility pole can break at any time. If they do, the pole can drop onto the wreckage, rescuers, emergency vehicles, and spectators with disastrous results.

If you arrive at the location of an accident and discover that a utility pole has been broken off close to the base but that all the conductors are intact:

- Park the ambulance at the edge of the danger zone.
- Notify your dispatcher of the situation.
- Remain at the edge of the danger zone until representatives of the power company can de-energize the conductors and stabilize the pole.

Pad-Mounted Transformer Damaged by a Vehicle

Pad-mounted transformers and underground cables supply electricity to homes in many developments throughout the country; they eliminate the need for unsightly utility poles and overhead wire installations. These above ground transformers are sometimes struck and damaged by vehicles, and when they are, they pose a serious threat to accident victims and emergency service personnel alike.

If you respond to an accident location and find that a vehicle has struck and come to rest against a pad-mounted transformer:

- Have your dispatcher advise the power company of the situation and request the immediate response of a power company representative.
- Do not touch either the vehicle or the transformer case, even if there is evidence that service to surrounding structures has been disrupted. Although secondary connections to the transformer may be broken, primary connections may be intact and energizing the transformer case and the accident vehicle with as much as 34,000 volts.
- Stand in a safe place until a power company representative can assure you that the transformer has been de-energized.
- Discourage occupants from leaving the vehicle.
- Keep spectators from the immediate area.
- Warn other emergency service personnel not to touch the vehicle or the transformer case.

EXTINGUISHING FIRES IN ACCIDENT VEHICLES

When you are first on the scene of an accident and see that a vehicle is on fire, always notify your dispatcher of the situation and request the response of firefighting units. Do not assume that someone else has called the fire department.

WARNING: Extinguishing a vehicle fire is the responsibility of persons who are trained and equipped for the job: firefighters.

Nonetheless there are some measures that *specially trained* EMS personnel can take when they arrive at the location of an accident before fire apparatus. Most ambulances carry some sort of portable fire extinguisher. Thus it is important for EMTs to know how extinguishers work and how they can be used to keep small fires from becoming big ones.

A 15- or 20-pound class A:B:C dry chemical fire extinguisher is a good choice because it can be used to extinguish virtually everything that is burning in a vehicle: upholstery and the ordinary combustible contents of the passenger compartment and trunk, fuel or other petroleum products in the engine compartment, fuel under the vehicle, and electrical components. The only things that cannot be extinguished by an A:B:C extinguisher are magnesium and other flammable metal parts.

Before you attempt to extinguish a fire in any part of an accident vehicle, even a small fire, put on a full set of protective gear. (See Scan 27-1.)

If the fire is in the engine compartment and the hood is open:

- Position yourself close to an A-pillar of the vehicle and, if possible, with your back to the wind. From this position there is less chance that the agent will enter the passenger compartment. Dry chemical extinguishing agent irritates the respiratory passages and may contaminate open wounds.
- Attack the fire with short bursts of agent. Use no more than is necessary to extinguish the fire. You will need what is left if there is a flare-up.

If the hood is open to the safety latch:

- Resist the temptation to fully raise the hood before discharging the agent. By keeping the hood closed, you will restrict the flow of air to the fire, and thus deprive it of oxygen.

- Direct the agent through the opening between the hood and the fender, through an opening around the grill, under a wheel well, or wherever there is an opening to the engine compartment. Again, don't use any more agent than is needed to extinguish the fire.

If the hood is closed tight and there is no apparent opening to the engine compartment:

- Quickly punch two or three holes in the hood with the pike of a forcible entry tool. Then discharge the agent through these openings. The resulting cloud of dry chemical in the engine compartment should quickly extinguish the fire.

If the fire is under the dash or in upholstery or other combustibles in the passenger compartment:

- Carefully apply the agent directly to the burning material. Apply it sparingly so the interior of the vehicle is not filled with a dense cloud of powder. Remember that the agent may be harmful to the occupants.

If there is fire in the trunk of the vehicle:

- Do not unlock and raise the trunk lid; the fire will intensify with a supply of fresh air. Moreover, if anything in the trunk explodes just as you raise the lid, you may be struck by a fireball or flying debris.
- With the wedge end of a combination forcible entry tool, punch a hole in one of the light wells and discharge agent through the opening into the trunk. The combination of agent and reduced oxygen supply should extinguish the fire.
- If you cannot break through the light well, make two or three holes in the trunk lid with the pike of the forcible entry tool and discharge agent through these openings.

Using a portable unit in an attempt to extinguish fuel that is burning under an accident vehicle may be an exercise in futility when the spill is large. But when there are people trapped in the vehicle, you must try nonetheless.

- Attempt to sweep the flames from under the passenger compartment as you apply the agent. If you are able to extinguish the fire, be sure that sources of ignition are kept away from the vehicle.

SCAN 27–1 EXTINGUISHING FIRES IN ACCIDENT VEHICLES

A

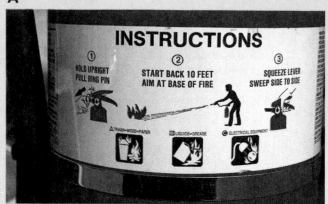

Markings that identify an extinguisher that can be used for Class A, B, and C fires.

B

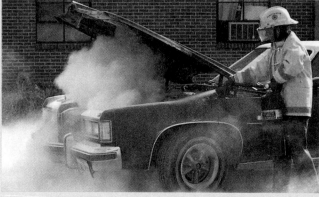

Extinguishing a fire in the engine compartment when the hood is fully open.

C

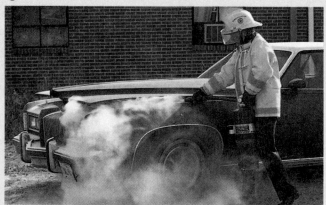

Extinguishing a fire in the engine compartment when the hood is partially open.

D

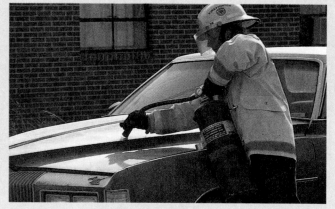

Extinguishing a fire in the engine compartment through an opening made in the closed hood.

E

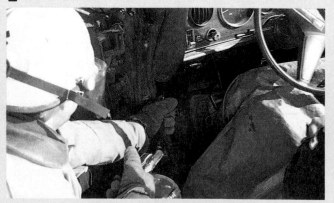

Extinguishing a fire under the dash. Care must be taken not to fill the vehicle's interior with a cloud of agent.

F

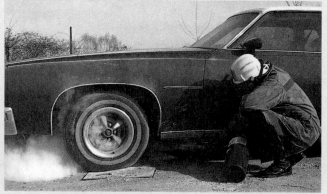

Extinguishing fuel burning under a vehicle. Flames are swept away from the vehicle.

NOTE: DO ONLY WHAT YOU ARE TRAINED TO DO.

An A:B:C extinguisher can also be used to combat tire fires. Burning truck tires are especially dangerous; flames can quickly spread to the body of the vehicle and to the cargo inside. Explosions that sometimes occur when a tire burns can cause debris and split rims to fly for a considerable distance.

WARNING: No matter how small the fire appears and how proficient you are with portable extinguishers, call for a fire department response as soon as you arrive at the location of an accident and discover that a vehicle is on fire.

COPING WITH SPILLED FUEL

There will undoubtedly be times during your career as an EMT when you will arrive at the scene of an accident and discover that fuel is leaking from a damaged vehicle, but is not on fire. Under-trunk fuel tanks are especially susceptible to damage. An under-truck tank may rupture when a vehicle is struck from behind or be penetrated when a vehicle rolls over debris. There is not much you can do when a tank has been ruptured in an accident; by the time you arrive on the scene the contents will probably have flowed from the tank.

- Call for a fire department response. The decision to continue with the rescue effort should be influenced by your perception of the danger. You should not be expected to carry out gaining access and disentanglement operations if gasoline is pooled under the vehicle or is flowing away from the vehicle toward a source of ignition.
- While you are waiting for fire units, warn spectators away from flowing fuel. This will at least minimize possible sources of ignition.

If you arrive at the scene of an accident and you see that a fuel tank has a slight leak or that a fuel line has been severed, you may be able to stop the leak if you are trained and equipped for the task, and if in attempting to do so you will not place yourself in an extremely dangerous position.

- Have your partner stand by with a class A:B:C dry chemical fire extinguisher ready for service. He should be in a position where he will be able to drive flames from under the passenger compartment if there is an ignition.
- Plug the hole in the tank with duct sealant or a sealant made for hazardus materials. Use golf tees to plug any leaking fuel lines.

STABILIZING UNSTEADY VEHICLES

Of all the hazard management procedures that might be necessary during a vehicle rescue operation, the least employed is stabilization. There are many reasons why rescuers fail to stabilize accident vehicles. They may not be trained in techniques of stabilization, or they may not be equipped for the task (or so they think). But the principal reason for not stabilizing accident vehicles is that in many accident situations the involved vehicles *appear* to be stable, especially in the eyes of untrained rescuers. Whether the vehicles *are* stable depends on factors such as the type of the vehicle, the nature and extent of damage, the position in which the vehicle has come to rest, and the character of the terrain under the vehicle.

WARNING: Rather than taking the chance of "reading" an accident vehicle wrong with regard to its stability and have the vehicle move during the rescue operation with disastrous results, we suggest that you consider *every* accident vehicle to be unstable and act accordingly.

Stabilizing a Vehicle on Its Wheels

The accident vehicle that is least likely to be stabilized because it looks stable is one that is upright on four inflated wheels, even one that is severely damaged as the result of a head-on or rear end collision.

Remember that serious injuries can happen to a vehicle's occupants during a head-on or rear-end collision. In addition to the usual cuts and bruises, the driver and occupants can suffer face and skull injuries, knee fractures and dislocations, fractured femurs, dislocated hips, broken ribs, flail chest, and a variety of internal injuries. But the injuries that can be aggravated most by the movements of an unstable vehicle are those to the cervical spine. The up-and-down, side-to-side, and back-and-forth motions caused by even careful rescuers in an attempt to gain access to trapped occupants can be easily transmitted to injured cervical spines.

Two easily accomplished steps will stabilize a vehicle on its wheels.

- Prevent forward and rearward movements by placing wheel chocks or cribbing ahead of one front wheel and behind the rear wheel on the same side. If you use cribbing, position it in the manner shown in Figure 27-4.

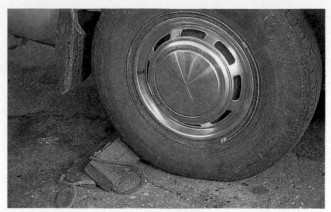

A. A wheel chock has been positioned to prevent forward movement.

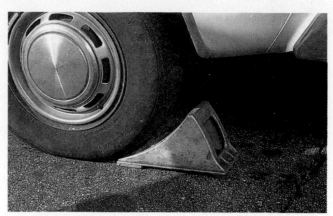

B. Cribbing has been placed in the manner of a wheel chock to prevent rearward movement.

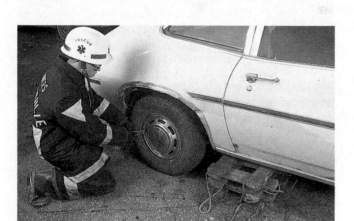

C. Cribbing has been positioned under the rocker panel to prevent up-and-down and side-to-side movements. The tires were deflated to allow the car to settle onto the cribs.

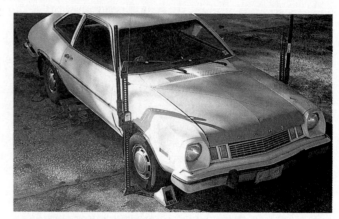

D. Hi-Lift® jacks can be used when there is not enough cribbing for four point stabilization.

FIGURE 27–4. Stabilizing a vehicle that is on its wheels.

- Prevent side-to-side and up-and-down movements by isolating the body of the vehicle from its springs. Build box cribs under the rocker panels, one just behind the front wheel and one just ahead of the rear wheel on both sides of the car. The box cribs must be rigid. Either insert the final layer of cribbing while your partner lifts a fender a short distance, or deflate the tires and allow the vehicle to settle onto the cribs.

If you do not have sufficient cribbing for four cribs, build two cribs, one under the rocker panel just ahead of the rear wheel on each side of the vehicle. Then eliminate the springing action by lifting the front fenders a short distance with Hi-Lift® or bumper jacks in the manner shown in Figure 27-4.

Lacking anything else, at least minimally stabilize a vehicle on its wheels by deflating all the tires.

Simply cut the valve stems or pull them from the wheels with pliers. It's surprising how much of a car's spring action is eliminated by deflating the tires. If you elect to deflate tires, let a police officer know that you have done so; thus investigators will not think that the tires are flat as a result of the accident.

Stabilizing a Vehicle on Its Side

A vehicle can roll over and come to rest on its side when it is struck broadside by another vehicle, when it is driven too fast around a corner or curve, or when the wheels of one side drop off the pavement onto a depressed shoulder and the driver attempts to bring it back onto the road by throwing the wheel to the side without slowing down.

There is a tendency for spectators and untrained rescuers to push a vehicle back onto its wheels after it has come to rest on its side as the result of a rollover accident. They fail to realize that during the rollover, persons inside the vehicle may have been subjected to bone-breaking forces, thrown against sharp metal edges, and rolled onto fragments of glass. They also fail to realize that if they roll the vehicle back onto its wheels they may duplicate whatever happened in the accident. Existing injuries may be aggravated and new injuries may be produced.

While a car that is on its side may appear stable, simply climbing onto the side in an attempt to open a door may cause the vehicle to drop onto its top or wheels. Moreover, you can be trapped under the vehicle if you do not jump far enough when the vehicle drops.

A vehicle that is on its side *can* be stabilized in the position found. However, it is a difficult procedure, and when the stabilization is accomplished, the only safe exitway for injured occupants will be through an opening made in the roof.

If a vehicle is stabilized in a vertical position, forces generated by someone standing on the side of the car are directed through the vehicle into the ground. Moreover, it is possible to access the entire interior of the passenger compartment by folding the top down, by folding a portion of the top back, or by removing the top altogether.

There are dozens of ways to stabilize a vehicle in a vertical position on its side, from using manpower alone to using hydraulic rams and pneumatic jacks. The techniques best and most easily accomplished by EMS personnel with the recommended equipment and some items that can be found on the scene are described here and illustrated in Figure 27-5.

Let's say that the car is on its side with the side and roof edge contacting the ground, the position in which a car is most likely to be after a rollover accident.

If you have sufficient cribbing:

- Build open box cribs under the front and rear wheels. The cribs should be just high enough that the wheels will settle on them when the car is moved to the vertical position; three or four layers of cribbing are usually sufficient for full-size cars; less for smaller cars.

- With the help of firefighters, police officers, or apparently responsible onlookers, ease the car to the vertical position. While your helpers hold the car vertical, build cribs under the A- and C-pillars. When you cannot fit another layer of cribbing under the pillars, have the helpers push gently on the roof. Insert a final piece of cribbing and instruct

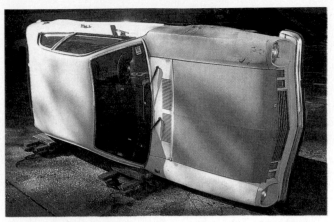

A. Cribbing was placed under the wheels. The car was then moved to the vertical position and cribs were built under the A- and C- pillars.

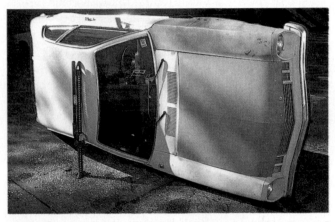

B. Cribbing was placed under the wheels and the car was moved to the vertical position. Stabilization was completed with a Hi-Lift® jack.

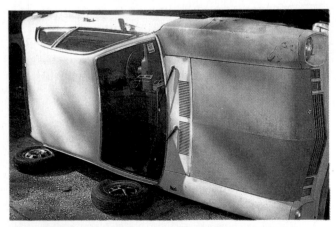

C. When no other equipment is available, a car can be effectively stabilized with spare wheels.

FIGURE 27–5. Stabilizing a vehicle on its side.

the helpers to quit pushing. The car will settle onto the cribs and lock them in place. Using cribbing in the manner just described provides four-point stabilization and is the ideal procedure because it leaves the entire roof of the vehicle accessible. Depending on needs, you can sever the uppermost roof pillars and fold the roof down. Or you can sever the A- and B-pillars, notch the roof edge just ahead of the C-pillars on each side of the car, and fold a section of the roof back. Or if the car is a small model with narrow C-pillars, you can cut all the pillars and remove the roof altogether.

If you do not have sufficient cribbing for four point stabilization:

- Use the available cribbing to build cribs under the wheels. Then have assistants ease the car to the vertical position and hold it there.
- Position a Hi-Lift® jack so that the lifting toe engages the drip molding just behind the A-pillar. Operate the jack until the car is vertical.

If you do not have any cribbing at all:

- Place a spare wheel under the rear wheel of the accident vehicle so that when the car is moved to the vertical position there will be wheel-to-wheel, not tire-to-tire, contact.
- Have helpers move the car to the vertical position and hold it while you position the lifting toe of a Hi-Lift® jack under the drip molding just behind the A-pillar.
- Operate the jack until the car is vertical.

An accident vehicle can be effectively stabilized vertically on its side even when the ambulance has no equipment at all for stabilization.

- Obtain two spare wheels. Place one under the rear wheel of the accident vehicle so there is metal-to-metal contact.
- While others are supporting the car in the vertical position, jam the other wheel under the A-pillar of the vehicle.

Using cribbing and a jack results in three-point stabilization, and using a spare wheel and a jack or two spare wheels affords only two-point stabilization. Don't be alarmed. It is no easier to push over a car that is stabilized vertically at two or three points than it is to push over a car that is stabilized

at four points. Remember, when a car is vertical, the weight of the vehicle is directed into the ground.

Stabilizing a Vehicle on Its Roof

Although stabilizing a vehicle on its roof is a little more difficult than stabilizing one that is on its wheels or side, it can be accomplished with items carried on the ambulance or available at the scene.

A vehicle that has come to rest on its roof after a rollover accident is likely to be in one of four positions:

1. Horizontal, with the roof crushed flat against the body of the vehicle and both the trunk lid and hood contacting the ground.
2. Essentially horizontal, resting entirely on the roof, with space between the hood and the ground and space between the trunk lid and the ground.
3. Front end down, with the front edge of the hood contacting the ground and the rear of the car supported by the C-pillars.
4. Front end up, with the trunk lid contacting the ground and much of the weight of the vehicle supported by the A-pillars.

When the roof of a car is crushed flat against the body of the vehicle, as when all the roof pillars have collapsed, the car is essentially a steel box that is resting on the ground with all the occupants completely trapped inside. Unless the vehicle is on a hill or perched precariously on debris or another vehicle, this is the one time when stabilization is unnecessary; the structure is rigid. Getting to the occupants will be difficult, however.

In each of the three situations illustrated in Figure 27-6, a major part of the body of the vehicle is supported by roof pillars. As long as the pillars remain intact, there will be an opening through which rescuers may be able to reach occupants. But if the pillars collapse because they were weakened during the rollover, the elevated portion of the vehicle may come crashing down. Woe be to a rescuer who is attempting to climb into the vehicle when the pillars collapse or one who has an arm in a window opening.

Stabilizing an upside-down car involves supporting the elevated portions of the vehicle. Use cribbing and jacks if you have them or a combination of cribbing, jacks, and spare wheels.

Regardless of the stabilization procedure, be sure to keep your arms from places where they might become trapped if the roof pillars collapse and the vehicle drops during the stabilization effort.

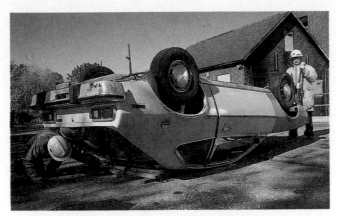

A. Cribbing, wedges, and Hi-Lift® jacks have been used to stabilize this car. Positioning the jacks with the lifting toes engaging the bumper is better than trying to engage the edge of the fender.

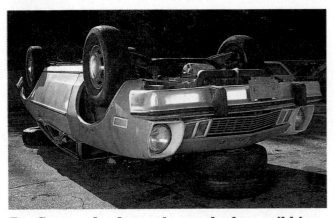

B. Spare wheels can be used when cribbing is not available or when there is not sufficient cribbing for the task.

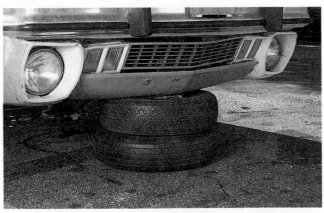

C. Lacking any other devices, an overturned vehicle can be stabilized with spare wheels. There must be enough people on hand to lift the front of the car so that one or two wheels can be slid under the hood.

FIGURE 27–6. Stabilizing an overturned vehicle.

Disabling an Accident Vehicle's Electrical System

It is standard operating procedure for many rescue units to permanently disable the electrical system of every accident vehicle by cutting a battery cable. This was a reasonable practice when vehicles had a great deal more combustible materials than they have today and when wiring did not have self-extinguishing insulation. Today, however, the situation is much different. **Unless gasoline is pooled under a vehicle, cutting the battery out of the electrical system may not only be a waste of time, it may actually hinder the rescue operation!** Remember that many cars have electrically powered door locks, window operators, seat adjustment mechanisms, and trunk latches. Being able to lower a window rather than breaking it will eliminate the likelihood that occupants will be sprayed with fragments of broken glass. Being able to operate a powered seat may save you the trouble of severing or displacing a steering column.

If for some reason you think it is necessary to disrupt an accident vehicle's electrical system, *disconnect the ground cable from the battery.* Thus you will not be likely to produce a spark that can drop onto spilled fuel or ignite battery gases. Such a spark can be created when the positive cable is pulled away from the battery terminal, or when a cutting tool or wrench touches a metal component while in contact with the positive cable.

WARNING: Take care when you are working under the hood of later-model passenger vehicles. The fans of some cars are driven by a motor that is actuated by a thermostat. Keep your hands away from this type of fan at all times.

SUMMARY

Vehicle accidents invariably produce traffic hazards, and police officers and firefighters are usually responsible for traffic control. When EMTs arrive first on the scene of an accident, however, they should initiate traffic control measures.

When at least one unobstructed lane is available, position flares or other warning devices so that vehicles are channeled safely past the danger zone. Set out flares so that the farthest one is at a distance from the edge of the danger zone equal to the stopping distance for the road's posted speed plus the distance in feet equal to the posted speed.

When an accident has occurred on a curved portion of a road, consider the start of the curve to be the edge of the danger zone when you are positioning flares or warning devices.

When an accident has occurred on a hill, consider the top of the hill to be an edge of the danger zone. Position flares or other warning devices so that vehicles approaching on the same side of the road as the accident vehicles are slowed before they reach the top of the hill.

Spectators can interfere with rescue and patient care activities if their movements are not limited. When there are no police officers or firefighters on the scene, ask apparently responsible bystanders to keep spectators away from the danger zone.

Downed wires threaten everyone at the location of an accident. **Do not attempt to move downed wires unless you are specially trained and have the proper equipment for the task.** Do not under any circumstances try to move a downed wire with a wooden pole, a tree limb, or other makeshift device.

Ground is sometimes energized for a considerable distance from the point of contact with downed wires; the condition is known as ground gradient. If a tingling sensation in your legs and groin warns that you have walked onto energized ground, turn around, grasp one leg with your hand, and hop on one foot to a safe place.

Pad-mounted transformers pose a problem in that virtually nothing can be done to reach and care for injured persons until the power flow is disrupted. **Do not touch an accident vehicle or the transformer case if the vehicle is contracting a pad-mounted transformer.** Keep spectators away, encourage occupants to stay in the vehicle, and stand by in a safe place until a power company representative arrives.

Use a portable fire extinguisher to combat fires in accident vehicles *after* you have made sure that the local fire department is respond-ing and after you have put on a full set of protective gear.

Attack an engine compartment fire by discharging agent through an opening between the hood and the fender, an opening in the grill, or an opening in the wheel well. Do not open the hood.

When fuel is burning under a vehicle, apply agent in such a way that the fuel is swept away from the vehicle.

Apply agent sparingly inside an accident vehicle so that occupants are not exposed to a cloud of dry chemical.

When there is fire in the trunk of an accident vehicle, discharge agent through openings made in the light wells or trunk lid.

Remember that there is no such thing as a stable accident vehicle when it is possible that an occupant has a cervical spine injury. Stabilize a vehicle that is on its wheels to prevent the back-and-forth, side-to-side, and up-and-down motions that are often associated with rescue efforts from being transmitted to injured occupants.

Stabilize a vehicle that is on its side to prevent it from dropping onto its wheels or top during the rescue operation. Stabilizing the vehicle in the vertical position ensures maximum stability and allows disposal of the roof in several ways.

Stabilize a vehicle that is on its roof to prevent the roof pillars from collapsing during the rescue effort.

Do not permanently disable a vehicle's electrical system unless there is a severe fire danger. Being able to operate powered seats, door locks, window operators, and trunk latches may be an advantage to the rescue effort. When you deem it necessary to disconnect the battery from a vehicle's electrical system, unbolt the ground cable.

SECTION THREE
Gaining Access to Vehicle Occupants

OBJECTIVES: **As an EMT trained in vehicle rescue procedures, you should be able to:**

1. List four ways in which the occupants of accident vehicles can be reached. (p. 640)
2. List three advantages to being able to open an accident vehicle's doors. (p. 640)
3. State the advantage of electric door locks to a rescue operation. (p. 640)
4. Describe a procedure for using a noose tool to open a door that has either a mushroom-head lock knob or a straight-shank lock knob. (p. 640 and p. 642)
5. Describe a procedure for using a hammer and awl to unlock a door that does not have an accessible lock knob. (p. 642)
6. Describe a procedure for exposing a door's locking and latching mechanism. (p. 642)
7. Describe the breaking characteristics of laminated and tempered glass. (p. 643)
8. Explain how a windshield or rear window can be identified as either mastic mounted or mounted in a U-shaped molding. (p. 643)

9. Describe steps that should be taken to protect the occupants of an accident vehicle from glass fragments produced during window removal operations. (p. 643)

10. Describe the procedure for removing intact a windshield or rear window that is set in a U-shaped molding. (p. 643)

11. Describe the procedure for removing a mastic-mounted windshield intact. (pp. 643–645)

12. Describe a procedure for removing a windshield (or a section of a windshield) that cannot be removed intact. (p. 645)

13. Describe the procedure for breaking tempered glass side windows with minimal particle spread. (p. 645)

14. State when it would be best to remove or fold back an accident vehicle's roof instead of attempting to reach occupants through door or window openings. (p. 646)

15. Describe a procedure for raising a crushed roof. (p. 647)

16. List three ways of gaining access to the occupants of an accident vehicle that is stabilized on its side. (p. 647)

17. Describe a procedure for entering an overturned accident vehicle when roof pillars are intact. (p. 647)

18. Describe a procedure for entering an overturned accident vehicle when the roof is crushed flat against the body of the vehicle. (p. 647)

19. Describe a procedure for unlocking the trunk of a car when the key is not available or when the key will not work. (p. 647)

20. Describe a procedure for reaching a person who is trapped underneath a vehicle. (pp. 647–649)

SKILLS As an EMT trained and equipped for vehicle rescue procedures, you should be able to:

1. Use a noose tool or other device in a nondestructive procedure for unlocking a vehicle door that has an accessible lock knob.

2. Unlock and unlatch an accident vehicle's doors by destructive means when a nondestructive technique is impossible or unsuccessful.

3. Remove mastic-mounted windshields and rear windows intact.

4. Remove intact windshields and rear windows that are set in a U-shaped molding.

5. Break tempered glass windows with a minimal spread of fragments to the interior of the vehicle.

6. Remove a windshield or a section of a windshield that cannot be removed intact.

7. Gain access to the occupants of an accident vehicle by removing or folding back the roof when opening doors will be difficult or time consuming.

8. Raise a crushed roof.

9. Enter a vehicle that is on its side by opening a door or removing the windshield or rear window.

10. Enter an overturned vehicle through door and/or window openings when the roof pillars are intact.

11. Make an opening in the floor in order to gain access to the occupants of an overturned vehicle when the roof is crushed flat against the body of a vehicle.

12. Open the trunk of a vehicle when the lock mechanism cannot be operated with the key.

13. Raise the side of a vehicle to reach a person who is trapped underneath.

GAINING ACCESS

The next step after eliminating or managing hazards is to gain access to the occupants of accident vehicles. Quick access is important if life-saving efforts are to be successful.

Not too long ago, it was the practice for rescuers to make an opening in a wrecked vehicle large enough for an EMT or paramedic to crawl through and reach the victims. While the idea was sound, the practice was flawed. EMS personnel were stomping on injured people. The problem became more acute as cars became smaller.

Today, improved tools and techniques enable

rescuers to gain access to vehicle occupants more quickly, so instead of making a single opening in a wrecked vehicle, rescuers can make multiple openings almost simultaneously. As a result, EMS personnel can carry out assessment procedures and initiate emergency care measures without being hindered by doors, windows, roof pillars, and the bodies of other victims.

Four procedures will be discussed in this section: gaining access through door openings, gaining access through window openings, gaining access by folding back or removing the roof, and gaining access by making openings in the body of the vehicle. All these tasks can be accomplished with the hand tools recommended for ambulances in Section Two.

GAINING ACCESS THROUGH DOOR OPENINGS

Today's cars are made with safety in mind. Doors are substantially stronger than in the past, and improved locking and latching mechanisms prevent doors from flying open when a vehicle collides with something. Nonetheless, the best way to gain access to the injured occupants of an accident vehicle is still to open doors. **There are three distinct advantages:**

- Opening doors allows rescuers to quickly evacuate uninjured persons and thus make injured persons more accessible.
- Opening a door exposes more of an injured person's body than does merely opening a window. A better assessment can be made and severe lower body injuries can be cared for quicker.
- Opening doors also creates an opening through which injured occupants can be removed after being secured to an immobilization device.

Many rescuers and EMS personnel have been conditioned to believe that vehicle doors cannot be opened with anything less than a powerful hydraulic rescue tool. This is simply not the case. In some situations you may be able to simply unlatch an unlocked door and pull it open even though the vehicle is severely damaged. **Remember: Try before you pry!**

When a vehicle's doors are locked, chances are good that you will be able to unlock them with a simple hand tool. If the doors are found to be jammed after being unlocked and unlatched, chances are that you will be able to open them with a pry bar or a forcible entry tool. Unlock, unlatch, and pry: that's the secret to opening vehicle doors with simple hand tools.

Unlocking Doors That Have Powered Locks

Before you go to the trouble of unlocking doors with tools, determine whether the vehicle has powered door locks. **If it does and the electrical system is intact, you will be able to unlock all doors simultaneously.**

- Look at the inside door panels and arm rests for the push buttons or toggle switches that operate the electric solenoids. If you see any, break a side window, reach in and operate the switches to unlock the doors. Take steps to minimize the spread of glass particles if you must break a window that is directly next to an occupant. The procedure is discussed later in this section.
- At the same time, operate the control switches to lower power-assist windows if the car is so equipped.

With all the windows rolled down, you will be able to reach at least the occupants who are seated next to doors. With all the doors unlocked, you may have to do nothing more than unlatch them and pull them open.

If the doors do not have electric locks, you will have to unlock them by using either a nondestructive or destructive procedure. When doors have an accessible lock knob, you may be able to unlock them with any of a number of simple tools. When doors do not have an accessible lock knob, you will have to use a destructive technique.

Unlocking and Unlatching Doors That Have an Accessible Lock Knob

While the doors of many modern cars have sliding lock operators set in the body of the door, tens of millions of cars still have accessible mushroom-head or straight-shank lock knobs. Mushroom-head lock knobs can be lifted with a wire flare stand or a length of bent wire and, if the door has an unframed window, a screwdriver or a windshield wiper arm. Antitheft lock knobs can be lifted with a wire-and-washer tool. However, both types of lock knobs can be lifted with the homemade noose tool shown in Scan 27-2.

Use the noose tool in the following manner:

- Move the window frame away from the body of the vehicle by alternately positioning and

SCAN 27–2 UNLOCKING VEHICLE DOORS

Using a Noose Tool

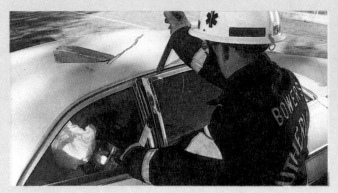

A An opening is made with pry bars.

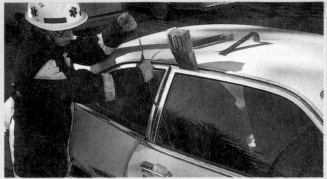

B While a wedge maintains the opening, the lock button is captured with the noose.

Using a Hammer and Awl

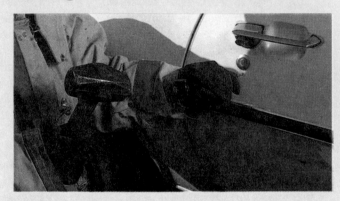

C The point of the awl is driven through the door panel.

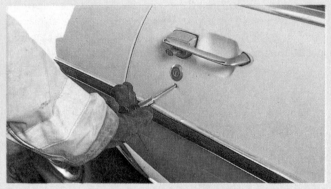

D After the opening is enlarged, the tail piece of the lock is captured with the point of the awl.

Exposing the Lock and Latch Mechanisms

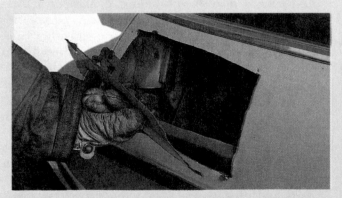

E A four-sided cut is made around the door handle and the panel is removed.

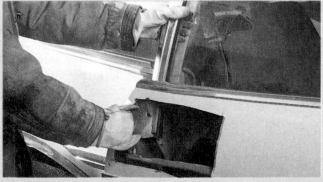

F The door is unlocked and unlatched by hand.

repositioning two short prybars until the desired gap is achieved. Maintain the gap with a wood wedge. Thus you will be able to operate the noose with both hands.

- Bend the copper tubing as necessary to capture the lock knob with the noose. While you hold the body of the tool with one hand, pull on the T-handle to tighten the noose snugly around the shank of the knob. Then pull up on the tool to lift the knob.
- Pry the window frame out slightly with a bar, remove the wedge, and open the door.

This technique works equally well on an older car that has unframed windows. Just remember that the most vulnerable part of an unframed tempered glass window is its exposed edge. Be careful not to strike the edge of the glass with the steel bar.

A word is in order about the use of locksmith tools. Many unlocking devices are available from locksmith supply houses and emergency service suppliers. One such device is a thin-blade tool that is slipped between the glass and the weather stripping of a door in an effort to reach and operate the lock mechanism. If the user does not know where to position the tool, the operation will be slow, and if the door has an antitheft device, the effort will fail.

Unlocking and Unlatching Doors That Do Not Have an Accessible Lock Knob

You will have to resort to a destructive technique when you have to open a door that does not have an accessible lock knob. One procedure enables you to operate the cylinder locks of most car doors quickly with a hammer and a steel awl.

- Drive the point of the awl through the metal skin of the door at a point about ⅜ inch below the lock cylinder. Move the awl handle in a circular fashion to widen the opening. Position the awl so that the point contacts the tail piece of the lock cylinder (usually a slotted piece of metal that is attached at a right angle to the cylinder). If the tail piece is not to the left of the lock cylinder, reposition the point of the awl to the right side. When the point has engaged the tail piece, move the awl handle (usually down) to unlock the door.

There will be times when you will not be able to open doors with either of the techniques described so far. You may have to open a door that is severely damaged or a door that is under such a strain that the latch cannot be operated in the conventional manner even though it has been unlocked. In such cases you will have to not only expose the lock and latch mechanisms, but disable or destroy them as well.

- Remove a section of the door panel by making four cuts around the handle and the lock cylinder with a panel cutter. When the cut section is free, carefully disconnect any rods that lead away from the latch and the lock cylinder.
- Locate the rod or bar that leads from the latch mechanism to the operator in the door panel. Move the rod to unlock the door. Then operate the portion of the mechanism that unlatches the door when a button is pushed or the door handle is lifted. While you maintain finger pressure on the latch, pull the door open.

If the door is jammed to the point where you cannot pull it open, drive the blade of a screwdriver into the mechanism to maintain it in the unlatched position and use a pry bar or forcible entry tool to open the door. In extreme cases you may have to remove the faceplate of the latch mechanism and then pry out the parts of the mechanism that keep the door latched. While it sounds difficult, the task can be easily accomplished with a ripping chisel.

ENTERING A VEHICLE THROUGH WINDOW OPENINGS

Conditions may prevail when it will be impossible to easily enter a vehicle through door openings, as when a car has been struck broadside by a truck and pushed against a building or another vehicle, or when there has been a multivehicle accident and cars are jammed together. In these and other cases you may be required to enter a vehicle through window openings.

There was a time in the history of vehicle rescue when breaking windows was just about the only known way of entering a vehicle when doors were either locked or jammed. The technique was simple. People simply bashed in windows with whatever tool was available. Firefighters used axes, rescue personnel used sledgehammers, ambulance attendants used jack handles, and police officers used riot sticks and even gun butts. Today, rescue operations are more "patient friendly." When possible, windshields and rear windows are removed rather than broken, and when breaking glass is absolutely necessary, it is done in such a way that the danger to occupants is minimal.

There's a reason for being careful. Large chunks of glass can be picked from an open wound, but very finely divided particles remain unnoticed deep in the wound. If they are not removed, as by debridement, they will continue to damage tissues even after the wound is closed.

All automotive glass is included in the category of *safety glass*. However, two types of safety glass are used in the manufacture of vehicle windows. **Windshields and some side and rear windows of trucks and vans are made with laminated glass. The rear and side windows of passenger cars are usually tempered glass.**

Laminated windows have two sheets of plate glass bonded to a sheet of tough plastic film. The resulting glass and plastic sandwich is tough, and even though the glass panes may break, a laminated windshield will usually prevent a person from flying through the windshield during a low- or moderate-speed crash. Moreover, the plastic inner layer prevents the glass from breaking into dangerous shards that can cause deep wounds.

A new form of laminated glass windshield is being installed in some cars and will probably be used in all passenger cars within a few years. Called an antilacerative windshield, it has a layer of clear plastic bonded to the interior surface of the glass. The plastic minimizes the soft tissue injuries that often result when a person's head strikes and breaks the windshield.

Most side and rear windows of passenger cars are tempered glass, a single sheet of glass that has been tempered much like steel. Tempered glass windows have a resilience that often keeps them from shattering even during broadside and rollover accidents. When tempered glass windows do break, they shatter into small fragments rather than long shards.

Window Installations

The fixed windows of motor vehicles (windshields, rear windows, and the nonmovable windows of trucks, vans, and recreational vehicles) are installed either in a U-shaped molding or against a mastic material. It is important that you learn to recognize the ways in which windshields and rear windows are installed. The method of removal is influenced by the manner of installation. You need not know the year, make, or model of a vehicle to determine how its windshield and rear window are installed. Simply look at the sides and top of the glass. If you see just glass and trim, the window is probably (but not necessarily) held in place with a mastic material.

If you see glass, then what appears to be black plastic or rubber, and then trim, the glass is set in a U-shaped rubber molding.

Protecting Occupants Before Removing or Breaking Glass

Every effort must be taken to protect the occupants of an accident vehicle from the flying fragments common to glass removal operations. If all of the doors are closed and locked and all of the windows are in place and tightly closed, then there is nothing you can do in the way of victim protection until at least one opening has been made in the vehicle. But if a door is open, or if a window is rolled down, try to cover at least the occupants' heads with sheets, disposable blankets, or lightweight tarps. Then as new openings are made in the vehicle, take additional victim protection measures as necessary.

Removing Windshields and Rear Windows That Are Set in a Molding

A window that is set in a U-shaped rubber molding can be easily and quickly removed with the linoleum knife that is included in the suggested tool inventory, although many other knives can be used.

- Remove the trim from the side and top of the window. Insert the point of the knife into the molding at the midpoint of the windshield or rear window. While you keep the blade as flat against the glass as possible, draw the knife across the top and down the side in such a way that the blade cuts away one side of the U-shaped molding and thus releases the glass. Repeat the procedure on the other side. Work the end of a short pry bar behind the glass and pry it from the frame. The window will pivot on its bottom edge.

Soapy water applied from one of the squirt bottles that are carried for saw blade lubrication will allow the knife blade to pass easily through the molding.

Removing Mastic-Mounted Windshields

The mastic-mounted windshields and rear windows of many cars can be removed quickly with an inexpensive glazier's knife.

- Remove the trim from the side and top of the windshield or rear window opening. Hold

SCAN 27–3 REMOVING WINDSHIELDS AND REAR WINDOWS

Removing a Mastic-Mounted Window

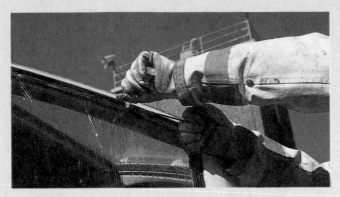

A After removing the trim, the knife is pushed into the mastic, turned 90°, and drawn across the top and down each side of the glass.

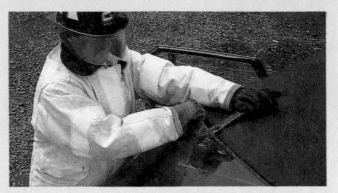

B The window is pried from the frame with a bar.

Removing a Molding-Mounted Window

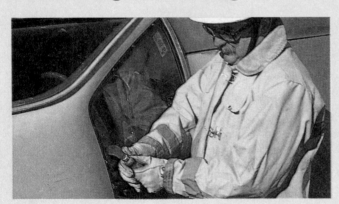

C After the trim has been removed from the top and sides of the window opening, the knife is drawn across the top and down the sides of the glass and the window is pried from the frame.

Using an Ax to Remove a Section of a Windshield

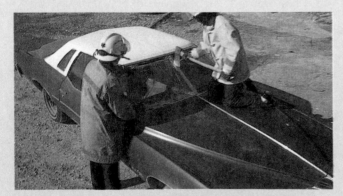

D Duct tape is applied to the glass to minimize debris, and four cuts are made with an ax.

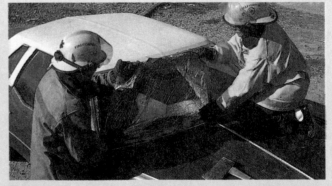

E The cut section of windshield is removed from the frame. Use the same procedure to remove the entire windshield.

the tool at about the midpoint of the window so the blade is between the edge of the glass and the window frame and parallel to the edges. Press the blade into the mastic and, at the same time, turn the tool handle so the point of the blade works its way under the glass. While you hold the tool handle perpendicular to the glass with one hand, use your other hand to pull the T-handle across the top of the glass and down the side. Repeat the procedure on the other side of the glass. Pry the glass from the frame with a short pry bar.

Many of today's cars have windshields and rear windows set against strips of mastic that are too wide for the standard blade of the glazier's knife. Unless you have a tool with a long blade, you will have no choice other than to cut a laminated windshield from its frame or break a tempered glass rear window.

Removing Sections of Windshields That Cannot Be Removed Intact

In addition to wide strips of mastic material, there are two other problems that often frustrate the attempts of rescuers to remove mastic mounted windshields intact: owner sealing and age.

Motorists often attempt to seal a leaking windshield or rear window with a silicone compound available in hardware and automotive supply stores. This sealant adheres so well and becomes so hard that the edge of the glazier's knife will neither separate the sealant from the glass nor cut through it. Windshield mastic hardens as time passes, sometimes to the point where it is impossible to separate it from the glass with a glazier's knife.

If, after you remove the trim from the window opening, you see evidence of home-sealing, or if you are unable to insert the blade of a windshield knife between glass and sealant, forget about removing the window intact. Remove the windshield by cutting the glass or a section of the glass from the frame, or simply break a rear window.

The ax that is included in the recommended inventory is an excellent tool for removing a windshield. It's a messy job, though, so take what steps you can to protect the occupants of the vehicle. Also, minimize the possibility that airborne glass powder will enter the unprotected eyes of people around the car by either coating the glass with an adhesive spray or putting down strips of duct tape where the ax blade will pass through the glass. Powdered glass can travel as much as 20 feet in a breeze. And, of course, put on a complete set of protective gear, in-

cluding wraparound safety goggles, before you cut a windshield.

- From a position on the hood, use short strokes to cut through the glass across the top, down the sides, and then across the bottom of the window frame. If you are removing only a section of the windshield in an effort to reach an injured driver, cut the glass from the top down at the midline of the windshield; then cut across the top, down the side, and across the bottom.

Breaking Tempered Glass Side and Rear Windows

You can use a hammer or any other striking tool to break a tempered glass window; but if you do, you will probably propel fragments into the vehicle with sufficient force to cut occupants. The correct way to break tempered glass is to shatter it in such a way that the fragments remain in the frame.

- Hold the point of a spring-loaded or manual center punch against a lower corner of the window where the glass is least resilient. Break the glass. Use the blunt end of the tool to carefully punch out fingerholds in the top of the window. Insert your leather-gloved fingers into the openings and pull fragments away from the window. Be sure to clean out the entire frame.

Minimizing the Spread of Tempered Glass Particles to the Interior of the Vehicle

Ideally, it is the windows that are distant from an accident vehicle's occupants that are broken during gaining access operations. In some cases, however, you may have no choice other than to break windows that are right next to occupants, as when there are three persons on the front seat of a car and three on the rear seat. You can minimize the spread of fragments to occupants by covering the window that must be broken with a special spray adhesive or strips of 2-inch duct tape.

- If you are using an adhesive spray, lay down two layers, the second at a right angle to the first. Give the spray a minute to dry before you break the glass. If you are using duct tape, overlap the strips to create a solid sheet of tape that covers the entire window.

It will be impossible to remove all the glass fragments with either technique. However, any fragments that do separate from the adhesive covering will drop straight down rather than be propelled into the vehicle.

GAINING ACCESS TO INJURED OCCUPANTS BY REMOVING THE ROOF OF AN ACCIDENT VEHICLE

When an accident vehicle has only one or two occupants, opening one or two doors or removing one or two windows is usually all that is necessary to reach them. But when an accident vehicle is filled with seriously injured people and opening doors will be difficult and time consuming because of structural damage, you will do better to dispose of the roof of the vehicle as soon as the hazard management operations are complete. In the time that it would take to open one or two severely damaged doors, you will probably be able to fold a section of the roof back, or if the car is a small one with narrow C-pillars, remove the roof altogether. With either technique, you will expose the entire interior of the vehicle and make the occupants immediately accessible.

Let's say that a compact car has been struck from behind and driven into a truck with considerable force. Because the car has been shortened by the long axis crash, you suspect that the doors are so badly jammed that opening them will require a hydraulic rescue tool. Collision forces have broken the side and rear windows. You can see that the occupants all have life-threatening injuries.

- While firefighters, First Responders, or police officers support the roof with their protected hands, sever the A-pillars, then the B-pillars, and then the C-pillars with hacksaws. You work on one side of the vehicle while your partner works on the other. Have someone continually lubricate the saw blades with the squirt bottles. When the final cut is made on each side, have the people who are supporting the roof lift it from the vehicle and carry it away from the wreckage.

When the car is a large model with C-pillars that are too wide to cut with hacksaws, make a cut in the roof edge ahead of each C-pillar with a hacksaw. The cut needs only to be as deep as the hacksaw frame will allow. Then fold the roof back convertible-style instead of removing it. You will be able to reach

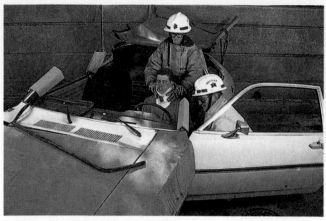

A. Folding back or removing the roof of a vehicle exposes the entire interior in one operation.

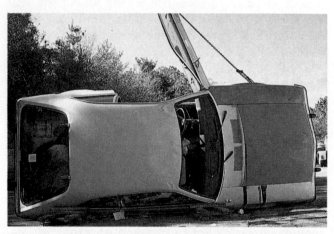

B. A vehicle that has been stabilized on its side can be entered through a door opening, through the windshield, or through the rear window opening.

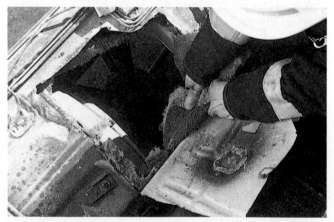

C. Entry into an overturned vehicle can be made through openings cut in the floor pan.

FIGURE 27–7. Gaining access to trapped occupants by making an opening in the vehicle.

all the rear-seat occupants even though the rear portion of the roof is still in place.

With the roof off or folded back out of the way, you will be able to carry out emergency care measures from positions at the sides of the vehicle while other rescuers open the doors.

Raising A Crushed Roof

A crushed roof will seriously impede attempts to either open doors or fold back or remove an accident vehicle's roof. Such might be the case when a car has rolled over several times and come to rest on its wheels. The Hi-Lift® jacks that are included in the recommended inventory of rescue tools are excellent devices for raising a crushed roof.

- Position the base of the jack on the door body and engage the upper part of the window frame and the roof edge with the lifting toe. Operate the jack and move the roof up just to the point where the roof pillars can be severed with a hacksaw.

ENTERING A VEHICLE THAT IS ON ITS SIDE

Depending on the location of the occupants, a car that is stabilized on its side can be entered through a door, windshield, or rear window opening. If you elect to open a door, chain it in the fully open position. Once inside, an EMT can initiate emergency care procedures (like establishing an open airway) and then protect the occupants while rescuers dispose of the roof.

Entering an Overturned Vehicle

You and your partner may arrive at the location of a rollover accident and discover that the overturned vehicle is resting on its top with the roof pillars intact. In this case, you may be able to use any of the procedures for gaining access discussed thus far.

Or you may find that the roof is crushed flat against the body of the vehicle and that the occupants are totally encapsulated in the wreckage. In this case it will be necessary for you to make an opening in the floor to reach the occupants, even though you may be able to do nothing more than insert your hand into the vehicle and help the patient maintain an open airway.

- After rigidly stabilizing the vehicle, use a

hammer and panel cutter to make a three-sided flap in the floor pan at the location of each foot well (the easily identified parts of the floor pan where passengers rest their feet). Fold the resulting flaps back and either pull out or cut the underlying insulation and floor mats. Use your handlight to look inside and assess the situation.

If there is room in the vehicle, it may be possible for a very small EMT or rescuer to either climb down through the opening or be lowered into the vehicle head first. But more likely than not, you will have to wait for rescue squad personnel to either lift the vehicle and remove the roof or force open jammed doors with hydraulic rescue tools.

Opening the Trunk of an Accident Vehicle

Trunk compartments are not usually thought of as passenger spaces; therefore, EMTs are seldom inclined to search trunks during vehicle rescue operations. Nonetheless, bodies have been discovered in trunk compartments long after the conclusion of rescue operations.

Include a trunk check as part of a routine vehicle rescue operation. Look not only for human cargo, but also hazardous materials that may pose a threat to you, the occupants of the vehicle, other emergency service personnel, and spectators.

The easiest way to enter a trunk is by unlocking the lid with the key. If the key is not available or if it does not work, you can quickly unlock most trunks with hand tools.

- Use a panel cutter to make a three-sided flap around the lock cylinder. Pry the flap down. The lock cylinder will come down with the flap, and when it does, a small bar will be pulled from a socket in the latch mechanism. Insert a 3/16-inch blade cabinet screwdriver or the point of a knife blade into the socket and turn it to unlock the trunk lid.

Reaching a Person Who Is Trapped Under a Vehicle

People become trapped under vehicles in a number of ways. A person who is struck by a car may become trapped underneath when both sets of wheels do not pass over him. A "Saturday mechanic" may become trapped when either the bumper jacks or milk jug crates that are supporting the vehicle fail while he is underneath.

Untrained persons often misunderstand the plight of a person who is trapped under a vehicle, so they do what seems to be the natural thing to do—pull the person out from under the vehicle by his feet or his shoulders. Not having been trained, they do not realize that their actions can aggravate skeletal injuries. Moreover, they fail to understand that if the person's body has been penetrated by a piece of the vehicle, fatal injuries can result if they try to pull him free.

This does not mean that you as a trained EMT should *never* pull someone from underneath a vehicle. If the vehicle is stable, if you can apply a cervical collar, and if you can be sure that the person is not impaled by a part of the vehicle, then there is no reason why you should not pull the person onto a long spine board with a rope sling. When you cannot do this safely, then you must lift the side of the vehicle. A procedure for using lift jacks is described below.

It is important that you lift the side of the vehicle closest to the person's head. Thus you will be able to apply a cervical collar and the rope sling. The procedure requires three people, so before you start, recruit a firefighter or a police officer.

- Prevent forward or rearward movement of the vehicle by placing chocks ahead of the front wheel and behind the rear wheel on the side opposite the one to be lifted.
- Build box cribs under the rocker panel of the side opposite the one that will be lifted. The cribbing will prevent that side from settling as the other side is lifted. Be sure the cribs are made rigid by inserting pieces as the side of the car is lifted, not by deflating the tires.
- Direct your partner to take a position on the ground next to the victim's head and apply a rigid cervical collar. At the same time, you and the third person position the Hi-Lift® jacks adjacent to the front and rear fender wells so the lifting toe will engage the lip of the fender.
- You and the third person operate the jacks to lift the side of the vehicle high enough to allow for the application of the rope sling.

Ideally, two cribs should be built under the rocker panel of the side that is being lifted, one just behind the front wheel and one just ahead of the rear wheel. However, chances are that you will not have enough cribbing for the task or the people to build the cribs. Because of their construction, the

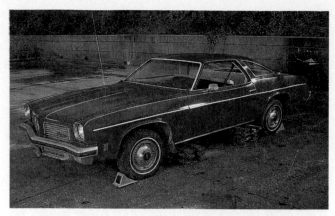

A. Wheel chocks are positioned to prevent forward and rearward movements and cribs are built under the side opposite the one to be lifted to prevent it from dropping down.

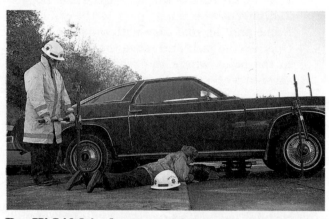

B. Hi-Lift® jacks are positioned under the edges of the front and rear fenders. The EMT on the ground will manage external bleeding if the victim is impaled.

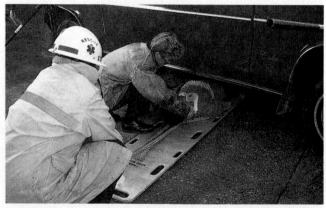

C. The side of the car has been lifted and is supported by the Hi-Lift® jacks. The EMTs are preparing to move the victim onto the long spine board with a rope sling.

FIGURE 27–8. Reaching a person who is trapped under a vehicle.

jacks will safely support the vehicle if corrosion or damage has not weakened the fenders. Steel pins slide into holes in the jack stand each time the handle is operated, and the resulting structure is able to support more than 7,000 pounds. If there is any question as to the integrity of the fenders, position the jacks so the lifting toes will engage the front and rear bumpers.

Your partner must watch carefully as the side of the vehicle moves up. If an object has penetrated the victim's chest or abdomen, your partner will have to apply manual pressure to the wound as the object is pulled free and maintain manual pressure until the person is pulled from under the vehicle. It will be impossible to cut the penetrating object.

As soon as you have reached the injured occupants of an accident vehicle, you can initiate emergency care measures according to your level of training.

SUMMARY

The injured occupants of an accident vehicle can be reached by opening doors, by removing windows, by removing the roof of the vehicle, and by making openings in the vehicle.

The initial effort should be to open doors, since to do so will create the largest openings without disposing of the roof. Even jammed vehicle doors can be quickly opened when they are unlocked and unlatched.

Before you use a tool to unlock a door, try to pull it open in the usual manner. Just because a vehicle is severely damaged does not mean that all the doors are locked and jammed shut.

Next, determine whether the vehicle has electric door locks. If so, break a window and operate the switches to unlock all the doors at one time. If the doors do not have electric locks, use a tool to unlock the doors.

If a door has an accessible lock knob, operate the knob with a noose tool. If the door does not have an accessible lock knob, attempt to unlock it with an awl and hammer. If neither method works, make an opening in the door panel and operate the locking and latching mechanisms. If a door remains jammed after being unlocked and unlatched, disable or destroy the latch mechanism and pry the door open with a bar or forcible entry tool.

All vehicle windows are safety glass. Windshields and some stationary windows of trucks, vans, and recreational vehicles are laminated glass. The rear windows and movable side windows of passenger cars are usually tempered glass. Laminated glass breaks into shards that are held together by a plastic inner layer. Tempered glass windows shatter into small fragments.

Vehicle windshields, rear windows, and the fixed windows of trucks, vans, and recreational vehicles are held in place with either a strip of adhesive material or a U-shaped molding. If you see only glass and trim, the glass is probably set against a mastic material. If you see glass, then what appears to be black rubber, then trim, the window is set in a U-shaped molding.

Remove windshields and rear windows intact when possible. Use a windshield knife to remove windows set against an adhesive material. Use a linoleum knife (or other knife) to remove windows that are set in a molding.

Use an ax to remove a windshield (or a section of a windshield) that cannot be removed intact. Break a tempered glass rear window that cannot be removed intact.

Use a spring-loaded or manual center punch to break tempered glass side windows; then pull fragments from the frame. Use an adhesive spray or duct tape to minimize the spread of fragments when it is necessary to break a window next to an occupant.

Remove the roof of a vehicle or fold back a section of the roof when it appears that occupants have life-threatening injuries and opening severely damaged doors will be difficult and time consuming.

Make an opening in a car that is stabilized on its side by opening a door or by removing the windshield or rear window.

When a car is overturned and the roof pillars are intact, stabilize the vehicle and gain access through door and/or window openings as if the car were on its wheels. When a car is overturned and the roof is crushed flat against the body, make openings in the floor pan. You will probably not be able to get into the vehicle, but you may be able to get close enough to occupants to establish open airways.

Always check the trunk of an accident vehicle for people and hazardous materials. If the trunk cannot be unlocked with a key, use a panel cutter to expose the lock mechanism and operate it with a small screwdriver or a knife.

Lift the side of a vehicle to reach a person who is trapped underneath whenever you cannot see whether the person has been impaled by an object that is projecting from the undercarriage, or when there is not enough room to secure a rope sling around the person so that he can be pulled onto a long spine board.

SECTION FOUR
Disentangling Trapped Persons

OBJECTIVES As an EMT trained for vehicle rescue procedures, you should be able to:

1. List the three parts of the disentanglement phase of a vehicle rescue operation. (p. 651)

2. List at least five ways in which an accident's victim can be shielded from contact with tools and debris during disentanglement operations. (p. 651)

3. Describe a way in which an accident victim can be protected from radiant heat and flames during a vehicle rescue operation. (p. 651)

4. Describe a way in which an accident victim's respiratory passages can be protected from dust during a vehicle rescue operation. (p. 651)

5. Describe at least five ways in which an accident victim can be protected from the elements during a rescue operation. (p. 652)

6. State the reason why the doors of an accident vehicle should be moved beyond their normal range of motion. (p. 652)

7. Describe a procedure for manually moving an accident vehicle's doors beyond their normal range of motion. (p. 652)

8. Describe a procedure for mechanically moving an accident vehicle's doors beyond their normal range of motion. (pp. 652–653)

9. Describe a procedure for folding back a section of the roof of a vehicle when the C-posts are too wide to cut with hacksaws. (p. 654)

10. Describe a procedure for folding down the B-post and rear door of a four-door sedan. (p. 655)

11. Describe a procedure for folding down the roof of a vehicle that has been stabilized on its side. (pp. 655–656)

12. Describe a procedure for folding back a section of the roof of a vehicle that has been stabilized on its side. (p. 656)

13. Describe a procedure for making an opening in the roof of a vehicle that has been stabilized on its side. (pp. 656–657)

14. Describe a procedure for shielding the sharp metal edges of severed roof pillars and openings made in a vehicle's roof. (p. 657)

15. Describe a procedure for safely unbuckling seat belts from around an injured person. (p. 657)

16. Describe a procedure for safely cutting seat belts that cannot be unbuckled. (p. 658)

17. List and describe a procedure for each of five steps that might be taken to create working space in front of an injured driver. (p. 658)

18. Describe at least four procedures for freeing a driver's foot from entrapment by a pedal. (pp. 660–663)

19. Describe a procedure for displacing the front bench seat of a passenger car. (pp. 663–665)

20. Describe a procedure for displacing the dash assembly of an accident vehicle. (p. 665)

SKILLS As an EMT trained and equipped for vehicle rescue procedures, you should be able to:

1. Protect the occupants of an accident vehicle from contact with tools and debris during disentanglement operations.

2. Protect accident victims from the elements during a vehicle rescue operation.

3. Manually move the doors of an accident vehicle beyond their normal range of motion.

4. Mechanically move the doors of an accident vehicle beyond their normal range of motion.

5. Dispose of the roof of a vehicle that is on its wheels by folding back a section of the roof or removing the roof altogether.

6. Dispose of the B-post and rear door of a four-door passenger car.

7. Dispose of the roof of a vehicle that is on its side by folding the roof down, folding back a section, or making an opening in the roof.

8. Remove seat belts from around an injured person in such a way that injuries will not be aggravated.

9. Create working space in front of an injured driver by disposing of parts of the steering column or disposing of the steering column altogether.

10. Free a driver's foot from entrapment by a pedal.

11. Displace the front bench seat of an accident vehicle.

12. Displace the dash assembly of an accident vehicle.

DISENTANGLEMENT

The disentanglement phase of a vehicle rescue operation has three parts: (1) protecting the occupants of the accident vehicle, (2) creating openings in the wreckage through which occupants can be removed, and (3) removing the mechanisms of entrapment from around the occupants.

There is great consternation among EMS and rescue personnel alike as to how much a vehicle should be disassembled in order to disentangle and remove injured occupants. The days of bending body parts around vehicle components and then dragging injured persons through whatever openings in the wreckage were available are gone.

If doors must be forced beyond their normal range of motion, if a vehicle's roof must be folded back or removed so that a person with a spinal injury can be properly immobilized, if the front seat of a vehicle must be displaced so that a person who is on the floor can be reached, properly cared for and then removed, then that is what must be done.

It is time we consider the damage that might be done to injured persons when there is not sufficient room for necessary patient care activities, not the damage that might be done to a vehicle that may already be beyond repair.

There will be times when you can gain access to an accident victim but not provide needed care because of the lack of working space. And there will be times when you can provide initial care for an accident victim, but not remove the person from the wreckage because of mechanisms of entrapment. These problems can be solved by the process of disentanglement.

Usually, disentanglement is accomplished by the members of a rescue squad. But if you are unable to undertake basic life support measures because of the proximity of mechanisms of entrapment, or if a person's condition is deteriorating too quickly to wait for appropriate help to arrive, you may have to begin the process of disentanglement with the supplies and equipment carried on the ambulance. Before you start however, be sure to check that a rescue unit is on its way. Then if you do not have the proper equipment or the skill needed to free the victims from the wreckage, there will not be a great interval from the time you must quit your efforts until the time that the rescuers begin theirs. Remember that the minutes of a seriously injured person's Golden Hour continue to tick away while the person is waiting for help to arrive.

PROTECTING THE OCCUPANTS

Many rescuers believe that merely throwing a soft covering of some sort over the occupants of an accident vehicle is sufficient to protect them from hazards during disentanglement operations. It is not a good idea for at least two reasons.

While a woven fiber blanket, a disposable paper blanket, or a lightweight tarp may protect the occupant of an accident vehicle from flying particles of glass or debris generated during a rescue operation, none of these items will adequately protect the person from forceful contact with a tool, a sharp metal edge, or a pointed object. Moreover, an already frightened accident victim may panic when his head is covered in this manner. Thrashing about wildly can aggravate existing injuries and cause new ones.

Following are some suggestions as to how you can protect the injured occupants of accident vehicles during disentanglement operations.

- Protect eyes with wraparound safety goggles.
- Protect ears with industrial hearing protectors. The rigid shells will shield the ear canals from flying particles and the external ears from contact by tools and debris.
- Use a hard hat to protect a person's scalp and skull.
- Use a short wood spine board to shield a person from contact by tools and debris, especially during roof and steering column removal operations.
- Insert a long spine board between the seat and the B-pillars when it is necessary to widen door openings or displace B-pillars.
- Cover the occupants of an accident vehicle with an aluminized blanket when there is any chance that they will be exposed to flames or radiant heat.
- Protect an accident victim's respiratory passages with a disposable dust mask when there is fine powder in the air (as when a bulk carrier has been involved in an accident).

Don't forget a hazard that is seldom thought of during vehicle rescue operations: the elements.

Body heat can be lost by radiation, conduction, convection, evaporation, and breathing, and waterchill and windchill can quicken heat loss.

- Cover an accident victim's head during disentanglement operations. Remember that at 40° F, an uncovered head can radiate up to one-half of the body's heat production.
- Place blankets under and around victims, as well as over them. Body heat is lost quickly to cold metal.
- Use plastic trash bags to prevent the loss of body heat through the effect of waterchill when a person's clothes are wet.
- Place a thermal mask over a person's mouth and nose during extremely cold weather so that breaths are warmed.

Heat, like cold, can be harmful to accident victims. Too much heat can quickly upset the body's temperature regulating mechanisms and even cause death.

- Shade an injured person's head if he is exposed to direct sunlight after the roof of a vehicle has been removed or folded back. Vital nerve centers for breathing and circulation lie close to the skull, and arteries that supply blood to the brain are close to the surface of the neck.

And, of course, have someone stand near the wreckage with a portable fire extinguisher during the disentanglement operations.

CREATING OPENINGS IN THE WRECKAGE

Three activities will make working space around the injured occupants of an accident vehicle while at the same time creating exitways through which the injured persons can be removed: Moving doors beyond their normal range of motion, disposing of the roof of the vehicle, and folding down the B-post and rear door (if the vehicle is a four-door sedan).

Moving Doors Beyond Their Normal Range of Motion

Undamaged vehicle doors seldom open a full 90 degrees, and damaged doors may not open more than a few inches. Thus doors may prevent you from work-

ing at the side of injured persons during assessment and emergency care activities. Moreover, when it is time to remove injured persons from a vehicle, doors often prevent the positioning of a long spine board at a right angle to the seat even when the doors are wide open.

Doors need not be impediments to rescue operations, however. They can be easily moved beyond their normal range of motion.

Manually Moving Doors

Few undamaged or slightly damaged vehicle doors can withstand the combined pushing and pulling efforts of two or three people. Following is a procedure you might use when the vehicle has been properly stabilized.

- Take a position where you can push on the open door. Instruct your partner to stand where he can pull on the door. If the car is an older, large model, have another person stand next to your partner so both can pull together. On your signal, you push the door while your partner pulls.
- If the door does not move the desired distance on the first effort, wait until any rocking motion has stopped before pushing and pulling again. Otherwise, a rhythmic movement may develop that is sufficient to cause the vehicle to ride over the wheel chocks.

Be aware that the cast hinges of some cars may break when the door is moved through 90 degrees. Be sure that your partner (and a helper) have their feet where they will not be struck if the door breaks away from its hinges and drops.

Using a Hand Winch

The combination of a hand winch and two chains can move a door beyond its normal range of motion even when the slightest rocking movement may be dangerous or when the door is so badly damaged that manual efforts will not move it. Following is a procedure that you and your partner might use to displace a door with a chain or cable hand winch.

- Secure the short rescue chain to the door. No special rigging is required. Simply catch the lower edge of the door with the slip hook, carry the chain up against the inner door panel, and lay the chain in the notch formed by the window frame and the door body. Do not catch the door handle with the slip hook, and do not secure the hook to the window

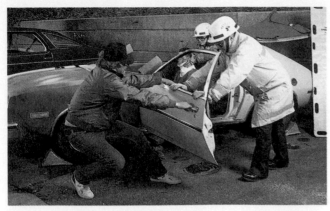

A. The EMTs are moving the door by hand. Wheel chocks and cribbing are preventing movements that may aggravate spinal injuries.

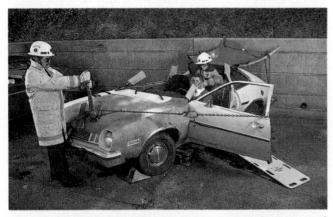

B. Moving a door beyond its normal range of motion with a hand winch. The forcible-entry tool is keeping the hand winch in position on the hood. Cribbing prevents the collapse of sheet metal.

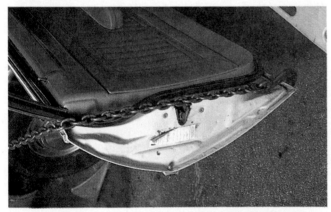

C. No special wrapping is necessary for the door chain. In this case, the slip hook has engaged the edge of the door, and the body of the chain is resting in the notch between the door and the window frame.

FIGURE 27–9. Moving vehicle doors beyond their normal range of motion.

frame. Neither may be strong enough to withstand the pull of the hand winch if the door is damaged and hard to move.

- Secure the slip hook end of the long rescue chain around a strong undercarriage component that is in line with the steering column.

- While your partner holds the anchor chain in place, place cribbing between the chain and any part of the front of the vehicle that is likely to collapse when pulling force is exerted by the hand winch.

- Use the grab hook to adjust the chain so that the ring is just behind the front edge of the hood. Capture the ring with the fixed hook of the hand winch. Pull out enough chain or cable to reach the ring of the chain that is around the door.

- Capture the ring of the short chain with the chain or cable hook of the hand winch.

- Operate the hand winch to move the door the desired distance.

- If you will not need the winch for another task, leave it attached to the anchor chain with the pulling line connected to the door chain. If you need the winch, secure the door in the wide open position with an elastic cargo strap.

When a hand winch is rigged in this manner, that is, in line with the steering column, the winch can be used later to displace the column or the dash, if necessary. And, of course, the winch can be used to move the passenger door beyond its normal range of motion if necessary.

A problem often encountered when moving a driver's door in this manner is that the hand winch will slip from the fender as the door swings open. Avoid this by having your partner drive the pike of a forcible entry tool into the fender so that the head of the tool will support the body of the hand winch during the pulling operation.

WARNING: Never use a "cheater bar" on a hand winch during this or any other pulling operation— a length of pipe slipped over the winch handle to lengthen it. The handles of hand winches are designed so that the user can just achieve maximum lifting or pulling power. A length of pipe over the handle affords greater mechanical advantage, but it also causes the winch to work beyond its rated capacity. Damage to the winch and injury to the user can result when a hand winch is forced to operate beyond its capacity.

Disposing of the Roof of a Vehicle That Is on Its Wheels

Folding back or removing the roof exposes the interior of an accident vehicle and provides the unrestricted working space that is so so important when there are seriously injured occupants.

Folding back the roof of even a full-size four-door sedan is neither a difficult nor lengthy operation for two persons to accomplish with hacksaws. In fact, two EMTs can usually fold back a roof in less than 3 minutes. When the vehicle is a compact passenger car that has narrow C-pillars, the roof can be removed altogether in about the same time.

The secrets to a quick and efficient operation are:

- Two rescuers working together, one on each side of the vehicle
- Not cutting trim and other components that can be easily removed
- Having unused high-speed shatterproof blades in the saw frames prior to starting the operation
- Having a spare saw that can be pressed into service immediately if one saw becomes inoperable for any reason
- Continually lubricating the saw blades during cutting efforts

---

Following is a procedure you might use to fold back the roof of a four-door sedan that has C-pillars that are too wide to cut with a hacksaw. The windshield and rear window have been removed, and the side windows have been rolled down or removed. Your partner is going to simultaneously carry out a similar procedure on the other side of the vehicle

- Use a short pry bar to strip plastic or chrome trim from the A-pillars. Pull away any U-shaped molding that has remained after the windshield was removed, or if the windshield was mastic-mounted, scrape off any gummy sealant where you will sever the A-pillar. This takes only a few seconds, and the effort may save valuable minutes. Chrome trim is difficult to cut, and plastic, rubber, and sealing materials tend to clog hacksaw blades.
- Cut the A-pillar first, as low as possible, but not so low that the front of the hacksaw will strike the dash. Hold the hacksaw firmly with both hands and make smooth, blade-

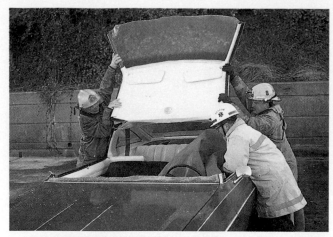

A. Folding back a section of a roof that has pillars too wide to sever with hacksaws.

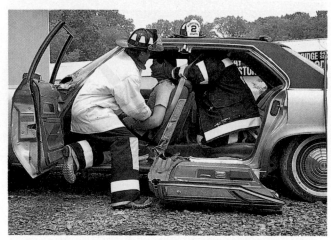

B. Disposing of the B-Pillar and Rear Door: More working space at the side of a four-door accident vehicle is gained by pulling down the B-pillar and rear door together.

FIGURE 27–10. Disposing of the roof of a vehicle that is on its wheels.

long cuts while exerting a steady downward force.

- As you cut, have someone lubricate the saw blade while supporting the roof edge with a hand or shoulder. Supporting the roof will keep the saw blade from binding.
- Next, cut the B-pillar. If you are going to displace the pillar and the rear door altogether, cut the pillar as high as possible; otherwise, cut the pillar as low as possible. More about this later.
- Climb onto the roof of the vehicle, kneel, and cut through the roof edge at a point just ahead of where the C-pillar starts. Cut as deep as the hacksaw frame will allow; then

tilt the saw down and again cut as deep as the saw frame will allow. Thus you will be sure that the rigid structure that makes up the edge of the roof is completely severed.

Cutting from a position on the roof is more efficient than cutting from a standing position at the side of the vehicle. When you are kneeling on the roof, your upper body weight and back and arm muscles will all be contributing to the cutting effort. When you finish making the right-angle cut into the roof edge, and when your partner has finished making a similar cut:

- Stand on the roof. Dimple the roof by placing your feet on an imaginary line between the two cuts and pressing down. At the same time, direct your partner and a person on the other side of the car to lift the cut section. When you can reach it, fold the cut section back into the uncut part. This will entail your stepping backward onto the trunk, so be careful.
- Secure the folded section in place with an elastic cargo strap, a length of rope, or a rescue chain if the chain set is not needed for another task.

If the car is a compact model with narrow C-pillars, simply cut through the pillars while other rescue personnel support the roof section. When the final cut is made, have them lift the cut section from the vehicle and carry it away.

Disposing of the B-Pillars and Rear Doors of a Four-Door Sedan

The rear doors of a four-door sedan will probably be in the way of patient removal efforts even if the doors are moved beyond their normal range of motion. You can dispose of a B-pillar and door in one operation by inserting the round edge of a 51-inch pinch bar into the stub of the severed pillar and pulling the pillar and the door down together. It is not a difficult operation, especially when the car is an intermediate-sized model or smaller.

Be aware that the technique will not work on older luxury cars that have massive, reinforced B-pillars, however. Before you spend any time attempting to displace the B-pillars and rear doors of a large, older car, look at the junction of the pillar with the rocker panel. If the pillar meets the rocker panel at a right angle, you will probably be able to pull the pillar down. If the bottom of the pillar curves inward, you will probably not be able to pull the pillar down.

Do not attempt to remove a rear door after pulling it down. It will serve as a convenient work platform.

Disposing of the Roof of a Vehicle That Is on Its Side

There are three ways in which injured persons can be removed from an accident vehicle that has been stabilized on its side: (1) through a door opening, (2) through a window opening, or (3) through an opening made in the vehicle.

Removing a person through a door opening when a vehicle is on its side is not an easy task, especially when the person is heavy and seriously injured. He has either to be pushed out by rescuers working inside the vehicle or pulled out by rescuers perched precariously atop the vehicle. In either case, the maneuvering that is necessary to get the person out is likely to aggravate existing injuries or cause new ones.

Removing a person through a windshield or rear window opening is possible only when the person is small enough to fit through the opening and may not be possible at all when the roof is partially crushed against the body of the vehicle.

Obviously, then, the proper procedure is to create a "doorway" in the vehicle by folding the roof down, folding the roof back, or making an opening in the roof. The first two procedures can be accomplished when a vehicle is stabilized with cribbing, while the third must be done when a jack has been used to stabilize the vehicle.

If you are thinking that a fourth technique is possible—removing the roof altogether—you are right. However, to do so is an unnecessary and difficult procedure. It's difficult to sever the roof pillars of the side of the vehicle that is closest to the ground.

In every case, the windshield and rear window must be out, the side windows must be rolled down or removed, and an EMT must be inside the vehicle to support and protect the occupants.

Folding the Roof Down

This procedure can be accomplished with hacksaws when the car has narrow C-pillars.

- Check to see that the cribs under the A- and C-pillars are tight. Make adjustments as necessary.
- Climb onto the vehicle so you can utilize your upper body weight and arm and back muscles while cutting.
- While one or two people support the roof and while someone lubricates your saw

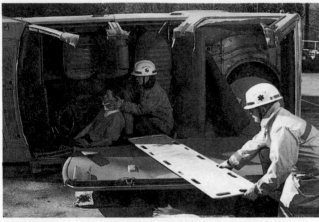

A. The roof has been folded down after the A-, B- and C-pillars were severed.

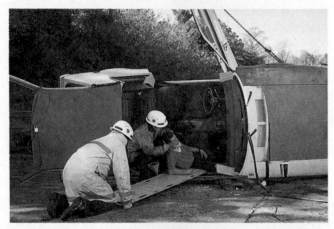

B. A section of the roof has been folded back. The C-pillars are too wide to sever with a hacksaw.

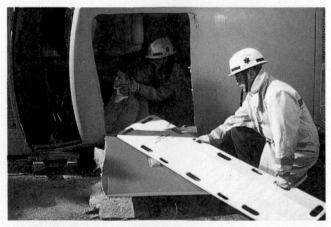

C. A three-sided flap was cut in the roof with a panel cutter. The roof could not be folded down or back because of the position of the stabilizing jack.

FIGURE 27–11. Disposing of the roof of a vehicle that is on its side.

blade, sever the A-, B-, and C-pillars in order. Climb down from the car.

- With your hands on the upper roof edge, gently pull the roof down. The points where the roof joins the A-, B-, and C-pillars on the uncut side will serve as hinges.

Don't be concerned about the vehicle becoming unstable. Remember that when a car is vertical the cribs are supporting very little weight. Moreover, the parts of the pillars that are being supported by the cribs are strong structural members.

Folding Back a Section of the Roof

Use this technique when a car's C-pillars are too wide to cut with a hacksaw.

- Make adjustments as necessary to assure that the cribs under the A- and C-pillars are tight.
- Sever the A- and B-pillars and make right-angle cuts into the roof edges just ahead of the C-pillars.
- While you dimple the roof between the right-angle cuts, instruct one or two assistants to fold the cut roof section back.
- Secure the cut section against the intact remainder of the roof with an elastic cargo strap, a length of rope, or a chain.

As you can imagine, the difficult part of this procedure will be severing the B-pillar that is closest to the ground. You may have to make the cut while standing in either the windshield or rear window opening.

Making an Opening in the Roof

If you have stabilized a vehicle on its side with a jack and cribbing or a spare wheel, you will have no choice other than to make an opening in the roof. The stabilizing jack will prevent you from folding the roof back or down.

- With the panel cutter, make a vertical cut downward from a point 5 inches from the side of the vehicle and 5 inches from the windshield opening. Drive the panel cutter down as far as you can.
- Have someone support the developing roof section so that it will not tend to drop down while you are making the second and third cuts.
- Next, make a horizontal cut along the upper-most side of the vehicle from a point about

6 inches from the rear window opening to the start of the first cut.

- Then make a vertical cut downward from the starting point of the second cut as far as you can drive the panel cutter.
- Dimple the metal and fold the cut section of roof down. You will probably have to stand on the crease to complete the fold.
- Cut the cloth headliner with a knife, pull out the headliner support rods, and cut the roof stiffeners with a hacksaw.

A problem common to all three techniques is that very sharp metal edges result from severing pillars and making an opening in the roof. Shield roof pillar stubs by making spiral wraps with 2-inch duct tape or by taping multitrauma dressings over the stubs. Shield sheet-metal edges by laying down strips of duct tape and folding the tape over the sharp edges.

Regardless of which technique you choose, when you are finished you will be able to quickly and easily move injured persons onto a long spine board with a rope sling.

REMOVING MECHANISMS OF INJURY FROM AROUND VICTIMS

After stabilizing a vehicle, removing the windshield and rear window, folding back or removing the roof, and either widening door openings or removing doors, you still may not be able to remove injured persons from an accident vehicle. Seat belts, the steering wheel and column, pedals, the seat, and the dash may individually, or in combination, be mechanisms of entrapment.

Removing Seat Belts from Injured Persons

While seat belts are seldom perceived as either mechanisms of injury or mechanisms of entrapment, they can be both. When a lap belt is buckled too high on a person's body, the abdominal organs and great vessels can be squeezed against the wearer's spine if the vehicle suddenly decelerates. A diagonal shoulder belt that is worn alone (not in conjunction with a lap belt, that is) can be particularly dangerous. The wearer is subject to a variety of injuries to the upper body from bruising to decapitation. As for being mechanisms of entrapment, seat belts will hold

a person in the wreckage of a vehicle until they are unbuckled or cut.

In their efforts to quickly help trapped and injured persons, untrained rescuers sometimes unbuckle seat belts without regard for the consequences of their hasty actions. They fail to realize that when the tension of a shoulder belt is suddenly released, the wearer's upper body may twist, and if there is a shoulder girdle injury, broken bone ends may override. When the tension of a lap belt is suddenly released, bleeding from an abdominal injury may become profuse.

Some emergency care procedures (the application of a cervical collar, for example) can be undertaken while a seat belt is still in place. Other proce-

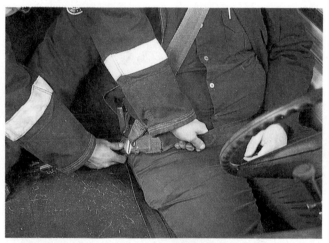

A. The seat belt is unbuckled and the parts are slowly separated so that pressure on internal injuries is not suddenly released.

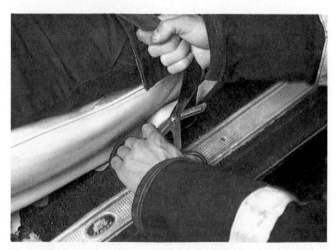

B. When it is not possible to unbuckle a seat belt, it should be cut close to the roller while manual tension is maintained on the lap belt.

FIGURE 27-12. Removing seat belts from around an injured person.

dures cannot be accomplished properly—or in some cases, at all—without first removing the seat belt. A sling and swathe cannot be applied when a shoulder belt is snug against the wearer's body. Unbuckling or cutting belts is the answer; but before you do, be sure that someone is supporting the victim.

Some operational guidelines call for the removal of a lap belt and the immediate securing of cravats around a person's body to maintain pressure on bleeding vessels when abdominal injuries are suspected. However, it may be better to leave a lap belt in place while carrying out the rest of the disentanglement procedures; then unbuckle or cut the belt just when you are ready to remove the injured person from the vehicle. Follow the protocol established for your EMS unit.

Unbuckling Seat Belts

As is the case for many other vehicle rescue operations, there's a right way and a wrong way to do something as simple as unbuckling a seat belt. Don't just push the release button with your finger. If the belt is under a great deal of tension, the ends will fly apart and pressure on the lower abdomen that was imposed by the belt will be released in a split second. Instead:

- Hold the buckle end of the belt with one hand and the mating part with your other hand. When you have a tight grip on both parts of the belt, depress the button with a thumb. Allow the belt parts to separate slowly.

A sudden deterioration of the person's condition upon release from a seat belt is a signal of increased abdominal bleeding. Be ready to take appropriate measures.

Cutting Seat Belts

While it's highly unlikely that the quick-release buckles of seat belts will not operate after an accident, it's possible. When you find that you cannot unbuckle a seat belt in the usual manner, don't simply cut through the webbing and allow the parts of the belt to spring apart. Instead:

- Grip the belt tightly with one hand close to the roller mechanism.
- Cut the webbing with your utility shears, a seat belt cutter, or a very sharp knife at a point between your hand and the roller mechanism. When the webbing is severed, move your hand slowly to release tension on the belt.

One final point about seat belts. Cutting seat belts need not always precede other disentanglement activities. A combination shoulder and lap belt restraint system may hold the wearer upright in the seat while you and your partner carry out other emergency care and rescue procedures. The "third pair of hands" that a seat belt offers will be welcome when there is much to do and few people to do it.

Coping with the Steering Column

The steering apparatus of an accident vehicle can be a major impediment to patient and rescue activities. The steering wheel can prevent you from effectively immobilizing a driver who may have a spinal injury. The steering column can prevent you from quickly freeing a driver's legs from mechanisms of entrapment under the dashboard.

The "Hollywood" approach to disposing of a vehicle's steering column (so-called because it is dramatic!) is to virtually pull the column through the windshield opening with a powerful hydraulic rescue tool. In reality, this procedure is time consuming and dangerous.

The practice is dangerous for several reasons. Pieces of metal and plastic invariably break away and fly for a considerable distance when a steering column is displaced upward. Tilt and telescoping steering columns have been known to break apart when displacing forces were applied. And when steering columns of front-wheel-drive cars are displaced, the joint that is on the passenger compartment side of the firewall can fail.

Displacing a steering column is often unnecessary. Some more easily accomplished steps may be all that are necessary to create working space in front of an injured driver.

Shortening the Steering Column and Raising the Steering Wheel

The first step in creating working space is to shorten a telescoping steering column if the vehicle has one. To have maximum leg room, tall motorists often drive with the seat all the way back and the steering column in the fully extended position. While some motorists drive with the steering wheel of a tilting column in the fully raised position, others drive with the wheel fully depressed.

- Before you do anything else to create working space in front of an injured driver, determine whether the vehicle has a tilt and telescoping steering column. If it does, disengage the friction lock mechanism. Push the steering wheel to its fully retracted position. Then operate the adjustment lever and tilt the wheel up as far as it will go.

Depending on the make and model of the car and the position of the wheel at the time of the accident, pushing the wheel toward the firewall may create 2 inches of working space in front of the driver, and tilting the wheel up may move the lower edge of the wheel almost 5 inches from the driver's lap. While this may not be enough room for the application of a spine immobilization device, it will at least make the wheel more accessible for subsequent steps.

Moving the Seat Backward

Moving the front seat backward takes only seconds and may create as much as 8 or 9 inches or working space between the steering wheel and an injured driver. It is not unusual for the seat adjustment mechanism to remain intact and operable and the seat tracks to remain undamaged even after a severe collision. If the vehicle has motorized seats and you have left the electrical system intact, moving the front seat backward may be a matter of merely operating the adjustment switch.

If the vehicle has a manually adjustable bench seat, use the following procedure after applying a rigid collar to minimize the chance that a cervical spine injury will be aggravated.

- While your partner supports the driver from behind or from the side, kneel at the driver's door opening. Direct another person to kneel at the passenger door opening.
- While you operate the seat adjustment lever with one hand and push on the front of the seat with your other hand, and while the person on the other side also pushes, carefully move the seat backward.

Always have another person help you move a manually adjustable bench seat. If you attempt to move the seat alone, the chance is good that it will angle on the tracks and thus become immovable.

Removing a Section of the Steering Wheel

When it is not possible to move the front seat backward, or when moving the seat does not provide adequate working space in front of an injured driver, removing a section of the steering wheel should be the next step. Before you do, however, make sure that the driver is protected by a rigid shield. A hacksaw blade will easily cut through the plastic covering and the iron core of a steering wheel.

- Rotate the wheel, if possible, to gain maximum space in front of the driver when you remove a portion of the wheel. If the wheel has only two spokes, rotate it so the spokes are horizontal.
- Direct another person to take a position on the seat next to the driver. Have him reach across the wheel and grip the rim at a point about 2 inches below the spoke. When the person has a firm grip on the wheel, sever the rim just below the spoke while he lubricates the saw blade.
- When you have finished the cut, pass the saw over the steering column to your assistant. Reach across the wheel and grip the rim at a point about 2 inches below the spoke. While you support the rim and lubricate the saw blade, have the person sever the rim at a point between the spoke and your hand. Remove the cut portion of the wheel.

At this point you may be wondering why you should make only one cut and then pass the saw to your assistant. Cutting the closest part of the rim while you are standing at the side of the vehicle will be no problem. Leaning across the wheel to sever the other part of the rim will put you slightly off balance, however. If you slip while you are cutting the wheel or if you drop the saw, the blade might cause injury to the driver's leg.

A large bolt cutter can be used to remove part of a steering column, but the technique is slower since it may be necessary to break away the plastic covering of the wheel at the cutting points so the iron core will fit in the jaws of the cutter. Moreover, the cutter is difficult to handle and can cause injury if dropped onto the driver's legs.

Removing the Steering Wheel Altogether

Unless a steering wheel has massive spokes, removal is seldom difficult. Protect the driver by placing a short spine board between him and the steering wheel.

- While another person holds the wheel steady and lubricates the saw blade, use a hacksaw to cut through each spoke of the wheel at a point close to the hub. Do not bother removing any of the metal or plastic trim from the wheel assembly; the task is usually time consuming and difficult. Simply cut through everything. Have a second hacksaw immediately available in case the first one becomes inoperable for any reason.

Severing the Steering Column

There may be times when you will not be able to employ any of the techniques suggested thus far. You may not be able to move a motor-operated seat because the vehicle's electrical system has been disrupted, and you may not be able to move a manually adjustable seat because of damage. For any of a number of reasons, you may decide that even removing a steering wheel will not provide sufficient working room for patient care activities.

To an untrained individual, severing a steering column sounds like a lengthy and difficult task. It really is not. Although many columns appear massive, most consist of nothing more than some concentric metal tubes around an iron shaft that has a diameter of less than 1 inch. If the diameter of the column assembly at a point where it can be cut is less than the distance between the blade and the back of the hacksaw frame, you can probably sever it with a hacksaw. In most accident situations, you should be able to sever a steering column with a hacksaw in less than 2 minutes—about half the time it takes to rig equipment for displacing the column.

- First, disconnect the battery from the vehicle's electrical system.

This is a step that must not be overlooked. As you move the saw blade through the column, it will sever wires that lead to and from the horn button, the turn signal control box, the ignition switch, and in some cars a cruise-control device, the windshield wiper controls, and the headlight and parking light controls. If the electrical system remains intact, arcing may occur when the wiring harness is severed. The vehicle may start as if someone has turned the ignition key, and if the transmission is engaged, the vehicle will lurch forward, perhaps with disastrous results!

- Next, have your partner or another person shield the driver's legs with a short wood spine board or other rigid device.
- While someone lubricates the saw blade, cut through the column at a convenient point just above the point where the steering column is attached to the underside of the dash.

Displacing the Column

Be aware that even though the techniques just described are faster and safer, there may be times when you have no choice other than to displace a steering column. There may not be sufficient working space for a hacksaw, or the column may be too large to sever with a hacksaw.

Scansheet 27-4 shows several techniques that can be used to displace a steering column from both outside and inside the vehicle. Two different chain wraps are shown—one for a nontilting column and one for a tilting column. Two different anchor chain rigs are also illustrated—one for a rear-wheel-drive car and one for a front-wheel-drive car that has a jointed column. Experiences with hydraulic rescue tools have shown that when a diagonal pull is exerted on a jointed column there is less chance that the joint just inside the firewall will fail.

Note that cribbing has been laid in the manner of a railroad track to cause the column chain to pull at a more efficient angle and to prevent the chain from cutting into the soft dash.

A Hi-Lift® jack can be used to displace a steering column when a hand winch is not available or inoperable. The jack is positioned so it exerts lift on the joined anchor and column chains. A Hi-Lift® jack can also be used to lift the column from inside the vehicle when the driver's legs are not in the way.

> AN IMPORTANT POINT: When you must displace a steering column, do not move it any more than is necessary to achieve the desired working space. The greater the force exerted on the column, the greater is the chance that it will break.

Freeing a Driver's Foot from Entrapment by a Pedal

When vehicles had brake and clutch pedals with shafts that passed through the floor pan, it was not unusual for a driver to have at least one foot trapped as the result of front end collision. The problem is not nearly as severe today since few cars have clutch pedals and since brake pedals are usually suspended from a pivot point. Nonetheless, you may respond to an accident location and discover that a driver's foot is trapped by a pedal or that a pedal will interfere with the movement of an injured foot. Several techniques can be used to deal with troublesome pedals.

Disassembling the Pedal

If damage to the firewall is not severe, you may be able to pull the pin from the pivot point with pliers and simply move the pedal out of the way.

Removing the Driver's Foot from the Shoe

More often than not it is a driver's shoe that is trapped by a pedal, not the foot. If the edge of the pedal has creased the leather or fabric over the point

A

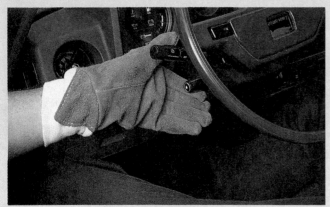

Shortening a tilt-and-telescoping steering column and raising the wheel is the first step.

B

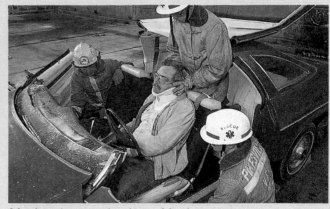

Moving the seat backward is the next step.

C

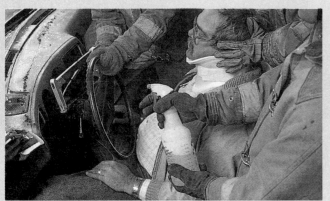

A section of the steering wheel should be cut away with a hacksaw if the first steps do not create the needed space.

D

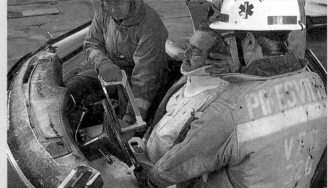

The next step is to remove the steering wheel altogether.

E

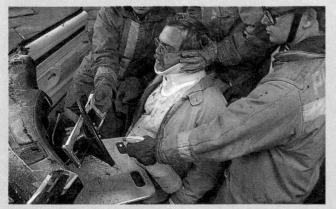

Severing the steering column provides maximum working space in front of an injured driver.

F

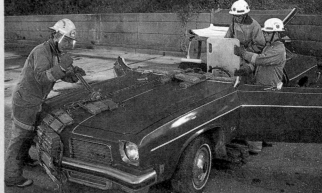

A column that cannot be severed must be displaced. In this case, the column is being moved with a hand winch.

where the toes join the instep, the person may not be able to withdraw the foot. This is especially true when the edge of a pedal is pressed into the leather just behind the steel toe cap of a work shoe.

- If a part of the pedal does not appear to be pressed so deeply into the shoe that the foot is injured, use pocket shears or aircraft snips to cut away the entire heel section of the shoe. Then carefully try to ease the foot from the shoe.

If you are unable to slide the foot from the shoe, or if you are hesitant to do so because of a possible injury to the foot, you will have to take steps to dispose of the pedal.

Severing the Pedal

If the pedal does not have the massive stamped shaft that is common to many older luxury cars and if there is sufficient working space, you should be able to sever a pedal shaft with the low-profile hacksaw that is suggested for the rescue tool inventory. It can be operated in a space that is too small for a full-sized hacksaw.

- While your partner or another person maintains a constant upward force on the pedal from a position at the driver's right side, sever the pedal shaft from behind.

If you attempt to sever the shaft by cutting from the top down in the usual manner, the saw blade will probably bind. If you cut the shaft from behind, the upward force on the pedal exerted by your partner will tend to separate the cut portion as the blade passes through the shaft. Moreover, your partner will be relieving any pressure that the pedal may have been imposing on the trapped foot.

Remember that lubricating the blade is important and that good illumination is necessary when it is necessary to work close to a body part in a confined space.

Displacing the Pedal

Displacing a pedal with a length of manila rope is a disentanglement technique that has been used for many years. A common practice was to secure one end of the rope to the pedal and the other end to the window frame of the right front door and then to pull the door to move the pedal. Today, doors are usually moved beyond their normal range of motion or removed altogether long before any attention is given to pedals. Nonetheless, a pedal can some-

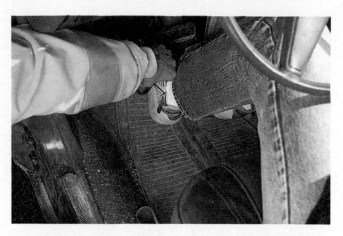

A. It may be possible to remove the pedal by disconnecting it from the point of attachment or cutting the back of the driver's shoe. Sliding the foot from the shoe may be possible if the pedal is not pressing into the foot.

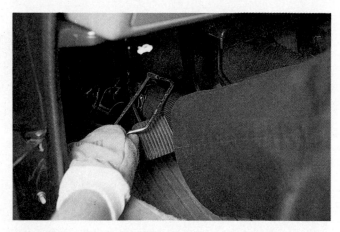

B. It may be possible to sever the pedal shaft with a low-profile hacksaw.

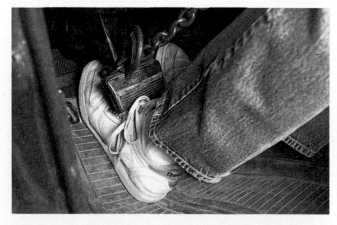

C. When all else fails, the pedal can be displaced with a hand winch rigged as for displacing the steering column.

FIGURE 27–13. Freeing a driver's foot from entrapment by a pedal.

times be displaced by a pulling effort, only now the effort is exerted by one or two people pulling on a rescue chain. Don't simply drop the slip hook of a chain over the pedal shaft and yank, however.

- First, examine the pedal and the trapped foot with the aid of a light. Visualize the path that the pedal will take when it is displaced. Determine whether the left lower corner of the pedal will drop down when the shaft is pulled toward the right door. If it does, even for just half an inch, it may aggravate an existing injury.
- If you feel that displacing the pedal will not be a problem, have your partner pass the end of the chain to you from a position at the right front door opening. Drop the slip hook of the chain over the pedal shaft with the throat facing down.
- While you support and protect the foot, instruct your partner to exert a slow, steady pull on the chain until the pedal is moved the desired distance. Then instruct your partner to secure the chain to the stub of the A-pillar or another convenient anchor point to keep the pedal from springing back to its original position.

If you feel that none of the techniques suggested so far will be successful or if they prove unsuccessful, use a hand winch to displace the pedal. The winch is rigged in the same manner suggested for displacing the steering column.

Displacing the Front Seat of a Passenger Car

You may arrive at the scene of an accident and find the driver on the floor ahead of the front seat. He may have dived there when he saw that the crash was inevitable, or he may have been thrown there upon impact.

One technique for removing a person from the floor of a vehicle has been used for years. Three or four people stand side-by-side behind the front seat (or crouch if the roof is in place). They lean over the seat, grip the person's clothing, and lift him like a sack of potatoes onto a long spine board that has been placed on the front seat.

By today's standards of emergency care, this procedure is unacceptable. If a rescuer's foot slips, or if a rescuer loses balance, or if the patient's clothing rips, the person may drop back onto the floor. Existing injuries can be worsened, and new injuries can be produced.

A better way is to displace the front seat backward and pull the injured person onto a long spine board with a rope sling while his body is maintained in a straight line.

Following is a procedure for displacing the one-piece bench seat of a passenger car with a hand winch and chain set. It is not a two-person procedure, however; recruit firefighters, first responders, or police officers to help you.

- Apply a rigid cervical collar while your partner manually stabilizes the victim's head from a position at the right front door. Your partner will have to remain in place throughout the remainder of the procedure.
- Have two assistants, one kneeling at the driver's door and the other kneeling at the right door, position a long spine board between the victim and the seat bottom. They, too, will remain in place throughout the procedure.
- Remove the bottom of the back seat so that the front seat can be moved backward for more than just a few inches.
- Rig the long rescue chain to a frame member under the right side of the vehicle as you would in preparation for displacing a steering column or moving a door. While an assistant holds the chain in place, position cribbing under parts of the vehicle that are likely to collapse when the chain is under tension.
- While the person continues to hold the chain in place, shorten the chain with the grab hook so that the ring is just resting on the trunk lid. Catch the ring with the fixed hook of the hand winch.
- Wrap the short chain around the seat in such a way that the chain will pull the seat backward on the tracks. Catch the ring of the chain with the running hook of the hand winch's chain or cable.
- Place cribbing under the hand winch and under the chain or cable at any point where the chain or cable is likely to snag or chafe.
- While the assistant that is kneeling at the driver's door holds the seat adjustment lever in the operating position, operate the hand winch until the right side of the seat breaks free.
- As soon as the spring that is part of the seat adjustment mechanism is visible, have someone use the bolt cutter to sever it.
- Continue to operate the hand winch until the seat is displaced the desired distance.

SCAN 27—5 DISPLACING THE BENCH SEAT OF A PASSENGER CAR

A

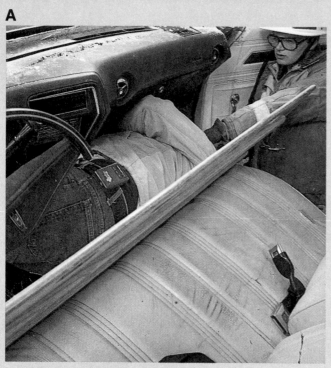

The victim is protected with a long spine board held by people on both sides of the vehicle.

B

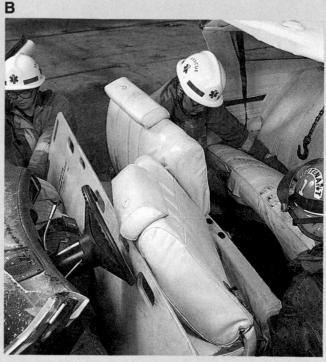

The bottom of the rear seat is removed so the front seat can be pulled back more than just a few inches.

C

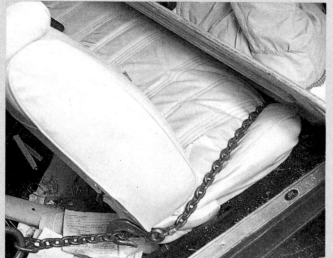

The chain is wrapped around the seat in such a way that pull will be exerted on the seat, not the tracks.

D

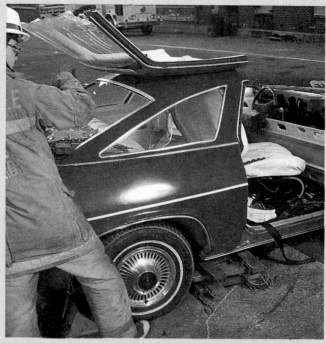

The hand winch is rigged to an anchor point under the car, joined to the seat chain, and operated to displace the seat.

Properly securing the short chain around the seat bottom is an important part of this procedure; pull must be exerted on the seat bottom, not the seat support. The 2-ton hand winch that is recommended for the ambulance inventory may not develop sufficient force to either shear the seat support bolts or pull the seat support from the floor. As the one side of the seat is pulled back, the other side may break loose from the track. If it does, cut the spring on that side, unhook the chain from the right side, and remove the seat from the vehicle. Instead of just a portion, the entire interior of the vehicle will become working space.

Displacing the Dash Assembly of an Accident Vehicle

In some unusual (but not impossible) head-on crash situations, it may be desirable to displace the dashboard upward away from a person who is either on the floor ahead of the front seat or rolled up against the firewall.

One of the more difficult tasks for EMTs working with hand tools is displacing a crushed dash. Even rescue squad personnel with power tools have trouble moving dashboards when victims are close to the crumpled metal. Nonetheless, you can move a dash with a hand winch and chain set and a little patience.

Proper victim protection is essential since the technique described below will cause plastic parts to shatter. Small pieces may fly for some distance with considerable velocity, and heavier pieces will drop when they break free.

- Rig the anchor strap and winch in the manner suggested for displacing a steering column.
- Use the wedge end of a forcible entry tool or a pinch bar to make an opening close to the center of the dash. Drive the tool downward through a "soft" spot in the dash, such as a speaker opening or a defroster vent.
- Pass the slip hook of the short rescue chain through the opening. Carry it up in front of the dash and join it to the grab hook to form a loop.
- While your partner or another person holds the chain in place, position two or three pieces of cribbing between the chain and the lower edge of the dash. Catch the ring of the short chain with the running hook of the hand winch.
- Arrange pieces of cribbing on the dash in the manner of a railroad track to give the

chain lift and to prevent the chain from snagging. Place cribbing under the hand winch.
- Operate the hand winch to collapse the dash and at the same time pull it upward.

With openings made in the vehicle and components removed from around the victims, the next step is to package the people and remove them from the wreckage.

SUMMARY

There are three parts to the disentanglement phase of a vehicle rescue operation:

- Protecting the occupants of the accident vehicle.
- Creating openings in the vehicle through which the occupants can be removed.
- Removing mechanisms of entrapment from around trapped occupants.

Accident victims must be shielded from contact with tools and debris generated during disentanglement efforts and from the elements.

Existing openings can be enlarged or new ones can be made in an accident vehicle. Doors can be moved beyond their normal range of motion, and the roof can be folded back or removed altogether.

Manually move undamaged doors when sufficient personnel are available. Use a hand winch to move doors beyond their normal range of motion when the doors are severely damaged or when you are working alone.

Fold back a section of the roof or remove the roof altogether when there are seriously injured people on both the front and rear seat, and whenever it is necessary to immobilize known or suspected spinal injuries.

Use one of two techniques to expose the interior of an accident vehicle that is on its side and at the same time create a large pathway through which injured persons can be removed. Fold the roof down or fold a section of the roof back when the vehicle is stabilized with cribbing. Make an opening in the roof when the vehicle is stabilized with a jack.

Remove seat belts from around an accident victim in such a way that pressure on injuries will not be suddenly released. If a seat belt is holding an unconscious person upright, consider leaving the belt in place while you carry out assessment, certain emergency care, and disentanglement operations. The belt will serve as a third pair of hands.

Follow this sequence of events when you need working space in front of an injured driver. First, shorten the steering column if it is a telescoping model. Then attempt to move the seat back. If this does not provide the room that you need, remove a section of the steering wheel or remove the steering wheel altogether. If there is still not enough room for patient care efforts, sever or displace the steering column.

Free a driver's foot from entrapment by a pedal by disassembling the pedal, removing the driver's foot from the shoe (if appropriate), and/or severing or displacing the pedal.

A person can be easily removed from the floor ahead of the bench seat of a vehicle after one side of the seat has been displaced backward with a hand winch. Be sure to remove the rear seat bottom so that the front seat can be moved the maximum distance.

Use a hand winch to displace the dash assembly when you need space to care for and remove an injured person who has rolled up against the firewall of an accident vehicle.

The Esophageal Obturator Airway

The esophageal obturator airway (EOA) is a primary airway adjunct that has been in use since 1973. One can be used to establish and maintain an airway in a person who is in respiratory or cardiac arrest or in a trauma patient who is unconscious with no gag reflex.

The principal advantage of an EOA is that it can be positioned without moving the patient's head; thus it is especially well suited for maintaining an airway in a person who may have a cervical spine injury. A disadvantage is that an EOA is ineffective if the face mask does not make a tight seal with the patient's face.

The plastic, semirigid tube of an esopageal obturator airway is 34 centimeters (cm) long and 13 millimeters (mm) in diameter; it has a smooth, rounded, closed lower end. The upper one-third of the tube has 16 holes that serve as passageways for the air that is intended for the lungs. When the tube is properly positioned, the holes are at the level of the pharynx and the lower two-thirds of the tube rests in the esophagus. A cuff at the lower end of the airway is inflated with air from a syringe to block the esophagus. The cuff prevents air from reaching the stomach and prevents stomach contents from being regurgitated up to the airway.

The inflatable face mask is designed to fit snugly over the patient's mouth and nose and make a tight seal. Air introduced through the opening in the face mask passes through the upper portion of the airway and exits through the holes in the tube. Ventilations can be delivered by the mouth-to-adjunct method, with a bag-valve-mask unit, or with a manually triggered, oxygen-powered ventilator.

Use of an EOA should be limited to deeply unconscious persons over the age of 16 years and over 5 feet tall. **An EOA should *not* be placed in:**

- Persons who are conscious or semiconscious, since the tube will trigger the gag reflex. Vomiting is likely, and with vomiting there is always the danger of vomitus being aspirated into the lungs.
- Children under the age of 16 years. There is only one size of EOA, and it is too large for children.
- Persons who have ingested a corrosive poison such as lye. The tip of the EOA may perforate the injured esophagus.
- Persons with a known esophageal disease such as cancer of the esophagus. Again, the tip of the airway may be pushed through the wall of the disease-weakened esophagus.
- Persons with significant upper airway bleeding. Blood flowing from nose or mouth injuries will pass directly into the lungs once the balloon has occluded the esophagus.

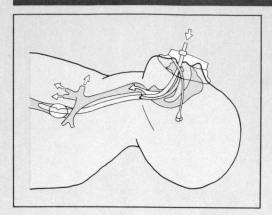

NOTE: If your medical advisor has approved the use of EOA, practice insertion in a manikin until you are proficient. The tube of an EOA is perforated in the upper third of its length. When tube is in place, the inflated cuff fills the area between tube and esophagus. Air forced through perforations is prevented from entering stomach. The inflatable face mask provides a tight seal over patient's mouth and nose.

DO NOT USE EOA WHEN PATIENT:

- Is conscious and/or breathing
- Has a gag reflex
- Is under 16 years old or under 5 ft. tall
- Has facial injury preventing tight seal
- Has known esophageal disease
- Has ingested known caustic

1

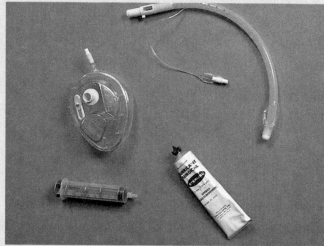

EOA kit with a water base surgical lubricant.

2

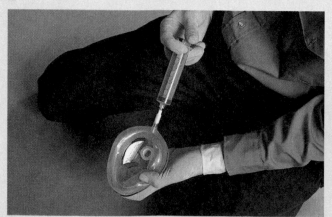

Draw 35 cc of air into syringe. Insert it into one-way valve of face mask. Inflate cushion.

3

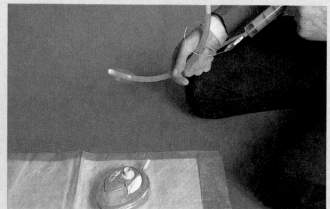

Test tube cuff by injecting 35 cc of air through valve. If cuff is usable, withdraw air and attach tube to mask. Lubricate tip of tube.

4

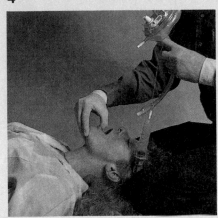

Lift jaw and tongue straight upward without hyperextending neck. Caution: A patient regaining consciousness may bite.

5

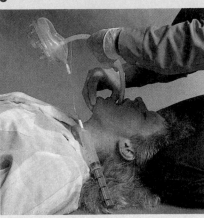

Advance airway carefully behind tongue and into pharynx and esophagus.

6

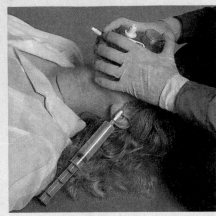

Hold mask in place with both hands.

7

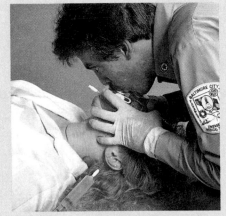

Test airway by blowing into mouth piece. Watch patient's chest rise. Remove and re-insert if chest does not rise.

8

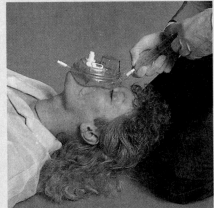

Inflate cuff with 35 cc of air from syringe. Remove syringe.

9

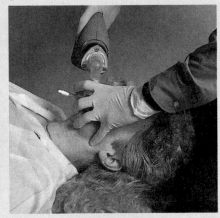

Ventilate by mouth-to-mask, bag-valve-mask, or positive pressure oxygen device.

REMOVING AN EOA: Be alert for vomiting. Do not deflate cuff or remove EOA until:

- Patient has resumed breathing
- Endotracheal tube is inserted and its cuff is inflated in trachea

When the tube is removed:
1. Have suction equipment ready for immediate use
2. Turn the patient on his side
3. Insert syringe into one-way valve and withdraw air slowly from the cuff
4. Carefully remove the tube

The EOA is intended for short-term use (up to 2 hours) and must be removed from a patient when spontaneous respirations resume.

Inserting and Using an EOA

As with any nonbreathing patient, no time must be lost in initiating basic life-support procedures while preparing an airway for use.

While your partner establishes an airway and ventilates the patient by the mouth-to-mouth technique or, better yet, with oxygen-enriched air from a bag-valve-mask unit:

- Inflate the tube cuff with 20 cubic centimeters (cc) of air (15 cc for new tubes) from the syringe and check the cuff for leaks. If the cuff is intact:
- Deflate the cuff with the syringe.
- Fill the syringe with 35 cc of air and set it aside where it will be immediately accessible.
- Connect the face mask to the tube. Rotate it into position until it locks in place.
- Check the face mask for proper inflation. The cushion of the face mask can be inflated to whatever pressure is desired; however, experience has shown that a soft cushion fits and seals better than one that is inflated to the point of being firm.
- Lubricate the lower two-thirds of the tube with a water-soluble gel such as K-Y Jelly. Do not use a silicone preparation, petroleum jelly, or another oil-based lubricant.

As soon as your partner has ventilated the patient:

- Insert your thumb deeply into the person's mouth and grasp the tongue and lower jaw between your thumb and index finger.
- Lift the tongue and jaw straight upward. This will remove the tongue from the back of the throat where it might prevent passage of the tube.

If your patient has been injured and there is the possibility of a cervical spine injury, have your partner maintain the person's head in a neutral position while you insert the tube.

If there is no likelihood of a cervical spine injury, resist any urge to tilt the head back with the objective of improving the airway and thus making insertion easier. The tube is designed to be inserted with the head in a neutral or slightly flexed position. Flexion will decrease the risk of passing the end of the tube into the larynx and trachea, while extension will increase the risk.

While you maintain an open airway:

- Grasp the airway with your other hand so it curves in the same direction as the natural curvature of the pharynx.
- Insert the tip of the airway into the patient's mouth and advance it carefully behind the tongue into the pharynx and esophagus. Do not use force.

If the tube does not advance easily:

- Either redirect the tube or withdraw it and start over after your partner ventilates the patient.

One reason for a tube not passing easily is excessive curvature, a problem that results from storing the EOA into too small a container where it remains bent for a long period. An EOA should always be stored in either the shipping box or a case designed especially for the device.

When the tube passes behind the tongue and into the pharynx:

- Advance the airway until the mask is seated on the patient's face.

To check for proper positioning of the tube:

- Hold the mask firmly on the patient's face with both hands and blow into the opening in the mask.

If the chest rises, the airway is in the esophagus. This occurs in most cases. If the chest does not rise, the airway has passed into and is blocking the trachea. If you suspect that this is the case, immediately remove the airway and have your partner continue artificial ventilation until you are ready to make another attempt at insertion. The position of the tube can also be determined with a stethoscope.

While you deliver breaths through the face mask, have your partner listen for breath sounds over both lung fields with a stethoscope. If the tube is in the esophagus, breath sounds will be heard over both lungs. If it is in the right mainstem bronchus, breath sounds will be heard only over the left lung. If the tube is in the trachea, your partner will not be able to hear any breath sounds. As with a visual determination, remove the EOA if there is any doubt as to whether the tube is in the esophagus, and reinsert the tube after your partner ventilates the patient.

When the airway is properly positioned in the esophagus:

- Inflate the tube cuff by injecting 15 cc of air through the one-way valve with the syringe. Do not overinflate the cuff; to do so may cause the esophagus to rupture.
- Remove the syringe. The one-way valve will keep the cuff inflated.

When the cuff is inflated:

- Ventilate the patient by the mouth-to-mask technique, with a bag-valve-mask unit or with a manually triggered, oxygen-powered ventilator.

It is vitally important that you hold the mask firmly against the patient's face during ventilations. If you are delivering breaths mouth-to-mask, this will be no problem; you can hold the mask in place with both hands. But if you are using a bag-valve-mask unit or an oxygen-powered ventilator, you will have only one hand free to hold the mask. Minimize the chance of air or oxygen leaking from under the cushion by using your thumb and index finger to hold the mask against the face and your other three fingers to hold the mandible against the mask.

Removing the EOA

Be prepared to remove the EOA if spontaneous respirations and the gag and swallowing reflexes return while a person is still in your care.

- Turn the patient onto one side.
- Have a suction unit ready for immediate use. Vomiting will usually occur when an EOA is removed.
- Deflate the cuff with the syringe.
- Remove the EOA.
- Suction the patient, if necessary, and support respirations with oxygen.

Using the Pharyngo-Tracheal Lumen (PtL®) Airway

An EMT's first concern while evaluating a patient must be the establishment of an open airway. If this is not accomplished, all further prehospital emergency care procedures may be useless.

Several adjunctive airways are available for use by emergency medical service personnel, including the simple oropharyngeal airway, the esophageal obturator airway (EOA), and the endotracheal tube (ETT).

The oropharyngeal airway is the most commonly used device for establishing and maintaining an open airway. Unfortunately, it is also the least effective, for it does little more than keep a person's tongue from occluding his airway.

The esophageal obturator airway (EOA) is an improvement over the oropharyngeal airway in that it prevents aspiration of gastric contents. Unfortunately, there are two problems associated with use of an EOA. First, tests have shown that an EOA delivers significantly less air than a face mask used in conjunction with an oropharyngeal airway and less air than an endotracheal tube. Second, an EOA does not protect the lower airway from upper airway hemorrhage and secretions.

The endotracheal tube offers the best method of airway management to date. It protects the patient's lungs from aspiration of either gastric contents or fluids from the upper airway, and it delivers effective ventilations. However, EMTs are not usu-

ally trained in the use of the ETT, skills degradation may be a problem when a trained individual must insert an ETT after a period of inactivity, and the use of an ETT is contraindicated in certain situations. For example, the hyperextension of the neck that is necessary when inserting an ETT in a person who may have a cervical spine injury may aggravate that injury.

The *pharyngo-tracheal lumen airway* (PtL®) is a device that can be easily inserted into the trachea or esophagus of a patient with minimum skill. The airway is designed as a tube within a tube, and for that reason is sometimes referred to as a double-lumen airway.

A long endotracheal-type tube is located within a short, large-diameter tube. The distal end of the long tube opens into either the trachea or the esophagus, while the short tube opens into the retropharynx above the epiglottis. Both tubes have low-pressure cuffs at their distal ends. On the long tube, the cuff provides a seal for either the trachea or esophagus, depending on placement. On the short tube, the larger-volume cuff seals off the oropharynx when fully inflated. When the PtL® is placed in the esophagus, the large cuff diverts air delivered through the short tube into the trachea. Both tubes are fitted with standard 15-mm adapters to allow universal connection to ventilatory devices. Inflation lines are provided in order that the cuffs may be inflated si-

Parts of the PtL® Airway:

A

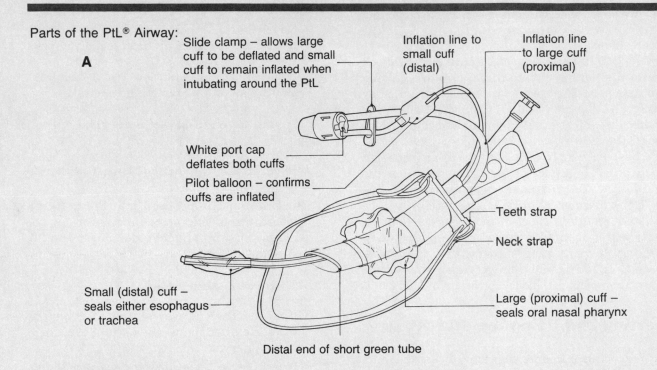

Slide clamp – allows large cuff to be deflated and small cuff to remain inflated when intubating around the PtL

Inflation line to small cuff (distal)

Inflation line to large cuff (proximal)

White port cap deflates both cuffs

Pilot balloon – confirms cuffs are inflated

Teeth strap

Neck strap

Small (distal) cuff – seals either esophagus or trachea

Large (proximal) cuff – seals oral nasal pharynx

Distal end of short green tube

B

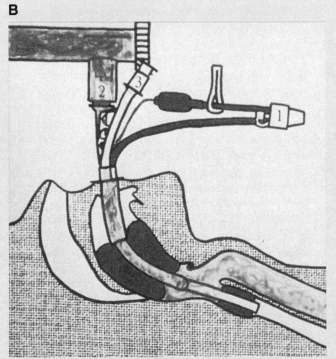

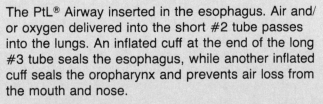

The PtL® Airway inserted in the esophagus. Air and/or oxygen delivered into the short #2 tube passes into the lungs. An inflated cuff at the end of the long #3 tube seals the esophagus, while another inflated cuff seals the oropharynx and prevents air loss from the mouth and nose.

C

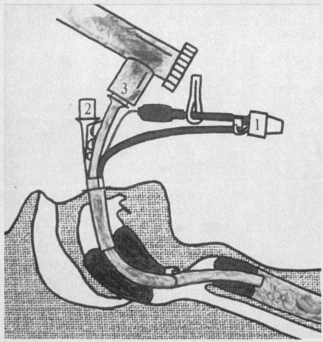

The PtL® Airway inserted in the trachea. Air and/or oxygen is delivered into the long #3 tube after the stylet is removed. The inflated cuff at the end of the long tube keeps air from leaking from the trachea into the esophagus. The large cuff that is sealing the oropharynx serves as a secondary seal.

multaneously or separately as desired. A stylet is provided to facilitate insertion, and a plastic bite block prevents the patient's teeth from occluding the airway. A neck strap secures the airway to the patient's head.

The PtL® airway is inserted until the bite block contacts the patient's teeth. Both cuffs are inflated simultaneously. The rescuer attempts ventilation by blowing into the short tube. If the chest rises, the long tube has entered the esophagus and ventilations through the airway can be initiated without delay. If the chest does not rise, the long tube has intubated the trachea. The stylet is then removed from the long tube and the patient is ventilated through this tube in the manner of an ETT. The patient may be ventilated mouth-to-tube, with a bag-valve-mask unit, or with a manually triggered, oxygen-powered ventilator. If ventilating through the short tube, catheters may be passed through the airways to suction the stomach, oral cavity, or bronchial tree.

Inserting and Using the PtL® Airway

Following is the procedure suggested for establishing an airway and ventilating an unconscious, non-breathing person with a PtL®.

While your partner initiates artificial ventilation or CPR and verifies an open airway:

- Prepare the PtL® airway. Insure that both cuffs are fully deflated, that the long clear #3 tube has a bend in the middle, and that the white cap is securely in place over the deflation port located under the #1 inflation valve.

To facilitate insertion:

- Lubricate the tube with a water-soluble jelly (such as K-Y jelly) if available. Do not use a silicone preparation, petroleum jelly, or another oil-based lubricant.

If the patient has facial injuries:

- Quickly sweep the mouth with your finger and remove broken teeth and dentures.

This is an important step that must not be overlooked. Broken teeth and/or broken dentures can interfere with the passing of the tube. Moreover, either can tear the cuffs.

When the patient and the airway are ready, insertion should be accomplished quickly between ventilations.

If the patient may have a cervical spine injury:

- Have your partner stabilize the person's head in the neutral position while you pass the well-lubricated PtL® airway with minimal cervical manipulation. Use a thumb-in-mouth, jaw-lift, or tongue-lift method.

If you have ruled out a cervical spine injury:

- Hyperextend the patient's head with one hand, then:
- Insert your thumb deep into the patient's mouth; grasp the tongue and lower jaw between your thumb and index finger and lift straight upward.

With your other hand:

- Hold the PtL® airway so that it curves in the same direction as the natural curvature of the pharynx.
- Insert the tip of the airway into the patient's mouth and advance it carefully behind the tongue until the teeth strap contacts the lips and teeth.

There will be modest resistance when making the right-angle bend at the back of the oropharynx. Do not use force! If the tube does not advance, either redirect it or withdraw it and start over.

Positioning the airway in this manner (teeth strap against the lips and teeth) is proper for an average-sized person. In the case of a very small patient, it may be necessary to withdraw the airway from the person's mouth as much as 1 inch (that is, so the teeth strap is 1 inch from the teeth). When the patient is a very large person, it may be necessary to insert the airway beyond the normal depth (that is, so the teeth strap is actually inside the person's mouth past the teeth).

When the tube is at the proper depth:

- Flip the neck strap over the patient's head, and:
- Tighten the strap with the hook and tape closures that are located on both sides of the strap.

The next step is to inflate the small cuff that seals either the esophagus or the trachea and the large cuff that seals the oral nasal pharynx.

A

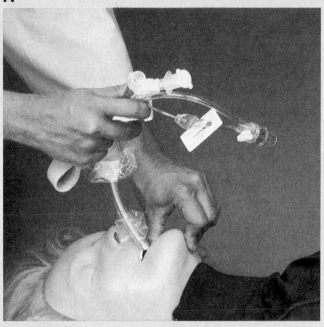

The patient's airway is opened by lifting the jaw, and the PtL® Airway is inserted so it follows the curve of the pharynx.

B

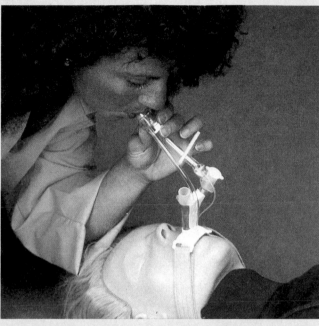

The neck strap is tightened to hold the airway in place. Then both cuffs are inflated simultaneously by blowing into the inflation valve.

C

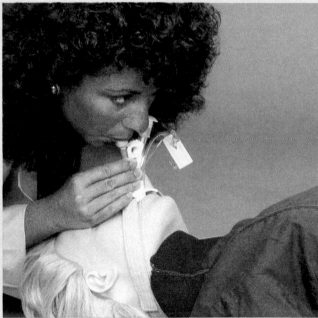

The location of the long tube is determined by blowing into the short #2 tube. If the tube is in the esophagus, air and/or oxygen is delivered through the #2 tube.

D

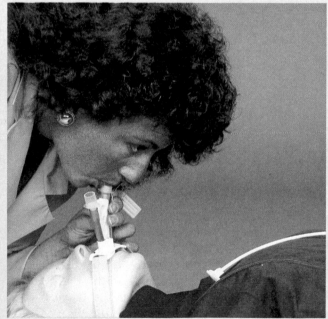

If the tube is in the trachea, the stylet is removed from the #3 tube. Air and/or oxygen is then delivered through the #3 tube.

First:

- Make sure that the white cap is in place over the port under the #1 inflation valve. It is through this valve that cuff air is exhausted.

To inflate both cuffs simultaneously:

- Deliver a sustained breath into the inflation valve.

If you are not able to inflate the cuffs, as evidenced by the failure of the pilot balloon to inflate, or your being able to hear and feel air escaping from the patient's mouth and nose, suspect that a cuff, most likely the large one, has been torn. Quickly remove the airway and replace it with a new PtL® or another airway.

When you see by the pilot balloon that the two cuffs are inflated:

- Deliver puffs of air from your cheeks to increase pressure in the cuffs and thus improve the seal.

To determine the location of the tube:

- Immediately blow forcefully into the short green #2 tube.

If the chest rises, the long clear #3 tube is in the esophagus. In this case:

- Initiate ventilations with breaths delivered through the green #2 tube, with air or oxygen delivered from a bag-valve-mask unit, or with oxygen delivered from a manually triggered ventilator.

If the chest does not rise, the long clear tube may be in the trachea. In this case:

- Remove the stylet and ventilate the patient through the long clear #3 tube.

If the tube is in the trachea and you are trained to do so, listen to both sides of the chest and over the stomach with a stethoscope during lung inflations. Also, verify chest rise with each breath, especially if the long clear tube is in the trachea of a small young female.

- Continue ventilations through the airway until the patient regains consciousness or protective airway gag reflexes return, or the patient is delivered to the care of emergency department personnel.

Dealing with Leaks

Continually monitor the appearance of the pilot balloon during ventilation efforts. Loss of pressure in the balloon will signal a loss of pressure in the cuffs. If you suspect that a cuff is leaking, increase cuff pressure by blowing forcefully into the #1 inflation valve or replace the airway. Repositioning the PtL® to ensure that the teeth strap is snug against the patient's teeth is another way of reducing leakage.

Monitoring the Patient During Ventilations

Continually watch for chest rise and listen for breath sounds while you ventilate a patient through a PtL® airway, especially in a patient who has facial trauma or burns of the face. Developing edema may gradually obstruct the airway.

Decompressing and Evacuating the Stomach

Patients who have received CPR or who have just eaten are candidates for the forceful or silent aspiration of stomach contents. Decompressing the stomach can reduce the possibility of aspiration. This can be accomplished by passing an 18 French Levine suction catheter into the nonairway tube. Remove the stylet of the long clear #3 tube only to pass the catheter. Catheters can be passed to suction the stomach, oral cavity, or bronchial tree. If suctioning is not indicated, do not remove the stylet from the #3 tube.

No Response to Ventilation Efforts

If your patient does not seem to be responding to ventilations delivered through the PtL® airway, or if there is any doubt in your mind as to whether the device is properly positioned, remove the PtL® airway and immediately replace it with a different airway device. Remember that your failure to provide an unconscious, nonbreathing patient with an adequate airway may result in severe injury or death.

Removing the PtL* Airway

Immediately remove the PtL® airway if the patient regains consciousness or if protective airway gag reflexes return. Turn the person onto his side and make

* PtL is a trademark of Resperonics, Inc.

sure that the stomach has been decompressed and that gastric contents have been evacuated. Remove the white cap from the deflation port of the #1 inflation valve to simultaneously deflate both cuffs. Carefully withdraw the PtL® airway and discard it. Continue to monitor the patient for adequate respirations.

NOTE: The PtL® airway is a single-patient-use device for short-term application. If you clean and retain a PtL® airway for future uses, you risk:

- Causing a small nick in one or both of the cuffs that will not be evident until the cuffs are inflated.
- Weakening the cuffs during the cleaning and disinfecting process.
- Contaminating the inflation valve, in which case the valve will leak during future operations.

Studies on the efficiency of the ReviveEasy PtL® Airway can be obtained from the manufacturer: Respironics, Inc., 530 Seco Road, Monroeville, PA 15146.

Intravenous Fluid Therapy

Adequate and uninterrupted circulation is essential to life. However, adequate and uninterrupted circulation can continue only when:

- The blood vessels constantly change in size.
- The cardiovascular system is full of blood.
- The heart continues to operate at maximum efficiency.

Shock is the collapse of the cardiovascular system. There are many types of shock, but that most commonly encountered by prehospital emergency care personnel is hypovolemic shock, that which results from the loss of blood or of plasma (the fluid portion of blood).

The first principle of emergency care for a person in shock is to elevate the lower extremities if there are no head or chest injuries. Thus, blood that may be pooled in the lower extremities is available to the heart and brain. This most basic procedure has undoubtedly saved countless lives that may have otherwise been lost because of shock.

However, blood loss may be so great in some injury situations that mere elevation of the feet will not be sufficient to maintain the cardiovascular system at the life sustaining level. If a seriously injured and hypovolemic patient is to be kept alive, he will have to be treated in a more definitive manner, as with intravenous therapy.

Two terms are associated with intravenous fluid therapy: transfusion and infusion. Transfusion is the introduction of whole blood or whole blood components into the cardiovascular system. It is a procedure that is seldom done outside a medical facility because of a number of complications that can arise. Thus, emergency medical service personnel seldom participate in a blood-transfusion effort.

Infusion is the introduction into the cardiovascular system of a fluid other than blood—a fluid that will fill the system sufficiently to allow the heart to operate efficiently while new blood is manufactured by the life processes or, in other words, a blood-volume expander. Infusion is a procedure that can be accomplished away from a medical facility by specially trained EMS personnel.

Supplies and Equipment for IV Therapy

There is a variety of sterile infusion sets available today for use by ambulance and rescue personnel. They are usually disposable and contain the following items:

- Connector (that joins the set to the fluid container) with a protective cap
- Drip chamber

- Flow adjustment valve
- Port (through which medications can be injected)
- Needle adapter that joins the set to the cannula

Other supplies and equipment associated with IV therapy are:

- Arm board, used for immobilizing the insertion site when necessary
- Tourniquet for restricting venous flow while an insertion site is selected
- Tape for securing tubing to the patient's arm and for securing the arm to the board
- Antiseptic solution for cleansing the insertion site
- Gauze pads for covering the insertion site
- Paper towels for cleaning up
- Pen and labels for identifying containers
- Prepared form or record book for recording information about the procedure

Depending on local policies, some ambulances and rescue units carry syringes in which blood can be collected, containers for the blood samples, and an antibiotic ointment that can be spread over the insertion site.

- Several fluids are available for intravenous therapy, including normal saline, Plasma-lyte, D5W (a 5% solution of dextrose in water), Dextran, and lactated Ringer's solution (a solution of salt, other electrolytes, and glucose in water). Lactated Ringer's solution does not have the red blood cells that carry life-sustaining oxygen to all parts of the body, but it can be used to replace up to two-thirds of the blood supply of a healthy individual before body functions start to fail.

THE IV INFUSION PROCEDURE

The infusion of an IV fluid is accomplished in several steps.

Preparing the Patient

As in any emergency care procedure, preparation of the patient is an important step.

While you are preparing the infusion equipment:

- In a calm and convincing manner, explain the procedure to your patient and why it is important. Emphasize that lost fluid must be replaced.

Even in the relative security of a doctor's office when they know that the resulting pain will be brief, most people become apprehensive when they know they are about to receive an injection. Thus you can be sure that your sick or injured patient in a prehospital setting will have some qualms when he sees you preparing the IV administration paraphernalia. Apprehension is heightened when a person has become conditioned to think that IV therapy is a "last ditch" effort made in an attempt to save a person's life.

Remember that a conscious, competent patient has a legal right to refuse your efforts to help him. Your explanation of the procedure will do much to instill confidence in a person who might otherwise be inclined to refuse your help. And don't lie to your patient! IV's hurt, so don't tell him they don't.

Selecting and Inspecting the Fluid

It is vitally important that you use only the fluid that has been ordered by medical command. A good practice is for you to repeat your instructions over the radio so the physician knows that you understand.

If you are using a fluid that is packed in a plastic bag:

- Remove the bag from the protective envelope.
- Check to ensure that the fluid is the one ordered and note the expiration date.
- Inspect the bag for leaks; gentle squeezing will force drops of liquid from pin-hole perforations that you might be able to see.

At the same time:

- Observe the fluid in the bag; it must be clear.

If you are using fluid that is in a glass bottle:

- Check the container for cracks and the fluid for clarity.

Preparing the Infusion Set

Remember that a macro-drip (standard) infusion set is needed for fluid replacement and that a micro-

A

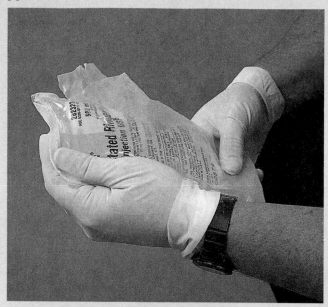

The fluid bag is removed from the protective container. At the same time, the patient can be told what is going to happen and why.

B

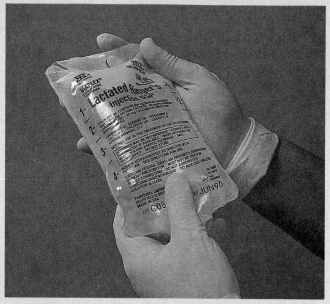

A check is made to ensure that the fluid is that which has been ordered. Then the bag is gently squeezed to determine whether there are any leaks. Check the expiration date on the bag.

C

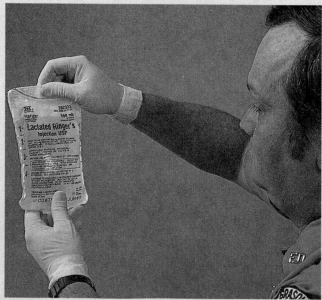

The fluid is checked for clarity.

D

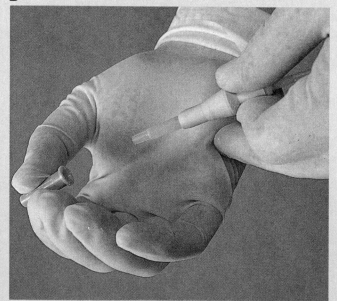

The protective covering is removed from the adapter, and the protective cap is removed from the extension tubing connector.

E

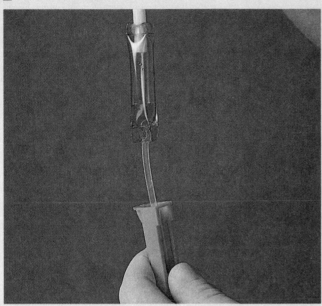

The extension tubing is joined to the infusion set, and the flow adjustment valve is closed.

F

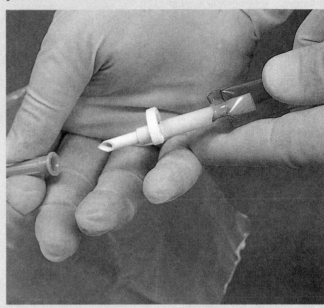

The protective covering is removed from the port of the fluid bag, and the protective covering is removed from the spiked end of the infusion tubing.

G

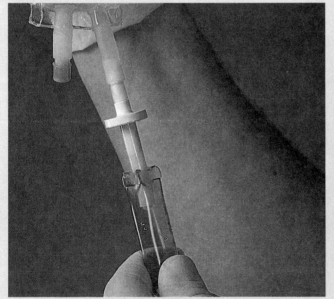

After the spiked end of the infusion set is inserted into the port of the fluid bag, the drip chamber is filled by alternately squeezing and releasing it.

H

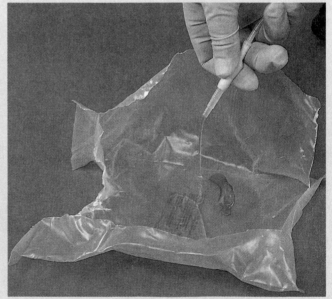

The protective covering is removed from the needle adapter, and air is flushed from the tubing by opening the flow adjustment valve.

(Scan continues on next page.)

I

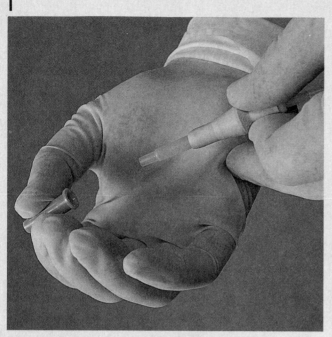

The flow adjustment valve is closed, and the needle adapter is recapped.

J

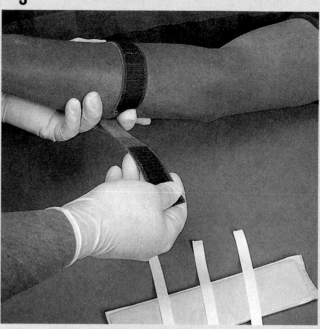

Strips of tape are torn and placed on the arm board or infusion set box, and a tourniquet is applied to the arm to cause venous distention.

K

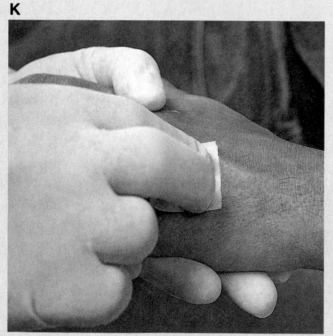

A vein that is well distended, fairly straight, and well fixed is chosen; then the insertion site is swabbed with a disinfectant.

L

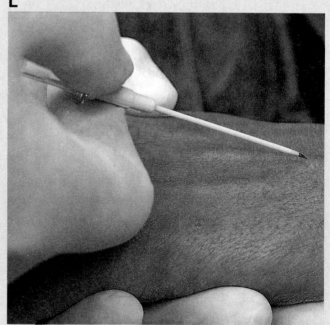

The skin is pierced at an angle of 30°, and the needle is inserted bevel up.

M

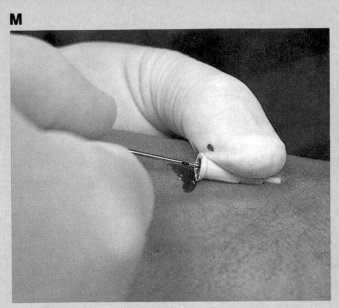

The catheter is slid into the vein; the tourniquet is loosened; and the needle is withdrawn.

N

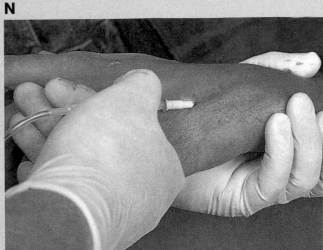

The vein is compressed with the thumb to prevent blood loss through the catheter while the needle adapter is attached to the cannula.

WARNING: No attempts should be made to recap; all needles should go to a designated container or marked medical waste.

O

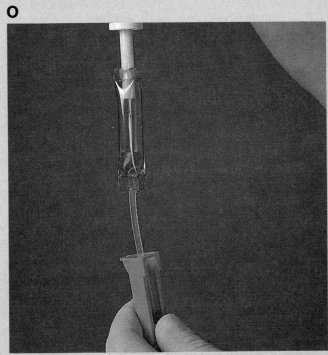

The flow adjustment valve is opened, and the fluid in the drip chamber is watched to see if it is flowing freely.

P

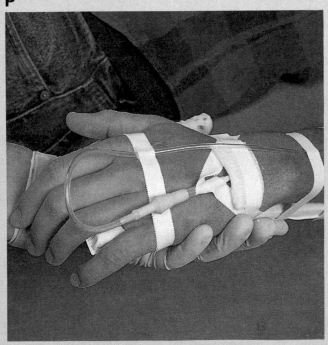

The insertion site is covered with a sterile dressing; the cannula is taped in place; and the arm is secured to an arm board.

drip set is used for maintenance of a life line and for infusing a child.

- Open the infusion set.
- Remove the protective covering from the adapter.
- Remove the protective cap from the extension tubing connector
- Join the extension tubing to the infusion set.
- Make sure that the flow adjustment valve is closed.
- Remove the protective covering from the port of the fluid bag.
- Remove the protective covering from the spiked end of the infusion tubing.
- Insert the spiked end of the infusion set into the port of the fluid bag.
- Fill the drip chamber by alternately squeezing and releasing it.
- Remove the protective covering from the needle adapter.
- Open the flow adjustment valve and allow a small amount of fluid to flow through the tubing, thus flushing air from it. Direct the fluid into the protective envelope to keep the work area dry.
- Close the flow adjustment valve.
- Recap the needle adapter.

Preparing the Tape That Will Secure the Cannula and Tubing

Once you start the insertion, you should not have to stop until the fluid is running. **Therefore:**

- Cut or tear strips of tape to the proper length *before* you start the insertion and place them on the arm board or the infusion set box where they will be handy.

Selecting the Cannula

An IV fluid can be infused in a number of ways: through a hollow needle inserted directly into a vein (as, for example, a "butterfly" needle); through a plastic catheter slipped over a hollow needle that has been inserted into a vein; or through a plastic catheter inserted into a vein through a hollow needle.

A 14-gauge over-the-needle catheter is generally recommended for trauma victims. It can handle large quantities of fluid and is more readily stabilized in place than a hollow needle. Smaller needles (18 or 20 gauge) are recommended for patients with med-

ical problems when large quantities of fluids are neither indicated nor desired.

- Select the proper cannula and keep it close at hand.

Selecting the Insertion Site

Any accessible vein in the body can be selected to receive an IV fluid. However, it is usually a vein in the forearm (below the crease of the elbow) that is selected since vessels there are large, straight, and easily entered. If possible, a vein in the left forearm should be selected since that area of the body is most accessible when the patient is on the ambulance stretcher.

To find a suitable vein:

- Apply a tourniquet to the arm to cause venous distention; a Velcro tourniquet can be used, or one can be fashioned from a length of soft rubber tubing.
- Palpate the radial pulse to be certain that you have not stopped arterial flow.
- Have the patient clench and unclench his fist several times to improve venous distention.

Once you have the tourniquet in place:

- Choose a vein that is well distended, fairly straight, well fixed (as opposed to one that rolls under your finger pressure), and springy when palpated.

Preparing the Insertion Site

Disinfecting the site directly over the vein that will be punctured is important.

- Scrub the area directly over the vein; then move the swab in ever-widening circles away from the puncture site.

If you are using an iodine swab:

- Follow the scrubdown with a wipedown with an alcohol sponge to reduce the possibility of an iodine reaction.

Preparing the Cannula

Hollow needles and plastic catheters are packaged in different ways. Sterility is ensured for as long as the packages remain unopened.

- Open the cannula package according to the manufacturer's directions, but do not touch the needle with your fingers.

Inserting the Cannula

Steady hands are most important during this step. If you are somewhat tense, take a deep breath and try to relax. If you don't puncture the vein the first try, you will subject your conscious patient to seemingly endless moments of agony while you poke and push in an effort to get the needle into the vein.

- Stabilize the vein by applying pressure on it distal to the point where the needle will enter.
- Hold the needle at an angle of 10 to 20 degrees with the bevel up and align it with the vein.
- Pierce the skin and insert the needle.

There will be little resistance as the needle passes through the skin, some resistance when the needle contacts the vein, and a loss of resistance when the needle passes through the wall of the vessel. The fact that the needle has entered the vein will be confirmed by a flashback of blood through the needle.

If you are using an over-the-needle or through-the-needle catheter:

- Continue to insert the needle for just a few millimeters more to make an opening sufficient for the catheter to pass through.

While holding the needle:

- Slide the catheter into the vein.
- Remove the tourniquet and withdraw the needle.

Compressing the vein with your thumb near the tip of the catheter as you support the patient's arm prevents blood loss through the catheter.

WARNING: Once you advance a plastic catheter over or through a needle, never pull it back. A piece of catheter may be sheared off by the sharp beveled edge of the needle point and become a plastic embolus that will interfere with circulation.

The procedure for inserting a hollow needle is essentially the same. The needle is inserted into the vein. It is then leveled until it is virtually parallel to the vessel and pushed forward until at least ½ inch, but less than ¾ inch of the needle is in the vein.

Blood Sampling

In some areas, it is the policy for emergency medical service personnel to draw blood samples at the time of an IV insertion.

If collecting blood is part of your standard operating procedures:

- Stabilize the catheter with one hand, attach a 20-milliliter (ml) syringe, draw the blood, and distribute blood among the required number of collection tubes.

Starting the Infusion

After making a quick visual check to see that the system is ready:

- Attach the needle adapter (of the infusion tubing) to the cannula.
- Open the flow adjustment valve.
- Observe the fluid in the drip chamber; it should flow freely.

If there is no free flow of fluid:

- Adjust the position of the catheter slightly; its tip may be pressing against the interior wall of the vein.

Securing the Catheter

Covering the puncture site is next. Whether the site is covered with an antiseptic ointment first is a matter of local policy.

In any case:

- Cover the insertion site with a sterile dressing.
- Tape the cannula in place by looping the tubing and securing the loop to the patient's arm with tape. Do not, however, cover the junction of the tubing and the cannula.
- Write on the tape the type of cannula used and the time and date of insertion. Do not write on the plastic fluid container, especially with a felt pen. Ink from a felt pen can permeate the bag and contaminate the fluid.

If necessary:

• Immobilize the patient's arm on an arm board, a flattened magazine, or the box that the infusion set came in.

Regulating the Flow Rate

The fluid flow rate must be adjusted according to the instructions of the physician. You must know (1) the volume of flow that is to be infused, (2) the time over which the volume is to be infused, and (3) the rate at which fluid is delivered to the drip chamber by the particular infusion set being used.

Calculate the fluid flow rate with this formula:

$$\text{Flow rate (drops per minute)} = \frac{(\text{volume of fluid to be infused}) \times (\text{drops per cc that the infusion set delivers})}{\text{time of infusion in minutes}}$$

For example, if the physician wants the patient to receive 1 liter (1000 ml) of a fluid in 2 hours and you have an infusion set that is capable of delivering 10 drops per cc, then:

$$\frac{1000 \text{ (ml)} \times 10 \text{ (drops per cc)}}{120 \text{ (min)}} = 83 \text{ drops per minute}$$

TROUBLESHOOTING AN IV

If it appears that the IV fluid is not running properly and there are no kinks in the tubing, take the following corrective measures, starting with the patient's arm and working back to the fluid container.

• Ensure that the tourniquet has been removed.

Sometimes a sleeve slips down over a tourniquet and obscures it while the cannula is being inserted. Thus, in a hasty operation, the tourniquet may be overlooked.

• Ensure that the patient's arm is not bent in such a way that circulation is impeded.
• Inspect the IV site for swelling.

Infiltration, the loss of blood into surrounding tissues, is not uncommon and occurs when a catheter or needle slips from the vein.

If you suspect infiltration:

• Lower the fluid container momentarily and watch for blood to appear in the tubing.

If blood does appear, the cannula is in the vein. If there is no sign of blood, the cannula has slipped from the vein. In either case, you must stop the infusion and remove the cannula.

If there is no indication of infiltration:

• Check to see that tape around the insertion site has not compressed any of the tubing.

If this is not the problem:

• Check to see that the flow adjustment valve has not been accidentally closed.

If it has not:

• Raise the fluid container to slightly increase the pressure of the fluid. Many times this is all that is necessary to cause a sluggish IV to run properly.

If these efforts do not result in a properly running fluid:

• Discontinue the IV and start one in another site with a new infusion set, a new cannula, and a new container of fluid. The new site should be above, not below, the original site.

COMPLICATIONS OF IV THERAPY

In addition to infiltration and plastic embolism, other local and systemic complications may arise during or after IV therapy.

Local Complications

Pain is common because of the skin puncture and should be expected. Intense and continuing pain should be regarded as an indication of infiltration.

Infection often results from the use of contaminated equipment or failure to use antiseptic procedures. Local infection is not usually evident until a few days after the infusion, however.

Accidental arterial puncture sometimes occurs when an artery lies close to the vein selected for puncture. Bright red blood spurting from the cannula indicates accidental arterial puncture. If you see this, quickly withdraw the cannula and apply pressure to the bleeding vessel until the flow stops, usually within a few minutes.

Nerve damage and **tissue sloughing** are rare local complications.

Systemic Reactions

Simple Fainting is usually nothing more than an emotional reaction to the insertion of the needle.

Pyrogenic reactions occur when foreign proteins capable of producing fever are introduced into the cardiovascular system. If your patient experiences a sudden rise in temperature (perhaps up to 106°F), headache, backache, chills, nausea, and vomiting within a half-hour or so after the start of IV therapy, discontinue the IV fluid immediately; the fluid may be contaminated. Start another IV in the other arm with a new infusion set, a new cannula, and a new container of fluid. You can reduce the likelihood of a fever-producing reaction by carefully inspecting IV fluid containers for leaks (through which contaminants can enter) and for contamination (evidenced by clouding).

Thrombophlebitis is inflammation of a vein and often occurs when IV therapy is prolonged. The problem may be caused by the solution itself (some IV solutions are more irritating than others) or by excessive movement of the cannula within the vein.

If you suspect thrombophlebitis because of pain along the vein and redness and swelling at the insertion site, stop the infusion and remove the cannula.

Air embolism, although more likely to occur when blood is being transfused under pressure, may occur during an IV fluid infusion. Air can enter the cardiovascular system in a number of ways, for example, when tubing fittings are not tight, when the fluid container is allowed to run dry, or when negative pressure is created in the tubing. When a bubble of air forms and is carried to a swollen vessel, it forms an obstruction to circulation. Suspect air embolism when circulatory collapse occurs while an IV is running properly.

Circulatory overload occurs when an excess of fluid is infused, perhaps because of miscalculation of the patient's needs. The symptoms of circulatory overload appear as those of congestive heart failure, dyspnea, rales, and distention of the jugular veins.

Anaphylactic reaction may occur in some patients. The reaction is generally due to a medication included with the IV solution rather than the IV solution itself.

Automated Defibrillation

This appendix was written by Kenneth R. Stults, M.S., Director of The University of Iowa Hospitals and Clinics, Emergency Medical Services Learning Resources Center, and modified for style by Harvey D. Grant.

The leading cause of death in the United States continues to be heart disease. Although many individuals have a chronic heart disease and die in a hospital following an extended illness, at least 300,000 people die suddenly each year with little or no warning. It should not be surprising that most sudden cardiac deaths occur outside a hospital, usually at home. This means that the epidemic of sudden cardiac death in this country is a problem that must be addressed by prehospital emergency care systems.

It is now clear that victims of sudden cardiac death have only a few minutes in which they can be successfully resuscitated and returned to a normal life. It is also clear that basic life support alone can rarely resuscitate these patients. Yet the vast majority of EMTs in the United States are trained only in basic cardiopulmonary resuscitation (CPR). This means that in most of the country our EMS systems are incapable of effectively managing the most common life-threatening emergency. It need not be this way.

The Importance of Early Defibrillation

Although many factors influence whether a person will survive an out-of-hospital cardiac arrest (the person's age and prior medical history, for example),

the most significant factor is the total time elapsed from collapse to defibrillation—the delivery of an electrical shock through the chest. Until recently, defibrillation was a skill performed only by medical personnel with hundreds or even thousands of hours of training. It has been demonstrated, however, that basic EMTs with only 10 to 20 hours of additional training can safely and effectively perform the skills of cardiac rhythm interpretation and defibrillation, even in rural communities where the frequency of cardiac arrest is very low. In one study, the survival rate of persons experiencing out-of-hospital cardiac arrest was more than five times higher in small communities where the EMTs had been trained to defibrillate than in communities where they could not. The reason for this has become increasingly clear: long-term survival is unusual in cases where more than 8 minutes have elapsed between collapse and defibrillation. Defibrillating a person this quickly (and even more quickly is ideal) will be possible only if the community emergency responders are trained and equipped to defibrillate in the field.

Automated Defibrillation

The user of a standard, manually operated defibrillator must be able to make rapid and correct decisions as to whether a shock is indicated. One drawback of using this type of defibrillator is the difficulty of maintaining crisp skills, especially in communities where the skills are rarely used in actual patient care activities. Frequent periodic recertification sessions that include thorough and strict evaluation of rhythm recognition and defibrillation skills are an absolute requirement when manual defibrillators are used.

Technological advances have now made it possible for a defibrillator itself to recognize rhythms that should be shocked and to either automatically charge up and deliver a shock or advise the rescuer to deliver a shock. These new defibrillators, called *automated external defibrillators* (AEDs), are so simple to operate that defibrillation should now be considered a skill well within the reach of every EMT and First Responder. The development of the AED has made effective emergency cardiac care outside a hospital a realistic goal for communities of all sizes.

Objectives

As an EMT who will be using an automated external defibrillator, you should be able to:

- Describe the effect of cardiac arrest on a person's heart and brain.
- State the principle of electrical defibrillation.
- Define the esential components of an effective community emergency cardiac care system.
- Describe the general procedures for the safe operation of a fully automatic defibrillator, or:
- Describe the general procedures for the safe operation of a semiautomatic (shock advisory) defibrillator, depending on the type of defibrillator available locally.
- State the importance of strict medical control and quality assurance in automated external defibrillation programs.

Cardiac rhythm recognition and the operation of a standard manual defibrillator will not be discussed in this appendix for two reasons. First, basic life-support ambulances and first-responder services are more likely to use one of the automated external defibrillators than a manually operated defibrillator. Second, textbooks devoted exclusively to the use of manually operated defibrillators are available. The in-depth discussions of cardiac rhythm interpretation and the more complex skill of manual defibrillation presented in a dedicated textbook are more appropriate to the needs of an EMT seeking certification in the use of a manual defibrillator than what could be included in the limited space of this appendix.

What Everyone Should Know About Defibrillation

Regardless of the type of device that you will use during your career as an EMT, there are certain facts you should know about cardiac arrest and defibrillation.

Cardiac Arrest

Cardiac arrest is a condition where the heart has stopped its life-sustaining function of pumping blood. Accordingly, cardiac arrest is diagnosed by confirming the absence of a pulse and regular respirations (although occasional gasping, or agonal, respirations sometimes continue). Usually, but not always, cardiac arrest results from the disturbance of the heart's electrical system, which must function normally if the heart is to continue to beat with a regular rhythm.

Ventricular Fibrillation

The primary electrical disturbance resulting in cardiac arrest is called ventricular fibrillation (VF). Between 50% and 60% of all cardiac arrest victims will be in VF by the time EMS personnel arrive. The heart in VF may have plenty of electrical energy, but it is totally disorganized. Chaotic electrical activity prevents the heart muscle from contracting normally and thus pumping blood. If you could see a heart in VF, it would appear to be quivering like a bag of worms. As you will see later, it is for this rhythm that defibrillation is indicated.

Ventricular Tachycardia

Automated external defibrillators are also designed to shock a rhythm known as ventricular tachycardia if it is very fast. In ventricular tachycardia (a very unusual cardiac arrest rhythm observed in less than 10% of all out-of-hospital cases), the heart beat is organized, but it is usually quite rapid. The faster the heart rate, the more likely it is that ventricular tachycardia will not allow the heart's chambers to fill with enough blood between beats to produce blood flow sufficient to meet the body's needs, especially that of the brain.

Electromechanical Dissociation

In 15% to 20% of cardiac arrest victims, the heart muscle itself fails even though the electrical rhythm remains relatively normal. As with any person in cardiac arrest, these individuals have no pulse or regular respirations. This condition of relatively normal electrical activity but no pumping action, called electromechanical dissociation because the electrical activity is dissociated, or separated, from the mechanical, or pumping activity, means that the heart muscle is severely and almost always terminally sick. Defibrillation cannot help these people because their heart's electrical rhythm is already organized and slow (unlike ventricular tachycardia, wherein the rhythm is organized but very fast). Automated defibrillators are designed not to shock patients experiencing electromechanical dissociation.

Asystole

In the remaining 20% to 25% of cardiac arrest victims, the heart has ceased generating electrical impulses altogether. When this happens, a condition called asystole, there is no repetitive electrical stimulus to cause the heart muscle to contract, and so it does not. As a result, there is no blood flow, and the patient has no pulse or regular respirations and is unconscious. As with electromechanical dissociation, defibrillation is not effective, and there is no other treatment known to be effective at this time except CPR. Automated defibrillators will not shock people in asystole.

If you have been adding up the numbers, you know by now that automated defibrillators will shock only about six of every ten cardiac arrest patients to whom they are attached.

Causes of Cardiac Arrest

Almost all victims of sudden cardiac death that has not resulted from an external cause such as drowning or trauma have some degree of atherosclerotic heart disease. That is, like most Americans, they have cholesterol plaques lining and narrowing the inside of their coronary arteries. These plaques reduce the amount of oxygen-carrying blood that can flow through the artery in a given period of time. This type of heart disease, common to most American adults but especially males, usually does not produce symptoms. Among people in whom the narrowing has reached more advanced stages, however, there are two primary mechanisms for initiating cardiac arrest: coronary artery spasm and myocardial infarction.

Coronary Artery Spasm

The more common mechanism involves a brief spasm of the muscular wall of a coronary artery. If the artery is already significantly narrowed due to the presence of cholesterol plaque, this spasm may result in a temporary interruption of blood flow to the part of the heart distal to the spasm. Even a brief interruption of blood supply in some people is enough to cause the heart to begin beating erratically and, ultimately, to fibrillate. These individuals may collapse suddenly with no warning symptoms.

Myocardial Infarction (Heart Attack)

A somewhat less common cause of cardiac arrest is actual blockage of a coronary artery, usually by a blood clot at a point where the artery is already narrowed by cholesterol plaque. When this happens, the interruption of the blood supply to the part of the heart distal to the blockage is prolonged and the deprived muscle begins to die. This condition is known as *myocardial infarction* or, more commonly, as heart attack.

While most people do not suffer cardiac arrest with their first heart attack, up to 45% of all cardiac arrests occur as the result of heart attacks. This means simply that there are many more heart attacks than there are cardiac arrests. A person experiencing a heart attack will generally complain of pain in the chest, jaw, left arm, or epigastric region, shortness of breath, diaphoresis, and so on, although the duration of symptoms prior to suffering a cardiac arrest is highly variable and may be short.

How Defibrillation Works

Contrary to popular opinion, defibrillation is *not* "jump-starting" a dead heart. In fact, it is just the opposite. The therapeutic action of a defibrillatory shock is the sudden *termination* of a heart's electrical activity.

For defibrillation to be of benefit to a person, the heart must have enough life left in it that it will be capable of beating on its own once the chaotic pattern of ventricular fibrillation has been disrupted. The amount of life left in a heart is evidenced by the coarseness (amplitude) of the ventricular fibrillation. The coarser the fibrillation the more likely it is that defibrillation will be successful. Since the coarseness of VF is determined in part by the total time in cardiac arrest, and since the extent of damage to the brain is certainly influenced by the total time in cardiac arrest, it should be clear that the sooner a person is defibrillated, the more likely he is to survive.

It should also be clear that delivering shocks to a person in asystole or even in very fine ventricular fibrillation will rarely result in the development of a spontaneous organized rhythm because there is simply not enough energy remaining in the heart to allow it to function on its own. It is of little, if any, clinical importance that AEDs do not shock asystole and sometimes fail to shock very fine VF.

The Importance of Speed

Recall that a major factor in the survival of a person who is in cardiac arrest is the amount of time that elapses from the moment of collapse until the start of defibrillation. This time period has four phases:

1. EMS access time
2. Dispatch time
3. Ambulance response time
4. Shock time

For an EMS system to be effective, each of these time segments must be as short as possible.

EMS Access Time

This is the time that passes from the time a person collapses in cardiac arrest until someone notifies the EMS system. A person who collapses in front of another person (witnessed arrest) should have a far greater chance of survival than a person who collapses in an isolated place away from other people; the person seeing the collapse can call for an ambulance.

That someone sees a person collapse in cardiac arrest is no guarantee that an ambulance will be called immediately, however. In fact, most witnesses to a collapse delay calling for an ambulance for 2 minutes or more, and many delay calling for 4 to 6 minutes and longer. The typical witness of a cardiac arrest is a woman 65 years old, alone with the patient at the time of collapse, and not trained in CPR. Even though CPR training programs are available for members of the public, few senior citizens attend.

Obviously, members of the public should be trained in CPR. But the public should also be trained to call for an ambulance immediately upon seeing someone collapse, even though they know CPR. Any delay in activating the community EMS system results in delayed defibrillation.

Dispatch Time

The second phase of a defibrillation effort begins with receipt of the call for help by a dispatcher and ends with the alerting of an ambulance crew, however that is accomplished in any given community. This time segment should be kept as short as possible. The dispatcher rapidly determines whether the call is for a cardiac problem (by asking the caller about difficult breathing, unconsciousness, unresponsiveness, and the like). Then the dispatcher immediately sends out an emergency service unit with a defibrillator. Once this is done, the dispatcher acquires additional information from the caller while the ambulance is on the way.

Ambulance Response Time

The third phase of the collapse-to-defibrillation period is the time from dispatch until the ambulance arrives at the location of the stricken person. Ambulance response time varies considerably from community to community, as well as from one area to another within large communities. Response times are often long in large cities where congested roads are a problem and in small communities where volunteers must respond to the ambulance garage from homes and places of businesses. The fastest ambulance response times are generally in towns and small cities that are large enough to have an ambulance service that is manned around the clock by paid personnel, but small enough that traffic and response distances are not problems.

One way to shorten the time from dispatch to the arrival of a defibrillator in communities with a volunteer ambulance service is to station an automated defibrillator with a trained EMT 24 hours a day. Thus, when a call for a potential cardiac problem is received, that trained individual can respond directly with the defibrillator while other EMTs respond with the ambulance. This approach works. In one group of small communities, the time it took to get a defibrillator on the road was reduced from 7.5 minutes to 2.5 minutes. Placing automated defibrillators with first responders in large cities has proved equally effective in reducing the response time of a trained individual with a defibrillator.

Shock Time

The final phase of a defibrillation period is the time that elapses from the time that a rescuer arrives at the side of the stricken person to the time the first shock is delivered. As with each of the other phases of the collapse to defibrillation period, this time segment must be kept as short as possible if life-saving efforts are to be effective—ideally 1.5 minutes or less.

The shorter the collapse-to-defibrillation time, the greater the chance for survival. A person who can be shocked in 6 minutes or less after collapse has a good chance of surviving. A person who cannot be shocked within 8 minutes of the moment of collapse has only a slim chance of surviving.

Because the ambulance response time alone approaches 8 minutes in many communities, the importance of implementing creative approaches to shortening the various components of the time from collapse to shock cannot be overemphasized. Following are some goals that, if achieved, should result in a witnessed VF survival rate of 25% or higher.

Time Component	Objective	Goal	Method
EMS access time	To minimize the time from collapse until someone places a call for help	1 min	An increased community awareness to the need for quickly calling for an ambulance; more public CPR programs
Dispatch time	To minimize the time it takes for an EMS dispatcher to elicit information from a caller and get a defibrillator-equipped unit on the road	0.5 min	Better dispatcher training, improved call handling procedures
Response time	To minimize the time it takes to get a trained defibrillator team to the patient	3.0 min	Strategic placement of automated defibrillators with first-response personnel
Shock time	To minimize the time it takes to deliver the first shock	1.5 min	Use automated defibrillators; continually practice to maintain peak efficiency

OPERATING AUTOMATED DEFIBRILLATORS

Ambulance and rescue services can choose between fully automatic and semiautomatic (shock advisory) defibrillators, depending on personal preference. The general operation of both types of defibrillator will be discussed here. The following "don'ts" apply to both types:

- Never activate an automated defibrillator unless the patient is in full cardiac arrest as evidenced by unconsciousness, the absence of a pulse, and the absence of other than agonal respirations.
- Never activate an automated defibrillator unless the patient is lying still and not in contact with rescuers or bystanders.
- Never activate an automated defibrillator in a moving ambulance.

Attaching the Defibrillator to the Patient

The basic steps for attaching an automated defibrillator to a patient are the same regardless of whether the unit is automatic or semiautomatic.

All automated external defibrillators use self-adhesive monitor/defibrillation pads rather than the standard monitoring electrodes and hand-held defibrillation paddles used with manual defibrillators. The self-adhesive pads allow for both monitoring of the patient's heart rhythm and for delivery of the shock. Correct placement of the pads is accomplished in the following manner.

While your partner initiates CPR:

- Expose the patient's chest and quickly wipe it dry, if necessary. Do not take the time to shave any chest hair from the pad sites. Every second counts.
- Remove two pads from their protective packages immediately upon arrival at the patient's side.
- Taking care not to tear the pad, remove the plastic backing from one pad and place it on the right upper chest with one edge of the pad next to, but not on, the sternum, and the top edge just touching the clavicle. Use a rolling motion when applying the pads to ensure that air is not trapped underneath.
- Press on the adhesive portion of the pad to ensure good contact with the skin. Do not press on the center of a pad that has a gel-sponge center; to do so will squeeze gel into the adhesion area and prevent the pad from sticking to the skin.
- Remove the backing from the second pad and place it over the apex of the heart (below and to the left of the nipple) in the same manner.
- Connect the cables that lead from the automated defibrillator according to the manufacturer's instructions and be sure that the connections are tight.

Although either pad may be attached to either cable, it is recommended for consistency that units employing color-coded cables or pads be placed as follows:

A

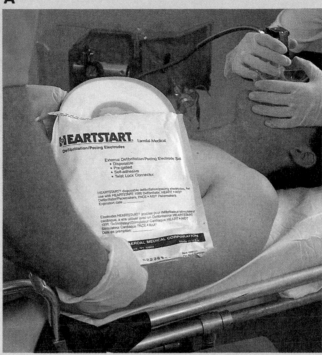

The patient's chest is exposed and the pads are removed from the protective covering.

B

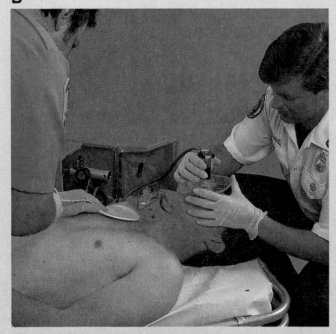

The plastic backing is removed from the first pad and the pad is placed on the chest.

C

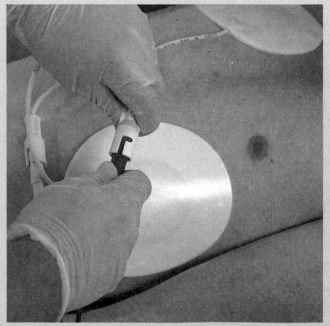

The second pad is placed on the patient's chest and the cables are connected.

- The red color (cable or pad, depending on the manufacturer) should be applied over the apex area.
- The white color (cable or pad, depending on the manufacturer) should be applied over the right border of the sternum.

This placement ensures correct positioning of the patient's ECG signal into the monitor circuitry.

If the pad/cable connections are not secure or if the pads are not firmly adhered to the patient's chest, all automated defibrillators will announce a warning to check the pad and cable monitoring system. An automated defibrillator will not function until the pads and cables are securely attached and properly connected.

Operating a Fully Automatic Defibrillator

A fully automatic defibrillator such as the Laredal Heartstart 1000 will assess the patient's rhythm and determine whether a shock is needed. If it senses that a shock is needed, a fully automatic defibrillator will automatically charge to a preset energy level and deliver the shock, all without any further action by the rescuer. The newest models of fully automatic defibrillators have only two controls: an ON button and an OFF button. Fully automatic defibrillators also make use of voice synthesizers to verbally announce instructions and warnings such as "STOP CPR" and "STAND BACK" and "CHECK BREATHING AND PULSE."

To operate a fully automatic defibrillator:

- Assess your patient's breathing and pulse.

If the person is not breathing and does not have a pulse, and you are working with a partner:

- Direct your partner to begin CPR while you prepare the defibrillator and attach the pads to the patient.

If you are working alone:

- Prepare the defibrillator, attach the pads to the patient, and then begin CPR to get some oxygenated blood moving.

When the defibrillator is attached to the patient:

- Clear everyone—including yourself—from contact with the patient.

- Press the ON button. The defibrillator will announce "STOP CPR" and begin analyzing the patient's rhythm. If a shock is indicated, the fully automatic defibrillator will repeatedly announce "STAND BACK," charge to 200 joules of energy, and deliver the shock. Do not touch or move the patient when you hear the warning "STAND BACK."
- Remain clear of the patient. Immediately following delivery of the first shock, the fully automatic defibrillator will again analyze the rhythm. If the patient still has a rhythm for which a shock is indicated, the defibrillator will once again warn "STAND BACK" and charge to 200 joules of energy. The second shock will be delivered as soon as the charging process is complete.
- Remain clear of the patient. The process continues automatically until three shocks have been delivered or until the patient has a rhythm for which shocking is not indicated. The energy level for the third shock will likely be higher than that of the first two shocks. With the newer fully automatic defibrillators, energy selection is not under the control of the rescuer.

After three shocks have been delivered or if the patient has a rhythm that should not be shocked, the defibrillator will announce "CHECK BREATHING AND PULSE" and then enter an inactive monitoring mode.

At this point:

- Check carefully for spontaneous pulses and respirations.

If a pulse is present:

- Immediately prepare the patient for transportation to a hospital. Leave the defibrillator connected to the patient. Continue life-support measures as necessary, including the administration of oxygen and assisting ventilations.

If there is no pulse:

- Leave the defibrillator connected and resume CPR.

In either case, after 60 seconds the fully automatic defibrillator will prompt you to "STOP CPR," following which it will again analyze the patient's rhythm. If a shock is indicated, the defibrillator will warn you to "STAND BACK" and then deliver up to three more shocks.

A

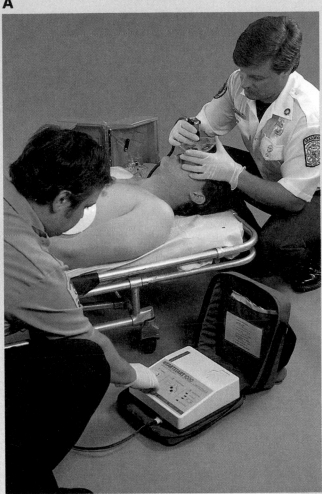

An EMT operating a fully automatic defibrillator.

B

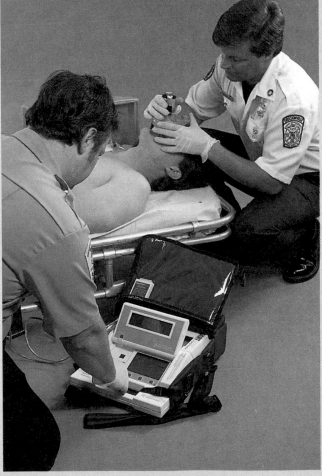

An EMT operating a semi-automatic defibrillator.

If a shock is not indicated or after the three additional shocks have been delivered, the fully automatic defibrillator will prompt you to "CHECK BREATHING AND PULSE," following which it will enter a perpetual monitoring mode. If CPR is indicated, perform it. If the patient has a pulse, continue preparations for transportation.

During the perpetual monitoring mode, the fully automatic defibrillator will continually assess the patient's heart rhythm, although it will not be able to deliver additional shocks without further action on your part, even if a rhythm develops for which a shock is indicated. If this should happen, you will hear a beep followed by the prompt "CHECK BREATHING AND PULSE." Stop immediately if you are performing CPR and carefully check for a spontaneous pulse and regular respirations. If there is no pulse, clear the area, press the ON button, and repeat the steps outlined above.

REMEMBER: Not all models of fully automatic defibrillators function in exactly the same manner as described here. Consult the user's manual for the defibrillator you will be using for accurate and detailed instructions.

Operating Semiautomatic Defibrillators

Semiautomatic, or shock advisory, defibrillators such as the Laerdal Heartstart 2000 require more rescuer interaction than do fully automatic models. Once attached and activated, a semiautomatic defibrillator will assess the patient's rhythm and, if a shock is indicated, begin charging to 200 joules. Once fully charged, however, a semiautomatic defibrillator will not automatically deliver the shock, but instead will prompt you to press a button and thus shock the patient. The safety precautions for fully automatic defibrillators also apply to semiautomatic models: before pressing the shock delivery button, ensure that everyone, including yourself, is clear from contact with the patient.

To operate a semiautomatic defibrillator:

- Assess your patient's breathing and pulse.

If the person is not breathing and does not have a pulse, and you are working with a partner:

- Direct your partner to begin CPR while you prepare the defibrillator and attach the pads to the patient.

If you are working alone:

- Prepare the defibrillator, attach the pads to the patient, and then begin CRP to get some oxygenated blood moving.

When the defibrillator is connected to the patient:

- Turn on the unit by lifting open the display module.

The LCD message screen will display a variety of information, including the command "PRESS TO ANALYZE" with an arrow pointing to the appropriate button. Pressing the button will cause the defibrillator to analyze the patient's rhythm.

If a shock is indicated, the semiautomatic defibrillator will begin charging to 200 joules of energy. The charging process may or may not be accompanied by a voice prompt to "STAND BACK," depending on the model of defibrillator being used. Once fully charged, a prompt will appear on the LCD screen to press the indicated button in order to deliver the shock.

When the prompt appears:

- Make sure that everyone is clear of the patient, including yourself; then press the indicated button.

Following delivery of the shock:

- Press the analyze button and repeat the procedure to deliver the second shock.

If a third shock is indicated, the energy level can be increased to 360 joules by pressing the indicated button during the charging process.

If no shock is indicated, a semiautomatic defibrillator will display a message to that effect.

When this occurs:

- Carefully check for spontaneous pulses and respirations.

If pulses and respirations are absent:

- Resume CPR.

If pulses and respirations are present:

- Prepare the patient for immediate transportation to a hospital.

The maximum number of shocks allowed and the energy levels to be used should be dictated by local physician-determined standing orders.

As with fully automatic defibrillators, differences exist in the operation of various models of semiautomatic defibrillators. Consult the user's manual for accurate and detailed operating instructions.

Medical Control and Quality Assurance

Although automated defibrillators are easy to operate and their use is encouraged in most EMS systems, no defibrillator should be used by EMS and rescue personnel unless authorized and monitored by a physician medical director. The physician must develop and/or approve a patient care protocol that defines exactly how the defibrillator is to be used in the field. Defibrillation is a potentially hazardous medical procedure that can be performed only under the direction of a licensed physician.

Because the necessity for speed requires that defibrillation-trained rescuers operate without direct medical control, there must be a mechanism for monitoring the performance of the rescuers and the automated defibrillator. Accordingly, all automated defibrillators are equipped with a dual-channel cassette tape recorder (or similar device) for recording the events of the resuscitation attempt. It is beyond the scope of this appendix to discuss the features or operation of the various recording devices currently available. You should be aware, however, that it is only through careful review of these recordings that the correct operation of the defibrillator can be ensured. Every effort must be made to ensure that complete recordings are made of each resuscitation effort and that these recordings are promptly reviewed by the physician medical director or his or her designee.

SUMMARY

The development of automated external defibrillators has made effective prehospital emergency cardiac care possible even in the smallest, most remote communities. However, placing an AED with trained rescuers in a community does not guarantee that the cardiac arrest survival rate will be improved. Having a defibrillator will help, but a significant number of "saves" will never be possible until steps are taken to reduce the time that elapses from the moment of collapse until the delivery of the first shock.

Helicopter Ambulance Operations

Helicopter medical evacuation first became popular during the Korean conflict. There, and later in Viet Nam, helicopters carried seriously wounded military personnel from front-line aid stations to Mobile Army Surgical Hospitals (M.A.S.H.) where "save" rates often exceeded 90%.

The first civilian hospital-based air medical team was established in Denver, Colorado, in 1972. Today more than 160 helicopter programs serve virtually all urban and rural areas of the United States. Modern air ambulances are safe and efficient, and their crews provide a high level of prehospital emergency care.

As helicopter ambulance programs continue to grow, so does the number of emergency medical service personnel who use them. More EMTs than ever before can request helicopter transportation of seriously sick and injured persons. For a helicopter program to be absolutely safe and effective, however, it must be integrated into the local EMS system.

This appendix has been prepared to acquaint you with helicopter ambulance operations in general. If your EMS system has a helicopter service, or if it utilizes a helicopter service from another EMS system, attend an orientation program as part of your training course. Then become completely familiar with the standard operating procedures developed for the system and follow those procedures when you become an EMT.

Helicopter Ambulances

The single-engine Bell Long Ranger is the rotary-wing aircraft that is most often used for helicopter evacuations. Long Rangers are usually configured and equipped for one patient. As helicopter programs grow and expand, twin-engine helicopters will probably become the standard. Among the larger aircraft that are popular now are the Aerospatiale Dauphin, the MBB BK117, the B0105, the Sikorsky S76, and the Bell 222.

Size, rotor lengths, loading systems, medical interiors, and other features vary among helicopters. Thus you should become familiar not only with the make and model that usually flies within your EMS response area, but also with the helicopters that might be called into your area in the event of a multiple-casualty incident.

Helicopter Ambulance Personnel

Hospital-based helicopters generally carry two advanced life-support personnel. One is usually a registered nurse; the other may be a paramedic, another nurse, or a physician. Specialty teams for neonates, organ donors, and complicated cardiac patients are also available in some areas.

Approximately 60% of helicopter operations involve transferring patients from one hospital to another. The remaining 40% are responses to the locations of sick or injured persons. It is during these responses that EMTs assist helicopter personnel with landing zone coordination, radio communications, patient packaging, and transfer to the aircraft.

Indications for Helicopter Ambulance Transport

Obviously, not every sick or injured person needs to be transported to a medical facility by helicopter. While local protocols vary, it is usually the patients who fit within the following categories that are considered for helicopter transportation when an ALS unit is unavailable or unable to reach the location of the patient within a reasonable time, and when travel time to a medical facility where the patient can be cared for properly will exceed 20 minutes.

Consider helicopter transportation when any patient exhibits:

- Respiratory distress
- A blood pressure of 90 systolic or less
- A heart rate greater than 110 in an adult
- Cyanosis
- Capillary refill greater than 2 seconds

Your ability to recognize potentially lethal mechanisms of injury is important. Consider an injured person to be a prime candidate for helicopter transportation when the individual was:

- In a motor vehicle accident that collided with another vehicle or object at a speed greater than 30 miles an hour
- In a motor vehicle where another person was killed
- In a motor vehicle that rolled over
- In a motor vehicle that exhibits passenger compartment intrusion greater than 1 foot
- Ejected from an accident vehicle
- Riding a motorcycle
- Trapped in an accident vehicle during a lengthy extrication procedure

A fall can be as deadly as a motor vehicle accident. Consider for helicopter transportation any person who has fallen for a distance greater than 12 feet.

The nature of the injury should also be considered when evaluating an injured patient for helicopter transportation. A person should be transported to a medical facility quickly when he or she has:

- A penetrating injury to the head, neck, or torso
- Severe blunt trauma to the head, neck, or torso
- Uncorrected complete or partial airway obstruction
- An amputation above the wrist or ankle
- Evidence of intrathoracic injury such as chest wall bruising or tenderness, absence of breath sounds, flail chest, or asymmetrical expansion of the chest
- A head injury with altered or a decreasing level of consciousness
- Fractures with absent distal pulses and/or a cold or cyanotic extremity
- Major burns, and major burns associated with injuries

Seriously injured young children are often transported by helicopter, as are persons over the age of 65 years who have multiple injuries.

A number of medical problems warrant helicopter transportation when an ALS unit is not available or when ground travel time is likely to be long, including:

- Chest pain with hypotension, delayed capillary refill, respiratory distress, or cardiac arrhythmias with or without cardiac history
- Suspected intracerebral emergency with altered level of consciousness or localizing neurologic findings
- Overdose with respiratory depression or seizures
- Obstetrical emergency or complicated delivery
- Suspected or diagnosed aortic aneurysm with severe pain, hypotension, pallor, or shock
- Uncontrolled seizure activity
- Respiratory emergency (asthma, COPD, airway obstruction, and the like) with respiratory distress.

Other times when rapid helicopter transportation may be instrumental in saving a life are when a sick or injured person is in a remote or inaccessible location, hazardous material emergencies, and multiple casualty incidents.

Your Role as an EMT in Helicopter Ambulance Operations

While you may not participate in the actual helicopter transportation of a sick or injured person to a medical facility, there is much you can do to prepare the person for transfer. You must initiate basic emergency care measures, and you may have to supervise the preparation or assist with the preparation of a landing zone suitable for the helicopter.

Preparing a Patient for Transfer by Air

Following are some of the steps that you might take to prepare the victim of a vehicle accident for helicopter transportation:

- Extricate the person in the safest and most expeditious manner.
- Apply a rigid cervical and an upper body immobilization device.
- Assure an open airway by inserting an endotracheal tube (ETT), an esophageal obturator airway (EOA or EGTA), a pharyngo-tracheal lumen airway (PtL®), or other device.
- Ventilate and suction the patient as necessary and administer oxygen
- Dress and bandage wounds and immobilize fractured parts.
- Put the patient in a pneumatic anti-shock garment, if its use is indicated.
- Completely immobilize the patient on a rigid, full-body patient-carrying device.

If the weather is cold:

- Protect the patient from hypothermia.
- Place the patient in a warm ambulance until the helicopter arrives.

If you are trained and authorized to do so:

- Start one or two 14- or 16-gauge IV infusions and draw blood samples. Be sure that the IV lines are well secured.

If your patient has a medical problem and is not injured, in addition to packaging the person for transportation:

- Obtain a history and the name of the patient's physician, if possible, and gather any medications.

Preparing the Landing Zone

Contrary to popular opinion, helicopters do not swoop down from the sky onto any piece of ground, scoop up a sick or injured person, and zoom off to a medical facility. They sit down on specially selected and prepared areas designated as landing zones.

Following are suggestions that you might use if you are in charge of preparing a landing zone for a helicopter ambulance.

- First, select a landing zone appropriate to the size of the helicopter.

During daylight hours, the landing zone for a small helicopter landing should be a square with 60-foot sides. At night, the square should have 100-foot sides. The landing zone for a medium-sized helicopter landing in daylight should be a square with 75-foot sides. The square should have 125-foot sides at night. A large helicopter needs even more room. The landing zone should be 120 feet square, and at night the sides should be increased to 200 feet.

The landing surface should be flat and firm and clear of people, vehicles, stumps, brush, posts, large rocks, and obstructions such as trees, poles, and wires. Rescuers and firefighters should pick up loose debris that might be blown up into the rotor system.

The landing zone should be at least 50 yards from the accident vehicles, if possible, so that noise and rotor wash will not be a problem for rescuers.

If the helicopter will land on a divided highway, traffic must be stopped in both directions even though the aircraft will land on only one side of the highway.

- Consider the wind direction when selecting a landing site.

Helicopters usually land and take off into the wind; they make vertical descents and ascents only when it is absolutely necessary. If the approach and departure path have obstructions such as wires, poles, antennas, and trees, notify the crew by radio during the initial radio transmission.

- Mark the touchdown area.

Each corner of the square touchdown area should be marked with a highly visible device (such as a flag or surveyor's tapes) during daylight hours and a flashing or rotating light at night. Flares can be used day or night, but only in areas where sparks from the flares will not ignite dry vegetation.

- Designate the wind direction.

Place a fifth warning device on the upwind side of the square to designate the wind direction.

- Create a safe environment.

Spectators should be kept at least 200 feet from the touchdown area and emergency service personnel

SCAN A5—1 DANGER AREAS AROUND HELICOPTERS

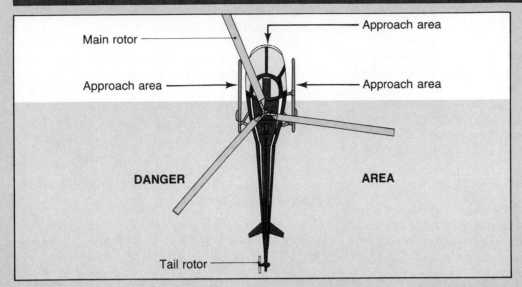

Main rotor

Approach area

Approach area

Approach area

Approach area

DANGER **AREA**

Tail rotor

A

The area around the tail rotor is extremely dangerous; a spinning rotor cannot be seen.

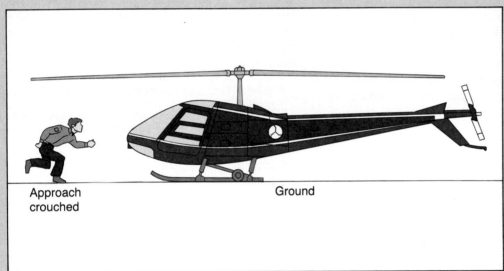

Approach crouched

Ground

B

A sudden gust of wind can cause the main rotor of a helicopter to dip to a point as close as 4 feet from the ground. Always approach a helicopter in a crouch when the rotor is moving.

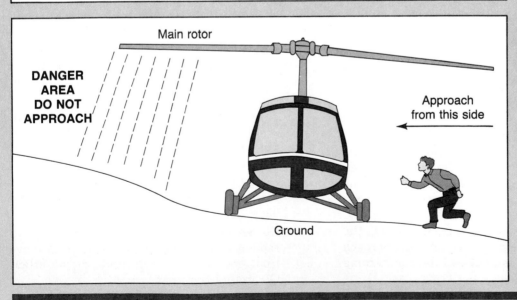

Main rotor

DANGER AREA DO NOT APPROACH

Approach from this side

Ground

C

Approach the aircraft from the downhill side when a helicopter is parked on a hillside.

who are not directly involved with the landing should remain at least 100 feet from the touchdown zone. A fire apparatus should be standing by in a safe place, and if the ground is extremely dusty, firefighters should wet down the touchdown area.

Personnel that will be near the helicopter when it touches down should be wearing protective clothing and safety goggles; debris dislodged by the rotor wash can blow under pull-down helmet shields. Helmet chin straps should be securely fastened. Baseball caps should not be worn; they can be blown from the wearer's head and drawn into the rotor system.

- Light the touchdown area at night.

Low-beam headlights, vehicle-mounted spotlights and floodlights and portable floodlights and handlights can be used to define the touchdown area at night. All other nonessential lights should be turned off, and no lights should be directed toward the helicopter. White lights can ruin a pilot's night vision and temporarily blind him. Prohibit photographers from using flashbulbs and video lights during landings and takeoffs.

- Assign personnel to keep spectators and nonessential emergency service personnel from wandering into the landing zone at any time until the helicopter departs.

Even when they have been asked to remain in a safe place, spectators and nonessential emergency service personnel have the tendency to approach the landing zone as a helicopter approaches, if for no other reason than to get a better view. Properly dressed (and thus easily identifiable) rescuers or firefighters should be assigned to locations around the landing zone to keep people from wandering into the danger area. These people should keep their eyes on the periphery of the landing zone, not the helicopter.

When you see the helicopter:

- Assign one person to guide the pilot to a safe landing.

The guide should wear eye protection, and he should stand at the location of the wind direction marker with his back to the wind and facing the touchdown area. He should stand with his arms raised over his head to indicate the landing direction.

As the helicopter turns into the wind, the ground guide should begin to direct the approach with appropriate hand signals while maintaining eye contact with the pilot.

Ground Operations

Safety remains the prime consideration even when the helicopter has landed.

- Do not approach the helicopter, and do not allow anyone else to approach it. The crew will leave the aircraft and approach you when it is safe to do so.
- Have the landing zone crew members prohibit smoking anywhere within 50 feet of the aircraft.

If the helicopter is to remain running while at the scene:

- Station a landing zone crew member near the tail of the helicopter to prevent anyone from approaching the tail rotor.

The tail rotor of a helicopter is generally 3 to 6 feet from the ground (if the ground is level) and spins so fast that it cannot be seen. Someone who inadvertently walks into a spinning rotor can be killed.

When the helicopter is ready for loading:

- Give the helicopter crew only the people they need to move the patient to the aircraft and assist with the loading.
- Instruct those people to follow the directions of the crew members without question.

If you are part of the transfer and loading team, or if you will accompany the team to the helicopter:

- Approach the helicopter only from the front or side, never from the rear. No one should ever be aft of the rear landing skid support tubes.
- Approach and depart from the helicopter on the downhill side if the helicopter is on uneven ground.
- Keep low when you are approaching the helicopter; a sudden gust of wind can cause the main rotor to suddenly dip to the point where the tip is only 4 feet off the ground.
- Do not carry anything to the helicopter that is over head high, including IV poles and bags.
- Do not duck under the body, boom, or tail section of the helicopter if you must move from one side of the aircraft to the other. Go around the front.

SCAN A5–2 HAND SIGNALS FOR HELICOPTER OPERATORS

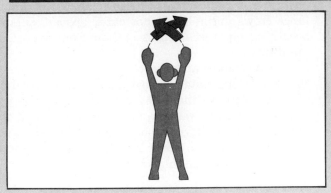

A   Landing zone unsafe

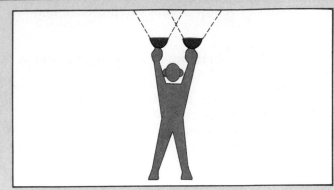

B   Night operations

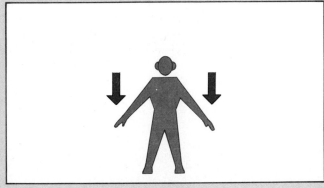

C   Go down

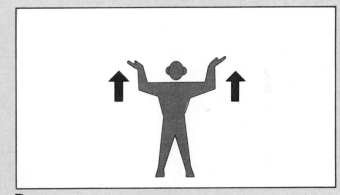

D   Go up

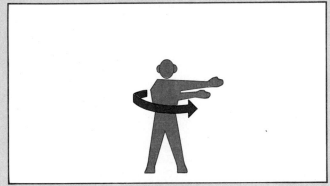

E   Move right

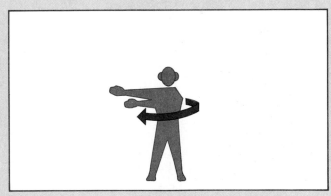

F   Move left

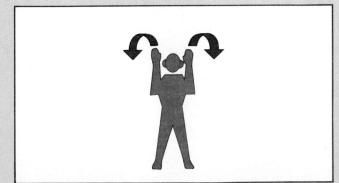

G   Move back

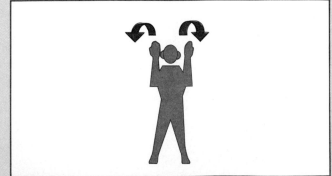

H   Move forward

When the patient is loaded:

- Allow only the flight crew to close and lock the doors. A broken door will prevent a takeoff.

When the helicopter is ready for departure:

- Be sure that the departure path is free from vehicles and spectators; if an emergency occurs during takeoff, the aircraft will land in that area.

HAZARDOUS MATERIAL SITUATIONS

Accidents involving hazardous materials require the special attention of fire and rescue units on the ground. The hazardous materials of concern are those that are toxic, poisonous, flammable, explosive, irritating, or radioactive in nature. Helicopter ambulance crews normally do not carry special suits or breathing apparatus to protect them from hazardous materials.

A helicopter ambulance crew must be warned that hazardous materials are present at the location of an accident so that they can take special steps to prevent contamination of crew members and the aircraft. Sick or injured persons who are contaminated by hazardous materials may require special protection before loading on the aircraft.

NOTE: Much of the information contained in this appendix has been compiled from the pamphlet *Preparing a Landing Zone*, edited by Jim Whitman and published by the National EMS Pilots Association. Information on the pocket sized pamphlet can be obtained by writing NEMSPA, P.O. Box 2354, Pearland, TX 77588.

Medical Terminology

As an EMT, you will probably never have to use more than a few medical terms in the course of your prehospital emergency care activities, and most of them will probably deal with parts of the body. Physicians and nurses prefer EMTs to speak in other than medical terms. But if you are an avid reader, much of what you read is likely to be freely sprinkled with medical terms, and if you cannot translate them, you may not understand what you are reading.

Medical terms are comprised of words, word roots, combining forms, prefixes, and suffixes—all little words, if you will, and each with its own definition.

Sometimes medical terms are made up of two whole words. For example, the word SMALL, is joined with the word POX to form the medical term SMALLPOX, the name of a disease. Would that it were all so simple!

Word roots are the foundations of words and are not used by themselves. THERM is a word root that means heat; to use it alone would make no sense. But when a vowel is added to the end of the word root to make it the combining form THERM/O, it can be joined with other words or word roots to form a compound term. THERM/O and METER (an instrument for measuring) combine to form THERMOMETER, an instrument for measuring heat or temperature.

More than one word root or combining form can be joined to form medical terms; ELECTROCARDIOGRAM is a good example. ELECTR/O (electric) is joined to CARDI (heart) and the suffix -GRAM (a written record) to form the medical term that means a written record of the heart's electrical activity.

Prefixes are used to modify or qualify the meaning of word roots. They usually tell the reader what kind of, where (or in what direction), or how many.

The term -PNEA relates to breathing, but it says nothing about the quality or kind of breathing. Adding the prefix DYS- qualifies it as difficult breathing.

ABDOMINAL PAIN is a rather broad term; it gives the reader no clue as to exactly where the pain is located either inside or outside the abdomen. Adding the prefix-INTRA to ABDOMINAL pinpoints the location of the pain, for INTRA-ABDOMINAL PAIN means pain within the abdomen. -PLEGIA refers to paralysis of the limbs. The prefix QUADRI-informs the reader as to how many limbs are paralyzed. QUADRIPLEGIA means paralysis of all four limbs.

Suffixes are word endings that form nouns, adjectives, or verbs. Medical terms can have more than one suffix, and a suffix can appear in the middle of a compound term affixed to a combining form. A number of suffixes have specialized meanings. -ITIS means inflammation; thus ARTHRITIS means inflammation of a joint. -IAC forms a noun indicating a person afflicted with a certain disease, as for example, HEMOPHILIAC.

Some suffixes are joined to word roots to form terms that indicate a state, quality, condition, procedure, or process. PNEUMONIA and PSORIASIS are examples of medical conditions, while APPENDECTOMY and ARTHROSCOPY are examples of medical procedures. The suffixes in each case are underlined.

Some suffixes combine with word roots to form adjectives, words that modify nouns by indicating quality or quantity or by distinguishing one thing from another. GASTRIC, CARDIAC, FIBROUS, ARTHRITIC, and DIAPHORETIC are all examples of adjectives formed by adding suffixes (underlined) to word roots.

Some suffixes are added to word roots to express reduction in size, -OLE and -ULE, for example. An ARTERIOLE is smaller than an ARTERY, and a VENULE is smaller than a vein.

When added to word roots, -E and -IZE form verbs. EXCISE and CATHETERIZE are examples.

Finally, some of what are commonly accepted as suffixes are actually the combination of a word root and a suffix. -MEGALY (enlargement) results from the combination of the word root MEGAL (large) and the suffix -Y (which forms the term into a noun). CARDIOMEGALY means enlargement of the heart.

Standard Terms

The following terms are used to denote direction of movement, position, and anatomical posture.

ABDUCTION: movement away from the body's midline.

ADDUCTION: movement toward the body's midline.

AFFERENT: conducting toward a structure.

ANTERIOR: the front surface of the body.

ANTERIOR TO: in front of.

CAUDAD: toward the tail.

CEPHALAD: toward the head.

CIRCUMDUCTION: circular movement of a part.

CRANIAD: toward the cranium.

DEEP: situated remote from the surface.

DISTAL: situated away from the point of origin.

DORSAL: pertaining to the back surface of the body.

DORSIFLEXION: bending backward.

EFFERENT: conducting away from a structure.

ELEVATION: raising a body part.

EXTENSION: stretching, or moving jointed parts into or toward a straight condition.

EXTERNAL: situated outside.

FLEXION: bending, or moving jointed parts closer together.

INFERIOR: situated below.

INTERNAL: situated inside.

LATERAD: toward the side of the body.

LATERAL: situated away from the body's midline.

LATERAL ROTATION: rotating outward away from the body's midline.

LEFT LATERAL RECUMBENT: lying horizontal on the left side.

MEDIAD: toward the midline of the body.

MEDIAL: situated toward the body's midline.

MEDIAL ROTATION: rotating inward toward the body's midline.

PALMAR: concerning the inner surface of the hand.

PERIPHERAL: away from a central structure.

PLANTAR: concerning the sole of the foot.

POSTERIOR: pertaining to the back surface of the body.

POSTERIOR TO: situated behind.

PRONATION: lying face downward or turning the hand so the palm faces downward or backward.

PRONE: lying horizontal, face down and flat.

PROTRACTION: a pushing forward, as the mandible.

PROXIMAL: situated nearest the point of origin.

RECUMBENT: lying horizontal, generally speaking.

RETRACTION: a drawing back, as the tongue.

RIGHT LATERAL RECUMBENT: lying horizontal on the right side.

ROTATION: turning around an axis.

SUPERFICIAL: situated near the surface.

SUPERIOR: situated above.

SUPINATION: lying face upward or turning the hand so the palm faces forward or upward.

SUPINE: lying horizontal, flat on the back and face up.

VENTRAL: the front surface of the body.

Planes

A plane is an imaginary flat surface that divides the body into sections.

CORONAL OR FRONTAL PLANE: an imaginary plane that passes through the body from side to side and divides it into front and back sections.

MIDSAGITTAL PLANE: an imaginary plane that passes through the body from front to back and divides it into right and left halves.

SAGITTAL PLANE: an imaginary plane parallel to the median plane. It passes through the body from front to back and divides the body into right and left sections.

TRANSVERSE PLANE: an imaginary plane that passes through the body and divides it into upper and lower sections.

Word Parts

Prefixes are generally identified by a following dash (AMBI-). Combining forms have a slash and a vowel following the word root (ARTHR/O). Suffixes are generally identified by a preceding dash (-EMIA).

A- (not, without, lacking, deficient); *afebrile*, without fever.

AB- (away from); *abduct*, to draw away from the midline.

-ABLE, -IBLE (capable of); *reducible*, capable of being reduced (as a fracture).

ABDOMIN/O (abdomen); *abdominal*, pertaining to the abdomen.

AC- (to); *acclimate*, to become accustomed to.

ACOU (hear); *acoustic*, pertaining to sound or hearing.

ACR/O (extremity, top, peak); *acrodermatitis*, inflammation of the skin of the extremities.

ACU (needle); *acupuncture*, the Chinese practice of piercing specific peripheral nerves with needles to relieve the discomfort associated with painful disorders.

AD- (to, toward); *adduct*, to draw toward the midline.

ADEN/O (gland); *adenitis*, inflammation of a gland.

ADIP/O (fat) *adipose*, fatty; fat (in size).

AER/O (air); *aerobic*, requiring the presence of oxygen to live and grow.

AF- (to); *afferent*, conveying toward.

AG- (to); *aggregate*, to crowd or cluster together.

-ALGESIA (painful); *hyperalgesia*, overly sensitive to pain.

-ALGIA (painful condition); *neuralgia*, pain that extends along the course of one or more nerves.

AMBI- (both sides); *ambidextrous*, able to perform manual skills with both hands.

AMBLY (dim, dull, lazy); *amblyopia*, lazy eye.

AMPHI-, AMPHO- (on both sides, around both); *amphigonadism*, having both testicular and ovarian tissues.

AMYL/O (starch); *amyloid*, starchlike.

AN- (without); *anemia*, a reduced volume of blood cells.

ANA- (upward, again, backward, excess); *anaphylaxis*, an unusual or exaggerated reaction of an organism to a substance to which it becomes sensitized.

ANDR/O (man, male); *android*, resembling a man.

ANGI/O (blood vessel, duct); *angioplasty*, surgery of blood vessels.

ANKYL/O (stiff); *ankylosis*, stiffness.

ANT-, ANTI- (against, opposed to, preventing, relieving; *antidote*, a substance for counteracting a poison.

ANTE- (before, forward); *antecubital*, situated in front of the elbow.

ANTERO- (front); *anterolateral*, situated in front and to one side.

AP- (to); *approximate*, to bring together; to place close to.

APO- (separation, derivation from); *apoplexy*, sudden neurologic impairment due to a cardiovascular disorder.

-ARIUM, -ORIUM (place for something); *solarium*, a place for the sun.

ARTERI/O (artery); *arteriosclerosis*, thickening of the walls of the smaller arteries.

ARTHR/O (joint, articulation); *arthritis*, inflammation of a joint or joints.

ARTICUL/O (joint); *articulated*, united by joints.

AS- (to); *assimilate*, to take into.

AT- (to); *attract*, to draw toward.

AUDI/O (hearing); *audiometer*, an instrument to test the power of hearing.

AUR/O (ear); *auricle*, the flap of the ear

AUT/O (self); *autistic*, self-centered

BI- (two, twice, double, both); *bilateral*, having two sides; pertaining to two sides.

BI/O (life); *biology*, the study of life.

BLEPHAR/O (eyelid); *blepharitis*, inflammation of the eyelid.

BRACHI/O (upper arm); *brachialgia*, pain in the upper arm.

BRADY- (slow); *bradycardia*, an abnormally slow heart rate.

BRONCH/O (larger air passages of the lungs); *bronchitis*, inflammation of the larger air passages of the lungs.

BUCC/O (cheek); *buccal*, pertaining to the cheek.

CAC/O (bad); *cacosmis*, a bad odor.

CALC/O (stone); *calculus*, an abnormal hard inorganic mass such as a gallstone.

CALCANE/O (heel); *calcaneus*, the heel bone.

CALOR/O (heat); *caloric*, pertaining to heat.

CANCR/O (cancer); *cancroid*, resembling cancer.

CAPIT/O (head); *capitate*, head-shaped.

CAPS/O (container); *capsulation*, enclosed in a capsule or container.

CARCIN/O (cancer); *carcinogen*, a substance that causes cancer.

CARDI/O (heart); *cardiogenic*, originating in the heart.

CARP/O (wrist bone); *carpal*, pertaining to the wrist bone.

CAT-, CATA- (down, lower, under, against, along with); *catabasis*, the stage of decline of a disease.

-CELE (tumor, hernia); *hydrocele*, a confined collection of water.

CELI/O (abdomen); *celiomyalgia*, a pain in the muscles of the abdomen.

-CENTESIS (perforation or tapping, as with a needle); *abdominocentesis*, surgical puncture of the abdominal cavity.

CEPHAL/O (head); *electroencephalogram*, a recording of the electrical activity of the brain.

CEREBR/O (cerebrum); *cerebrospinal*, pertaining to the brain and spinal fluid.

CERVIC/O (neck, cervix); *cervical,* pertaining to the neck (or cervix).

CHEIL/O, CHIL/O (lip); *cheilitis,* inflammation of the lips.

CHEIR/O, CHIR/O (hand); *cheiralgia,* pain in the hand.

CHLOR/O (green); *chloroma,* green cancer, a greenish tumor associated with myelogenous leukemia.

CHOL/E (bile, gall); *choledochitis,* inflammation of the common bile duct.

CHONDR/O (cartilage); *chondrodynia,* pain in a cartilage.

CHROM/O, CHROMAT/O (color); *monochromatic,* being of one color.

CHRON/O (time); *chronic,* persisting for a long time.

-CID- (cut, kill, fall); *insecticide,* an agent that kills insects.

CIRCUM- (around); *circumscribed,* confined to a limited space.

-CIS- (cut, kill, fall); *excise,* to cut out.

-CLYSIS (irrigation); *enteroclysis,* irrigation of the small intestine.

CO- (with); *cohesion,* the force that causes various particles to unite.

COL- (with); *collateral,* secondary or accessory; a small side branch such as a blood vessel or nerve.

COL/O (colon, large intestine); *colitis,* inflammation of the colon.

COLP/O (vagina); *colporrhagia,* bleeding from the vagina.

COM- (with); *comminuted,* broken or crushed into small pieces.

CON- (with); *congenital,* existing from the time of birth.

CONTRA- (against, opposite); *contraindicated,* inadvisable.

COR/E, CORE/O (pupil); *corectopia,* abnormal location of the pupil of the eye.

COST/O (rib); *intercostal,* between the ribs.

CRANI/O (skull); *cranial,* pertaining to the skull.

CRY/O (cold); *cryogenic,* that which produces low temperature.

CRYPT/O (hide, cover, conceal); *cryptogenic,* of doubtful origin.

CYAN/O (blue); *cyanosis,* bluish discoloration of the skin and mucus membranes.

CYST/O (urinary bladder, cyst, sac of fluid); *cystitis,* inflammation of the bladder.

-CYTE (cell); *leukocyte,* white cell.

CYT/O (cell); *cytoma,* tumor of the cell.

DACRY/O (tear); *dacryorrhea,* excessive flow of tears.

DACTYL/O (finger, toe); *dactylomegaly,* abnormally large fingers or toes.

DE- (down); *descending,* coming down from.

DENT/O (tooth); *dental,* pertaining to the teeth.

DERM/O, DERMAT/O (skin); *dermatitis,* inflammation of the skin.

DEXTR/O (right); *dextrad,* toward the right side.

DI- (twice, double); *diplegia,* paralysis affecting like parts on both sides of the body.

DIA- (through, across, apart); *diaphragm,* the partition that separates the abdominal and thoracic cavities.

DIPL/O (double, twin, twice); *diplopia,* double vision.

DIPS/O (thirst); *dipsomania,* alcoholism.

DIS- (to free, to undo); *dissect,* to cut apart.

DORS/O (back); *dorsal,* pertaining to the back.

-DYNIA (painful condition); *cephalodynia,* headache.

DYS- (bad, difficult, abnormal, incomplete); *dyspnea,* labored breathing.

-ECTASIA (dilation or enlargement of an organ or part); *gastrectasia,* dilation (stretching) of the stomach.

ECTO- (outer, outside of); *ectopic,* located away from the normal position.

-ECTOMY (the surgical removal of an organ or part); *appendectomy,* surgical removal of the appendix.

ELECTR/O (electric); *electrocardiogram,* the written record of the heart's electrical activity.

-EMIA (condition of the blood); *anemia,* a deficiency of red blood cells.

EN- (in, into, within); *encapsulate,* to enclose with a container.

ENCEPHAL/O (brain); *encephalitis,* inflammation of the brain.

END-, ENDO- (within); *endotracheal,* within the trachea.

ENT-, ENTO- (within, inner); *entopic,* occurring in the proper place.

ENTER/O (small intestine); *enteritis,* inflammation of the intestine.

EP-, EPI- (over, on, upon); *epidermis,* the outermost layer of skin.

ERYTHR/O (red); *erythrocyte,* a red blood cell.

ESTHESIA (feeling); *anesthesia,* without feeling.

EU (good, well, normal, healthy); *euphoria,* an abnormal or exaggerated feeling of well-being.

EX- (out of, away from); *excrement,* waste material discharged from the body.

EXO- (outside, outward); *exophytic,* to grow outward or on the surface.

EXTRA- (on the outside, beyond, in addition to); *extracorporeal,* outside the body.

FACI/O (face, surface); *facial,* pertaining to the face.

FEBR/I (fever); *febrile,* feverish.

-FERENT (bear, carry); *efferent,* carrying away from a center.

FIBR/O (fiber, filament); *fibrillation,* muscular contractions due to the activity of muscle fibers.

-FORM (shape); *deformed,* abnormally shaped.

-FUGAL (moving away); *centrifugal,* moving away from a center.

GALACT/O (milk); *galactopyria,* milk fever.

GANGLI/O (knot); *ganglion,* a knotlike mass.

GASTR/O (stomach); *gastritis,* inflammation of the stomach.

GEN/O (come into being, originate); *genetic,* inherited.

-GENESIS (production or origin); *pathogenesis,* the development of a disease.

-GENIC (giving rise to, originating in); *cardiogenic,* originating in the heart.

GLOSS/O (tongue); *glossal,* pertaining to the tongue.

GLYC/O (sweet); *glycemia,* the presence of sugar in the blood.

GNATH/O (jaw); *gnathitis,* inflammation of the jaw.

-GRAM (drawing, written record); *electrocardiogram,* a recording of the heart's electrical activity.

-GRAPH (an instrument for recording the activity of an organ); *electrocardiograph,* an instrument for measuring the heart's electrical activity.

-GRAPHY (the recording of the activity of an organ); *electrocardiography,* the method of recording the heart's electrical activity.

GYNEC/O (woman); *gynecologist,* a specialist in diseases of the female genital tract.

GNOS/O (knowledge); *prognosis,* a prediction of the outcome of a disease.

HEM/A, HEM/O, HEMAT/O (blood); *hematoma,* a localized collection of blood.

HEMI- (one-half); *hemiplegia,* paralysis of one side of the body.

HEPAT/O (liver); *hepatitis,* inflammation of the liver.

HETER/O (other); *heterogeneous,* from a different source.

HIDR/O, HIDROT/O (sweat); *hidrosis,* excessive sweating.

HIST/O (tissue); *histodialysis,* the breaking down of tissue.

HOM/O, HOME/O (same, similar, unchanging, constant); *homeostasis,* stability in an organism's normal physiological states.

HYDR/O (water, fluid); *hydrocephalus,* an accumulation of cerebrospinal fluid in the skull with resulting enlargement of the head.

HYPN/O (sleep); *hypnotic,* that which induces sleep.

HYAL/O (glass); *hyaline,* glassy, transparent.

HYPER- (beyond normal, excessive); *hypertension,* abnormally high blood pressure.

HYPO- (below normal, deficient, under, beneath); *hypotension,* abnormally low blood pressure.

HYSTER/O (uterus, womb); *hysterectomy,* surgical removal of the uterus.

-IASIS (condition); *psoriasis,* a chronic skin condition characterized by lesions.

IATR/O (healer, physician); *pediatrician,* a physician that specializes in children's disorders.

-ID (in a state, condition of); *gravid,* pregnant.

IDI/O (peculiar, separate, distinct); *idiopathic,* occurring without a known cause.

IL- (negative prefix); *illegible,* cannot be read.

ILE/O (ileum); *ileitis,* inflammation of the ileum.

ILI/O (ilium); *iliac,* pertaining to the ilium.

IM- (negative prefix); *immature,* not mature.

IN- (in, into, within); *incise,* to cut into.

INFRA- (beneath, below); *infracostal,* below a rib, or below the ribs.

INTER- (between); *intercostal,* between two ribs.

INTRA- (within); *intraoral,* within the mouth.

INTRO- (within, into); *introspection,* the contemplation of one's own thoughts and feelings; self-analysis.

IR/O, IRID/O (iris); *iridotomy,* incision of the iris.

ISCHI/O (ischium); *ischialgia,* pain in the ischium.

-ISMUS (abnormal condition); *strabismus,* deviation of the eye that a person cannot overcome.

ISO- (same, equal, alike); *isometric,* of equal dimensions.

-ITIS (inflammation); *endocarditis,* inflammation within the heart.

KERAT/O (cornea); *keratitis,* inflammation of the cornea.

KINESI/O (movement); *kinesialgia,* pain upon movement.

LABI/O (lip); *labiodental,* pertaining to the lip and teeth.

LACT/O (milk); *lactation,* the secretion of milk.

LAL/O (talk); *lalopathy,* any speech disorder.

LAPAR/O (flank, abdomen, abdominal wall); *laparotomy,* an incision through the abdominal wall.

LARYNG/O (larynx); *laryngoscope,* an instrument for examining the larynx.

LEPT/O (thin); *leptodactylous,* having slender fingers.

LEUC/O, LEUK/O (white); *leukemia,* a malignant disease characterized by the increased development of white blood cells.

LINGU/O (tongue); *sublingual,* under the tongue.

LIP/O (fat); *lipoma,* fatty tumor.

LITH/O (stone); *lithotriptor,* an instrument for crushing stones in the bladder.

-LOGIST (a person who studies); *pathologist,* a person who studies diseases.

LOG/O (speak), give an account; *logospasms,* spasmodic speech.

-LOGY (study of); *pathology,* the study of disease.

LUMB/O (loin); *lumbago,* pain in the lumbar region.

LYMPH/O (lymph); *lymphoduct,* a vessel of the lymph system.

-LYSIS (destruction); *electrolysis,* destruction (of hair, for example) by passage of an electric current.

MACR/O (large, long); *macrocephalous,* having an abnormally large head.

MALAC/O (a softening); *malacia*, the morbid softening of a body part or tissue.

MAMM/O (breast); *mammary*, pertaining to the breast.

-MANIA (mental aberration); *kleptomania*, the compulsion to steal.

MAST/O (breast); *mastectomy*, surgical removal of the breast.

MEDI/O (middle); *mediastinum*, middle partition of the thoracic cavity.

MEGA- (large); *megacolon*, an abnormally large colon.

MEGAL/O (large); *megalomaniac*, a person impressed with his own greatness.

-MEGALY (an enlargement); *cardiomegaly*, enlargement of the heart.

MELAN/O (dark, black); *melanoma*, a tumor comprised of darkly pigmented cells.

MEN/O (month); *menopause*, cessation of menstruation.

MES/O (middle); *mesiad*, toward the center.

META- (change, transformation, exchange); *metabolism*, the sum of the physical and chemical processes by which an organism survives.

METR/O (uterus); *metralgia*, pain in the uterus.

MICR/O (small); *microscope*, an instrument for magnifying small objects.

MON/O (single, only, sole); *monoplegia*, paralysis of a single part.

MORPH/O (form); *morphology*, the study of form and shape.

MULTI- (many, much); *multipara*, a woman who has given two or more live births.

MYC/O, MYCET/O (fungus); *mycosis*, any disease caused by a fungus.

MY/O (muscle); *myasthenia*, muscular weakness.

MYEL/O (marrow, also often refers to spinal cord); *myelocele*, protrusion of the spinal cord through a defect in the spinal column.

MYX/O (mucus, slimelike); *myxoid*, resembling mucus.

NARC/O (stupor, numbness); *narcotic*, an agent that induces sleep.

NAS/O (nose); *oronasal*, pertaining to the nose and mouth.

NE/O (new); *neonate*, a newborn infant.

NECR/O (corpse); *necrotic*, dead (when referring to tissue).

NEPHR/O (kidney); *nephralgia*, pain in the kidneys.

NEUR/O (nerve); *neuritis*, inflammation of nerve pathways.

NOCT/I (night); *noctambulism*, sleep walking.

NORM/O (rule, order, normal); *normotension*, normal blood pressure.

NULL/I (none); *nullipara*, a woman who has never given birth to a child.

NYCT/O (night); *nycturia*, excessive urination at night.

OB- (against, in front of, toward); *obturator*, a device that closes an opening.

OC- (against, in front of, toward); *occlude*, to obstruct.

OCUL/O (eye); *ocular*, pertaining to the eye.

ODONT/O (tooth); *odontalgia*, toothache.

-OID (shape, form, resemblance); *ovoid*, egg-shaped.

OLIG/O (few, deficient, scanty); *oligemia*, lacking in blood volume.

-OMA (tumor, swelling); *adenoma*, tumor of a gland.

O/O- (egg); *ooblast*, a primitive cell from which an ovum develops.

ONYCH/O (nail); *onychoma*, tumor of a nail or nail bed.

OOPHOR/O (ovary); *oophorectomy*, a surgical removal of one or both ovaries.

-OPSY (a viewing); *autopsy*, postmortem examination of a body.

OPTHALM/O (eye); *opthalmic*, pertaining to the eyes.

OPT/O, OPTIC/O (sight, vision); *optometrist*, a specialist in adapting lenses for the correcting of visual defects.

OR/O (mouth); *oral*, pertaining to the mouth.

ORCH/O, ORCHID/O (testicle); *orchitis*, inflammation of the testicles.

ORTH/O (straight, upright); *orthopedic*, pertaining to the correction of skeletal defects.

-OSIS (process, an abnormal condition); *dermatosis*, any skin condition.

OSTE/O (bone); *osteomyelitis*, inflammation of bone or bone marrow.

OT/O (ear); *otalgia*, earache.

OVARI/O (ovary); *ovariocele*, hernia of an ovary.

OV/I, OV/O (egg); *oviduct*, a passage through which an egg passes.

PACHY- (thicken); *pachyderma*, abnormal thickening of the skin.

PALAT/O (palate); *palatitis*, inflammation of the palate.

PAN- (all, entire, every); *panacea*, a remedy for all diseases, a "cure-all."

PARA- (beside, beyond, accessory to, apart from, against); *paranormal*, beyond the natural or normal.

PATH/O (disease); *pathogen*, any disease-producing agent.

-PATHY (disease of a part); *osteopathy*, disease of a bone.

-PENIA (an abnormal reduction); *leukopenia*, deficiency in white blood cells.

PEPS/O, PEPT/O (digestion); *dyspepsia*, poor digestion.

PER- (throughout, completely, extremely); *perfusion*, the passage of fluid through the vessels of an organ.

PERI- (around, surrounding); *pericardium*, the sac that surrounds the heart and the roots of the great vessels.

-PEXY (fixation); *splendopexy,* surgical fixation of the spleen.

PHAG/O (eat); *phagomania,* an insatiable craving for food.

PHARYNG/O (throat); *pharyngospasms,* spasms of the muscles of the pharynx.

PHAS/O (speech); *aphasic,* unable to speak.

PHIL/O (like, have an affinity for); *necrophilia,* an abnormal interest in death.

PHLEB/O (vein); *phlebotomy,* surgical incision of a vein.

-PHOBIA (fear, dread); *claustrophobia,* a fear of closed spaces.

PHON/O (sound); *phonetic,* pertaining to the voice.

PHOR/O (bear, carry); *diaphoresis,* profuse sweating.

PHOT/O (light); *photosensitivity,* abnormal reactivity of the skin to sunlight.

PHREN/O (diaphragm); *phrenic nerve,* a nerve that carries messages to the diaphragm.

PHYSI/O (nature); *physiology,* the science that studies the function of living things.

PIL/O (hair); *pilose,* hairy.

-PLASIA (development, formation); *dysplasia,* poor or abnormal formation.

-PLASTY (surgical repair); *arthroplasty,* surgical repair of a joint.

-PLEGIA (paralysis); *paraplegia,* paralysis of the lower body, including the legs.

PLEUR/O (rib, side, pleura); *pleurisy,* inflammation of the pleura.

-PNEA (breath, breathing); *orthopnea,* difficult breathing except in an upright position.

PNEUM/O, PNEUMAT/O (air, breath); *pneumatic,* pertaining to the air.

PNEUM/O, PNEUMON/O (lung); *pneumonia,* inflammation of the lungs with the escape of fluid.

POD/O (foot); *podiatrist,* a specialist in the care of feet.

-POIESIS (formation); *hematopoiesis,* formation of blood.

POLY- (much, many); *polychromatic,* multicolored.

POST- (after, behind); *postmortem,* after death.

PRE- (before); *premature,* occurring before the proper time.

PRO- (before, in front of); *prolapse,* the falling down, or sinking of a part.

PROCT/O (anus); *proctitis,* inflammation of the rectum.

PSEUD/O (false); *pseudoplegia,* hysterical paralysis.

PSYCH/O (mind, soul); *psychopath,* one who displays aggressive antisocial behavior.

-PTOSIS (abnormal dropping or sagging of a part); *hysteroptosis,* sagging of the uterus.

PULMON/O (lung); *pulmonary,* pertaining to the lungs.

PY/O (pus); *pyorrhea,* copious discharge of pus.

PYEL/O (renal pelvis); *pyelitis,* inflammation of the renal pelvis.

PYR/O (fire, fever); *pyromaniac,* compulsive fire setter.

QUADRI- (four); *quadriplegia,* paralysis of all four limbs.

RACH/I (spine); *rachialgia,* pain in the spine.

RADI/O (ray, radiation); *radiology,* the use of ionizing radiation in diagnosis and treatment.

RE- (back, against, contrary); *recurrence,* the return of symptoms after remission.

RECT/O (rectum); *rectal,* pertaining to the rectum.

REN/O (the kidneys); *renal,* pertaining to the kidneys.

RETRO- (located behind, backward); *retroperineal,* behind the perineum.

RHIN/O (nose); *rhinitis,* inflammation of the mucus membranes of the nose.

-RRHAGE (abnormal discharge); *hemorrhage,* abnormal discharge of blood.

-RRHAGIA (hemorrhage from an organ or body part); *menorrhea,* excessive uterine bleeding.

-RRHEA (flowing or discharge); *diarrhea,* abnormal frequency and liquidity of fecal discharges.

SANGUIN/O (blood); *exsanguinate,* to lose a large volume of blood either internally or externally.

SARC/O (flesh); *sarcoma,* a malignant tumor.

SCHIZ/O (split); *schizophrenia,* any of a group of emotional disorders characterized by bizarre behavior (erroneously called split personality).

SCLER/O (hardening); *schleroderma,* hardening of connective tissues of the body, including the skin.

-SCLEROSIS (hardened condition); *arteriosclerosis,* hardening of the arteries.

SCOLI/O (twisted, crooked); *scoliosis,* sideward deviation of the spine.

-SCOPE (an instrument for observing); *endoscope,* an instrument for the examination of a hollow body, such as the bladder.

-SECT (cut); *transsect,* to cut across.

SEMI- (one-half, partly); *semisupine,* partly, but not completely, supine.

SEPT/O, SEPS/O (infection); *aseptic,* free from infection.

SOMAT/O (body); *psychosomatic,* both psychological and physiological.

SON/O (sound); *sonogram,* a recording produced by the passage of sound waves through the body.

SPERMAT/O (sperm, semen); *spermacide,* an agent that kills sperm.

SPHYGM/O (pulse); *sphygmomanometer,* a device for measuring blood pressure in the arteries.

SPLEN/O (spleen); *splenectomy,* surgical removal of the spleen.

-STASIS (stopping, controlling); *hemostasis,* the control of bleeding.

STEN/O (narrow); *stenosis,* a narrowing of a passage or opening.

STERE/O (solid, three-dimensional); *stereoscopic,* a three-dimensional appearance.

STETH/O (chest); *stethoscope,* an instrument for listening to chest sounds.

STHEN/O (strength); *myasthenia,* muscular weakness.

-STOMY (surgically creating a new opening); *colostomy,* surgical creation of an opening between the colon and the surface of the body.

SUB- (under, near, almost, moderately); *subclavian,* situated under the clavicle.

SUPER- (above, excess); *superficial,* lying on or near the surface.

SUPRA- (above, over); *suprapubic,* situated above the pubic arch.

SYM-, SYN- (joined together, with); *syndrome,* a set of symptoms that occur together.

TACHY- (fast); *tachycardia,* a very fast heart rate.

-THERAPY (treatment); *hydrotherapy,* treatment with water.

THERM/O (heat); *thermogenesis,* the production of heat.

THORAC/O (chest cavity); *thoracic,* pertaining to the chest.

THROMB/O (clot, lump); *thrombophlebitis,* inflammation of a vein.

-TOME (a surgical instrument for cutting); *microtome,* an instrument for cutting thin slices of tissue.

-TOMY (a surgical operation on an organ or body part); *thoracotomy,* surgical incision of the chest wall.

TOP/O (place); *topographic,* pertaining to special regions (of the body)

TRACHE/O (trachea); *tracheostomy,* an opening in the neck that passes to the trachea.

TRANS- (through, across, beyond); *transfusion,* the introduction of whole blood or blood components directly into the bloodstream.

TRI- (three); *trimester,* a period of three months.

TRICH/O (hair); *trichosis,* any disease of the hair.

-TRIPSY (surgical crushing); *lithotripsy,* surgical crushing of stones.

TROPH/O (nourish); *hypertrophic,* enlargement of an organ or body part due to the increase in the size of cells.

ULTRA- (beyond, excess); *ultrasonic,* beyond the audible range.

UNI- (one); *unilateral,* affecting one side.

UR/O (urine); *urinalysis,* examination of urine.

URETER/O (ureter); *ureteritis,* inflammation of a ureter.

URETHR/O (urethra); *urethritis,* inflammation of the urethra.

VAS/O (vessel, duct); *vasodilator,* an agent that causes dilation of blood vessels.

VEN/O (vein); *venipuncture,* surgical puncture of a vein.

VENTR/O (belly, cavity); *ventral,* relating to the belly or abdomen.

VESIC/O (blister, bladder); *vesicle,* a small, fluid-filled blister.

VISCER/O (internal organ); *visceral,* pertaining to the viscera (abdominal organs).

XANTH/O (yellow); *xanthroma,* a yellow nodule in the skin.

XEN/O (stranger); *xenophobia,* abnormal fear of strangers.

XER/O (dry); *xerosis,* abnormal dryness (as of the mouth or eyes).

ZO/O (animal life); *zoogenous,* acquired from an animal.

Glossary

A

A-pillar first roof pillar from the windshield of a vehicle.

Abandonment to leave an injured or sick patient before care is assumed by an equally or more highly trained person. Leaving the scene without giving patient information may be viewed as a form of abandonment.

ABC Method sequence of operations required in cardiopulmonary resuscitation. 'A' stands for airway, 'B' for breathe, and 'C' for circulate.

Abdomen (AB-do-men) area of the body between the diaphragm and the pelvis.

Abdominal Cavity the anterior body cavity located between the diaphragm and the ring of the pelvis. It houses and protects the abdominal organs, glands, and the major abdominal blood vessels and nerves.

Abdominal Quadrants the four zones assigned to the anterior abdominal wall that are used for quick reference.

Abdominal Thrusts manual thrusts delivered to the abdominal region between the navel and xiphoid process to create pressure to help expel an airway obstruction.

Abdominopelvic (AB-dom-i-no-PEL-vik) anterior body cavity inferior to the diaphragm.

Abduction movement *away* from the vertical midline of the body.

Abortion (ah-BOR-shun) spontaneous (miscarriage) or induced delivery of the fetus and placenta before the 28th week of pregnancy.

Abrasion (ab-RAY-zhun) *see* Scratch.

Abruptio (ab-RUP-she-o) **Placentae** (plah-SEN-ti) the premature separation of the placenta from the uterus wall.

Abscess (AB-ses) a limited structure containing the collecting pus associated with tissue death and infection.

Accident Zone *see* Danger Zone.

Acetabulum (AS-i-TAB-u-lem) the socket of the pelvis that receives the head of the femur to form the ball and socket joint of the hip.

Acetone Breath sweet breath with a fruit-like odor. A sign associated with diabetic coma.

Achilles (ah-KEL-ez) **Tendon** the common term for the tendon that connects the posterior lower leg muscles to the heel. The anatomical term is calcaneal (kal-KA-ne-al) tendon.

Acid being acidic, as opposed to being neutral or basic (alkaline). Associated with free hydrogen ions.

Acidosis (AS-i-DO-sis) condition of increased acidity.

Acromioclavicular (ah-KRO-me-o-cla-VIK-u-lar) **Joint** the superior joint of the shoulder formed by the scapula and clavicle.

Acromion (ah-KRO-me-on) **Process** the part of the spine of the scapula that forms the superior shoulder.

Actual Consent consent by the adult patient, usually in oral form, accepting emergency care. This must be informed consent.

Acute to have a rapid onset. Sometimes used to mean severe.

Acute Abdomen inflammation in the abdominal cavity producing intense pain.

Acute Myocardial Infarction (AMI) (my-o-KARD-e-al in-FARK-shun) heart attack. The sudden death of heart muscle due to oxygen starvation. Usually caused by a narrowing or blockage of a coronary artery supplying the myocardium.

Adduction movement *toward* the vertical midline of the body.

Afterbirth the placenta, membranes of the amniotic sac, part of the umbilical cord, and some uterine lining tissues that are delivered after the birth of the baby.

Air Embolism gas bubbles in the bloodstream.

Airway the passageway for air from the nose and mouth to the exchange levels of the lungs. Can also mean artificial airways, such as an oropharyngeal airway.

Airway Adjunct a device placed in a patient's mouth or nose in order to help maintain an open airway. Those inserted in the mouth help to hold the tongue clear of the airway.

Alkali a substance that is basic, as opposed to being acid or neutral.

Alkalosis (AL-ke-LO-sis) condition of an increase in base (alkaline).

Allergen (AL-er-jin) any substance capable of inducing an allergic reaction.

Alveoli (Al-VE-o-li) microscopic air sacs of the lungs where gas exchange takes place with the circulatory system.

Ambulance vehicle for emergency care with a driver compartment and a patient compartment, carrying all equipment and supplies needed to provide basic EMT-level emergency care at the scene and en route to the emergency department.

Amnesia the short- or long-term loss of memory. Usually associated with a sudden onset.

Amniotic Sac fluid-filled sac that surrounds the fetus.

Amputation the surgical removal or traumatic severing of a body part. The most common usage in emergency care refers to the traumatic amputation of an extremity or part of an extremity.

Analgesic pain reliever.

Anaphylactic (an-ah-fi-LAK-tik) **Shock** allergy shock. The most severe type of allergic reaction in which a person goes into shock when he comes into contact with a substance to which he is allergic.

Anatomical Position standard reference position for the body in the study of anatomy. The body is erect, facing the observer. The arms are down at the sides and the palms of the hands face forward.

Aneurysm (AN-u-riz'm) blood-filled sac caused by the localized dilation of an artery or vein. The dilated or weakened section of an arterial wall.

Angina Pectoris (an-JI-nah PEK-to-ris) chest pains often caused by an insufficient blood supply to the heart muscle.

Angulation angle formed above and below a break in a bone. The fracture changes the straight line of a bone into an angle.

Anoxia absence of oxygen. *See* Hypoxia.

Anterior front surface of the body or body part.

Antiseptic substance that will stop the growth of, or prevent the activities of, germs (microorganisms).

Anus (A-nus) outlet of the large intestine.

Aorta (a-OR-ta) major artery of systemic circulation that carries blood from the heart out to the body.

Aphasia (ah-FAY-zhe-ah) the complete loss or impairment of speech usually associated with a stroke or brain lesion.

Apical Pulse heartbeat felt over the lower portion of the heart.

Apnea (ap-NE-ah) temporary suspension of breathing.

Apoplexy (AP-o-plek-see) loss of consciousness, movement, and sensation that is caused by a stroke.

Appendicular (AP-pen-dik-u-ler) **Skeleton** clavicles, scapulae, bones of the upper limbs, pelvis, and the bones of the lower limbs.

Arm body part from shoulder to elbow.

Arrhythmia (ah-RITH-me-ah) disturbance of heart rate and rhythm.

Arteriosclerosis (ar-TE-re-o-skle-RO-sis) "hardening of the arteries" caused by calcium deposits.

Artery any blood vessel carrying blood away from the heart.

Articulate to unite to form a joint.

Ascites (a-SI-tez) noticeable distention of the abdomen caused by accumulation of excessive fluids.

Aseptic clean, free of particles of dirt and debris, but not necessarily sterile.

Asphyxia (as-FIK-si-ah) suffocation resulting in the loss of consciousness caused by too little oxygen reaching the brain. The functions of the brain, heart, and lungs will cease.

Aspiration to inhale materials into the lungs. Often used to describe the breathing in of vomitus.

Asthma (AS-mah) condition that constricts the bronchioles, causing a reduction of air flow and congestion. Air usually enters to the level of the alveoli, but it cannot be expired easily.

Asystole (a-SIS-to-le) cardiac standstill.

Atelectasis (at-i-LEK-tah-sis) the partial or complete collapse of the alveoli of the lungs.

Atherosclerosis (ATH-er-o-skle-RO-sis) build-up of fatty deposits and other particles on the inner wall of an artery. This build-up is called "plaque." Calcium may deposit in the plaque, causing the wall to become hard and stiff.

Atrium (A-tree-um) superior chamber of the heart (plural—atria).

Auscultation (os-skul-TAY-shun) the process of listening to sounds that occur within the body.

Autonomic Nervous System parts of the central nervous system, structures that parallel the spinal cord, and shared peripheral nerve pathways that combine to form a system involved with the involuntary control of the heart, blood vessel diameter, organs, and glands.

Avulsion (ah-VUL-shun) piece of tissue or skin that is torn loose or pulled off by injury.

Axial (AK-si-al) **Skeleton** skull, spine, sternum, and ribs.

Axilla (ak-SIL-ah) the armpit.

B

B-pillar second roof pillar from a vehicle's windshield.

Bag-Valve-Mask Device aid for artificial ventilation. It has a face mask, a self-inflating bag, and a valve that allows the bag to refill while the patient exhales. It can be attached to an oxygen line.

Bandage material such as gauze or tape used to hold a dressing in place.

Basal Skull Fracture a fracture to the bones of the cranial floor (base of the skull).

Bilateral existing on both sides.

Bile fluid produced by the liver and sent to the small intestine. It may be stored in the gallbladder. Bile has many functions, including changing intestinal motility and helping to digest fatty foods.

Biological Death when lung and heart activity stops and brain cells die. Changes in the brain cells and blood vessels usually begin within 4 to 6 minutes after breathing stops. Brain cell death typically begins within 10 minutes after respiratory arrest.

Bladder usually referring to the urinary bladder located in the pelvic cavity.

Blanch become pale.

Blood Pressure pressure caused by blood exerting force on the walls of blood vessels. Usually, arterial blood pressure is measured.

Bolus mass of chewed or partially chewed food that is ready to be swallowed.

Bourdon (bore-DON) **Gauge** a gauged flowmeter that indicates the flow of a gas in liters per minute.

Bowel intestine.

Brachial (BRAY-key-al) **Artery** the major artery of the arm.

Brachial (BRAY-key-al) **Pulse** pulse produced by compressing the major artery of the upper arm. Used to detect heart action and circulation in infants.

Bradycardia (bray-de-KAR-de-ah) abnormal condition where the heart rate is very slow. The pulse rate will be below 50 beats per minute.

Breech Birth delivery where the buttocks or both legs of the baby are born first.

Bronchiole (BRONG-key-ol) small branches of the airway that carry air to and from the alveoli.

Bronchus (BRONC-kus) the portion of the airway connecting the trachea to the lungs (plural—bronchi).

Bruise contusion.

C

C-pillar third roof pillar from a vehicle's windshield.

Cannula hollow tube that can be inserted into a cavity to allow for fluid drainage.

Capillary microscopic blood vessel where exchange takes place between bloodstream and body tissues.

Cardiac (KAR-de-ak) refers to the heart.

Cardiac Arrest when the heart stops beating.

Cardiogenic (KAR-de-o-JEN-ik) **Shock** failure of the cardiovascular system brought about when the heart can no longer develop the pressure needed to circulate blood to all parts of the body.

Cardiopulmonary Resuscitation (KAR-de-o-PUL-mo-ner-e re-SUS-ci-TA-shun) **(CPR)** heart-lung resuscitation where there is a combined effort to restore or maintain respiration and circulation.

Carotid (kah-ROT-id) **Artery** large neck artery.

One is found on each side of the neck. Its pulse is of prime importance in the primary survey and CPR.

Carpals (KAR-pals) wrist bones.

Catheter flexible tube passed through body channels to allow for the drainage or withdrawal of fluids.

Cephalic (ce-FAL-ik) refers to the head.

Cerebrospinal (ser-e-bro-SPI-nal) **Fluid** clear watery fluid that surrounds and helps to protect the brain and spinal cord.

Cerebrovascular Accident (CVA) a stroke. The rupturing or blockage of a major blood vessel supplying or draining the brain.

Cervical (SER-ve-kal) relating to the neck or to the inferior end of the uterus. The first seven vertebrae.

Cervix (SER-vicks) inferior portion of the uterus, where it enters the vagina.

Child Abuse assault of the infant or child that produces physical and/or emotional injuries. Sexual assault is included as a form of child abuse. The victim of physical assault is often called a battered child.

Chronic opposite of acute. It can be used to mean long and drawn out or recurring.

Chronic Heart Failure *see* Congestive Heart Failure.

Chronic Obstructive Pulmonary Disease (COPD) group of diseases and conditions in which the lungs decline in their ability to exchange gases. COPD includes emphysema, chronic bronchitis, and miner's black lung.

Clavicle (KLAV-i-kul) collarbone.

Clinical Death state when breathing and heart action cease.

Clonic Phase second phase of a convulsive seizure, with the patient exhibiting violent body jerks, drooling, and possibly cyanosis. Most convulsions last 1 to 2 minutes.

Closed Fracture simple fracture where the skin is not broken by the fractured bones.

Closed Wound injury where the skin is not broken, as in the case of a contusion.

Clot formation of fibrin and entangled blood cells that act to stop bleeding from a wound.

Coccyx (KOK-siks) lowermost bones of the vertebral column. They are fused into one bone in the adult.

Collarbone clavicle.

Coma state of complete unconsciousness, the depth of which may vary.

Comminuted (KOM-i-nu-ted) **Fracture** fracture where the bone is fragmented or turned to powder.

Concussion mild state of stupor or temporary unconsciousness caused by a blow to the head. There is no laceration or bleeding in the brain.

Condyles (KON-dials) the large, rounded projections at the distal end of the femur and the proximal end of the tibia. Often called the sides of the knees by the layperson.

Congestive Heart Failure associated with lung conditions and diseases (e.g., COPD) or heart disease. Excessive fluid build-up occurs in the lungs and/or body organs. The heart fails in its efforts to properly circulate blood and the lungs fail in their effort to properly exchange gases.

Constricting Band used to restrict the flow of venom.

Contraindicated condition, sign, or symptom that makes a particular course of treatment or procedure inadvisable.

Contusion (kun-TU-zhun) bruise. The simplest form of closed wound where blood flows between tissues causing a discoloration.

Convulsion uncontrolled skeletal muscle spasm, often violent.

COPD chronic obstructive pulmonary disease.

Core Temperature body temperature measured at a central point, such as within the rectum.

Cornea (KOR-ne-ah) transparent covering over the iris and pupil of the eye.

Coronary (KOR-o-nar-e) refers to the blood vessels that supply blood to the heart muscle. Many people use this term to mean heart attack.

Coronary (KOR-o-nar-e) **Artery** a blood vessel that supplies the myocardium.

Coronary Artery Disease (CAD) the narrowing of a coronary artery brought about by atherosclerosis. Occlusion (blockage) occurs in many cases.

CPR cardiopulmonary resuscitation.

CPR Compression Site mid-sternal point approximately two finger-widths superior to the xiphoid process. During CPR of adults, compressions are delivered to this site. In children, this site is along the midline of the breastbone, between the nipples. In infants, the site is one finger-width below the intermammary line.

Cranial (KRAY-ne-al) pertaining to the braincase of the skull.

Cranium (KRAY-ne-um) braincase of the skull. Many people use the term skull when they mean cranium.

Crepitus (KREP-i-tus) grating noise or the sensation felt caused by the movement of broken bone ends rubbing together.

Crisis any event seen as a crucial moment or turning point in the patient's life.

Croup (Kroop)   the general term for a group of viral infections that produce swelling of the larynx.

Crowing   atypical sound made when a patient breathes. It usually indicates airway obstruction.

Crowning   when the presenting part of the baby first bulges out of the vagina opening. It is usually in reference to a normal head-first delivery.

Cryotherapy   to treat with cold.

Cut   an open wound with smooth edges (incision) or jagged edges (laceration).

Cyanosis (sign-ah-NO-sis)   when the skin, lips, tongue, and/or nailbed color changes to blue or gray because of too little oxygen in the blood.

D

Danger Zone   at the scene of an accident, a circle with a 50-foot radius with the wreckage at the center of the circle. Special danger zones must be formed if the accident involves downed electrical wires, gas leaks, hazardous materials, fire, possible explosions, or radiation.

Debridement   surgical removal of dead, injured, or infected tissue from around a wound or a burn.

Decompression Sickness   the "bends." Usually associated with SCUBA divers who have returned too rapidly to the surface. Nitrogen is trapped in the body's tissues, possibly finding its way into the bloodstream.

Deep Frostbite   *see* Freezing.

Delerium Tremens (DTs)   a severe reaction that can be part of alcohol withdrawal. The patient's hands tremble, hallucinations may occur, the patient displays atypical (unusual) behavior, and convulsions may take place. Severe alcohol withdrawal accompanied by the DTs can lead to death.

Demand Valve Resuscitator   a device that will automatically deliver oxygen when the patient attempts an inspiration.

Dermis (DER-mis)   the inner (second) layer of skin, found beneath the epidermis. This layer is rich in blood vessels, nerves, and skin structures.

Diabetes (di-ah-BE-teez)   disease caused by the inadequate production of insulin.

Diabetic Coma   result of an inadequate insulin supply that leads to unconsciousness, coma, and eventually death unless treated.

Diabetic Ketoacidosis (KEY-to-as-i-DOH-sis)   the condition that occurs when the diabetic's body attempts to break down an excessive amount of fats to obtain energy-rich compounds. This causes ketones to collect in the blood. There is an excessive loss of fluids and glucose through the kidneys associated with this condition.

Diaphoresis (DI-ah-fo-RE-sis)   profuse perspiration. The patient is said to be diaphoretic (DI-ah-fo-RET-ik).

Diaphragm (DI-ah-fram)   dome-shaped muscle that separates the thoracic cavity from the abdominopelvic cavity. It is the major muscle of respiration.

Diaphragmatic (di-a-FRAG-mat-ik) **Breathing**   weak and rapid respirations with little movement of the chest wall and slight movement of the abdomen. An attempt to breathe with the diaphragm alone.

Diastolic (di-as-TOL-ik) **Pressure**   pressure exerted on the internal walls of the arteries when the heart is relaxing.

Dilation   to enlarge, expanding in diameter.

Disaster   any emergency involving illness or injury that taxes the resources of the EMS System.

Disinfect   to destroy harmful microorganisms, but not necessarily their resistant spores.

Dislocation   displacement (pulling out) of a bone end that forms part of a joint.

Distal   away from a point of reference, such as the shoulder or the hip joint. More distant to. *See* Proximal.

Distended   inflated, swollen, or stretched.

Dressing   protective covering for a wound that will aid in the stoppage of bleeding and help to prevent contamination.

Duodenum (du-o-DE-num or du-OD-e-num)   first portion of the small intestine, connected to the stomach. More rigid than the other portions, causing it to receive greater injury in accidents.

Duty to Act   typically a local law that identifies which agencies have a legal responsibility to provide emergency care. If an EMT is a member of such an agency, he or she has a legal responsibility to render care while on duty.

Dynamic Pressure   energy released as an airborne shock wave.

Dyspnea (disp-NE-ah)   difficult or labored breathing.

E

Ecchymosis (EK-i-MO-sis)   discoloration of the skin because of internal bleeding. A "black and blue" mark.

Eclampsia (e-KLAM-se-ah)   convulsive state during pregnancy due to toxemia.

-ectomy (EK-toe-me)   word ending meaning surgical removal.

Ectopic (ek-TOP-ik) **Pregnancy**   when embryo implantation is not in the body of the uterus, occurring instead in the oviduct (fallopian tube), cervix, or abdominopelvic cavity.

Edema (e-DE-mah) swelling due to the accumulation of fluids in the tissues.

Embolism (EM-bo-liz-m) movement and the lodgement of a blood clot or foreign body (fat or air bubble) inside a blood vessel. The foreign body is called an embolus (EM-bo-lus).

Emergency Care at the EMT-level, this is usually the prehospital assessment and basic treatment of the sick or injured patient. The care is initiated at the emergency scene and is continued through transport and transfer to a medical facility. The physical and emotional needs of the patient are considered and attended to during care.

Emergency Medical Services System EMS System. A chain of services linked together to provide care for the patient at the scene, during transport to the hospital, and upon entry at the hospital.

Emergency Medical Technician (EMT) professional-level provider of emergency care. This individual has received formal training and is state certified.

Emesis vomiting.

Emotional Emergency a situation in which a patient behaves in a manner that is not considered to be typical for the occasion. The patient's behavior is often not considered to be socially acceptable. The patient's emotions are strongly evident, interfering with his or her thoughts and behavior.

Emphysema (EM-fi-SEE-mah) chronic disease where the lungs progressively lose their elasticity. *See* Chronic Obstructive Pulmonary Disease.

Epidermis (ep-i-DER-mis) the outer layer of skin.

Epiglottis (EP-i-GLOT-is) flap of cartilage and other tissues that is the superior structure of the larynx. It closes off the airway and diverts solids and liquids down the esophagus.

Epiglottitis (ep-i-glo-TI-tis) a bacterial infection that causes a swelling of the epiglottis.

Epilepsy (EP-i-lep-see) episodic medical disorder characterized by sudden attacks of unconsciousness, with or without convulsions.

Episodic a medical problem that affects the patient at irregular intervals.

Epistaxis (ep-e-STAK-sis) nosebleed.

Erect the body is in the upright position.

Esophageal Obturator Airway (EOA) breathing tube inserted into the esophagus. The vents in the tube are positioned at the opening into the larynx.

Esophagus (e-SOF-ah-gus) muscular tube leading from the pharynx to the stomach.

Eviscerate (e-VIS-er-ate) usually applies to the intestine or other abdominal organ protruding through an incision or wound.

Expiration breathing out. To exhale.

Extension act of straightening.

External Auditory Canal the opening of the external ear and its pathway to the middle ear.

Extrication any actions that disentangle and free from entrapment.

Extruded when an organ, bone, or vessel is pushed out of position.

F

Facial Artery a major artery supplying blood to the face.

Fainting simple form of shock, occurring when the patient has a temporary, self-correcting, loss of consciousness caused by a reduced supply of blood to the brain. Also called psychogenic (SI-ko-JEN-ic) shock.

False Motion movement of an extremity where there should be no motion, such as at the point of a fracture.

Febrile feverish.

Femoral (FEM-o-ral) **Artery** main artery of the thigh. A major pulse location and pressure point site.

Femoral Hernia when an abdominal membrane and perhaps part of an intestine push through the opening where blood vessels and nerves pass into the thigh. This is usually an injury of the female.

Femur (FE-mer) thigh bone.

Fetus (FE-tus) developing unborn. It is an embryo until the third month, when it becomes a fetus until birth.

Fibrillation uncoordinated contractions of the myocardium resulting from independent individual muscle fiber activity.

Fibrin (FI-brin) fibrous protein material formed and utilized to produce a blood clot.

Fibula (FIB-yo-lah) lateral leg bone.

First-degree Burn mild, partial thickness burn, only involving the outer layer of skin.

First Responder a person who is part of the EMS System, having been trained in a First Responder course, and where it is policy, having the appropriate certification. Such an individual is trained below the level of an EMT. The basic training emphasizes first arrival and initial assessment and care.

Flail Chest condition where the ribs and/or the sternum are fractured in such a way as to produce a loose section of the chest wall that will not move with the rest of the wall during breathing.

Flexion bending. To lessen the angle of a joint.

Flowmeter a Bourdon or pressure-compensated

device used to indicate the flow of oxygen in liters per minute.

Formed Elements red blood cells, white blood cells, and platelets.

Fracture break, crack, split, or crumbling of a bone.

Freezing deep frostbite. An injury due to cold involving the skin and subcutaneous layers. Deep structures such as bone and muscle can be involved.

Frostbite *see* Superficial Frostbite.

Frostnip incipient frostbite. Minor injury to the epidermis caused by exposure to cold.

G

Gallbladder organ that attaches to the lower back of the liver. It stores bile.

Gastro- (GAS-tro) used as a beginning of words in reference to the stomach.

Genitalia (jen-i-TA-le-ah) external reproductive organs.

Good Samaritan Laws series of laws written to protect emergency care personnel. These laws require a standard of care to be provided in good faith, to the level of training, and to the best of ability.

Grand Mal severe epileptic seizure.

Greenstick Fracture split along the length of a bone, giving the appearance of a green stick bent to its breaking point.

Gurgling atypical sound of breathing made by patients having airway obstruction, lung disease, or lung injury due to heat.

H

Handoff orderly transfer of the patient, patient information, and patient valuables to more highly trained personnel.

Hare Traction Splint lower extremity splint that will apply a set amount of tension along the long axis of a lower extremity. This tension is limited by the windlass mechanism.

Heart Attack usually the sudden blockage of a coronary vessel that can cause death to the heart muscle.

Heat Cramps condition brought about by loss of body fluids and possibly salts. Usually occurs in people working in hot environments. Muscle cramps occur in the lower extremities and abdomen.

Heat Exhaustion condition where blood pools in the vessels of the skin. This is an attempt by the body to give off excessive heat. It causes an inadequate return of blood to the heart that can lead to collapse.

Heatstroke true emergency caused by a failure of the body's heat-regulating mechanisms. The patient cannot cool his overheated body.

Hematemesis (HEM-ah-TEM-e-sis) vomiting bright red blood.

Hematoma (hem-ah-TO-mah) collection of blood under the skin or in the tissues as a result of an injured or broken blood vessel. Sometimes referred to as a "blood tumor."

Hematuria (HEM-ah-TU-ri-ah) passing blood in the urine.

Hemorrhage (HEM-o-rej) internal or external bleeding.

Hemorrhagic (HEM-o-RIJ-ic) **Shock** *see* Hypovolemic Shock.

Hemothorax (he-mo-THO-raks) condition of blood and bloody fluids in the area between the lungs and the walls of the chest cavity.

Hiatal (hi-A-tal) **Hernia** occurs when part of the stomach bulges upward through the opening (hiatus, hi-A-tus) that allows the esophagus to pass through the diaphragm.

Hip joint made between the pelvis and the femur.

Hives slightly elevated red or pale areas of skin that often itch. Hives are transient, and often a reaction to certain foods, drugs, infection, or stress.

Humerus (HU-mer-us) arm bone.

Humidifier a device connected to the flowmeter to add moisture to the dry oxygen that is coming from the cylinder.

Hydroplaning when a film of water develops between a vehicle's tires and the road surface so that the vehicle is riding in an uncontrolled fashion upon the water.

Hyperextension overextension of a limb or body part.

Hyperglycemia (hi-per-gli-SEE-me-ah) excess of sugar in the blood.

Hyperthermia greatly increased body temperature.

Hyperventilation increased rate and depth of breathing.

Hypoglycemia (hi-po-gli-SEE-me-ah) too little sugar in the blood.

Hypothermia general cooling of the body.

Hypovolemic Shock state of shock brought about by an excessive loss of whole blood or plasma.

Hypoxia (hi-POK-se-ah) inadequate supply of oxygen to the body tissues.

I

Iliac (IL-e-ak) **Crest** the upper, curved boundary of the ilium.

Ilium (IL-e-um) the upper portions of the pelvis, forming the wings of the pelvis.

Implied Consent legal position that assumes an unconscious patient, or one so badly injured or ill that he cannot respond, would consent to receiving emergency care. Implied consent applies to children, developmentally disabled, and mentally or emotionally disturbed patients, when parents or guardians are not at the scene.

Incipient Frostbite *see* Frostnip.

Incision *see* Cut.

Infarction localized death of tissue resulting from the discontinuation of its blood supply.

Inferior away from the top of the body. Usually compared with another structure which is closer to the top (superior).

Inflammation pain, heat, redness, and swelling of tissues as they react to infection, irritation, or injury.

Informed Consent actual consent given after the patient knows your level of training and what you are going to do.

Inguinal (IN-gwin-al) **Canal** the passageway from the scrotum into the pelvic cavity that carries the blood vessels, nerves, and cord of the testis.

Inguinal (IN-gwin-al) **Hernia** a "rupture." A soft tissue injury in which the lining of the abdominopelvic cavity ruptures and a portion of the small intestine protrudes through the opening into the inguinal canal.

Inspiration breathe in, inhale.

Insulin (IN-su-lin) hormone produced in the pancreas that is needed to move sugar from the blood into cells.

Insulin Shock state of shock from too much insulin in the blood causing low sugar levels for the brain and nervous system. The high level of insulin can be due to overdose or from too low of a sugar intake (hypoglycemia).

Intercostal (in-ter-KOS-tal) **Muscles** the muscles found between the ribs. When they contract during an inspiration, the ribs are lifted to increase the volume of the thoracic cavity.

Intermammary Line an imaginary line that is drawn to connect the nipples.

Interposed Ventilation artificial ventilations provided during CPR after a fixed set of compressions.

Intravenous (IV) into a vein.

Iris the colored portion of the anterior eye that adjusts the size of the pupil.

Ischium (IS-ke-em) the lower, posterior portions of the pelvis.

-itis (I-tis) word ending used to mean inflammation.

J

Jaundice yellowing of the skin, usually associated with liver or bile apparatus injury or disease.

Jaw-Thrust method of opening the airway without lifting the neck or tilting the head.

Jugular Veins large veins in the neck that drain blood from the head.

K

Ketoacidosis (KE-to-as-i-DO-sis) when a diabetic's body breaks down too many fats trying to obtain energy, ketone bodies build in the blood and the blood becomes acid.

Kidneys excretory organs located high in the back of the abdominal region. They are behind the abdominal cavity.

L

Labor three stages of childbirth, including the beginning of contractions, delivery of the child, and delivery of the afterbirth (placenta, umbilical cord and some tissues of the lining of the uterus).

Laceration jagged-edged, open wound. *See* Cut.

Lacrimal (LAK-ri-mal) **Gland** tear gland.

Laryngeal Edema fluids invading the tissues of the larynx causing swelling.

Laryngectomy (lar-in-JEK-toe-me) total or partial removal of the larynx. The patient is called a neck breather or a laryngectomee.

Larynx (LAR-inks) airway situated between the pharynx and the trachea. Contains the voice box.

Lateral to the side, away from the vertical midline of the body.

Lateral Recumbent lying on the side.

Lateral Rotation to turn the foot or hand outward, away from the midline.

Ligament fibrous tissue that connects bone to bone.

Liter (LE-ter), **Litre** metric measurement of liquid volume that is equal to 1.057 quarts. One pint is almost equal to one-half liter.

Liver largest gland in the body, having many functions. Located in the upper right abdominal region, extending over to the central abdominal region.

Lumbar (LUM-bar) **Spine** vertebrae of the lower back, consisting of 5 bones.

M

Manual Thrusts abdominal or chest thrusts provided to expel an object causing an airway obstruction.

Mechanical Pump Failure inability of the heart to function properly due to damaged myocardial tissue.

Mechanism of Injury what forces caused the injury, allowing you to relate types of accidents to certain types of injuries. You must consider the kind of force, its intensity and direction, and the area of the body that is affected.

Medial toward the vertical midline of the body. *See* lateral.

Medial Rotation to turn the foot or hand inward toward the midlinc.

Mediastinum (me-de-as-TI-num or me-de-ah-STI-num) central portion of the chest cavity (thoracic cavity) containing the heart, its greater vessels, part of the esophagus, and part of the trachea.

Medical Practices Act laws requiring an individual to be licensed or certified in order to practice medicine or to provide certain levels of care.

Meninges (me-NIN-jez) three membranes surrounding the brain and spinal cord.

Metabolic Shock state of shock due to a loss of body fluids (dehydration) and a change in body chemistry.

Metacarpals (meta-KAR-pals) hand bones.

Metatarsals (meta-TAR-sals) foot bones.

Midline an imaginary vertical line drawn down the center of the body, dividing it into right and left halves.

Morbidity the occurrence of illness.

Mortality the occurrence of death.

Myocardium (mi-o-KAR-de-um) heart muscle.

N

Nasopharyngeal (na-zo-fah-RIN-je-al) **Airway** a flexible breathing tube that is inserted through the patient's nostril into the pharynx.

Negligence at the EMT level, this is the failure to provide the expected care at the standard of care.

Neurogenic Shock caused when the nervous system fails to control the diameter of the blood vessels. The vessels remain widely dilated, providing too great a volume to be filled by available blood.

O

Objective Examination a part of the secondary survey. This is a hands-on survey of the patient during which you determine vital signs and perform a head-to-toe examination.

Occlusion blockage, as in the blockage of an artery.

Occlusive Dressing covering a wound and forming an airtight seal.

Open Fracture when a bone is broken and bone ends or fragments cut through the skin. Listed in older references as a compound fracture.

Open Wound when the skin is broken.

Oropharyngeal (or-o-fah-RIN-jee-al) **Airway** curved breathing tube inserted into the patient's mouth. It will hold the base of the tongue forward.

Oxygen Delivery Device typically one of four face masks or a nasal cannula.

Oxygen Toxicity uncommon, rarely fatal effect of oxygen on a patient who has received too high a concentration of the gas for too long a period of time.

P

Packaging part of the procedure of preparation for removal in an accident. It can involve applying splints, dressings, and stabilizing impaled objects.

Palpate, Palpation to feel any part of the body, as to palpate the carotid pulse; also, to use the blood pressure cuff while feeling the radial pulse in order to determine the approximate patient systolic pressure.

Pancreas (PAN-cre-as) gland in the back of the upper portion of the abdominal cavity, behind the stomach. It produces insulin and digestive juices.

Patient Assessment the systematic gathering of information in order to determine the nature of a patient's illness or injury.

Paradoxical Motion (Movement) associated with flail chest, where a loose segment of chest wall moves in the opposite direction to the rest of the chest during respiratory movements.

Paralysis complete or partial loss of the ability to move a body part. Sensation in the area may also be lost.

Patella (pah-TEL-lah) kneecap.

Pedal Pulse foot pulse; dorsalis pedis and posterior tibial.

Penetrating Wound puncture wound with only an entrance wound.

Perforating Wound puncture wound with an entrance and an exit wound.

Perfusion the constant flow of blood through the capillaries.

Pericardium (per-e-KAR-de-um) the membranous sac that surrounds the heart.

Perineum (per-i-NE-um) region of the body located between the genitalia and the anus.

Peritoneum (per-i-toe-NE-um) membrane that lines the abdominal cavity.

Periosteum (per-e-OS-te-um) the white fibrous membrane covering a bone.

Petit Mal minor epileptic attack noted by a momentary loss of awareness.

Phalanges (fah-LAN-jez) bones of the toes and fingers.

Pharynx (FAR-inks) throat.

Pinna (PIN-nah) the external ear; also called the auricle (AW-re-kal).

Placenta (plah-SEN-tah) organ made of both maternal and fetal tissues to allow for exchange between the circulatory systems of the mother and fetus without having a mixing of blood.

Plasma (PLAZ-mah) fluid portion of the blood. It is blood minus blood cells and other structures (formed elements).

Platelet (PLATE-let) formed elements of the blood that release factors needed to form blood clots.

Pleura (PLOOR-ah) double-membrane sac. The outer layer lines the chest wall and the inner layer covers the outside of the lungs.

Pleura Cavities the right and left portions of the thoracic cavity that contain the lungs.

Pneumothorax (NU-mo-THO-raks) collection of air in the chest cavity to the outside of the lungs, caused by punctures to the chest wall or the lungs.

Pocket Face Mask (with a one-way valve) a device to aid in mouth-to-mouth resuscitation to prevent contact with the patient's mouth. It may be used with supplemental oxygen when fitted with an oxygen inlet.

Positive Pressure Resuscitation delivering oxygen to the nonbreathing patient using a oxygen-powered, manually triggered ventilating device.

Posterior the back of the body or body part.

Postictal (post-IK-tal) third phase of a convulsive seizure. Convulsions stop and the patient may be drowsy or remain unconscious for hours.

Pressure Regulator a device connected to an oxygen cylinder to reduce the cylinder pressure to a safe working level (a safe pressure for delivery of oxygen to the patient).

Priapism (PRE-ah-pizm) persistent erection of the penis associated with spinal damage.

Primary Survey first examination of a patient to detect life-threatening problems dealing with breathing, heartbeat, and profuse bleeding.

Prolapsed Cord abnormal delivery where the umbilical cord is presented first.

Prone lying face down.

Proximal close to a point of reference such as the shoulder or hip joint. Used with distal, meaning away from.

Psychogenic Shock (SI-ko-JEN-ic) *see* Fainting.

Pubic (PYOO-bik), **Pubis** (PYOO-bis) the middle (medial), anterior portion of the pelvis.

Pulmonary (PUL-mo-ner-e) refers to the lungs.

Pulmonary (PUL-mo-ner-e) **Arteries** the blood vessels that transport blood from the right ventricle to the lungs.

Pulmonary Circulation circuit of blood traveling from the right ventricle of the heart to the lungs and returning to the left atrium.

Pulmonary (PUL-mo-ner-e) **Resuscitation** (re-SUS-si-TAY-shun) providing ventilations (rescue breathing) to a patient in an attempt to artificially restore normal lung function.

Pulmonary (PUL-mo-ner-e) **Veins** the vessels that transport oxygenated blood from the lungs to the left atrium.

Pulse alternate expansion and contraction of arterial walls as the heart pumps blood.

Puncture Wound open wound tearing through the skin and destroying tissue in a straight line. *See* Penetrating Wound and Perforating Wound.

R

Radial Pulse wrist pulse.

Radius lateral forearm bone.

Rales (rahlz) abnormal sound produced in the lungs as air moves through fluids in the bronchiole tree. The sound is like that made when you rub the hair near your ears.

Rectum (REK-tum) lower portion of the large intestine ending with the anus.

Red Blood Cells also called erythrocytes and RBCs. These are the circulating blood cells that carry oxygen to the tissues and pick up carbon dioxide for return to the lungs.

Referred Pain pain felt in a part of the body other than where the source or cause of the pain is located. For example, an inflamed gallbladder may have referred pain over the right scapula.

Respiratory Arrest when the patient stops breathing.

Respiratory Shock state of shock caused by too little oxygen in the blood. Usually due to lung failure, where the patient is unable to adequately fill the lungs.

Resuscitation (re-SUS-ci-TA-shun) any effort to artificially restore or provide normal heart and/or lung function.

Rhonchi (RONG-ki) coarse loud rales resulting from a partial obstruction of the bronchi or bronchioles.

S

Sacrum (SA-krum) fused vertebrae of the lower back, inferior to the lumbar spine.

Sanitize rigid standard of cleaning, often to the point of practical sterilization.

Scapula (SKAP-u-lah) shoulder blade.

Sclera (SKLE-rah) the "whites of the eyes."

Scratch abrasion (ab-RAY-shun). An open wound that damages the surface of skin without breaking all the skin layers.

Secondary Survey patient interview, vital signs, and the physical examination performed after the primary survey.

Second-degree Burn partial thickness burn where the epidermis is burned through and the dermis is damaged.

Septic Shock form of shock caused by severe infection. Toxins from the infection cause the blood vessels to dilate and plasma to be lost through vessel walls.

Shock failure of the circulatory system to provide an adequate blood supply to all parts of the body.

Shoulder Dystocia (dis-TO-she-ah) when a delivering baby with large shoulders wedges between its mother's sacrum and pubic bones.

Sign any observed evidence of injury or illness.

Sphygmomanometer (SFIG-mo-mah-NOM-e-ter) instrument used to measure blood pressure.

Spinal Cavity the area within the spinal column that contains the spinal cord and its protective membranes, the meninges.

Spleen organ located to the left of the upper abdominal cavity, behind the stomach. It stores blood and destroys old blood cells.

Splint any device that will immobilize a fracture.

Sprain injury in which ligaments are partially torn.

Standard of Care the minimum accepted level of emergency care to be provided as set forth by law, administrative orders, guidelines published by emergency care organizations and societies, local protocols and practice, and what has been accepted in the past (precedent).

Sterile free of all life forms.

Sternum (STER-num) breastbone.

Stethoscope instrument used to amplify body sounds.

Stoma (STO-mah) opening in the neck of a neck breather. Any permanent opening surgically made.

Strain injury to muscles caused by overexertion.

Subclavian (sub-CLA-vi-an) **Artery** the major artery located under the clavicle.

Subcutaneous (SUB-ku-TA-ne-us) beneath the skin. Usually refers to the fatty and connective tissue layer found beneath the dermis.

Subcutaneous (SUB-ku-TA-ne-us) **Emphysema** (EM-fi-SEE-mah) air under the skin. This is observed most frequently when a lung is punctured and air escapes into the surrounding tissues of the thorax.

Subjective Interview a part of the secondary survey that uses the patient and bystanders as sources of information by having them answer specific questions.

Substernal Notch a general term for the lowest region on the sternum to which the ribs attach.

Suction Device a vacuum-, air-, or oxygen-powered device that is used to remove blood, secretions, or other fluids from a patient's mouth, throat, or stoma. Electrical, oxygen, and manually powered units are available.

Superficial Frostbite injury due to cold involving the skin and the subcutaneous layers. The upper layers are frozen, but some elasticity remains in the tissues below the skin.

Superior toward the top of the body. Often used in reference with inferior, meaning away from the top of the body.

Supine lying flat on the back.

Sympathetic Eye Movement the coordinated movement of both eyes in the same direction. If one eye moves, the other eye will carry out the same movement, even if it is covered or the eyelid is shut.

Symptom evidence of injury or illness told to you by the patient.

Systemic (sis-TEM-ik) refers to the entire body.

Systemic (sis-TEM-ik) **Circulation** the portion of the circulatory system that transports blood from the left ventricle out to the body tissues and back to the right atrium.

Systemic Hypothermia generalized cooling of the body.

Systolic (sis-TOL-ik) **Blood Pressure** force exerted by the blood on the artery walls when the heart is contracting.

T

Tachycardia (tak-e-KAR-de-ah) rapid heartbeat, usually 100–120 or more beats per minute.

Tarsals (TAR-sals) ankle bones.

Temporal Artery the major artery in the region of the temple.

Tendon fibrous tissue that connects muscle to bone.

Thigh Bone femur (FE-mur).

Third-degree Burn full thickness burn, where all layers of the skin are damaged. Deep structures may also be burned.

Thoracic (tho-RAS-ik) **Cavity** anterior body cavity above the diaphragm. It protects the heart and lungs.

Thoracic (tho-RAS-ik) **Spine** the 12 vertebrae of the upper back to which the ribs attach.

Thoracic (tho-RAS-ik) **Vertebrae** the 12 vertebrae of the thoracic spine.

Thorax (THO-raks) chest.

Thrombosis (throm-BO-sis) formation of a blood clot in a blood vessel or within a chamber of the heart.

Thyroid (THY-roid) **Cartilage** the Adam's apple.

Tibia (TIB-e-ah) medial lower leg bone.

Tonic Phase first stage of a convulsive seizure where the patient's body can become rigid for up to 30 seconds per episode.

Tourniquet last resort used to control bleeding. A band or belt is used to constrict blood vessels to stop the flow of blood.

Trachea (TRA-ke-ah) windpipe.

Tracheostomy (TRA-ke-OS-to-me) a surgical opening made through the anterior neck, entering into the trachea (windpipe).

Traction part of the action taken to stabilize a broken bone to prevent any additional injury. To pull gently along the length of a limb.

Traction Splinting to use a special splint to apply a constant pull along the length of a lower extremity. This helps to stabilize a fractured femur and may reduce muscle spasms.

Trauma injury caused by violence, shock, or pressure.

Traumatic Asphyxia condition that arises from a broken sternum and ribs forcing blood out of the right side of the heart into the veins of the neck. Acute thoracic compression syndrome.

Triage method of sorting patients according to the severity of their injuries or illnesses.

Tympanic (tim-PAN-ik) **Membrane** the eardrum.

U

Ulna (UL-nah) medial forearm bone.

Umbilical (um-BIL-i-kal) **Cord** structure that connects the body of the fetus to the placenta.

Umbilicus (um-BIL-i-kus) navel.

Uterus (U-ter-us) muscular structure in which the fetus develops. The womb.

V

Vagina (vah-JI-nah) canal leading from the vulva to the cervix. The birth canal.

Vascular referring to the blood vessels.

Vein any blood vessel that returns blood to the heart.

Venae (VE-ne) **Cavae** (KA-ve) the superior vena cava and the inferior vena cava. These two major veins return blood from the body to the right atrium.

Ventilation supplying air to the lungs.

Ventral front of the body or body part. *See* Anterior.

Ventricle inferior chamber of the heart. Ventricles pump blood from the heart.

Vertebra (VER-te-brah) bone of the spinal column.

Viscera (VIS-er-ah) internal organs. Usually refers to the abdominal organs.

Vital Signs in basic EMT-level care, pulse rate and character, breathing rate and character, blood pressure, and relative skin temperature.

Vitreous Fluid transparent jelly-like substance filling the posterior cavity of the eye.

Vulva (VUL-vah) external female genitalia.

W

Wheal localized accumulation of fluid under the skin that may be accompanied by itching. A hive.

Wheeze whistling respiratory sound. It can be caused in asthma when air is trapped in the alveoli and cannot be expired easily.

White Blood Cells also called leukocytes and WBCs. These are the blood cells that are involved with destroying microorganisms and producing antibodies to fight off infection.

Womb *See* Uterus.

X

Xiphoid (ZI-foyd) inferior process of the sternum.

Z

Zygomatic (zi-go-MAT-ik) **Bone** cheek bone. Also called the malar (MA-lar).

Index

Page numbers followed by the letter f indicate illustrations;
those followed by the letter t indicate tables

Advance Your Career With JEMS And Rescue

Let Jems Publishing Company be your companion in the ever-changing world of prehospital care by subscribing to *JEMS* and *Rescue* magazines. In each issue of *JEMS* and *Rescue* you'll find exciting and informative stories to help keep your skills sharp and your senses keen. Stay ahead of the "learning curve" with two of the most respected journals for emergency responders.

JEMS & Rescue: Practical Information for Career-Minded Emergency Responders.

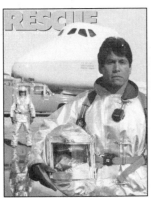

Uniting Rescue and Basic Life Support

Rescue Magazine is for the people of rescue—rescuers and EMTs who care for the sick and injured, who locate and extricate those in peril. *Rescue* educates and entertains, building basic skills while introducing innovations and information that bring rescue and basic life support together.

Rescue is edited by experts, to provide reliable and updated information on a wide variety of topics.

With your subscription to *Rescue* you get:

- full coverage of basic life support topics
- features on rescue and extrication techniques and equipment, with special articles on heavy rescue
- full-color photographs and insider reports on technical rescue innovations
- special reports covering the emergency response to major disasters around the world
- provacative commentary and humor from the field
- tips and "how to" articles designed to make your job easier and better

Take the Sting out of Continuing Education

Though your formal education may be finished, continuing education is a reality in emergency medical services and rescue. Jems Publishing makes earning continuing education units easy with the Jems CEU Program. You can earn CEUs in the comfort of your own home just by reading selected articles in *JEMS* and *Rescue* and successfully completing the test at the end. The program is recognized by the National Registry of EMTs, the National Association of State EMS Training Coordinators, and the National Association of State EMS Directors.

The Journal of Emergency Medical Services

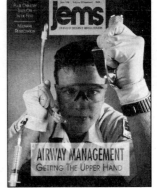

For more than a decade, *JEMS* has set the standard for news, information and education related to prehospital advanced life support and EMS systems. Paramedics, nurses, physicians, instructors and administrators look to *JEMS* for the articles and columns that will give them the edge in patient care and their careers. Nearly 100,000 readers in more than 30 countries around the world enjoy *JEMS* every month.

With your subscription to *JEMS* you get:

- full coverage of advanced life support topics
- special reports on the critical issues facing EMS systems
- columns and features aimed at helping instructors and administrators with legal questions, management techniques and system design
- original research and surveys, including our annual salary survey, Almanac of EMS, and Buyer's Guide
- Thom Dick's Tricks of the Trade column
- news, commentary and editorials from the leaders of EMS

To subscribe, call our toll-free number 1-800-334-8152 (in Calif., call 1-800-255-3302), or send $19.97 for *JEMS* (12 issues) or $9.95 for *Rescue* (6 issues) to Jems Publishing Company, P.O. Box 3730, Escondido, CA 92033.